American Medical Association

Physicians dedicated to the health of America

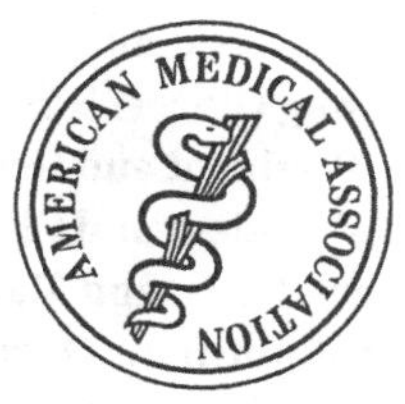

Guides to the Evaluation of Permanent Impairment

Fourth Edition

Guides the Evaluation of Permanent Impairment, Fourth Edition

Fourth Edition—First Printing: June 1993
Second Printing: January 1994
Third Printing: August 1995
Fourth Printing: October 1999
Fifth Printing: August 2001
Sixth Printing: April 2003
Seventh Printing: April 2004
Eighth Printing: December 2006
Ninth Printing: October 2008
Tenth Printing: April 2015
Eleventh Printing: August, 2018
Twelfth Printing, March, 2021
Thirteenth Printing: August 2022

Printed in the United States of America. 22 23 24 / LSC / 15 14 13

Internet address: www.ama-assn.org
The American Medical Association ("AMA") and its authors and editors have consulted sources believed to be knowledgeable in their fields. However, neither the AMA nor its authors or editors warrant that the information is in every respect accurate and/or complete. The AMA, its authors, and editors assume no responsibility for use of the information contained in this publication. Neither the AMA nor its authors or editors shall be responsible for, and expressly disclaims liability for, damages of any kind arising out of the use of, reference to, or reliance on, the content of this publication. This publication is for informational purposes only. The AMA does not provide medical, legal, financial, or other professional advice and readers are encouraged to consult a professional advisor for such advice.

Additional copies of this book may be ordered by calling 800-621-8335 or AMA|Store at amastore.com. Refer to product number OP 025493.

AMA publication and product updates, errata, and addendum can be found at amaproductupdates.org.

ISBN: 0-89970-553-7
BP61: 08/22

Table of Contents

Foreword

The Fourth Edition of the *Guides to the Evaluation of Permanent Impairment (Guides)* continues an activity begun by the American Medical Association (AMA) almost four decades ago, the purpose of which was to bring greater objectivity to estimating the degree of long-standing or "permanent" impairments. The rationale for this new edition is that the pace of progress and advance in medicine continues to be rapid, and that a new look at the impairment criteria for all organ systems is advisable. This edition has been prepared under the auspices of the AMA's Council on Scientific Affairs.

In preparing the Fourth Edition, the *Guides*' editors, AMA staff members, and the Council's liaison members first selected well-qualified individuals who, as chairs, would be responsible for preparing the chapters on organ system impairments and other subjects. Then the AMA staff requested nominations of knowledgeable, interested physicians from all the state medical societies and the medical specialty societies that make up the AMA federation. Thereafter, the chairs and committee members selected by them and the AMA staff prepared the text.

All of the chapters of this edition have undergone peer review, either by the committees who prepared them or by other knowledgeable persons. In March 1992, representatives of 11 medical specialty societies, the Social Security Administration, the US Department of Veterans Affairs, the American Bar Association, and the Oklahoma State Workers' Compensation Agency, a representative agency that mandates the *Guides*' use, met to consider a draft of the Fourth Edition and provide further peer review. After this meeting, the chairs made appropriate changes. A multidisciplinary *ad hoc* committee provided special assistance with the musculoskeletal system.

The Fourth Edition has some new features. Case reports or examples are included in most of the parts dealing with the different organ systems. A chapter on pain is included. Organ transplantation and the adverse effects of pharmaceuticals are considered. The Glossary contains informative material on the Americans with Disability Act (ADA) of 1992. New data are cited in Chapter 1 on the widespread use of the *Guides* by state workers' compensation agencies.

The Fourth Edition continues to convey several basic principles. A key tenet is that the book applies only to permanent impairments, which are defined as adverse conditions that are stable and unlikely to change. Evaluating the magnitude of these impairments is in the purview of the physician, while determining disability is usually not the physician's responsibility. This edition emphasizes that impairment percentages derived by using *Guides* criteria represent *estimates* rather than precise determinations. Permanent impairments are evaluated in terms of how they affect the patient's daily activities, and this edition recognizes that one's occupation constitutes part of his or her daily activities.

Many persons helped with the Fourth Edition. The authors of and the contributors to the *Guides*, reviewers, and responsible AMA staff members are listed after the Foreword. The editors acknowledge especially the research and assistance of Alfred B. Swanson, MD, and Genevieve de Groot Swanson, MD, whose work was essential in preparing the hand and upper extremity section in the chapter on the musculoskeletal system.

The editors also wish to acknowledge the hundreds of *Guides* users who have written the AMA in past years and offered their suggestions. While the editors' goal has been to prepare the best *Guides* yet, we realize there still is room for improvement. The *Guides* readers and users can contribute to this process. Therefore, we invite all to continue offering their comments and advice.

Theodore C. Doege, MD, MS, Editor

Thomas P. Houston, MD, Associate Editor

Chairs, Contributors, Reviewers, and Participants

Chairs

C. Eugene Carlton, MD, Baylor College of Medicine, Houston, Texas
—The Urinary and Reproductive Systems

Francis I. Catlin, MD, ScD, Houston, Texas
—Ear, Nose, Throat, and Related Structures

Paul E. Epstein, MD, The Graduate Hospital, Philadelphia, Pennsylvania
—The Respiratory System

Don E. Flinn, MD, US Department of Veterans Affairs Medical Center West Los Angeles, Los Angeles, California
—Mental and Behavioral Disorders

Robert H. Haralson III, MD, Maryville Orthopedic Clinic, Maryville, Tennessee
—The Musculoskeletal System, The Spine

William S. Haubrich, MD, La Jolla, California
—The Digestive System

David L. Horwitz, MD, PhD, SciClone Pharmaceuticals, San Mateo, California
—The Endocrine System

Philipp M. Lippe, MD, San Jose, California
—Pain

James V. Luck, Jr., MD, Orthopaedic Hospital, Los Angeles, California
—The Lower Extremity (In: The Musculoskeletal System)

Nelson G. Richards, MD, Associated Neurologists and US Department of Veterans Affairs McQuire Hospital, Richmond, Virginia
—The Nervous System

Joseph Sataloff, MD, DSc, Jefferson Medical College, Philadelphia, Pennsylvania
—Impairment Evaluation and Records and Reports

George M. Smith, MD, MPH, GM Smith Associates, Bethesda, Maryland
—Glossary

John A. Spittell, Jr., MD, Mayo Clinic, Rochester, Minnesota
—The Cardiovascular System

Alfred B. Swanson, MD, Michigan State University, Grand Rapids, Michigan
—The Hand and Upper Extremity (In: The Musculoskeletal System)

James S. Taylor, MD, Cleveland Clinic Foundation, Cleveland, Ohio
—The Skin

Ralph O. Wallerstein, Sr., MD, University of California, San Francisco, California
—The Hematopoietic System

Nancy Webb, MD, Kelsey-Seybold Clinic, Houston, Texas
—The Visual System

Contributors

Roy D. Altman, MD, University of Miami School of Medicine, Miami, Florida

Douglas R. Anderson, MD, Bascom-Palmer Eye Institute, Miami, Florida

Thomas P. Ball, Jr., MD, University of Texas Health Sciences Center, San Antonio, Texas

Stanley J. Bigos, MD, University of Washington School of Medicine, Seattle, Washington

E. Richard Blonsky, MD, Rehabilitation Institute of Chicago, Chicago, Illinois

Lewis E. Braverman, MD, University of Massachusetts Medical School, Worcester, Massachusetts

James E. Culver, MD, Cleveland Clinic Foundation, Cleveland, Ohio

William E. Davis, MD, University of Missouri School of Medicine, Columbia, Missouri

Theodore C. Doege, MD, MS, American Medical Association, Chicago, Illinois

John A. Dowdle, Jr., MD, St. Paul, Minnesota

Loren H. Engrav, MD, University of Washington, Harborview Medical Center, Seattle, Washington

Gary R. Epler, MD, New England Baptist Hospital, Boston, Massachusetts

E. Harvey Estes, Jr., MD, Raleigh, North Carolina

Blair C. Filler, MD, Los Angeles, California

Gregory Firman, MD, JD, US Department of Veterans Affairs Medical Center West Los Angeles, Los Angeles, California

John J. Gerhardt, MD, Milwaukie, Oregon

Sherwin Goldman, MD, Mayo Clinic, Rochester, Minnesota

William Jason Groves, JD, Rapid City, South Dakota

Donald Hammersley, MD, Bethesda, Maryland

Stephen C. Hammill, MD, Mayo Clinic, Rochester, Minnesota

Jeanne E. Hicks, MD, National Institutes of Health, Bethesda, Maryland

Thomas P. Houston, MD, American Medical Association, Chicago, Illinois

Paul E. Kaplan, MD, Ohio State University, Columbus, Ohio

Arthur H. Keeney, MD, University of Louisville, Louisville, Kentucky

David G. Kline, MD, Louisiana State University, New Orleans, Louisiana

Joseph E. Kutz, MD, Louisville Hand Surgery, Louisville, Kentucky

Paul R. Lambert, MD, University of Virginia School of Medicine, Charlottesville, Virginia

Philip Levy, MD, Phoenix Endocrinology Clinic, Phoenix, Arizona

Donlin M. Long, MD, PhD, Johns Hopkins University School of Medicine, Baltimore, Maryland

L. Russell Malinak, MD, Baylor University College of Medicine, Houston, Texas

John H. Mather, MD, Social Security Administration, Baltimore, Maryland

C. G. Toby Mathias, MD, Group Health Associates, Cincinnati, Ohio

Tom G. Mayer, MD, PRIDE Research Foundation, Dallas, Texas

J. Michael McWhorter, MD, Bowman Gray School of Medicine, Winston-Salem, North Carolina

William Melnick, PhD, University Hospital Clinic, Ohio State University, Columbus, Ohio

Arthur T. Meyerson, MD, Hahnemann University, Philadelphia, Pennsylvania

Ernest H. Neighbor, MD, JD, Bisko, Fee, and Parkins, Kansas City, Missouri

James R. Nethercott, MD, Johns Hopkins University School of Hygiene and Public Health, Baltimore, Maryland

Rick A. Nishimura, MD, Mayo Clinic, Rochester, Minnesota

George E. Omer, Jr., MD, University of New Mexico, Albuquerque, New Mexico

John T. Purvis, MD, Knoxville, Tennessee

Herbert E. Rosenbaum, MD, Washington University, St. Louis, Missouri

Karen S. Rucker, MD, Medical College of Virginia, Richmond, Virginia

Joel R. Saper, MD, Michigan Headache and Neurological Institute, Ann Arbor, Michigan

Robert T. Sataloff, MD, DMA, Jefferson Medical College, Philadelphia, Pennsylvania

Labe C. Scheinberg, MD, Albert Einstein College of Medicine, New York, New York

William S. Shaw, MD, Billings Clinic, Billings, Montana

Elizabeth F. Sherertz, MD, Bowman Gray School of Medicine, Winston-Salem, North Carolina

William Douglas Skelton, MD, Mercer University School of Medicine, Macon, Georgia

Thomas R. Sprenger, MD, Bradenton, Florida

Genevieve de Groot Swanson, MD, Michigan State University, Grand Rapids, Michigan

Sridhar V. Vasudevan, MD, Elmbrook Memorial Hospital, Brookfield, Wisconsin

Kenneth M. Viste, Jr., MD, Oshkosh, Wisconsin

Paul Volberding, MD, San Francisco General Hospital, San Francisco, California

Robert A. Wise, MD, Francis Scott Key Medical Center, Baltimore, Maryland

Edwin T. Wyman, Jr., MD, Massachusetts General Hospital, Boston, Massachusetts

Reviewers

Russell F. Allen, MD, Oklahoma Workers' Compensation Court, Oklahoma City, Oklahoma

Fern E. Asma, MD, Chicago, Illinois

Philip L. Barney, MD, Community Medical Center, Missoula, Montana

Mark E. Battista, MD, Unum Life Insurance Company, Portland, Maine

E. Richard Blonsky, MD, Rehabilitation Institute of Chicago, Chicago, Illinois

Marcus B. Bond, MD, Golden, Colorado

Bernard B. Bradley, MD, The University of Texas Medical School, Pasadena, Texas

Sergio Delgado, MD, Topeka, Kansas

Joseph L. Demer, MD, PhD, University of California at Los Angeles, Los Angeles, California

John W. Ellis, MD, Oklahoma City, Oklahoma

Alan L. Engelberg, MD, Monsanto Company, St. Louis, Missouri (Editor of the Second and Third Editions, *Guides to the Evaluation of Permanent Impairment*)

Kenneth G. Gould, Jr., MD, Exxon USA Company, Houston, Texas

Elwood J. Headley, MD, Department of Veterans Affairs, Washington, DC

Alfred Healy, MD, University Hospital, Iowa City, Iowa

Keith S. Henley, MD, University Hospitals, Ann Arbor, Michigan

Ronald Klein, MD, University of Wisconsin Hospital, Madison, Wisconsin

Myron Lewis, MD, Memphis Gastroenterology Group, Memphis, Tennessee

John A. Linfoot, MD, Oakland, California

John H. Mather, MD, Social Security Administration, Baltimore, Maryland

Siza Mekky, MD, Mekky Associates, Bethesda, Maryland

William T. Rumage, Jr., MD, Louisville, Kentucky

William S. Shaw, MD, Billings Clinic, Billings, Montana

Ralph E. Yodaiken, MD, US Department of Labor, Washington, D.C.

Don J. Young, MD, Sandusky, Ohio

Council on Scientific Affairs

Yank D. Coble, Jr., MD, Jacksonville, Florida (Vice Chair)

E. Harvey Estes, Jr., MD, Raleigh, North Carolina (Chairman)*

C. Alvin Head, MD, Tucker, Georgia

Mitchell S. Karlan, MD, Beverly Hills, California

William R. Kennedy, MD, University of Minnesota Hospitals, Minneapolis, Minnesota

Patricia J. Numann, MD, State University of New York Health Science Center, Syracuse, New York

William C. Scott, MD, University Medical Center, Tucson, Arizona

W. Douglas Skelton, MD, Mercer University School of Medicine, Macon, Georgia*

Richard M. Steinhilber, MD, Cleveland Clinic Foundation, Cleveland, Ohio

Jack P. Strong, MD, Louisiana State University Medical Center, New Orleans, Louisiana

Christine C. Toevs, Medical Student Representative, Greenville, North Carolina

Henry N. Wagner, Jr., MD, Johns Hopkins University School of Hygiene and Public Health, Baltimore, Maryland

---

*Liaison Council members for *Guides*

American Medical Association Staff

Department of Preventive Medicine and Public Health

Theodore C. Doege, MD, MS, Senior Scientist, Editor, *Guides to the Evaluation of Permanent Impairment*, Fourth Edition

Thomas P. Houston, MD, Director, Associate Editor, *Guides to the Evaluation of Permanent Impairment*, Fourth Edition

Mary D. Haynes, Senior Secretary

Sharon E. Major, Secretary

Michiko Sidney, Senior Secretary

Division of Health Science

Robert C. Rinaldi, PhD, Director

Eileen Keane, Administrative Assistant

Group on Science, Technology, and Public Health

James R. Allen, MD, MPH, Vice President

Jerod M. Loeb, PhD, Assistant Vice President

Leatha A. Tiggelaar, Assistant to the Vice President

Medical Education and Science

M. Roy Schwarz, MD, Senior Vice President

Marketing Services

Walter J. Kaban, Jr.

Denise M. McGill

Louis G. Schaaf

Boon Ai Tan

Marketing Management

R. Todd Bake

Sharna Fetman

Lewis W. Jenkins

Barry S. Litwin

Jane E. Piro

Scientific Indexing

Norman Frankel

George Kruto

Office of the General Counsel

Betty Jane Anderson, JD

Veda L. Britt, JD

Executive Vice President

James S. Todd, MD

Participants

Copy Editor

Nicole Netter, Lake Bluff, Illinois

List of Tables and Figures

The Lower Extremity

The Spine

Chapter 4
The Nervous System

Chapter 5
The Respiratory System

Chapter 1

Impairment Evaluation

Is it possible to improve estimates of the severity of human impairments, basing them on accepted medical standards? Can those estimates be used in comparing, evaluating, and adjudicating claims of ill health and impairment arising in workers' compensation cases, Social Security Administration cases, and other types of cases?

This book, *Guides to the Evaluation of Permanent Impairment (Guides)*, began to take form during the 1950s under the premise that the answer to the first question is "yes." An ad hoc committee appointed by the Board of Trustees of the American Medical Association (AMA) gave impetus to the effort. The first edition of the *Guides* was published in 1971, and those involved with succeeding editions have sought to improve and refine it, to the end that it could be useful anywhere when questions arise about people's physical and mental functioning and capabilities.

The *Guides* provides a standard framework and method of analysis through which physicians can evaluate, report on, and communicate information about the impairments of any human organ system. The book uses up-to-date information on impairment and illness provided by knowledgeable clinicians and scholars. In the physician's office, the book can be an aid to making the diagnosis of an impairment and following the course of therapy.

1.1 Impairment, Disability, Handicap

Impairment is defined in the *Guides* as an alteration of an individual's health status. Impairment, according to the *Guides*, is assessed by medical means and is a medical issue. An impairment is a deviation from normal in a body part or organ system and its functioning. The *Guides* defines "permanent impairment" as one that has become static or stabilized during a period of time sufficient to allow optimal tissue repair, and one that is unlikely to change in spite of further medical or surgical therapy.

The *Guides* definition of an impairment closely parallels that of the World Health Organization (WHO), which has defined an impairment as "any loss or abnormality of psychological, physiological, or anatomical structure or function."[1]

In the *Guides*, impairments are defined as conditions that interfere with an individual's "activities of daily living," some of which are listed in the Glossary (p. 315). Activities of daily living include, but are not limited to, self-care and personal hygiene; eating and preparing food; communication, speaking, and writing; maintaining one's posture, standing, and sitting; caring for the home and personal finances; walking, traveling, and moving about; recreational and social activities; and work activities.

An impairment percentage derived by means of the *Guides* is intended, among other purposes, to represent an informed estimate of the degree to which an individual's capacity to carry out daily activities has been diminished.

The *Guides* recognizes that "normal" is not a fine point or an absolute in terms of physical and mental functioning and good health. More often, normality is a range or a zone, as with vision and hearing. The normal can vary with age, sex, and other factors. For example, the physical abilities and the visual capabilities of a 21-year-old almost certainly will differ from those of a 75-year-old person. An interpretation of normal that is too strict can result in an overestimation or underestimation of impairment. What is normal must be determined by sufficient studies of representative populations carried out with valid methods.

Disability may be defined as an alteration of an individual's capacity to meet personal, social, or occupational demands, or statutory or regulatory requirements, because of an impairment. Disability refers to an activity or task the individual cannot accomplish.[2] A disability arises out of the interaction between impairment and external requirements, especially those of a person's occupation. Disability may be thought of as the gap between what a person *can* do and what the person *needs* or *wants* to do.

The WHO defines a disability as "any restriction or lack [resulting from an impairment] of ability to perform an activity in the manner or within the range considered normal for a human being."[1]

An "impaired" individual is not necessarily "disabled." For example, loss of the distal phalanx of the little finger of the right hand will impair the functioning of the digit and hand of both a concert pianist and a bank president. However, the bank president is less likely to be disabled than the pianist. A surgeon who loses a hand will be impaired and will be disabled in terms of the ability to operate; but the surgeon may be fully capable of being the chief of a hospital medical staff and may not be at all disabled with respect to that occupation.

Millions of people have slight hearing losses that deviate from the normal and can be classified as impairments. However, this does not mean all of those individuals are disabled. An individual who is able to meet life's demands is not disabled, even if a medical examination discloses an impairment. An impaired individual may or may not have sufficient ability or capacity to meet the demands or requirements of a particular position or occupation.[3]

A recent review of disability in the U.S. indicated that about 7.1 million persons living in the community at large and in long-term care institutions, about 3% of the nation's population, have disabilities in performing daily activities. About 60% of the disabled are older than 65 years, and the prevalence is substantially higher among women.[4]

The concept of "handicap" is related to but different from the concepts of disability and impairment. Under federal law, an individual is handicapped if he or she has an impairment that substantially limits one or more of life's activities, has a record of such impairment, or is regarded as having such an impairment. This definition is so broad that, under it, almost any person may be considered to be handicapped.

For the purposes of the *Guides*, when an impairment is associated with an obstacle to useful activity, a handicap may exist. An impaired individual is handicapped if there are obstacles to accomplishing life's basic activities that can be overcome only by compensating in some way for the effects of the impairment. Such compensation or accommodation often entails the use of assistive devices, such as crutches, wheelchairs, elevators, hearing aids, optical magnifiers, protheses, or special tools or equipment. Accommodation may include modification of the environment.

If an impaired individual is not able to accomplish a specific task or activity despite accommodation, or if no accommodation exists that will enable completion of the task, then that individual is both handicapped and disabled. However, an impaired individual who is able to accomplish a specific task with or without accommodation is neither handicapped nor disabled with regard to that task.

In general, it is a physician's responsibility to evaluate a patient's health status and determine the presence or absence of an impairment. The physician may work in one of several settings, including a clinic or hospital, in the workplace as an occupational medicine specialist, or as an independent medical examiner. If the physician is well acquainted with the patient's activities and needs, he or she may also express an opinion about the presence or absence of a disability or handicap. Some physicians in occupational medicine, for example, have acquired enough experience and knowledge about workers and workplaces that they can provide useful insights on workers' disabilities and handicaps.

1.2 Structure and Use of the *Guides*

Using the *Guides* requires integrating previously gathered medical information with the results of a current medical evaluation. The evaluation should be carried out in accordance with the directions in the *Guides*, and it should be based on three components.

First, certain types of information, described in Chapter 2, are needed to document the nature of an impairment and its consequences. Chapter 2 specifies how to acquire information and defines a format for analyzing, recording, and reporting the information. Second, the *Guides* chapters on the organ systems contain protocols or descriptions of ways to evaluate a particular body part, function, or system. Third, the chapters contain tables relating to the evaluation protocols. If the physician has followed the protocols and tables, then the reported findings will be congruent with the *Guides* criteria.

In practice, the first key to effecting an accurate impairment evaluation is a review of office and hospital records maintained by the physicians who have cared for the patient since the onset of the medical condition. Such records include clinical notes, medical consultation reports, hospital records, admission and discharge summaries, notes on operations, pathology and laboratory test reports, and reports on special tests and diagnostic procedures. Using multiple sources of information and attempting to ensure that the sources are objective can help eliminate bias, an error introduced by selecting or encouraging one outcome over another.

Before judgments according to the *Guides* are accepted, the history and course of the medical condition must be analyzed. This analysis should include findings from previous examinations, the treatment and responses to treatment, and the impact of the condition on the patient's activities. Before a judgment regarding impairment is made, it must be shown that the problem has been present for a period of time, is stable, and is unlikely to change in future months in spite of treatment.

In evaluating an impairment, it is important to obtain enough clinical information to characterize it in accordance with the *Guides* requirements. Once this task is accomplished, the evaluator's findings may be compared with the clinical information already available about the individual. If the evaluator's findings are consistent with the results of previous clinical studies, the findings may be compared with the *Guides* criteria to estimate the impairment. If the findings are not consistent with those of earlier studies, there should be communication between the involved physicians and clinical studies as needed to resolve any disparities.

1.3 Are the *Guides* Criteria Objective and Authoritative?

The contributors to the *Guides* understand the importance of having objective data on the functioning of normal persons' organ systems in order to evaluate those of impaired individuals. For many systems (eg, the respiratory, cardiovascular, visual, auditory, endocrine, hematologic, and digestive systems), medically accepted and scientifically derived data on normal functioning are available. The *Guides* generally makes use of these data and references their sources.

If the *Guides* contributors have been unable to identify objective data on the normal functioning of an organ system, they have estimated the extent of impairments on the basis of clinical experience, judgment, and consensus. The estimates of the well qualified persons contributing to this book, most of them physicians, would be more convincing than those of most others in estimating the severity of people's impairments.

It should be understood that the *Guides* does not and cannot provide answers about every type and degree of impairment, because of the considerations noted above and the infinite variety of human disease, and because the field of medicine and medical practice is characterized by constant change in understanding disease and its manifestations, diagnosis, and treatment. Further, human functioning in everyday life is a highly dynamic process, one that presents a great challenge to those attempting to evaluate impairment.

The physician's judgment and his or her experience, training, skill, and thoroughness in examining the patient and applying the findings to *Guides* criteria will be factors in estimating the degree of the patient's impairment. These attributes compose part of the "art" of medicine, which, together with a foundation in science, constitute the essence of medical practice. The evaluator should understand that other considerations will also apply, such as the sensitivity, specificity, accuracy, reproducibility, and interpretation of laboratory tests and clinical procedures, and variability among observers' interpretations of the tests and procedures.

1.4 Is the *Guides* Widely Used?

In a word, yes. Recently compiled data from a 1991 AMA survey indicate that in 40 of 53 jurisdictions (38 states and two territories), use of the *Guides* is *mandated* or *recommended* by law in workers' compensation cases, or the book is frequently used in such cases. In the survey, the chief executives of the 50 state workers' compensation agencies and those of two trust territories (Puerto Rico and the Virgin Islands) and the District of Columbia received letter questionnaires asking whether use of the *Guides* was (1) mandated by state laws or regulations; (2) recommended by state laws or regulations; (3) not mentioned in state laws or regulations; or (4) usual or frequent. More than one response was permissible.

The results of the survey are shown below in the Table. It may be seen that use of the *Guides* is mandated or recommended by laws or regulations in 29 (55%) of 53 workers' compensation jurisdictions. In 11 jurisdictions (21%) that do not mention the *Guides* in their laws, the book is frequently used. In 13 jurisdictions (24%), the book was reported *not* to be used frequently or mentioned in the statutes. These were Alabama, California, the District of Columbia, Illinois, Michigan, Minnesota, Missouri, New Jersey, New York, North Carolina, Pennsylvania, West Virginia, and Wisconsin. In Texas, mandatory use of the book was in litigation.

Table. Status of *Guides to the Evaluation of Permanent Impairment (Guides)* According to 53 Workers' Compensation Agencies.

Use of *Guides*	No. of states and territories
Mandated by state or territory's law	19
Recommended by state or territory's law	10
Not mentioned in state or territory's law	21*
Usual or frequent in workers' compensation cases	19
Not mentioned in state or territory's law; and use is *not* usual or frequent in workers' compensation cases	13

*Eleven states in this category are included also in the "usual or frequent" category of the table.

1.5 Impairment and Workers' Compensation

In general, state and federal workers' compensation laws are based on the concept that a worker who either sustains an injury or incurs an illness arising during and because of employment is entitled to protection against financial loss without being required to sue the employer. In exchange for workers' having lost the right to sue, state workers' compensation systems guarantee benefits to the covered workers who meet the law's requirements.

The types of payments that may be made when a claim is approved fall into three categories: payments to the claimant to compensate for lost wages due to temporary total disability; payment of medical bills; and payment of an award for permanent partial, or total, disability. Under the workers' compensation laws, disability, whether temporary or permanent, is equivalent to economic loss for which the individual is to be compensated. Temporary partial disability occurs when the individual with impairment returns to work but earns less than before.

Normally, a permanent disability associated with a permanent medical impairment is independent of an individual's capacity to work and is formulated in terms of expected long-term economic loss. The award may be paid according to a schedule that associates impairments of certain body parts, functions, or systems with specific awards. Examples are amputations, loss of sight, and loss of hearing. Usually, a schedule in the workers' compensation law equates the disability with a maximum number of weeks for which benefits are to be paid at a rate based on average weekly wages.

Rating permanent partial disability is necessary when the law, in recognition that the loss of the body part, function, or system may be less than total, requires a determination of the proportion or percentage of loss. Many states stipulate, for example, that if a worker has incurred partial amputation or loss of the use of a part, the Workers' Compensation Commission must allow compensation in proportion to the number of weeks' compensation allowed for total amputation or loss of use of the part.

Because schedules usually do not cover all conditions arising out of injuries, there is likely to be a provision in the law that, in cases of permanent disability other than those that are specifically listed, the Workers' Compensation Commission must determine the percentage by which the "industrial use" of the employee's body was impaired. The Commission also must consider the nature of the injury and the employee's occupation, experience, training, and age and then award proportional compensation. Medical information is essential for the decision process in all of these cases, and a critical problem arises in the interpretation and use of the medical information.

The critical problem is that no formula is known by which knowledge about a medical condition can be combined with knowledge about other factors to calculate the percentage by which the employee's industrial use of the body is impaired. Accordingly, each commissioner or hearing official must come to a conclusion on the basis of assessment of the available medical and nonmedical information. The *Guides* may help resolve such a situation, but it cannot provide complete and definitive answers. Each administrative or legal system that uses permanent impairment as a basis for disability ratings should define its own means for translating knowledge about an impairment into an estimate of the degree to which the impairment limits the individual's capacity to meet personal, social, occupational, and other demands or to meet statutory requirements.

It must be emphasized and clearly understood that impairment percentages derived according to *Guides* criteria should not be used to make direct financial awards or direct estimates of disabilities.

The physician performing an impairment evaluation must provide more than a number or percentage. The physician should provide as comprehensive a medical picture of the patient as possible, using the Report of Medical Evaluation form (p. 11) as an outline. If this is done, the person receiving the evaluation will be able to determine how the medical information fits with the nonmedical information and will have the basis for an improved understanding of how the impairment may affect the patient's employability and daily activities.

The American Medical Association strongly discourages the use of any but the most recent edition of the *Guides,* because the information in it would not be based on the most recent and up-to-date material.

The Minnesota Medical Association prepared a guide to conditions that may cause "temporary disability," that is, disability lasting less than 52 weeks. The guide estimated the durations of short-lived conditions for persons performing clerical or administrative, light manual, or heavy manual work.[5]

1.6 Railroad and Maritime Workers' Compensation

State workers' compensation laws are not the only means by which employees are compensated for injuries or illnesses. In 1908, Congress provided for railroad workers, passing the Federal Employer's Liability Act (FELA), which put in place a comprehensive injury compensation system. The FELA is an exclusive remedy for injured railroad workers, and it supercedes state workers' compensation laws. The Jones Act, passed in 1920, covers compensation for maritime workers who are injured because of a ship owner's negligence. That law provides for the same rights and remedies that were extended through FELA.

A lawsuit under FELA must be based on the negligence of the railroad in failing to provide the employee with a safe workplace. An injured employee must prove that the railroad should have foreseen that a condition or activity might have caused the injury or disease. The test used is to determine whether the employer's negligence played any part in producing the injury. Recoverable amounts include those for necessary medical expenses, pain and suffering, loss of past earnings, and future losses due to diminished earning capacity. An important stipulation is that the effects of the injury must be diagnosed by a physician.

Under FELA, all cases must go before a jury or judge, and there are no limits to the amounts of awards. This is in contrast to awards under state workers' compensation systems, which are fixed and limited. Under FELA the jury decides on the degree of the injured person's disability and handicap. In a case under FELA, as in any workers' compensation case, the physician has the obligation of obtaining a reliable history and accurately determining the extent of the worker's impairment. The physician should confirm past employment by obtaining others' records and should collect all available medical information.

1.7 Usefulness of the *Guides* for Claims and Litigation

The growing emphasis on workers' compensation claims and litigation makes it increasingly important to use the *Guides* extensively and properly. Even though rating or estimating impairments cannot be totally objective, use of the *Guides* increases objectivity and enables physicians to evaluate and report medical impairment in a standardized manner, so that reports from different observers are more likely to be comparable in content and completeness. The *Guides* helps minimize abuses and unrealistic verdicts that may arise from unjustified claims.

In recent years, workers' claims involving hearing losses or exposures to asbestos have reached the tens of thousands. Judges would be able to render decisions in the cases more expeditiously and equitably, if physicians prepared impairment evaluations according to the methods and criteria of the *Guides.*

Compensation claims may be adjudicated by referees, commissioners, or court judges if the claims fall within state workers' compensation laws; or they may be decided by a judge or jury in federal or state courts. Occasionally, decisions are made by administrators, as with the Social Security Administration, U.S. Department of Veterans Affairs, and some insurance companies. Most individuals making these decisions have specialized training in evaluating and deciding claims. In some instances the claims are evaluated by one or more arbitrators, who may be attorneys or others with special training. The backgrounds and work experience of the adjudicators vary widely; following the *Guides* might improve the quality and equity of their decisions.

Among the many factors that contribute to inequities in workers' compensation cases are inaccurate or incomplete responses from patients, especially with regard to medical and work histories. Frequently the information in the medical report differs from that in a deposition taken during the legal proceedings. Physicians will save time in the long run by gathering adequate, accurate information about the onset, duration, symptoms, and treatment of illnesses; work histories and workplaces; and the usual activities of patients.

1.8 Employability: Management and Administrative Considerations

The concept of employability deserves special attention, especially since physicians, and particularly occupational physicians, are frequently called on to determine whether an individual can be employed or should be allowed to continue the job. If an individual with a medical abnormality has the capacity, with or without accommodation, to meet job demands and the conditions of employment as defined by the employer, the individual is employable and is not necessarily disabled.

Employability is critically related to an individual's capacity to travel to and from work, be at work, and perform assigned tasks and duties for which the employer is willing to pay wages. If the individual has that capacity, even in the presence of impairment, he or she is not disabled for those tasks. Disability results when the individual lacks, among other capabilities, the prerequisites of employability. Emphasis in the United States on hiring the handicapped and making it possible for individuals with impairments and disabilities to continue their work satisfactorily should receive sensitive and sympathetic attention from physicians. Information from the physician's standpoint on the recently passed Americans with Disabilities Act appears in the Glossary (p. 315).

In determining the employability of individuals with impairments, it is important to establish their status as safety risks to themselves or other employees. The first step in carrying out a medical determination related to employability is to learn about the job, including the employer's expectations with respect to performance, physical activity, reliability, availability, productivity, expected duration of useful service, and any other criteria associated with job qualification and suitability. A sufficiently detailed job analysis can provide the basis on which a physician can determine the kinds of medical information needed to assess an individual's health with respect to the job's demands.

Quite often an individual who alleges disability may already be under the care of a physician, especially if the medical condition is interfering with workplace activities. The physician's medical records are important in the determination of employability. During the assessment of employability, the physician and other responsible persons should keep in mind the potential for aggravation of an impairment and the possibility of changing an individual's job responsibilities.

With respect to employability, the medical questions to be answered are whether or not the documentation supports the conclusion that the individual's medical condition precludes travel to and from work, being at work, and performing assigned tasks and duties, and, in the case of a deficiency in service at work, whether or not the medical condition has contributed to the deficiency. It is important to verify all of the clinical findings and history to be sure they are reliable and valid.

In general, two physicians who are given the same information gathered from previous records and who examine the same patient for employment under the same protocol should obtain approximately the same findings. The results of their evaluations then may be compared with the criteria for the position. When approached in this way, the physician's participation in an employability determination will be independent of the individual's motivation to work.

References

1. World Health Organization. *International Classification of Impairments, Disabilities, and Handicaps.* Geneva, Switzerland: World Health Organization; 1980.

2. Luck JV Jr, Florence DW. A brief history and comparative analysis of disability systems and impairment rating guides. *Orthop Clin North Am.* 1988;19:839-844.

3. Battista ME. Assessing work capacity. *J Insurance Med.* 1988;20:16-22.

4. LaPlante MP. *Disability in Basic Life Activities Across the Life Span.* Washington, DC: National Institute on Disability and Rehabilitation Research, U.S. Department of Education; 1991.

5. Minnesota Medical Association. *Revised Temporary Disability Duration Guide.* Minneapolis, Minn: Minnesota Medical Association; 1984.

For information on this subject contact the Minnesota Department of Labor and Industry, 443 Lafayette Rd., St. Paul, MN 55155; tel. no. (612) 296-6107.

Chapter 2

Records and Reports

Estimating the extent of permanent impairments is most effective when there is sufficient medical and nonmedical information to justify the estimates and minimize adversarial situations. This chapter describes how the *Guides* can help provide consistent and reliable acquisition, analysis, communication, and utilization of medical information.

The major objective of the *Guides* is to define the assessment and reporting of medical impairments so that physicians can collect, describe, and analyze information about impairments in accordance with a single set of standards. Two physicians, following the methods of the *Guides* to evaluate the same patient, should report similar results and reach similar conclusions. Moreover, if the clinical findings are fully described, any knowledgeable observer may check the findings with the *Guides* criteria.

If two physicians who examine a patient and use the methods of the *Guides* do not obtain similar results and reach similar conclusions, then the book can be used to resolve the discrepancies. Analysis of the records and reports in question will disclose the disparities, which should be in matters of fact rather than opinion. If the patient's medical condition is stable, then different physicians should reach the same general conclusion. If widely disparate evaluations occur, then the stability of the medical condition and the matter of permanent impairment would be in question.

Compare this approach with some impairment evaluations wherein physicians examine and report on patients without a standard protocol. In such instances, it is impossible to compare reports, because there is no assurance that the physicians have examined the same body parts or systems in the same way. For example, one physician may measure flexion of the hip or knee, but another may not mention those movements. Or one physician may report that the patient can flex the arm 90°, while another may not measure the range of motion. Without standardization of evaluations and reporting procedures, an individual reading these reports would have difficulty deciding which report to believe. This outcome is neither reasonable nor fair, and it tends to give rise to avoidable confrontation.

When physicians follow the *Guides* to measure and report their impairment estimates, the persons who receive the evaluations may be held accountable for assessing the results in accordance with the *Guides* recommendations. Because issues of medical fact should have been settled by this stage in the process, the recipients of the evaluations should not find it necessary to choose among conflicting opinions.

By consulting the standardized medical evaluation protocols and reference tables and reviewing the recommendations of the *Guides*, the recipient may verify whether or not all necessary information was collected. If it was, the correctness of the evaluation may be ascertained by comparing it with the *Guides* tables. If there is disagreement about the clinical findings, further medical evaluation may be necessary. The recipient should not give one inadequately supported medical evaluation greater weight than another.

The impairment estimate or rating is a simple number. Although it may have been derived from a well structured set of thorough observations, it does not convey any information about the person or the impact of the impairment on the person's capacity to meet personal, social, or occupational demands. In fact, one may lose sight of important information in viewing the number. The strength of the medical support for an impairment estimate depends on the completeness and reliability of the medical documentation. The scope of the documentation needed for a reliable report is indicated in the Report of Medical Evaluation (p. 11).

Knowledge of the course of an individual's medical condition over time is essential in reaching an understanding of the individual's health status. Thus, within legal constraints, copies of existing medical office and hospital records should be attached to the evaluation report, even if the report itself discusses the medical history and course of the condition.

Impairment evaluation involves not only an examination, but also the management of a medical condition. Having complete information about the impairment will enable a reviewer to determine whether or not a claim makes sense and to approach the question of disability and economic loss in a logical and systematic fashion.

2.1 Medical Assessment of Impairment

According to the *Guides*, the first step in assessing an individual's impairment is gathering thorough and complete historical information on the medical condition(s) and then carrying out a medical evaluation supported by appropriate tests and diagnostic procedures.

A proper medical evaluation accurately documents the individual's clinical status. If the current findings are consistent with the results of previous clinical evaluations, the findings may be compared with the appropriate *Guides* tables to estimate the individual's impairment. If the current findings do not agree with the recorded information, there should be further clinical evaluation to resolve the disparities.

The second step in assessing the impairment is analyzing the history and the clinical and laboratory findings to determine the nature and extent of the impairment or dysfunction of the affected body part or system.

The third step is comparing the results of the analysis with the criteria specified in the *Guides* for the particular body part, system, or function. This comparison is distinct from the preceding clinical evaluation and need not be performed by the physician who did that evaluation; rather, any knowledgeable person can compare the clinical findings with the *Guides* criteria and determine whether or not the impairment estimates reflect those criteria.

2.2 Rules for Evaluations

In general, the physician should estimate the extent of the patient's primary impairment or impairing condition, that is, the condition that seems to be of most concern to the patient. The estimate should be based on current findings and evidence. It may be necessary to refer to the criteria and estimates in several chapters if the impairing condition involves several organ systems. In that case, each organ system impairment should be expressed as a whole-person impairment; then the whole-person impairments should be combined by means of the Combined Values Chart (p. 322). The general philosophy of the Combined Values Chart is explained in Section 3.1, Chapter 3 (p. 15).

If the physician believes that the patient has two significant, unrelated conditions and that the extent of each should be estimated, this may be done. The whole-person impairment estimates for the two separate conditions then would be combined into an overall impairment estimate using the Combined Values Chart.

Tests of consistency, such as the one described to check the patient's lumbosacral spine range of motion (Chapter 3, Section 3.3j p. 113), are good but imperfect indicators of patients' efforts. The physician must utilize the entire gamut of clinical skill and judgment in assessing whether or not the results of measurements or tests are plausible and relate to the impairment being evaluated. If in spite of an observation or test result the medical evidence appears not to be of sufficient weight to verify that an impairment of a certain magnitude exists, the physician should modify the impairment estimate accordingly, describing the modification and explaining the reason for it in writing.

In this book, a 95% to 100% whole-person impairment is considered to represent almost total impairment, a state that is approaching death.

Interpolating, Measuring, and Rounding Off

In general, an impairment value that falls between those appearing in a table or figure of the *Guides* may be adjusted or interpolated to be proportional to the interval of the table or figure involved, unless the book gives other directions.

Unless generally accepted standards exist, as with many laboratory tests, two measurements made by the same examiner and involving a patient or a patient's functions may be expected to lie within 10% of each other.

Measurements should be consistent between two trained observers; if they have been made by one observer on separate occasions, they also should be consistent. Repeating measurements may increase their credibility.

A final estimated whole-person impairment percent, whether it is based on the evaluation of one organ system or several organ systems, may be rounded to the nearer of the two nearest values ending in 0 or 5.

Pain

In general, the impairment percents shown in the chapters that consider the various organ systems make allowance for the pain that may accompany the impairing conditions. Chronic pain, also called the chronic pain syndrome, is evaluated as described in the chapter on pain (p. 303).

Using Prostheses in Evaluations

The general view of the *Guides* is that if an individual's prosthesis or assistive device can be removed or its use eliminated relatively easily, the organ system should be tested and evaluated without the device. For example, a hearing aid should be removed before auditory acuity is tested. However, the examiner may choose to test the system with the assistive device in place also and then report both sets of results.

If the assistive device is not easily removable, as with an implanted lens, the organ system's functioning should be evaluated with the device in place. The visual system should be tested with the patient's glasses or contact lenses in place if they are used.

Adjustments for Effects of Treatment or Lack of Treatment

In certain instances, the treatment of an illness may result in apparently total remission of the patient's signs and symptoms. Examples include the treatment of hypothyroidism with levothyroxine and the treatment of type I diabetes mellitus with insulin. Yet it is debatable as to whether the patient has regained the previous status of normal good health. In these instances, the physician may choose to increase the impairment estimate by a small percentage (eg, 1% to 3%), combining that percent with any other impairment percent by means of the Combined Values Chart (p. 322).

In some instances, as with the recipients of transplanted organs who are treated with immunity-suppressing pharmaceuticals or persons treated with anticoagulants, the pharmaceuticals themselves may lead to impairments. In such an instance, the physician should use the appropriate parts of the *Guides* to evaluate the impairment related to the pharmaceutical. If information in the *Guides* is lacking, the physician may combine an estimated impairment percent, the magnitude of which would depend on the severity of the effect, with the primary organ system impairment, by means of the Combined Values Chart.

A patient may decline treatment of an impairment with a surgical procedure, a pharmacologic agent, or other therapeutic approach. The view of the *Guides* contributors is that if a patient declines therapy for a permanent impairment, that decision should neither decrease nor increase the estimated percentage of the patient's impairment. However, the physician may wish to make a written comment in the medical evaluation report about the suitability of the therapeutic approach and describe the basis of the patient's refusal.

2.3 General Comments on Evaluation

The *Guides* attempts to take into account all relevant considerations in estimating or rating the severity and extent of permanent impairment and the effects of the impairment in terms of the individual's everyday activities. An impairment should not be considered "permanent" until the clinical findings, determined during a period of months, indicate that the medical condition is static and well stabilized.

A physician who is asked to reevaluate an individual's impairment must realize that change may have occurred, even though a previous evaluator considered the impairment to be permanent. For instance, the condition may have become worse as a result of aggravation or clinical progression, or it may have improved. The physician should assess the *current* state of the impairment according to the criteria in the *Guides*.

Valid assessment of a change in the impairment estimate would depend on the reliability of the previous estimate and the reliability of the evidence on which it was based. If there were no valid previous evaluation, information gathered earlier could be used to estimate impairment according to *Guides* criteria. However, if there were insufficient information to document the change accurately, then the evaluator ought not attempt to estimate the change but should explain that decision.

If "apportionment" is needed, the analysis must consider the nature of the impairment and its possible relationship to each alleged factor, and it must provide an explanation of the medical basis for all conclusions and opinions. Apportionment and causation are considered more fully in the Glossary (p. 315).

For example, in apportioning a spine impairment, first the current spine impairment would be estimated, and then impairment from any preexisting spine problem would be estimated. The estimate for the preexisting impairment would be subtracted from that for the present impairment to account for the effects of the former. Using this approach to apportionment would require accurate information and data on both impairments.

Even when the impairment is well localized, its consequences cannot be understood without taking an individual's activities into account. Attention to full and complete reporting will provide the best opportunity for physicians to explain the health status of patients and the nature of their impairments to reviewers, claims examiners, and hearing officials; for attorneys to understand impairments; and for individuals to pursue any benefits to which they are entitled.

2.4 Preparing Reports

A clear, accurate, and complete report is essential to support a rating of permanent impairment. The following kinds of information are expected.

Medical Evaluation

1. Medical evaluation includes a narrative history of the medical condition(s) with specific reference to onset and course of the condition, symptoms, findings on previous examination(s), treatments, and responses to treatment, including adverse effects. Information that may be relevant to onset, such as an occupational exposure, should be included.

2. It also includes results of the most recent clinical evaluation, including any of the following:
• physical examination
• laboratory tests
• electrocardiograms
• radiographic studies
• rehabilitation evaluation
• mental status examination, including testing of intellectual functioning and evaluation of character traits
• other tests or diagnostic procedures

3. Current clinical status is assessed, and a statement of plans for future treatment, rehabilitation, and reevaluation is included.

4. Diagnoses and clinical impressions are reported.

5. The expected date of full or partial recovery is estimated.

Analysis of the Findings

1. An explanation of the impact of the medical condition(s) on life activities should be given. The types of activities affected should be listed.

2. The medical basis for concluding that the condition and the patient's symptoms have or have not become stable should be explained.

3. An explanation should be given of the medical basis for concluding that the individual is or is not likely to suffer sudden, subtle, or other incapacitation as a result of a change in the condition.

4. An explanation should be given of the medical basis for concluding that the individual is or is not likely to suffer injury or harm or further impairment by engaging in activities of daily living or other activities necessary to meet personal, social, and occupational demands.

5. Any conclusion that restrictions or accommodations are or are not warranted with respect to daily activities or activities that are required to meet personal, social, and occupational demands should be explained. If restrictions because of risks to the patient or others, or accommodations, are necessary, an explanation of their expected outcome and value should be provided.

Comparison of the Results of Analysis with the Impairment Criteria

1. A description should be given of specific clinical findings related to each impairment, with reference to how the findings relate to and compare with the criteria described in the applicable *Guides* chapter; reference should be made to the absence of, or the examiner's inability to obtain, pertinent data.

2. An explanation of each impairment value with reference to the applicable criteria of the *Guides* should be included.

3. A summary list of impairment estimates in percents should be included.

On the following two pages is a standard form that may be used by the evaluator as a cover sheet for a medical report and report on permanent impairment. The form may be reproduced without permission from the American Medical Association.

In determining the approximate location in the *Guides* of material concerning a particular kind of organ system impairment, the evaluator may find it useful to refer to the List of Tables and Figures (p. xi) as well as the Index.

Report of Medical Evaluation (Permanent Medical Impairment)

To:

Re:

Case number:

Report date:

Onset of injury or illness:

1. Medical history		Yes	No
a. Medical office records	Reviewed		
	Enclosed		
b. Hospital records	Reviewed		
	Enclosed		
c. From other source (describe)			
d. From patient			

2. Clinical evaluation		Yes	No
a. Physical examination	Reports enclosed		
b. Laboratory tests	Reports enclosed		
c. Special tests and diagnostic procedures	Reports enclosed		
d. Specialist's evaluation	Reports enclosed		

3. Diagnoses
a.
b.
c.
d.

4. Stability of the medical condition	Yes	No
a. The clinical condition is stabilized and not likely to improve with surgical intervention or active medical treatment; medical maintenance care only is warranted.		
b. The degree of impairment is not likely to change substantially within the next year.		
c. The patient is not likely to suffer sudden or subtle incapacitation.		

Report of Medical Evaluation (Permanent Medical Impairment) Page 2

5. Other analyses

a. Explain briefly the impact(s) of the medical condition(s) on the patient's activities of daily living, including occupation (see Chapter 1 and Glossary, p. 315).

List types of daily activities affected:

1.

2.

3.

4.

5.

6.

b. Is there a medical reason to believe the patient is likely to suffer injury, harm, or further medical impairment by engaging in usual activities of living or other activities necessary to meet personal, social, or occupational demands? Explain briefly.

_____Yes No_____

c. Is there a medical reason to believe restrictions, accommodations, or assistive devices are necessary to help the patient carry out usual activities or meet personal, social, and occupational demands? If so, briefly describe them and explain their therapeutic, risk-avoidance, or other kind of value.

_____Yes No_____

6. Impairment evaluation according to *Guides*–Attach a complete report of findings and narrative comments for each body part or system. Each organ system impairment estimate should be expressed in terms of percent impairment of the whole person.

Body part or system	Chapter No.	Table No.	% Impairment of the whole person
a.			
b.			
c.			
d.			

7. Final estimated whole-person impairment: __________________%.

8. _____ This patient has been under my care from ________________ to ________________.

_____ I have not provided care for this patient. I have seen this patient _______ time(s) for the purpose of evaluating medical impairment.

9. I (do) (do not) believe there is inconsistency among the history, physical examination, laboratory finding, and other studies (cross out the nonapplicable verb phrase). If an inconsistency exists, explain it in writing.

____, MD

(Signature)

____ ____________________

(Print name) (Date)

Chapter 3

The Musculoskeletal System

This chapter includes sections on the upper extremity, the lower extremity, the spine, and the pelvis. The sections describe and recommend methods and techniques of determining impairments due to amputation, restriction of motion or ankylosis, sensory or motor deficits, peripheral nerve disorders, and peripheral vascular diseases. Also included are tables with impairment estimates relating to specific disorders of the upper extremity, lower extremity, and spine. Each section describes appropriate methods and considers issues applicable to that section.

In general, the impairment percents shown in this chapter make allowance for the pain that may accompany the musculoskeletal system impairments. The chapter also considers pain related to peripheral nerve disorders. Chronic pain and the chronic pain syndrome are evaluated as described in the *Guides* chapter on pain (p. 303).

Description: The upper extremity, the lower extremity, the spine, and the pelvis are each to be considered a unit of the whole person. The upper extremity has four parts: hand, wrist, elbow, and shoulder. The normal hand has five digits: the thumb and the index, middle, ring, and little fingers (Figs. 1 through 3, pp. 16 through 18). The thumb has three joints: the interphalangeal (IP), metacarpophalangeal (MP), and carpometacarpal (CMC) joints. Each finger has three joints: the distal interphalangeal (DIP), proximal interphalangeal (PIP), and MP joints.

The lower extremity has six sections: the foot, the hindfoot, the ankle, the leg, the knee, and the hip. The foot has five digits: the great toe and the second, third, fourth, and fifth toes. The great toe has two joints: the interphalangeal (IP) and the metatarsophalangeal (MTP) joints. The second, third, fourth, and fifth toes all have three joints: the DIP, PIP, and MTP joints.

Normally the spine has 24 vertebrae. The cervical region has seven vertebrae, C 1 through C 7; the thoracic region has 12 vertebrae, T 1 through T 12; and the lumbar region has five vertebrae, L 1 through L 5.

The pelvis is composed of the pubis, ischium, and ilium, which form its side and front, and the sacrum and coccyx, which form its posterior portion.

Examinations for determining musculoskeletal system impairments are based on traditional approaches for recording the medical history and performing the physical examination. The impairment examination and report should not be separated from the generally accepted principles of medical practice or the consensus of medical knowledge and experience.

The measurement techniques recommended in this chapter are current and are as simple, practical, and scientifically sound as possible. The tests should be done accurately and precisely. For evaluating ranges of motion of the upper and lower extremities, small and large goniometers are needed. For evaluating the spine, either two mechanical inclinometers are needed, or a single, computerized inclinometer is needed that is capable of calculating compound joint motion. These instruments are described further in Section 3.3j (p. 113).

The tables of Chapter 3 are based on the *active* range of motion, which is determined with the patient's full effort and cooperation. The recommended tests should be performed and reported according to *Guides* recommendations, so they can be repeated by others and the results compared. Comparing the patient's active range of motion with the passive range of motion provides useful information.

Evaluating the range of motion of an extremity or of the spine is a valid method of estimating an impairment. To some extent, however, the range of motion is subject to the patient's control. The results of such evaluations should be consistent and concordant with the presence or absence of pathologic signs and other medical evidence.

Ancillary tests and professional opinions that help delineate the impairing condition may contribute to the musculoskeletal system evaluation. Useful diagnostic procedures may include roentgenographic studies, arthrography, computed tomographic (CT) scans, or magnetic resonance imaging (MRI). Such procedures should be done only if necessary and relevant, and they should not be ordered without consideration of costs as well as benefits.

The electrodiagnostic examination may provide useful information and includes electromyography, nerve conduction, or neurophysiologic evaluations. It should be performed by a physician with knowledge and experience in the field, preferably one who is certified by the American Board of Electrodiagnostic Medicine, and it should be done in a laboratory meeting the guidelines of the American Association of Electrodiagnostic Medicine.[1]

Before using the information in this chapter, the reader should study Chapters 1 and 2 and the Glossary (p. 315), which discuss the purposes of the *Guides*, the situations in which they are useful, and basic definitions relating to impairments. Chapters 1 and 2 also discuss methods of examining patients and preparing reports. An impairment evaluation report should include information such as that shown below.

A. Medical Evaluation

- History of medical condition
- Results of most recent clinical evaluation
- Assessment of current clinical status and statement of further medical plans
- Diagnosis

B. Analysis of Findings

- Impact of medical condition on daily activities
- Explanation for concluding that the condition is stable and stationary and unlikely to change
- Explanation for concluding the individual is or is not likely to suffer further impairment by engaging in usual activities
- Explanation for concluding that accommodations or restrictions related to the impairment are or are not warranted

C. Comparison of Analysis with Impairment Criteria

- Description of clinical findings and how these findings relate to *Guides* criteria
- Explanation of each estimated impairment
- Summary list of all impairment percents
- Estimated whole-person impairment percent

3.1 The Hand and Upper Extremity

3.1a Evaluation

Methods for evaluating impairments of the upper extremity may be described as having anatomic, cosmetic, or functional bases. The *physical evaluation* is based on a detailed examination of the patient and the upper extremity and is necessary to determine anatomic aspects of the impairment. The *cosmetic evaluation* concerns the patient's and society's reaction to the impairment or the results of surgical treatment. The *functional evaluation* is a measure of the individual's ability to carry out an expected function or task within a set time frame. Evaluation of anatomic impairment is considered to be the most reproducible and reliable system and is the approach recommended in this section. Using a combination of these approaches would be ideal.

A system for evaluating impairment of the hand and upper extremity due to amputation, sensory loss, abnormal motion, and ankylosis was developed and approved by the International Federation of Societies for Surgery of the Hand in association with the American Society for Surgery of the Hand. That approach forms the basis of the tests and procedures recommended in the *Guides* for evaluating the hand and upper extremity.

The most practical and useful approach to evaluating impairment of a digit is to compare it with the loss of function resulting from amputation. Total loss of motion and sensation of a digit, or ankylosis with severe malposition that renders the digit essentially useless, is considered to be about the same as amputation of the part. Ankylosis of the digit or joint in the optimal functional position is given the least impairment. Impairment due to total sensory loss only is considered to be 50% of that due to amputation.

In evaluation of restriction of motion of the hand and upper extremity, the full range possible of *active* motion should be carried out by the subject and measured by the examiner. Several repetitions may be performed to obtain reliable results. The examiner may check the range of *passive* motion by applying moderate pressure to the joint. However, in the *Guides*, the range of *active* motion takes precedence. If a joint cannot be moved actively by the subject or passively by the examiner, the position of ankylosis should be recorded.

In general, range of motion measurements are rounded to the nearest 10°. The measurements are converted to impairment estimates by referring to the appropriate tables.

For accurate impairment evaluation, a complete and detailed examination of the upper extremity is necessary. This is facilitated by the use of a printed chart or figure that lists the various tests and measurements in an orderly fashion, such as the Upper Extremity Impairment Evaluation Record, Fig. 1 (pp. 16 and 17).

Part 1 of Fig. 1 (p. 16) has been designed to assist evaluation of hand impairment due to abnormal motion, amputation, sensory loss, and other disorders. Part 2 (p. 17) has been designed to assist evaluation of wrist, elbow, and shoulder impairment due to abnormal motion, amputation, and other disorders, and upper extremity impairments related to the peripheral nerve system, the peripheral vascular system, and other disorders that are not included in regional impairments. As Fig. 1 indicates, the hand, wrist, elbow, and shoulder impairments are *combined* using the Combined Values Chart (p. 322) to determine the total upper extremity impairment. The latter is converted to a whole-person impairment using Table 3 (p. 20).

The hand and upper extremity section considers evaluation of the thumb, finger, wrist, elbow, and shoulder regions. Each part considers techniques of measurement and includes values for impairments due to amputation, sensory loss, and abnormal motion. In addition, impairments of the upper extremity due to peripheral nerve, brachial plexus and spinal nerve lesions, vascular problems, loss of strength, and other conditions receive consideration in this section. Also, combining two or more impairments and relating them to the individual as a whole ("the whole person") is illustrated.

Figure 1. Upper Extremity Impairment Evaluation Record**–**Part 1 (Hand)** Side☐R ☐L

Name________________ Age____ Sex ☐M ☐F Dominant hand ☐R ☐L Date________

Occupation________________ Diagnosis________________

			Abnormal motion Record motion, ankylosis, and impairment %				**Amputation** Mark level & impairment %	**Sensory loss** Mark type, level, & impairment %	**Other disorders** List type & impairment %	**Hand impairment%** • Combine digit IMP% *Convert to hand IMP%	
			Flexion	Extension	Ankylosis	IMP%					
Thumb	IP	Angle°									
		IMP%									
	MP	Angle°									
		IMP%									
				Motion	Ankylosis	IMP%					
	CMC	Radial abduction Angle°								Abnormal motion [1]	
		Radial abduction IMP%								Amputation [2]	
		Adduction CMS								Sensory loss [3]	
		Adduction IMP%								Other disorders [4]	
		Opposition CMS					R L	R L		Digit impairment % • Combine 1, 2, 3, 4	
		Opposition IMP%									
	Add impairment % CMC + MP + IP =					[1]	[2] **IMP % =**	[3] **IMP % =**	[4] **IMP % =**	**Hand impairment % *Convert above**	

			Flexion	Extension	Ankylosis	IMP%					
Index	DIP	Angle°								Abnormal motion [1]	
		IMP%								Amputation [2]	
	PIP	Angle°								Sensory loss [3]	
		IMP%								Other disorders [4]	
	MP	Angle°								Digit impairment % • Combine 1, 2, 3, 4	
		IMP%									
	• Combine impairment % MP + PIP + DIP =					[1]	[2] **IMP % =**	[3] **IMP % =**	[4] **IMP % =**	**Hand impairment % *Convert above**	
Middle	DIP	Angle°								Abnormal motion [1]	
		IMP%								Amputation [2]	
	PIP	Angle°								Sensory loss [3]	
		IMP%								Other disorders [4]	
	MP	Angle°								Digit impairment % • Combine 1, 2, 3, 4	
		IMP%									
	• Combine impairment % MP + PIP + DIP =					[1]	[2] **IMP % =**	[3] **IMP % =**	[4] **IMP % =**	**Hand impairment % *Convert above**	
Ring	DIP	Angle°								Abnormal motion [1]	
		IMP%								Amputation [2]	
	PIP	Angle°								Sensory loss [3]	
		IMP%								Other disorders [4]	
	MP	Angle°								Digit impairment % • Combine 1, 2, 3, 4	
		IMP%									
	• Combine impairment % MP + PIP + DIP =					[1]	[2] **IMP % =**	[3] **IMP % =**	[4] **IMP % =**	**Hand impairment % *Convert above**	
Little	DIP	Angle°								Abnormal motion [1]	
		IMP%								Amputation [2]	
	PIP	Angle°								Sensory loss [3]	
		IMP%								Other disorders [4]	
	MP	Angle°								Digit impairment % • Combine 1, 2, 3, 4	
		IMP%									
	• Combine impairment % MP + PIP + DIP =					[1]	[2] **IMP % =**	[3] **IMP % =**	[4] **IMP % =**	**Hand impairment % *Convert above**	

Total hand impairment (Add hand impairment % for thumb + index + middle + ring + little finger) = %
Upper extremity impairment (†Convert total hand impairment % to upper extremity impairment %) = %; enter on Part 2, Line II
If hand region impairment is only impairment, convert upper extremity impairment to whole-person impairment:‡ = %

• Combined Values Chart; (p. 322-324) *Use Table 1 (Digits to hand p. 18); †Use Table 2 (Hand to upper extremity p. 19) ‡Use Table 3 (p. 20)

** Courtesy of G. de Groot Swanson, MD

Figure 1. Upper Extremity Impairment Evaluation Record–**Part 2 (Wrist, elbow, and shoulder)** Side ☐ R ☐ L

Name________ Age____ Sex ☐ M ☐ F Dominant hand ☐ R ☐ L Date________

Occupation________ Diagnosis________

		Abnormal motion				Other disorders	Regional impairment %	Amputation
		Record motion, ankylosis and impairment %				List type & impairment %	• Combine [1] + [2]	Mark level & impairment %
Wrist		Flexion	Extension	Ankylosis	IMP%			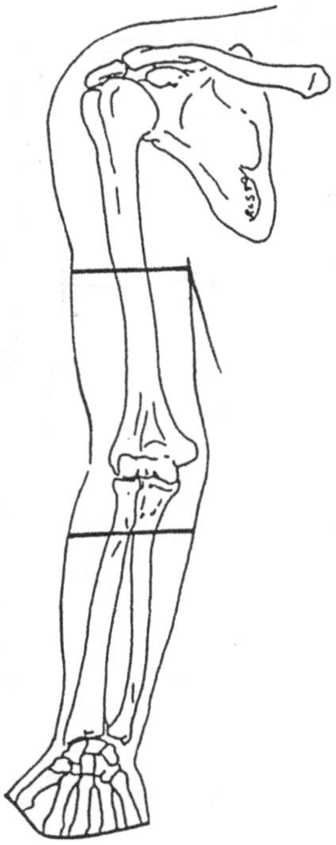
	Angle°							
	IMP%							
		RD	UD	Ankylosis	IMP%			
	Angle°							
	IMP%							
	Add IMP% F/E + RD/UD =				[1]	**IMP% =** [2]		
Elbow		Flexion	Extension	Ankylosis	IMP%			
	Angle°							
	IMP%							
		Pro	Sup	Ankylosis	IMP%			
	Angle°							
	IMP%							
	Add IMP% F/E + PRO/SUP =				[1]	**IMP% =** [2]		
Shoulder		Flexion	Extension	Ankylosis	IMP%			
	Angle°							
	IMP%							
		Add	Abd	Ankylosis	IMP%			
	Angle°							
	IMP%							
		Int Rot	Ext Rot	Ankylosis	IMP%			
	Angle°							
	IMP%							
	Add IMP% F/E + Add/Abd + IR/ER =				[1]	**IMP% =** [2]		**IMP %**

I. Amputation impairment (other than digitis)	=
II. Regional impairment of upper extremity • (Combine hand ____% + wrist ____% + elbow ____% + shoulder ____%)	=
III. Peripheral nerve system impairment	=
IV. Peripheral vascular system impairment	=
V. Other disorders (not included in regional impairment)	=

Total upper extremity impairment (• Combine I + II + III + IV + V)	=
Impairment of the whole person (Use Table 3 p. 20)	=

If both limbs are involved, calculate the whole-person impairment for each on a separate chart and *combine* the percents (Combined Values Chart).

Figure 2. Impairments of Upper Extremity from Amputation at Various Levels.*

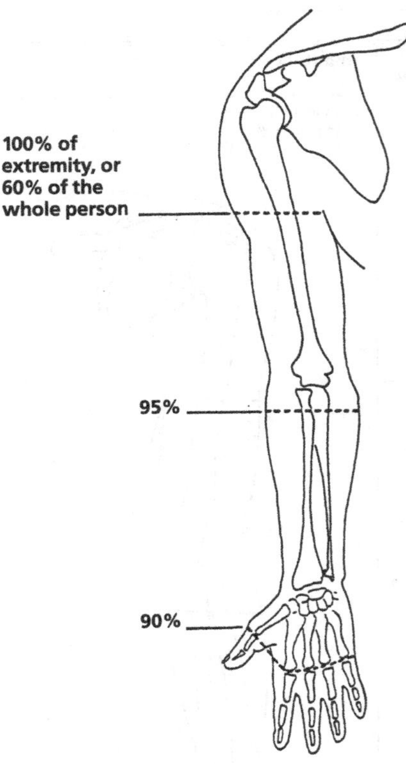

*With permission from Swanson, AB[34], p. 926, Fig. 1.

Figure 3. Impairments of the Digits (percents outside digits) and of Hand (percents inside digits) for Amputations at Various Levels.*

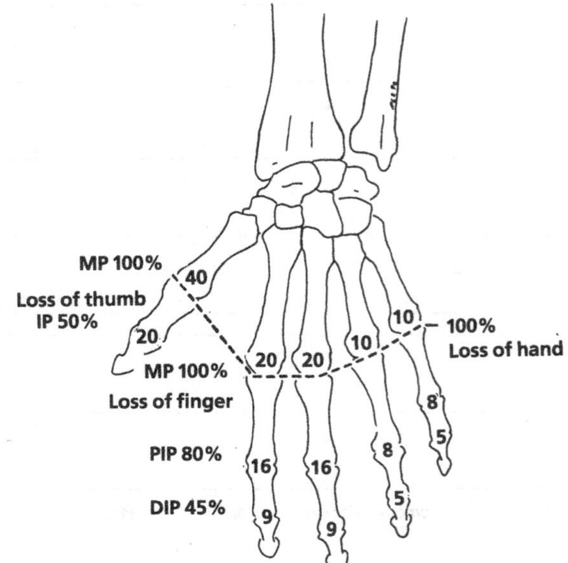

*With permission from Swanson, AB[34], p. 926, Fig. 1.

Table 1. Relationship of Impairment of the Digits to Impairment of the Hand.*

% Impairment of		% Impairment of		% Impairment of	
Thumb	**Hand**	**Index or middle finger**	**Hand**	**Ring or little finger**	**Hand**
0- 1	= 0	0- 2	= 0	0- 4	= 0
2- 3	= 1	3- 7	= 1	5- 14	= 1
4- 6	= 2	8- 12	= 2	15- 24	= 2
7- 8	= 3	13- 17	= 3	25- 34	= 3
9- 11	= 4	18- 22	= 4	35- 44	= 4
12- 13	= 5	23- 27	= 5	45- 54	= 5
14- 16	= 6	28- 32	= 6	55- 64	= 6
17- 18	= 7	33- 37	= 7	65- 74	= 7
19- 21	= 8	38- 42	= 8	75- 84	= 8
22- 23	= 9	43- 47	= 9	85- 94	= 9
24- 26	= 10	48- 52	= 10	95-100	= 10
27- 28	= 11	53- 57	= 11		
29- 31	= 12	58- 62	= 12		
32- 33	= 13	63- 67	= 13		
34- 36	= 14	68- 72	= 14		
37- 38	= 15	73- 77	= 15		
39- 41	= 16	78- 82	= 16		
42- 43	= 17	83- 87	= 17		
44- 46	= 18	88- 92	= 18		
47- 48	= 19	93- 97	= 19		
49- 51	= 20	98-100	= 20		
52- 53	= 21				
54- 56	= 22				
57- 58	= 23				
59- 61	= 24				
62- 63	= 25				
64- 66	= 26				
67- 68	= 27				
69- 71	= 28				
72- 73	= 29				
74- 76	= 30				
77- 78	= 31				
79- 81	= 32				
82- 83	= 33				
84- 86	= 34				
87- 88	= 35				
89- 91	= 36				
92- 93	= 37				
94- 96	= 38				
97- 98	= 39				
99-100	= 40				

*See Table 2 (p. 19) for converting hand impairment to upper extremity impairment.

Table 2. Relationship of Impairment of the Hand to Impairment of the Upper Extremity.*

% Impairment of		% Impairment of		% Impairment of		% Impairment of		% Impairment of		% Impairment of	
Hand	Upper extremity	Hand	Upper extremity	Hand	Upper extremity	Hand	Upper extremity	Hand	Upper extremity	Hand	Upper extremity
0 =	0	18 =	16	35 =	32	53 =	48	70 =	63	88 =	79
1 =	1	19 =	17	36 =	32	54 =	49	71 =	64	89 =	80
2 =	2	20 =	18	37 =	33	55 =	50	72 =	65	90 =	81
3 =	3	21 =	19	38 =	34	56 =	50	73 =	66	91 =	82
4 =	4	22 =	20	39 =	35	57 =	51	74 =	67	92 =	83
5 =	5	23 =	21	40 =	36	58 =	52	75 =	68	93 =	84
6 =	5	24 =	22	41 =	37	59 =	53	76 =	68	94 =	85
7 =	6	25 =	23	42 =	38	60 =	54	77 =	69	95 =	86
8 =	7	26 =	23	43 =	39	61 =	55	78 =	70	96 =	86
9 =	8	27 =	24	44 =	40	62 =	56	79 =	71	97 =	87
10 =	9	28 =	25	45 =	41	63 =	57	80 =	72	98 =	88
11 =	10	29 =	26	46 =	41	64 =	58	81 =	73	99 =	89
12 =	11	30 =	27	47 =	42	65 =	59	82 =	74	100 =	90
13 =	12	31 =	28	48 =	43	66 =	59	83 =	75		
14 =	13	32 =	29	49 =	44	67 =	60	84 =	76		
15 =	14	33 =	30	50 =	45	68 =	61	85 =	77		
16 =	14	34 =	31	51 =	46	69 =	62	86 =	77		
17 =	15			52 =	47			87 =	78		

*Consult Table 3 (p. 20) to convert upper extremity impairment to whole-person impairment.

Previous Injury or Illness

An impairment evaluation should be based on the examiner's actual findings. A prior injury or illness should receive consideration only if valid evidence, such as a roentgenogram or laboratory test result, exists that it was present before the impairment being evaluated was incurred. Apportionment is discussed in Chapter 2 and the Glossary.

Cumulative Trauma Disorder

A patient with wrist or hand pain or other symptoms may not have evidence of a permanent impairment. Alteration of the patient's daily activities or work-related tasks may reduce the symptoms. Such an individual should not be considered to be permanently impaired under *Guides* criteria.

Example: A 43-year-old woman assembly-line worker who carried out repetitive motion activities with her hands complained of a 3-month history of pain and swelling in the hand and wrist with occasional radiation to the elbow and shoulder. Results of physical examination, including range of motion assessment and electrodiagnostic studies, were negative. The woman was treated with splints and flexibility exercises, and a 3-week leave of absence was advised.

On follow-up evaluation she had no symptoms. She returned to work and 2 weeks later complained of recurrence of the same symptoms. The physical examination and laboratory studies were still normal. The same conservative therapy was prescribed, and after 3 weeks the symptoms were relieved.

It was clear the woman should not return to her former job. After several months, she returned to be evaluated for permanent impairment. The physical examination remained normal.

Impairment: 0% whole-person impairment.

3.1b Evaluating Amputation

Amputation of the entire upper extremity, or 100% loss of the limb, is considered to be a 60% impairment of the whole person (Fig. 2, p. 18). Amputation at a level below the elbow, distal to the biceps insertion and proximal to the metacarpophalangeal joint level, is considered to be a 95% loss of the upper extremity or a 57% impairment of the whole person. Each digit is given a value relative to the whole hand: thumb, 40%; index and middle fingers, 20% each; and ring and little fingers, 10% each. Amputation through each portion of a digit is given a relative value of loss to the entire digit: digit metacarpophalangeal joint, 100%; thumb interphalangeal joint, 50%; finger proximal interphalangeal joint, 80%; and finger distal interphalangeal joint, 45% (Fig. 3, p. 18).

Amputation of all digits at the metacarpophalangeal joint level is considered to be 100% impairment of the hand or a 90% impairment of the upper extremity. Since loss of the entire upper extremity is equivalent to a 60% impairment of the whole person, 90% impairment of the upper extremity is equivalent to a 54% impairment of the whole person. By multiplying with the appropriate percent, the impairment of each digit or portion thereof can be related to the hand, to the upper extremity, and to the whole person (Tables 1 through 3, pp. 18 through 20).

A summary of steps in evaluating impairments of the upper extremity appears in Section 3.1o (p. 66).

3.1c Evaluating Sensory Loss of the Digits

Any sensory loss or deficit that is believed to contribute to permanent impairment must be unequivocal and permanent. Impairments are estimated according to the sensory quality and its distribution on the palmar aspect of the digits. Sensory loss on the distal dorsal surface of the digits is not considered to be an impairment. Sensory losses proximal to the digits are evaluated according to Section 3.1k (p. 46).

Sensibility Assessment Method

Evaluation of sensory function in the hand considers all sensory modalities, including perception of pain, heat, cold, and touch. The system introduced by the Nerve Injuries Committee of the British Medical Research Council in 1954 (S0, S1, S2, S3, S3+, S4) grades the sensory recovery after nerve injury as follows: first, there is no sensibility; then a spectrum of protective sensations ensues, including perception of pain, heat and cold, and some degree of light touch; finally, recovery of fine discriminative touch functions occurs. If a patient has normal two-point discrimination, it is not necessary to test sensory submodalities; rather, they are assumed to be present.

A test for sudomotor function, including the Ninhydrin test, may be useful in documenting interruption of digital nerves. However, such a test has limitations in evaluating the recovering nerve, because there is no direct relationship between the return of sudomotor function and the return of tactile gnosis. The moving two-point discrimination test may be useful in evaluating the regenerating nerve, because this sense recovers before static two-point discrimination.

Objective tests for sensory impairments are scarce, and the examiner must rely on the patient's truthfulness. If malingering is suspected, a test for sudomotor function can be used as well as antegrade or orthograde electrodiagnostic testing of nerve and muscle function.

The classic Weber static two-point discrimination test is of most value. Moberg originally described the use of a paper clip opened and bent into a caliper (Fig. 4, p. 21). More accurate instruments are listed below.*

Table 3. Relationship of Impairment of the Upper Extremity to Impairment of the Whole Person.

% Impairment of			% Impairment of			% Impairment of		
Upper extremity		Whole person	Upper extremity		Whole person	Upper extremity		Whole person
0	=	0	35	=	21	70	=	42
1	=	1	36	=	22	71	=	43
2	=	1	37	=	22	72	=	43
3	=	2	38	=	23	73	=	44
4	=	2	39	=	23	74	=	44
5	=	3	40	=	24	75	=	45
6	=	4	41	=	25	76	=	46
7	=	4	42	=	25	77	=	46
8	=	5	43	=	26	78	=	47
9	=	5	44	=	26	79	=	47
10	=	6	45	=	27	80	=	48
11	=	7	46	=	28	81	=	49
12	=	7	47	=	28	82	=	49
13	=	8	48	=	29	83	=	50
14	=	8	49	=	29	84	=	50
15	=	9	50	=	30	85	=	51
16	=	10	51	=	31	86	=	52
17	=	10	52	=	31	87	=	52
18	=	11	53	=	32	88	=	53
19	=	11	54	=	32	89	=	53
20	=	12	55	=	33	90	=	54
21	=	13	56	=	34	91	=	55
22	=	13	57	=	34	92	=	55
23	=	14	58	=	35	93	=	56
24	=	14	59	=	35	94	=	56
25	=	15	60	=	36	95	=	57
26	=	16	61	=	37	96	=	58
27	=	16	62	=	37	97	=	58
28	=	17	63	=	38	98	=	59
29	=	17	64	=	38	99	=	59
30	=	18	65	=	39	100	=	60
31	=	19	66	=	40			
32	=	19	67	=	40			
33	=	20	68	=	41			
34	=	20	69	=	41			

*Instruments for testing two-point discrimination: Aesthesiometer, Fred Sammons, Inc., Box 32, Brookfield, IL 60513; Disk-Criminator, P.O. Box 16392, Baltimore, MD 21210; De Mayo 2-Point Discrimination Device, Padgett Instrument Co., 2838 Warwick Traffic Way, Kansas City, MO 64108.

Figure 4. Two-point Discrimination Test for Determining Sensory Loss.

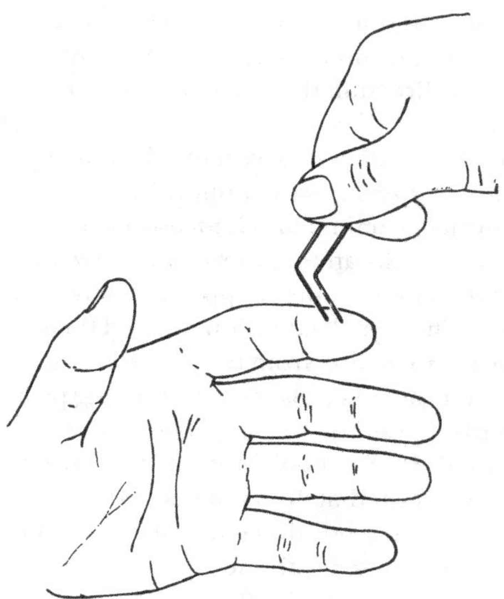

With the patient's eyes closed, the tips of the testing device are touched lightly to the digit in the longitudinal axis without producing an ischemic area or indentation of the skin. A series of touches with one or two points is made, and the subject indicates whether one or two points are felt. The distance of the tips is set first at 15 mm, and this distance is progressively decreased if the patient's responses are accurate. Testing is started distally and proceeds proximally to determine the level of involvement. The minimum distance at which the patient can discriminate between one- and two-point applications in two of three trials is recorded.

The sensory quality impairment for a digit is based on the results of the two-point discrimination test carried out over the distal palmar (volar) area, that is, from the distal phalangeal flexion crease to the distal part. If there is a partial amputation, the most distal part of the digital stump is evaluated for sensory quality impairment.

The *sensory quality* is classified and the impairment for the digit is estimated as follows:

1. Two-point discrimination greater than 15 mm: ***total sensory loss***, or 100% sensory impairment. *No* response is present to touch, pin, pressure, or vibratory stimulus.

2. Two-point discrimination 15 through 7 mm: ***partial sensory loss***, or 50% sensory impairment. *Poor* localization and abnormal response are present to touch, pin, pressure, or vibratory stimulus.

3. Two-point discrimination equal to or less than 6 mm: ***normal sensibility***, or 0% sensory impairment. *Normal* localization and response are present to touch, pin, pressure, or vibratory stimulus.

The *distribution of the sensory loss* is determined by the level of involvement of one or both digital nerves and is classified as follows:

1. ***Transverse sensory loss:*** both digital nerves are involved.

2. ***Longitudinal sensory loss:*** one digital nerve is involved, on either the radial or the ulnar side of the digit.

The level of involvement is calculated as a percentage of the length of the digit.

Sensory Impairment Rating

Total transverse sensory loss (greater than 15 mm two-point discrimination) is a 100% sensory loss and receives 50% of the amputation impairment value for that level (Figs. 3, 5, 7, and 17, pp. 18, 22, 24, and 30). *Partial transverse sensory loss* (15 through 7 mm two-point discrimination) is a 50% sensory loss and receives 25% of the amputation impairment value (Tables 4, and 9, pp. 25 and 31).

Longitudinal sensory loss impairments are based on the relative importance of the side of the digit for sensory function in hand activities: thumb and little finger, radial side 40% and ulnar side 60%; index, middle, and ring fingers, radial side 60% and ulnar side 40%.

Hand impairments for total transverse and longitudinal sensory losses of the fingers and thumb are shown in Fig. 5 (p. 22).

Figure 5. Impairment of Hand Due to Total Transverse Sensory Loss of Digits (numbers at tips of digits) and Longitudinal Sensory Loss of Radial and Ulnar Sides of the Digits (numbers at sides of digits).*

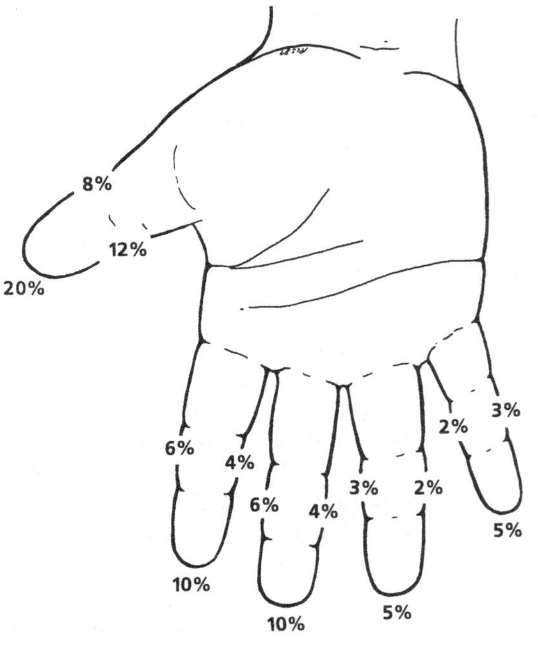

*Redrawn with permission from Swanson, AB[34], p. 931, Fig. 5.

Impairment percents of digits for total and partial longitudinal sensory losses are calculated according to the level of involvement and the relative value of the side of the digit involved. The percents for the thumb and little finger are shown in Table 4 (p. 25), and those for the index, middle, and ring fingers are shown in Table 9 (p. 31).

Sensibility on the outer aspect of a border digit is rated more highly. If the ring finger becomes a border digit due to amputation of the little finger, loss of sensibility along the ulnar border would be 3% and that along the radial border would be 2%.

Loss of palmar cutaneous nerve sensibility is considered to be a 5% impairment of the hand. Zero to 10% impairment of the upper extremity may be given for loss of sensibility of the palmar or dorsal ulnar cutaneous nerve, the palmar branch of the median nerve, or the superficial branch of the radial nerve (Fig. 45, p. 50).

Section 3.1k (p. 46) on impairment of the upper extremity due to peripheral nerve disorders considers evaluation of sensory losses proximal to the digit level and motor losses of the upper extremity.

3.1d Evaluating Abnormal Motion

The range of motion should be recorded on the principle that the neutral position equals 0°. In this method, all joint motions are measured from 0° as the starting position, and the degrees of motion are added in the direction the joint moves from that point.

Active motion is obtained with full flexion or extension muscle force. Passive motion may be carried out by the examiner and is measured after normal soft-tissue resistance to movement is overcome; in the finger joints, this is approximately 0.5 kg of force. The term "extension" is used for a motion opposite to flexion from the zero starting position. If extension exceeds the zero starting position, it is referred to as "hyperextension" and is expressed with the "+" symbol. Motion of extension from a flexed position that does not reach the neutral or zero starting position is defined as "extension lag" and is expressed with the "–" symbol.

For example, a finger joint flexion contracture of 15° with flexion to 45° would be recorded as –15° to 45°. The motion of a finger joint that has 15° of hyperextension and 45° of flexion would be recorded as +15° to 45° (Fig. 6, p. 23). The plus and minus signs are used to indicate, respectively, hyperextension and extension lag and have no mathematical significance.

The "position of function" or "functional position" of a joint is the position that is considered least impairing when the joint is ankylosed.

A = E + F Method for Impairment Evaluation

The range of motion of a joint is the total number of degrees of movement traced by an arc between the extreme angles of motion of the joint, for example, from maximum extension to maximum flexion. When there is complete loss of joint motion, or ankylosis, the total number of motion degrees lost (A) equals the sum of extension degrees lost (E) and flexion degrees lost (F).

The symbol "V" represents an angle. The measured angle of extension is represented by V_{ext}, and the measured angle of flexion is represented by V_{flex}. Assuming that a joint, which normally has a range of motion of 0° extension to 90° flexion, has a measured V_{ext} at 0° and V_{flex} at 90°, there is no loss of motion.

When the joint flexion is decreased, F (lack of flexion degrees) equals the theoretically largest V_{flex} minus the measured V_{flex}.

Figure 6. Illustration of MP Joint Positions in Flexion, Extension, Extension Lag, and Hyperextension. Full extension or the neutral position is considered to be 0°.

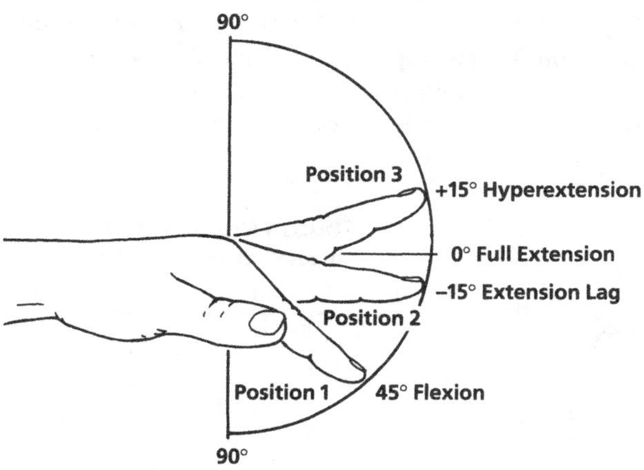

Example: A joint that would normally flex to 90° has measured V_{flex} at 60°:

F = 90° – 60° = 30° lack of flexion.

When joint extension is decreased, E (lack of extension degrees) equals the measured V_{ext} minus the theoretically smallest V_{ext}.

Example: A joint that would normally extend to 0° has a measured V_{ext} at –20°, or 20° of extension lag:

E = 20° – 0° = 20° lack of extension.

With decreasing flexion, V_{flex} decreases, and with greater impairment of extension, V_{ext} increases; as motion is lost, these values will finally meet at the same point on the arc of motion, or V_{flex} will equal V_{ext}. When this occurs, there is ankylosis, or total loss of the potential arc of motion (A).

Example: A joint that would normally extend to 0° and flex to 90° is ankylosed at 40°:

$V_{ext} = V_{flex} = 40°$
E = 40°– 0° = 40°; F = 90° – 40° = 50°
By definition, A = 40° (E) + 50° (F) or 90°, and there is total loss of the potential arc of motion. Note that A always equals the potential full arc of motion of a joint.

Impairment of finger function may be caused by loss of extension (E) with or without loss of flexion (F), or by ankylosis (A). The restricted motion impairment percents are called $I_E\%$, $I_F\%$, and $I_A\%$, respectively, and are functions of the angle (V) measured at examination.

$I_E\%$ is a function of V_{ext} and goes to 0% when V_{ext} reaches its smallest theoretical value.

$I_F\%$ is a function of V_{flex} and goes to 0% when V_{flex} reaches its largest theoretical value.

$I_A\%$ is a function of V when $V_{ext} = V_{flex}$; similarly, $I_A\% = I_E\% + I_F\%$. Note that $I_A\%$ varies according to the angle at which V_{ext} equals V_{flex}, even as A always equals the full range of motion of the joint. $I_A\%$ reaches its lowest value when the angle of the ankylosis corresponds to the "functional position" of the joint.

The formula A = E + F can also be written E = A –F; therefore, impairment values for lack of extension ($I_E\%$) can be derived for any measured extension angle on the basis that $I_E\% = I_A\% - I_F\%$.

Example: A patient's wrist is ankylosed in 10° extension. Figure 26 (p. 36) shows that wrist ankylosis in 10° extension corresponds to an ankylosis impairment of 21%. The flexion loss impairment is indicated by the $I_F\%$ row: $I_F\%$ is 13%. The extension impairment is derived according to the formula above: $I_E\% = I_A\% - I_F\%$, $I_E\% = 21\% - 13\%$, or 8%.

Impairment curves based on the formula A = E + F were derived on a 100% scale for each motion unit of each upper extremity joint, taking into consideration the functional position of each joint as recommended in the literature for fusion. The impairment curves then were converted to impairment graphs by applying the relative values of the respective motion units as conversion factors. An ankylosis impairment reaches its maximum, 100%, at the two extreme positions of the arc of motion and drops to its lowest percent when the ankylosis occurs in the joint's functional position.

Impairment curves for loss of motion of the fingers, thumb, wrist, elbow, and shoulder are given in Sections 3.1f through 3.1j (pp. 24 through 45).

3.1e Combining Impairment Values

When there is more than one impairment of a member, such as abnormal motion, sensory loss, and amputation of a finger, the impairments must be *combined* before the conversion to the next larger unit, in this case the hand, is made.

The method for *combining* impairments is based on the idea that a second or a succeeding impairment should apply not to the whole, but only to the part that remains after the first and other impairments have been applied. The *combined value* determination is based on the following formula: A% + B% x (100% –A%) equals the *combined value* of A% plus B%.

The Combined Values Chart on p. 322 may be used to determine the combined value of two impairment percents or, in succession, any number of impairment percents.

Example: An index finger shows amputation at the DIP joint (45% finger impairment, Fig. 17, p. 30) and 90° flexion ankylosis at the PIP joint (75% finger impairment, Fig. 21, p. 33). To estimate the index finger's impairment, the two percentages should be *combined.* The *combined* impairment is calculated as follows: 45% + 75% (100% –45%) = 86% impairment of the finger. This number may be found using the Combined Values Chart (p. 322), at the intersection of the row representing 75% and the column representing 45%.

Multiple regional impairments, as with those of the hand, wrist, elbow, and shoulder, are expressed in terms of impairment of the upper extremity and are *combined* using the Combined Values Chart. The chart is used also to *combine* impairments of two or more organ systems and express these as a whole-person impairment.

3.1f Thumb

Amputation of Thumb

1. Determine the length of thumb remaining after amputation and consult Fig. 7 (top scale) to find the thumb impairment. Amputations through the metacarpal bone are considered to be 100% impairments of the thumb and are not given extra values.

2. Relate the thumb impairment to the hand, upper extremity, and whole person (Tables 1 through 3, pp. 18 through 20).

Example: A thumb amputation through the proximal metaphysis of the proximal phalanx is equivalent to 90% impairment of the thumb (Fig. 7, below).

Figure 7. Impairment of Thumb Due to Amputation at Various Levels (top scale) or Total Transverse Sensory Loss (bottom scale). Total transverse sensory loss impairments correspond to 50% of amputation values.*

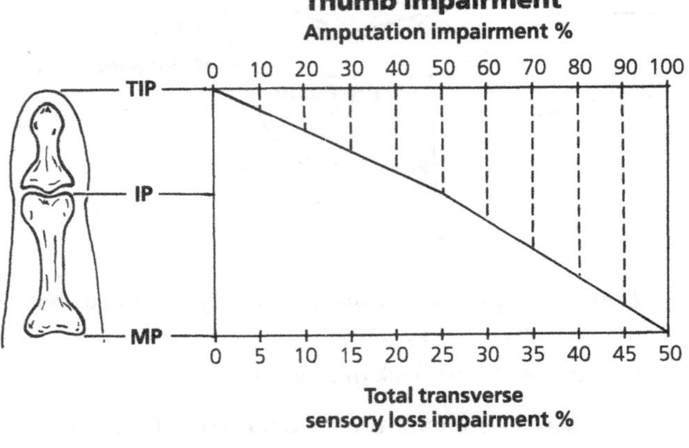

*Redrawn with permission from Swanson, AB[34], p. 927, Fig. 2.

Sensory Loss of Thumb

Transverse Sensory Loss (both digital nerves involved)

1. Determine the type of transverse sensory loss and the percent of the digit's length involved, using the two-point discrimination test.

A two-point discrimination value greater than 15 mm is considered to be a *total sensory loss* and is given 50% of the amputation impairment estimate.

Two-point discrimination values of 15 through 7 mm are considered to be *partial sensory losses* and are given 50% of the total sensory loss values or 25% of the amputation impairment values.

Two-point discrimination of 6 mm or less is considered to be normal and not an impairment.

2. Consult Fig. 7 (above), bottom scale, to determine the thumb impairment percent for *total transverse* sensory loss according to the level of occurrence. A *partial transverse* sensory loss is given 50% of the bottom scale values.

Example: A patient has two-point discrimination of more than 15 mm over the palmar surface of the thumb from the IP joint in a distal direction (50% digit length). Based on Fig. 7, bottom scale, a total transverse sensory loss over 50% of the thumb's length is estimated to be a 25% thumb impairment, or a 10% hand impairment (Table 1, p. 18).

Example: Two-point discrimination from 15 through 7 mm over the palmar surface of the thumb from the MP joint in a distal direction (100% thumb length) represents a 25% impairment of the thumb or 10% impairment of the hand (Table 1, p. 18).

Table 4. Longitudinal Sensory Loss Impairment for the *Thumb* and *Little Finger* Based on Percent of Digit Length Involved (values are expressed in percent of digit impairment).

	Longitudinal sensory loss %			
	Ulnar digital nerve		Radial digital nerve	
% of digit length	Total loss	Partial loss	Total loss	Partial loss
100	30	15	20	10
90	27	14	18	9
80	24	12	16	8
70	21	11	14	7
60	18	9	12	6
50	15	8	10	5
40	12	6	8	4
30	9	5	6	3
20	6	3	4	2
10	3	2	2	1

Longitudinal Sensory Loss (one digital nerve involved)

1. Determine the type and level of *longitudinal sensory loss* with the two-point discrimination test.

2. Use Fig. 7 (p. 24) to determine the percent of the thumb length involved according to the amputation impairment (top) scale.

3. Thumb impairment values for *total and partial longitudinal sensory loss* are determined according to the level of involvement or the percent of the digit's length involved (Table 4, above).

Example: A total sensory loss (>15 mm) over the ulnar palmar surface of the thumb from the MP joint level (100% of digit length) in a distal direction is equivalent to 30% impairment of the thumb (Table 4, above), or 12% impairment of the hand (Table 1, p. 18).

Example: A partial sensory loss (15 through 7 mm) over the radial palmar surface of the thumb from the IP joint level (50% of digit length) in a distal direction gives a 5% impairment of the thumb (Table 4, last column) or a 2% impairment of the hand (Table 1).

Abnormal Motion of Thumb

The thumb has five functional units of motion, each contributing a relative value to thumb motion as follows: flexion and extension of the IP joint, 15%; flexion and extension of the MP joint, 10%; adduction, 20%; radial abduction, 10%; and opposition, 45%.

Impairment percents for each of these units of motion were derived and expressed in graphs on a 100% scale (Figs. 9, 12, 14, and 16, pp. 26 through 29) and then expressed in charts or pie graphs of thumb impairment by applying the relative value of each functional unit as a conversion factor (Figs. 10 and 13, Tables 5, 6 and 7, pp. 26, 27, 28, and 29).

Thumb Interphalangeal (IP) Joint: Flexion and Extension

1. Measure the maximum flexion and extension, and record the goniometer readings (Fig. 8, below). Round the readings to the nearest 10°. Normal flexion is to 80°. Functional position is 20° flexion.

Figure 8. Neutral Position (top) and Flexion (bottom) of Thumb IP Joint.

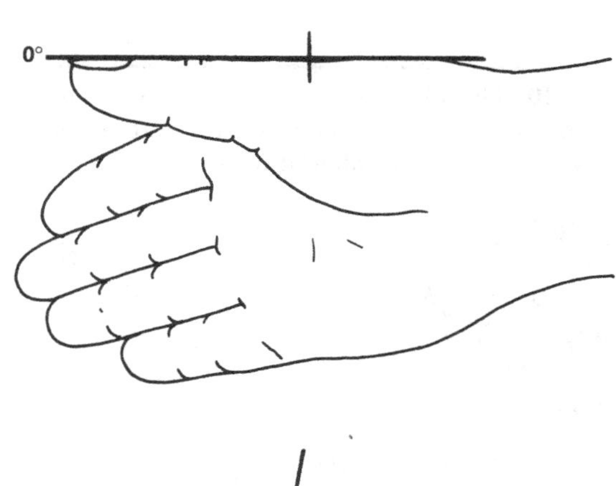

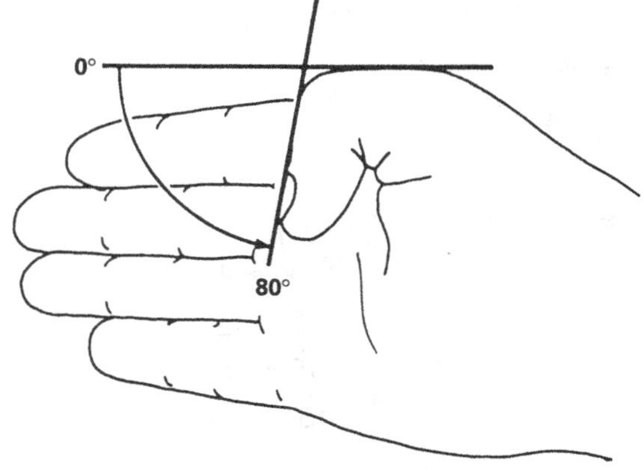

Figure 9. Impairment Curves for Ankylosis (I_A%), Loss of Flexion (I_F%), and Loss of Extension (I_E%) of IP Joint of Thumb. Ankylosis in functional position (20° flexion) receives lowest I_A% value (50%).

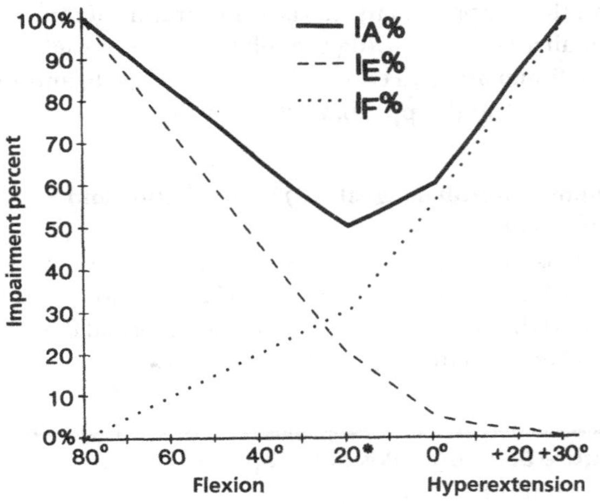

Figure 10. Thumb Impairments Due to Abnormal Motion at the IP Joint. Relative value of functional unit is 15% of total thumb motion.†

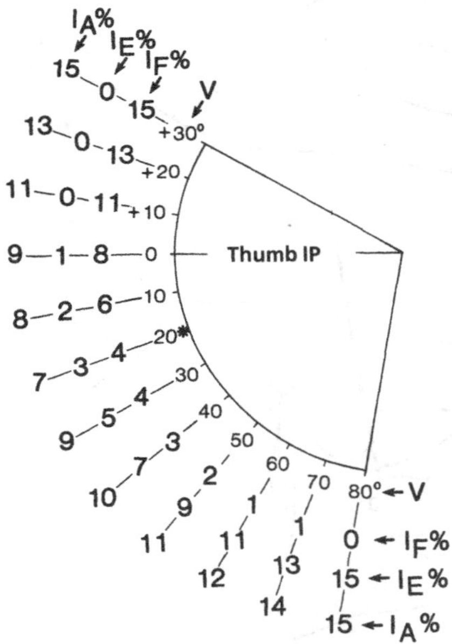

I_A% = Impairment due to ankylosis
I_E% = Impairment due to loss of extension
I_F% = Impairment due to loss of flexion
V = Measured angles of motion
* = Position of function

†Adapted from Swanson, AB, Goran-Hagert, C, de Groot Swanson, G[31], p. 62, Fig. 4-22.

2. Using Fig. 10 (at left), match the measured angle (V) of flexion and of extension to the corresponding impairment of flexion (row headed I_F%) and of extension (row headed I_E%). Impairment percents for positions of hyperextension are read above the 0° neutral position.

3. *Add* the flexion and extension impairment percents to obtain thumb impairment for loss of motion at the IP joint.

4. If the IP joint is ankylosed, measure the position and match the angle (V) to the corresponding impairment of ankylosis under the row headed I_A% (Fig. 10). Ankylosis in the functional position (20° flexion) is given the lowest ankylosis impairment value (7%).

Example: A thumb IP joint has –10° extension and 50° flexion:
I_E% = 2%; I_F% = 2% (Fig. 10);
2% + 2% = 4% thumb impairment.

Example: A thumb IP joint has ankylosis in 80° flexion:
I_A% = 15% thumb impairment (Fig. 10).

Thumb Metacarpophalangeal (MP) Joint: Flexion and Extension

1. Measure the maximum flexion and extension and record the goniometer readings (Fig. 11, p. 27). Round the readings to the nearest 10°. Normal flexion is 60°. The functional position is 20° flexion.

2. Using Fig. 13 (p. 27), match the measured angle (V) of flexion and of extension to the corresponding impairment of flexion (row headed I_F%) and of extension (row headed I_E%). Impairment percents for positions of hyperextension are read above the 0° neutral position.

3. *Add* the percents for flexion and extension impairments to obtain thumb impairment for loss of motion at the MP joint.

4. If the MP joint is ankylosed, measure the position and match the angle (V) to the corresponding impairment of ankylosis under the row headed I_A% (Fig. 13, p. 27). Ankylosis in the functional position (20° flexion) is given the lowest ankylosis impairment value (5%).

Example: A thumb MP joint has +10° hyperextension and 40° flexion:
I_E% = 0%; I_F% = 2% (Fig. 13, p. 27);
0% + 2% = 2% thumb impairment.

Figure 11. Neutral Position (bottom) and Flexion (top) of Thumb MP Joint.

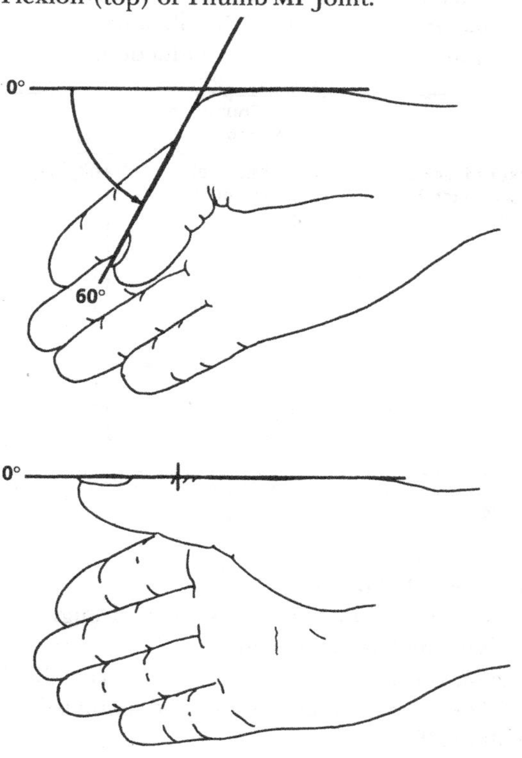

Figure 12. Impairment Curves for Ankylosis ($I_A\%$), Loss of Flexion ($I_F\%$), and Loss of Extension ($I_E\%$) of Thumb MP Joint. Ankylosis in functional position (20° flexion) receives lowest $I_A\%$ value (50%).

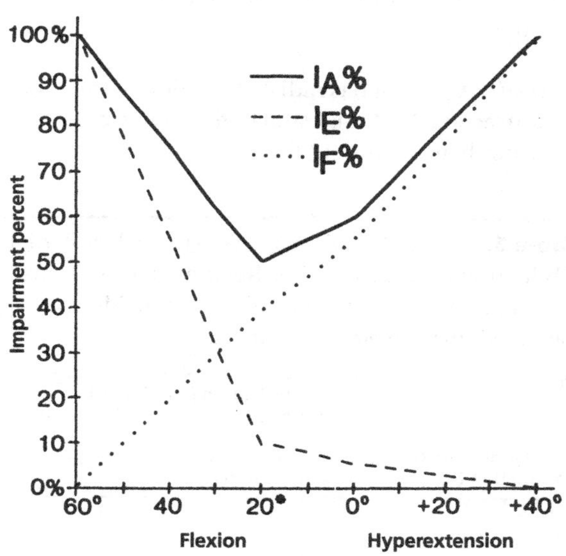

Figure 13. Thumb Impairments Due to Abnormal Motion at the MP Joint. Relative value of functional unit is 10% of total thumb motion.†

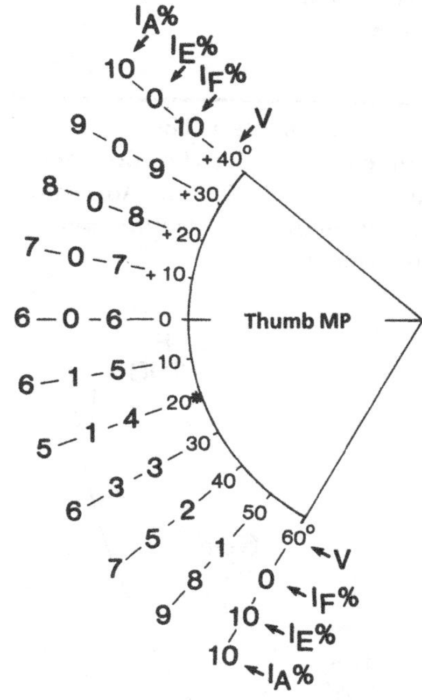

$I_A\%$ = Impairment due to ankylosis
$I_E\%$ = Impairment due to loss of extension
$I_F\%$ = Impairment due to loss of flexion
V = Measured angles of motion
* = Position of function

†Adapted from Swanson, AB[31], p. 61, Fig. 4-21.

Example: A thumb MP joint has –20° extension lag and 60° flexion:
$I_E\%$ = 1%; $I_F\%$ = 0% (Fig. 13, above);
1% + 0% = 1% thumb impairment.

Example: A thumb MP joint is ankylosed in 60° flexion:
$I_A\%$ = 10% thumb impairment (Fig. 13).

Involvement of Thumb IP and MP joints

Add the thumb impairment percents at the IP and MP joints to obtain the thumb flexion and extension impairment. *Add* ankylosis impairment values in a similar fashion.

Example: Thumb impairment due to motion loss is 2% at the IP joint and 2% at the MP joint:
2% + 2% = 4% thumb impairment.

Example: Thumb impairment due to ankylosis of the IP joint is 15% and that due to ankylosis of the MP joint is 10%: 15% + 10% = 25% thumb impairment.

Thumb Adduction

1. Measure and record the smallest possible distance in centimeters from the flexor crease of the thumb IP joint to the distal palmar crease over the MP joint of the little finger (Fig. 14, below). The normal range is from 8 to 0 cm.

Figure 14. Linear Measurements of Thumb Adduction in Centimeters at Various Positions and Impairment Curve for Lack of Adduction. Adduction to 0 cm gives 0% impairment; 8 cm of adduction *lack* gives 100% impairment

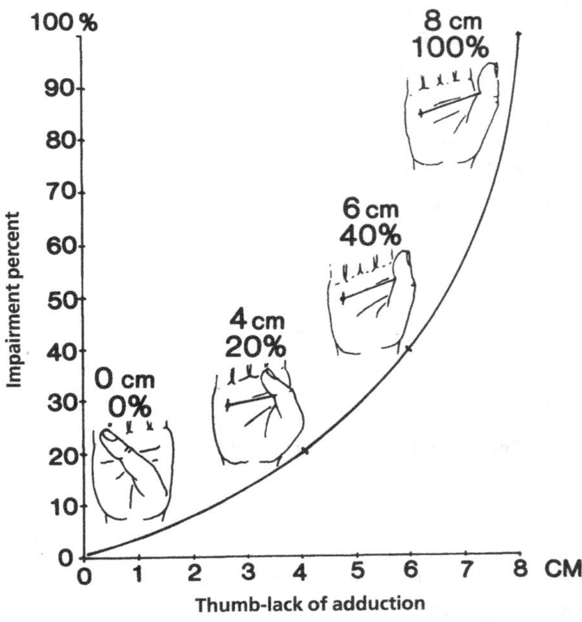

*Redrawn with permission from Swanson, AB, Goran-Hagert, C, de Groot Swanson, G[31], p. 59, Fig. 4-19.

2. Consult Table 5 (right) to determine the percent of thumb impairment contributed by adduction lack or ankylosis.

Example: A patient has a 4-cm thumb adduction lack; this is equivalent to a 4% thumb impairment (Table 5, at right).

Example: Ankylosis of the thumb in a position of either 0- or 8-cm adduction lack is equivalent to a 20% thumb impairment (Table 5).

Table 5. Thumb Impairment Values Due to Lack of Adduction and to Ankylosis. Relative value of functional unit is 20% of total thumb motion. Motion ranges from 8 to 0 cm of adduction.*

Measured lack of adduction (cm)	% Thumb impairment due to	
	Abnormal motion	Ankylosis
8	20	20
7	13	19
6	8	17
5	6	15
4	4	10
3	3	15
2	1	17
1	0	19
0	0	20

*Adapted from Swanson, AB, Goran-Hagert, C, de Groot Swanson, G[28], p. 124, Table 8-11.

Thumb Radial Abduction

1. Measure and record the largest possible angle in degrees formed by the first and second metacarpals during maximum active radial abduction (Fig. 15, p. 29). The normal range of radial abduction is from 0° to 50°.

2. Consult Table 6 (below) to determine the percentage of thumb impairment that is contributed by radial abduction loss or ankylosis.

Ankylosis in any position of radial abduction corresponds to complete impairment of this function (10% thumb impairment, see Table 6), because prehension is not possible without some abduction component.

Example: A patient has radial abduction of the thumb measured at 20°; this is estimated to represent a 7% thumb impairment (Table 6).

Table 6. Thumb Impairments Due to Lack of Radial Abduction and to Ankylosis. Relative value of functional unit is 10% of total thumb motion. Motion ranges from 0° to 50° radial abduction.

Measured radial abduction (°)	% Thumb impairment due to	
	Abnormal motion	Ankylosis
0	10	10
10	9	10
20	7	10
30	3	10
40	1	10
50	0	10

Figure 15. Radial Abduction of Thumb, Measured in Degrees.

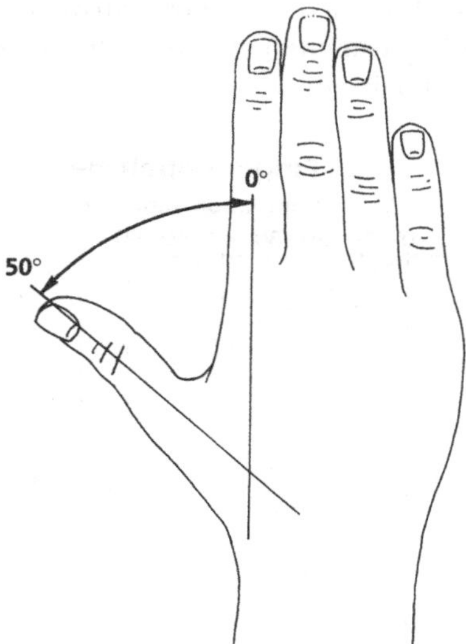

Thumb Opposition

1. Measure and record the largest possible distance in centimeters from the flexor crease of the thumb IP joint to the distal palmar crease directly over the third MP joint (Fig. 16, below). The normal range of opposition is from 0 to 8 cm.

2. Consult Table 7 (at right) to determine percent of thumb impairment contributed by opposition loss or ankylosis.

Figure 16. Linear Measurements of Thumb Opposition (cm) at Various Positions and Impairment Curve for Lack of Opposition.*

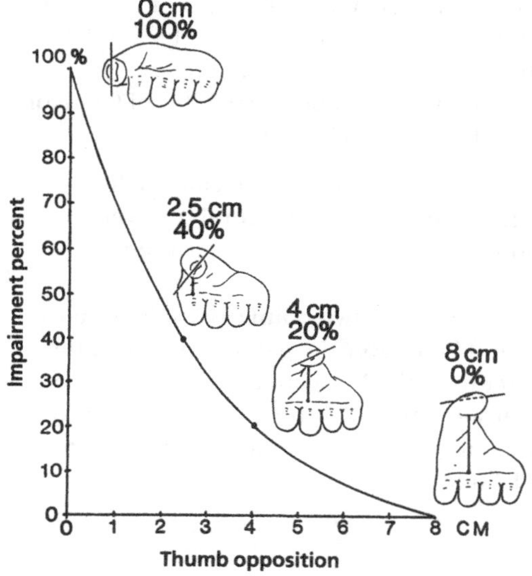

*With permission from Swanson, AB, Goran-Hagert, C, de Groot Swanson, G[31], p. 60, Fig. 4-20.

Table 7. Thumb Impairments Due to Lack of Opposition and to Ankylosis. Relative value of functional unit is 45% of total thumb motion. Motion ranges from 0 to 8 cm of opposition.*

Measured opposition (cm)	% Thumb impairment due to: Abnormal motion	% Thumb impairment due to: Ankylosis
0	45	45
1	31	40
2	22	36
3	13	31
4	9	27
5	5	22
6	3	24
7	1	27
8	0	29

*Data from Swanson, AB, Goran-Hagert, C, de Groot Swanson, G[28], p. 124, Fig. 8-20.

Example: Opposition of a thumb measured at 4 cm is equivalent to 9% thumb impairment (Table 7).

Example: Ankylosis of the thumb in a position of 4 cm of opposition is estimated to be a 27% thumb impairment.

Two or More Abnormal Thumb Motions

1. Measure and record the thumb motion impairments of flexion and extension, adduction, radial abduction, and opposition as described above.

2. *Add* these values to determine abnormal thumb motion impairment.

Because the relative value of each thumb functional unit has been taken into consideration in the impairment values of the entire thumb, *impairments of thumb motions are added, while those for the fingers are combined* (Combined Values Chart, p. 322). If there were maximum impairment of each type of motion of the thumb, the sum of the impairments would be 100%.

Example: A patient has a thumb IP joint flexion and extension impairment of 4%, adduction impairment of 4%, radial abduction of 0%, and opposition impairment of 10%. *Add* the impairments:
4% + 4% + 0% + 10% = 18% thumb impairment.

Example: A patient has thumb flexion and extension impairment totaling 25% for the IP and MP joints, adduction impairment of 20%, radial abduction impairment of 10%, and opposition impairment of 45%:
25% + 20% + 10% + 45% = 100% or total thumb impairment.

Combining Thumb Amputation, Sensory, and Abnormal Motion Impairments

1. Measure separately and record the impairment of the thumb that is contributed by amputation, sensory loss, and abnormal motion.

If an amputation affects the measurement of abnormal motion, then only the amputation impairment is acknowledged. For example, amputation proximal to the MP joint will affect measurements of adduction and opposition. However, only the impairment due to amputation is given.

2. *Combine* the impairment values using the Combined Values Chart (p. 322) to obtain the thumb impairment.

3. Use Tables 1, 2, and 3 (pp. 18 through 20) to relate thumb impairment to impairments of the hand, the upper extremity, and the whole person.

Example: A patient has a thumb amputation impairment of 30%, a sensory impairment of 10%, and an abnormal motion impairment of 10%.
From the Combined Values Chart (p. 322):
30% *combined* with 10% = 37%; 37% *combined* with 10% = 43% thumb impairment.

A 43% thumb impairment is estimated to be a 17% impairment of the hand, a 15% impairment of the upper extremity, and a 9% impairment of the whole person (Tables 1, 2, and 3, pp. 18 through 20).

3.1g Fingers

Amputation of Fingers

1. Determine the length of the finger remaining after amputation and consult Fig. 17, top scale, to determine the impairment.

2. Relate the finger impairment to the hand, upper extremity, and whole person (Tables 1, 2, and 3, pp. 18 through 20). An amputation through the metacarpal bone is considered to be a 100% impairment of the finger.

Example: Amputation of the index finger through the PIP joint is equivalent to an 80% finger impairment.

Figure 17. Finger Impairment Due to Amputation at Various Lengths (top scale) and Total Transverse Sensory Loss (bottom scale). Total transverse sensory loss impairments correspond to 50% of amputation impairments.*

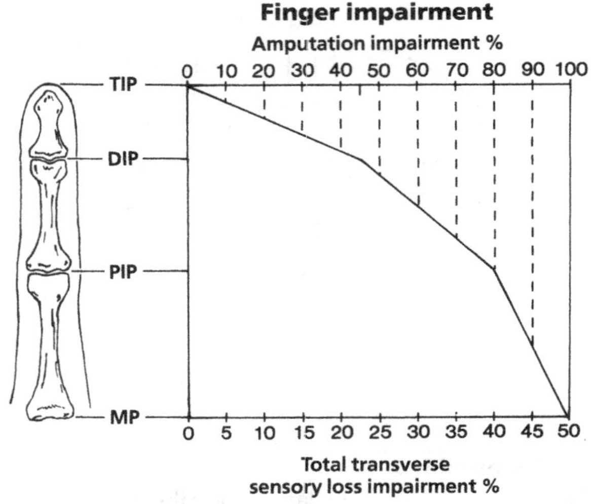

*Redrawn with permission from Swanson, AB[34], p. 927, Fig. 2.

Sensory Loss of Fingers

Transverse Sensory Loss (both digital nerves involved)

1. Determine the type and level of *transverse sensory loss* with the two-point discrimination test (Section 3.1c, p. 20).

Two-point discrimination values greater than 15 mm are considered to be *total sensory losses* and receive 50% of the impairment amount for amputation.

Two-point discrimination values from 15 through 7 mm represent partial sensory losses and receive 50% of the total sensory loss value, or 25% of the amputation impairment value.

Two-point discrimination sensibility of 6 mm or less is normal and not an impairment.

2. Consult Fig. 17 (above), bottom scale, to determine the finger impairment for total transverse sensory loss according to level of occurrence.

Example: A patient has two-point discrimination greater than 15 mm over the palmar surface of the index finger from the PIP joint in a distal direction. This is equivalent to a 40% impairment of the finger and an 8% impairment of the hand (Fig. 17, bottom scale, and Table 1, p. 18).

Example: Two-point discrimination values from 15 through 7 mm over the palmar surface of the entire index finger from the MP joint in a distal direction give a 25% impairment of the finger (Fig. 17, p. 30) and a 5% impairment of the hand (Table 1, p. 18).

Longitudinal Sensory Loss (one digital nerve involved)

1. Determine the type and level of *longitudinal sensory loss* with the two-point discrimination test.

2. Use Fig. 17 (p. 30) to determine the relative value of the finger length involved according to the amputation impairment scale (top scale).

3. Finger impairments due to *total and partial longitudinal sensory loss* are determined according to the level of involvement (percent of finger length) using Table 8 (below) for the thumb and little finger and Table 9 (at right) for the index, middle, and ring fingers.

Example: A patient has total sensory loss (>15 mm) over the ulnar palmar surface of the index finger from the MP joint level in a distal direction:
MP joint level = 100% relative value (Fig. 17, p. 30, top scale).
Index ulnar side = 40% relative value (Fig. 5, p. 22).
Total sensory loss is equivalent to a 50% amputation impairment.
100% x 40% x 50% = 20% finger impairment.

To ease determination, use Table 9 (at right), row headed "Ulnar Digital Nerve" and column headed "Total Loss," to find the finger impairment for 100% of the digit's length, which is 20%.

Table 8. Longitudinal Sensory Loss Impairment for the *Thumb* and *Little Finger* Based on Percent of Digit Length Involved (values are expressed as percent of digit impairment).

	Longitudinal sensory loss %			
	Ulnar digital nerve		Radial digital nerve	
Percent of digit length	Total loss	Partial loss	Total loss	Partial loss
100	30	15	20	10
90	27	14	18	9
80	24	12	16	8
70	21	11	14	7
60	18	9	12	6
50	15	8	10	5
40	12	6	8	4
30	9	5	6	3
20	6	3	4	2
10	3	2	2	1

Example: A partial sensory loss (15 through 7 mm) over the radial palmar surface of the index finger from the PIP joint level (80% length) in a distal direction gives a 12% impairment of the index finger (Table 9), or a 2% impairment of the hand (Table 1, p. 18).

Table 9. Longitudinal Sensory Loss Impairment of *Index, Middle,* and *Ring Fingers* Based on the Percent of Digit Length Involved (values are expressed as percent of finger impairment).

	Longitudinal sensory loss (%)			
	Ulnar digital nerve		Radial digital nerve	
Percent of digit length	Total loss	Partial loss	Total loss	Partial loss
100	20	10	30	15
90	18	9	27	14
80	16	8	24	12
70	14	7	21	11
60	12	6	18	9
50	10	5	15	8
40	8	4	12	6
30	6	3	9	5
20	4	2	6	3
10	2	1	3	2

Abnormal Motion of Fingers

The fingers have three functional units of motion, each having the same relative value as that found in amputation impairments: DIP, 45%; PIP, 80%; and MP, 100% (Figs. 3 and 17, pp. 18 and 30).

Impairment values for each of these units of motion have been derived according to the basic formula, A = E + F (p. 22), and expressed in a chart or pie graph showing finger impairments by applying the relative value of each functional unit as a conversion factor (Figs. 19, 21, and 23, pp. 32 through 34).

Distal joints are evaluated with the proximal joints in the neutral (straight line) position.

Distal Interphalangeal (DIP) Joint: Flexion and Extension

1. Measure the maximum flexion and extension, and record the goniometer readings (Fig. 18, p. 32). Round the readings to the nearest 10°. Normal flexion is 70°. Functional position is 20° flexion.

2. Using Fig. 19, p. 32, match the measured angles (V) of flexion and extension to their corresponding impairments of flexion (row headed I_F%) and extension (row headed I_E%). Impairment percents for positions of hyperextension are read above the 0° neutral position.

3. *Add* the flexion and extension impairments to obtain the finger impairment due to loss of motion at the DIP joint.

4. If the DIP joint is ankylosed, measure the position and match the angle (V) to the corresponding ankylosis impairment (row headed $I_A\%$) in Fig. 19. Ankylosis in the functional position (20° flexion) is given the lowest ankylosis impairment value (30%).

Figure 18. Neutral Position (top) and Flexion (bottom) of Finger DIP Joint.

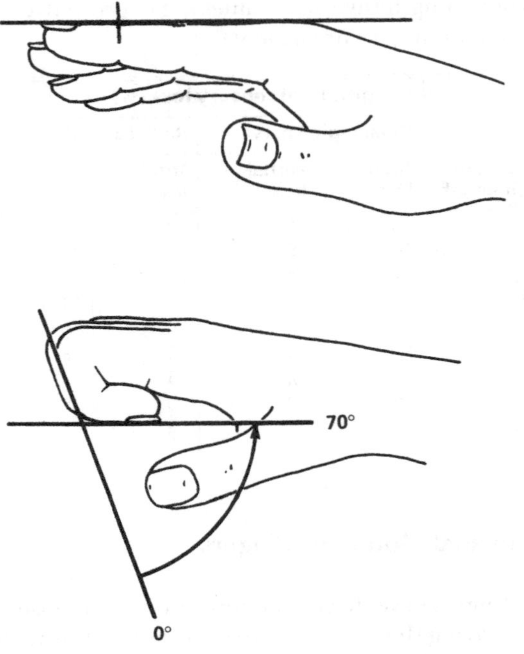

Figure 19. Finger Impairments Due to Abnormal Motion at the DIP Joint. Relative value of functional unit is 45%.†

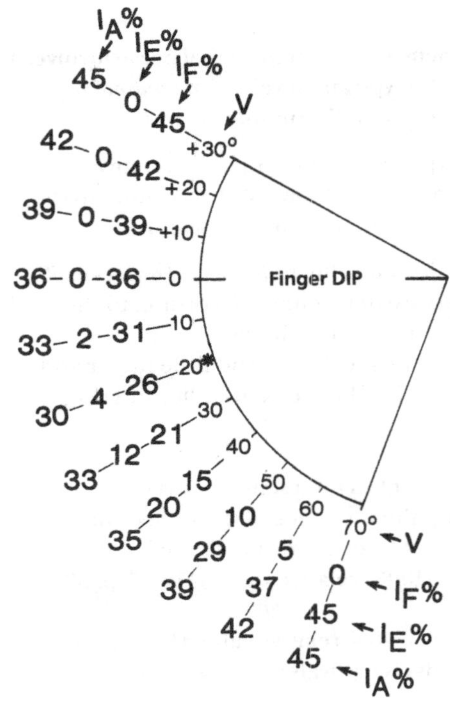

$I_A\%$ = Impairment due to ankylosis
$I_E\%$ = Impairment due to loss of extension
$I_F\%$ = Impairment due to loss of flexion
V = Measured angles of motion
* = Position of function

†Redrawn with permission from Swanson, AB, Goran-Hagert, C, de Groot Swanson, G[31], p. 58, Fig. 4-18.

Example: A middle finger DIP joint has –10° extension lag and 50° flexion:
$I_E\%$ = 2%, $I_F\%$ = 10% (Fig. 19, above);
2% + 10% = 12% impairment of the middle finger.

Example: A patient's DIP joint has +30° extension and 0° flexion;
$I_E\%$ = 0%, $I_F\%$ = 36% (Fig. 19, above);
0% + 36% = 36% finger impairment.

Example: A DIP joint has ankylosis in 30° flexion:
$I_A\%$ = 33% finger impairment.

Proximal Interphalangeal (PIP) Joint: Flexion and Extension

1. Measure the maximum flexion and extension and record the goniometer readings (Fig. 20, below). Round the figures to the nearest 10°. Normal flexion is 100°. Functional position is 40° flexion.

2. Using Fig. 21 (at right), match the measured angles (V) of flexion and extension to their corresponding impairments of flexion (row headed I_F%) and extension (row headed I_E%). Impairment percents for positions of hyperextension are read above the 0° neutral position.

Figure 20. Neutral Position (top) and Flexion (bottom) of Finger PIP Joint.

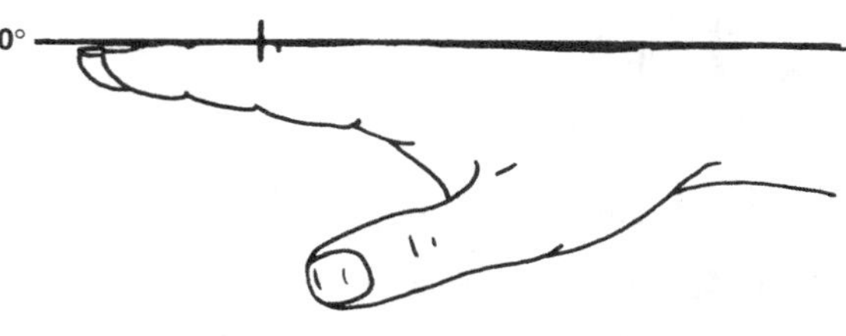

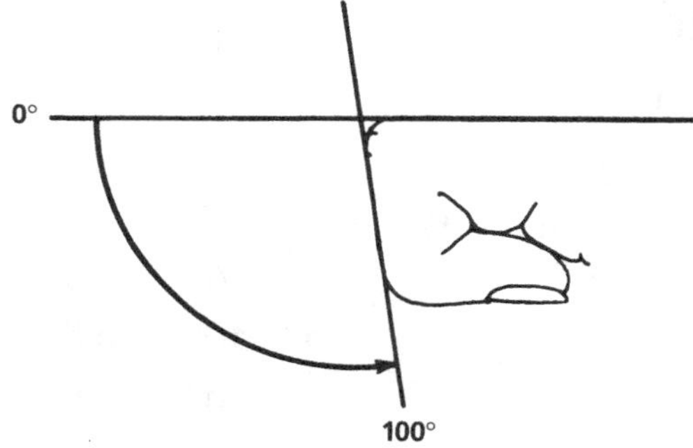

Figure 21. Finger Impairments Due to Abnormal Motion at PIP Joint. Relative value of functional unit is 80%.†

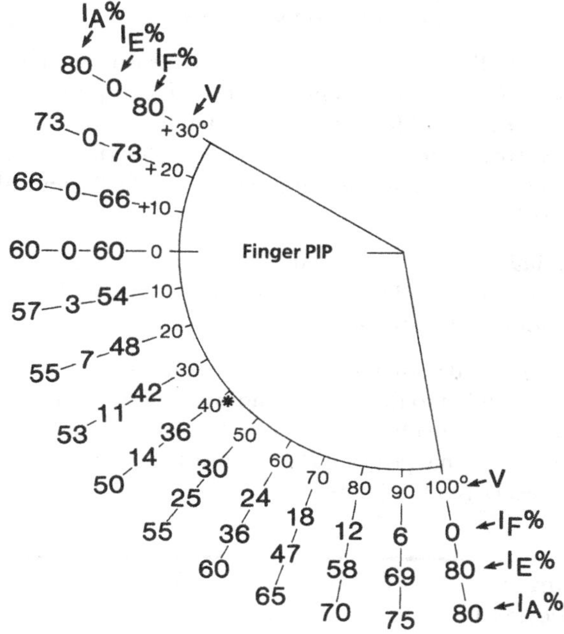

I_A% = Impairment due to ankylosis
I_E% = Impairment due to loss of extension
I_F% = Impairment due to loss of flexion
V = Measured angles of motion
* = Position of function

†Redrawn with permission from Swanson, AB, Goran-Hagert, C, de Groot Swanson, G[31], p. 57, Fig. 4-17.

3. *Add* the flexion and extension impairment percents to obtain the estimated finger impairment due to loss of motion at the PIP joint.

4. If the PIP joint is ankylosed, measure the angle (V) and match it to the corresponding ankylosis impairment (row headed I_A%) in Fig. 21. Ankylosis in the functional position (40° flexion) is given the lowest ankylosis impairment percent (50%).

Example: A patient's middle finger PIP joint has –20° extension lag and 60° flexion:
I_E% = 7%; I_F% = 24% (Fig. 21); 7% + 24% = 31% impairment of the middle finger.

Example: A patient has ankylosis of the PIP joint in 40° flexion:
I_A% = 50% finger impairment (Fig. 21).

Metacarpophalangeal (MP) Joint: Flexion and Extension

1. Measure the maximum flexion and extension, and record the goniometer readings (Fig. 22, below). Round the figures to the nearest 10°. Normal flexion is 90°. Functional position is 30° flexion.

2. From Fig. 23 (at right), match the measured angles (V) of flexion and extension to their corresponding impairments of flexion (row headed I_F%) and extension (row headed I_E%). Impairment values for positions of hyperextension are read above the 0° neutral position.

3. *Add* the flexion and extension impairment percents to obtain finger impairment due to loss of motion at the MP joint.

4. If the MP joint is ankylosed, measure the angle (V) and match it to the corresponding ankylosis impairment (row headed I_A%) in Fig. 23. Ankylosis in the functional position (30° flexion) is given the lowest I_A% value (45%).

Figure 22. Neutral Position (top) and Flexion (bottom) of Finger MP Joint.

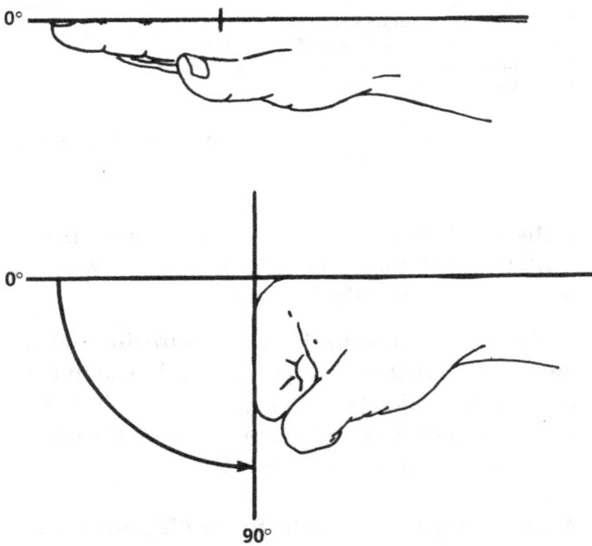

Example: A middle finger MP joint has 0° extension and 50° flexion:
I_E% = 5%; I_F% = 22% (Fig. 23, at right);
5% + 22% = 27% impairment of the middle finger.

Example: A patient's MP joint is ankylosed in 30° flexion:
I_A% = 45% finger impairment (Fig. 23).

Abnormal Motion of More Than One Finger Joint

1. Determine the flexion and extension impairments of each joint as described in the preceding pages.

2. Use the Combined Values Chart (p. 322) to *combine* the joint impairments, thereby estimating impairment of the entire finger.

3. Express the finger impairment in terms of the hand, upper extremity, and whole person (Tables 1 through 3, pp. 18 through 20).

Figure 23. Finger Impairments Due to Abnormal Motion at the MP Joint. Relative value of functional unit is 100%.†

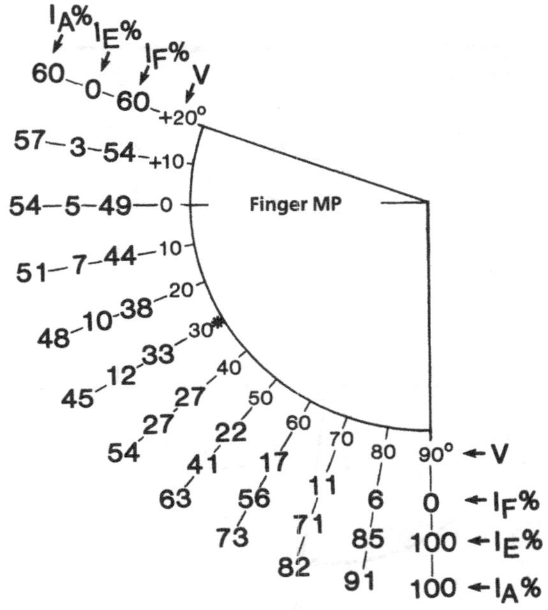

I_A% = Impairment due to ankylosis
I_E% = Impairment due to loss of extension
I_F% = Impairment due to loss of flexion
V = Measured angles of motion
* = Position of function

†Redrawn with permission from Swanson, AB, Goran-Hagert, C, de Groot Swanson, G[31], p. 56, Fig. 4-16.

Example: A patient's middle finger shows DIP joint impairment of 12%, PIP joint impairment of 31%, and MP joint impairment of 27%:
12% *combined* with 31% = 39% (Combined Values Chart, p. 322);
39% *combined* with 27% = 55%, which is the motion impairment of the finger.

Combining Finger Amputation, Sensory, and Abnormal Motion Impairments

1. Determine as described above the impairments of the finger contributed by amputation, sensory loss, and abnormal motion.

2. *Combine* the impairment percents using the Combined Values Chart (p. 322) to ascertain total finger impairment.

3. Use Tables 1 through 3 (pp. 18 through 20) to relate the finger impairment in succession to impairment of the hand, the upper extremity, and the whole person.

Example: A patient has a middle finger amputation impairment of 20%, a sensory impairment of 10%, and an abnormal motion impairment of 10%:
20% *combined* with 10% = 28% (Combined Values Chart, p. 322);
28% *combined* with 10% = 35% finger impairment; the latter is considered a 7% impairment of the hand, a 6% impairment of the upper extremity, and a 4% impairment of the whole person (Tables 1 through 3).

Determining Impairments of Several Digits

1. If two or more digits of the hand are involved, evaluate them separately and calculate the impairment for each digit.

2. Using Table 1 (p. 18), find the hand impairment contributed by each digit.

3. *Add* the hand impairments contributed by each digit to obtain the total hand impairment.

4. Using Tables 2 and 3 (pp. 19 and 20), the hand impairment is related to impairment of the upper extremity and the whole person.

Example:

% Impairment of digit	% Impairment of hand
10, thumb	4
20, index finger	4
30, middle finger	6
40, ring finger	4
50, little finger	5
Total hand impairment	23

Tables 2 and 3 (pp. 19 and 20) indicate that a 23% hand impairment is equivalent to a 21% impairment of the upper extremity and a 13% impairment of the whole person.

3.1h Wrist

Amputation About the Wrist

1. Determine the level of amputation about the wrist (Fig. 2, p. 18).

2. An amputation at a level below the biceps insertion and proximal to the MP joint is a 90% to 95% impairment of the upper extremity, depending on the location.

3. Use Table 3 (p. 20) to relate impairment of the upper extremity to impairment of the whole person.

Example: An amputation at the wrist joint level is a 92% impairment of the upper extremity (Fig. 2, p. 18) and a 55% impairment of the whole person (Table 3, p. 20).

Abnormal Motion at Wrist

The wrist functional unit represents 60% of the upper extremity's function. The wrist has two units of motion, each contributing a relative value to its function. The wrist motion impairments are converted to upper extremity impairments by multiplying these values by 60% as follows:

1. Flexion and extension represent 70% of wrist function: 70% x 60% = 42% of upper extremity function.

2. Radial and ulnar deviation represent 30% of wrist function: 30% x 60% = 18% of upper extremity function.

Impairment values for each functional unit of motion have been derived according to the basic formula described on p. 22, A = E + F, and expressed in graphs on a 100% scale (Fig. 25 and 28, pp. 36 and 37). These graphs have been expressed in charts of upper- extremity impairment by multiplying the relative value of each functional unit as a conversion factor (Figs. 26 and 29, pp. 36 and 38).

Figure 24. Wrist Flexion (above) and Extension (below):*

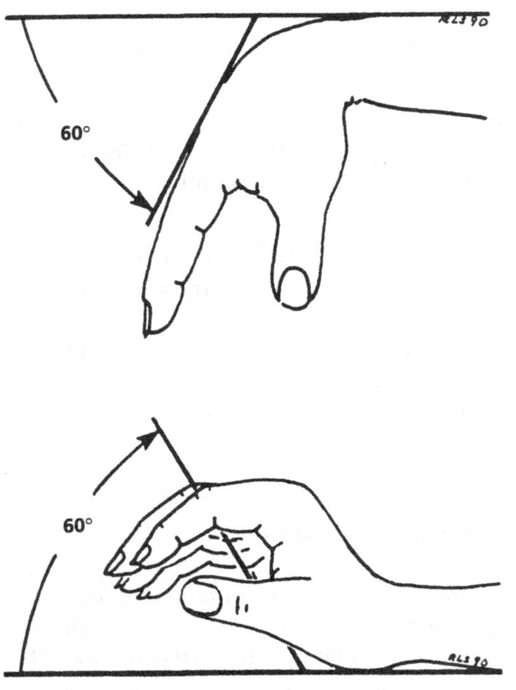

*Redrawn with permission from Swanson, AB, Goran-Hagert, C, de Groot Swanson, G[31], p. 63, Fig. 4-23.

Figure 25. Impairment Curves for Ankylosis (I_A%), Loss of Flexion (I_F%), and Loss of Extension (I_E%) of Wrist Joint. Ankyloses in functional positions (10° extension to 10° flexion) are given the lowest I_A% value (50%):*

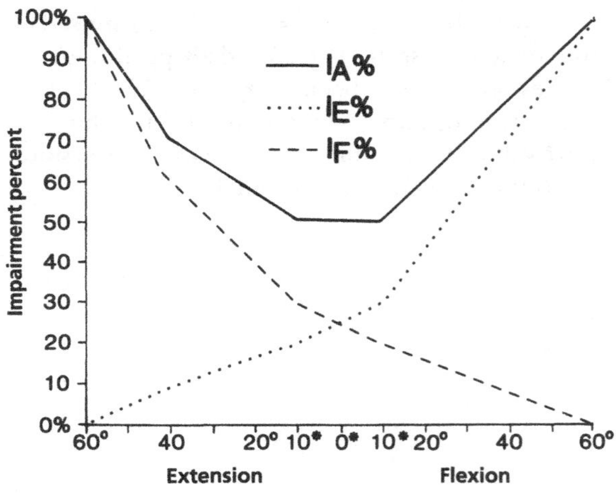

*Redrawn with permission from Swanson, AB, Goran-Hagert, C, de Groot Swanson, G[31], p. 63, Fig. 4-23.

Figure 26. Upper Extremity Impairments Due to Lack of Flexion and Extension of Wrist Joint. Relative value of this functional unit to upper extremity impairment is 42%.†

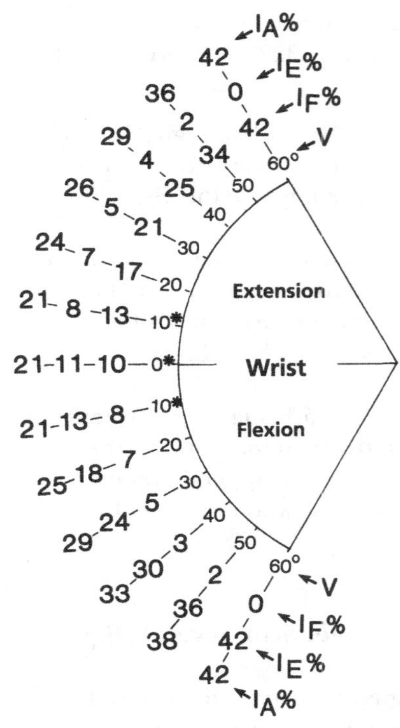

I_A% = Impairment due to ankylosis
I_E% = Impairment due to loss of extension
I_F% = Impairment due to loss of flexion
V = Measured angles of motion
* = Positions of function

†Data from Swanson, AB, Goran-Hagert, C, de Groot Swanson, G[31], p. 63, Fig. 4-23.

Wrist: Flexion and Extension

1. Measure maximum wrist flexion and extension and record the goniometer readings (Fig. 24, at left). Round the measurements to the nearest 10°. The normal range of motion is from 60° extension to 60° flexion. The position of function is from 10° extension to 10° flexion.

2. In Fig. 26 (above), match the measured angles (V) of flexion and of extension to the corresponding impairments of flexion (row headed I_F%) and extension (row headed I_E%).

3. *Add* the flexion and extension impairment percents to obtain the percent of upper extremity impairment.

4. If the wrist is ankylosed, measure the position and match the angle (V) to the corresponding ankylosis impairment (row headed I_A%) in Fig. 26 (above). Ankyloses in functional positions (10° extension to 10° flexion) are given the lowest ankylosis impairment value, 21% impairment of the upper extremity.

Wrist ankylosis in 60° flexion or 60° extension represents 100% loss of wrist extension and flexion function. This is equivalent to a 70% impairment of wrist function, or 42% impairment (70% x 60%) of the upper extremity.

Example: A patient has wrist extension of 10° and flexion of 10°:
I_E% = 8% impairment of the upper extremity (Fig. 26, p. 36);
I_F% = 8% impairment of the upper extremity;
8% + 8% = 16% impairment of the upper extremity.

Example: A patient's wrist has ankylosis in 40° flexion: Fig. 26 (p. 36) indicates this is a 33% impairment of the upper extremity (I_A% = 33%).

Wrist: Radial and Ulnar Deviation

1. Measure maximum radial and ulnar deviation and record the goniometer readings (Fig. 27, at right). Round the figures to the nearest 10°. The normal range of motion is from 20° radial deviation to 30° ulnar deviation. The position of function is from neutral to 10° ulnar deviation.

2. From Fig. 29 (p. 38), match the measured ulnar and radial deviation angles (V) to the corresponding impairments of radial deviation (row headed I_{RD}%) and ulnar deviation (row headed I_{UD}%).

3. *Add* the impairment values for radial and ulnar deviation loss to obtain the upper extremity impairment value.

4. If the wrist is ankylosed, measure the position and match the angle (V) to the corresponding ankylosis impairment value (row headed I_A%) in Fig. 29 (p. 38). Ankyloses in functional positions (0° to 10° ulnar deviation) receive the lowest ankylosis impairment values, or 9% impairment of the upper extremity.

Wrist ankylosis in either 30° ulnar deviation or 20° radial deviation represents 100% loss of wrist lateral deviation. This is equivalent to a 30% impairment of wrist motion and 18% impairment (60% x 30%) of the upper extremity (Fig. 29).

Example: A patient has wrist ulnar deviation to 0° and radial deviation to 10°:
I_{UD}% = 5% impairment of the upper extremity (Fig. 29, p. 38);
I_{RD}% = 2% impairment of the upper extremity;
5% + 2% = 7% impairment of the upper extremity.

Figure 27. Radial Deviation (left) and Ulnar Deviation (right) of Right Wrist.*

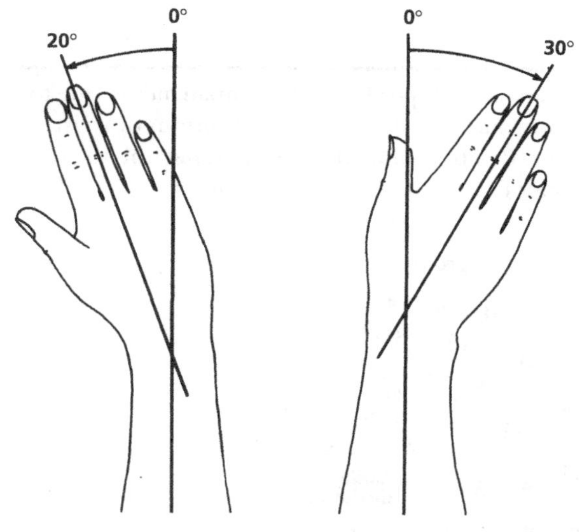

*Redrawn with permission from Swanson, AB, Goran-Hagert, C, de Groot Swanson, G[31], p. 64, Fig. 4-24.

Figure 28. Impairment Curves for Ankylosis (I_A%), Loss of Radial Deviation (I_{RD}%), and Loss of Ulnar Deviation (I_{UD}%) of Wrist Joint. Ankyloses in functional positions (0° to 10° ulnar deviation) are given the lowest ankylosis impairment (50%).*

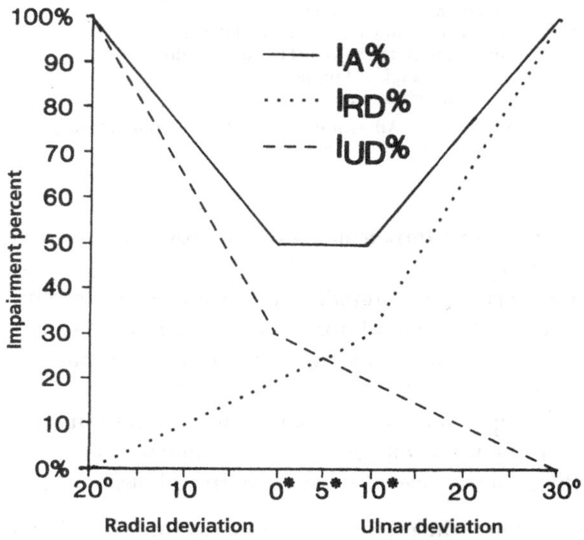

*Redrawn with permission from Swanson, AB, Goran-Hagert, C, de Groot Swanson, G[31], p. 64, Fig. 4-24.

Example: A patient's wrist has ankylosis in 15° radial deviation:
$I_A\%$ = 16% impairment of the upper extremity (Fig. 29).

Figure 29. Upper Extremity Impairments Due to Abnormal Radial and Ulnar Deviations of Wrist Joint. Relative value of this functional unit to upper extremity impairment is 18%.†

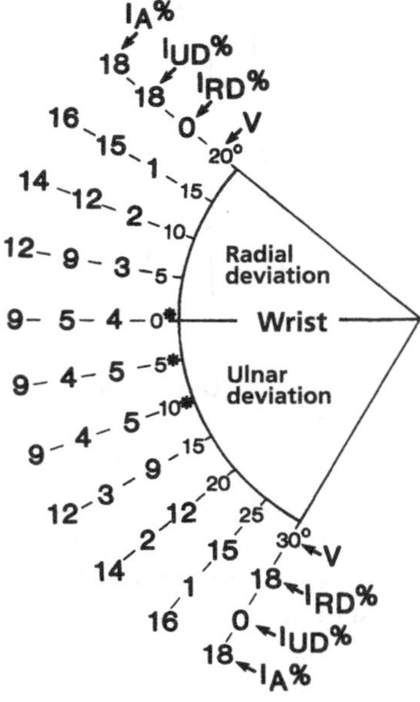

$I_A\%$ = Impairment due to ankylosis
$I_{RD}\%$ = Impairment due to loss of radial deviation
$I_{UD}\%$ = Impairment due to loss of ulnar deviation
V = Measured angles of motion
* = Positions of function

†Data from Swanson, AB, Goran-Hagert, C, de Groot Swanson, G[31], p. 64, Fig. 4-24.

Determining Impairments Due to Abnormal Motion of the Wrist Joint

1. Determine the impairments of the upper extremity contributed by abnormal wrist motions relating to flexion and extension and to radial and ulnar deviation.

Impairments of pronation and supination are ascribed to the elbow, because the major muscles for this function are inserted about the elbow.

2. Because the relative value of each wrist functional unit has been taken into consideration in the impairment charts, impairments of flexion and extension and of radial and ulnar deviation are *added* to determine the impairment of the upper extremity.

3. Use Table 3 (p. 20) to relate impairment of the upper extremity to impairment of the whole person.

Example: A patient has an upper extremity impairment of 16% due to loss of wrist flexion and extension and an impairment of 7% due to loss of wrist radial and ulnar deviation:
16% + 7% = 23% impairment of the upper extremity, or 14% impairment of the whole person (Table 3, p. 20).

Example: A patient has wrist ankylosis in 0° flexion and 0° lateral deviation:
flexion $I_A\%$ = 21%; lateral deviation $I_A\%$ = 9% (Figs. 26 and 29, pp. 36 and left);
21% + 9% = 30% impairment of the upper extremity, or 18% impairment of the whole person (Table 3).

3.1i Elbow

Amputation About the Elbow

1. Determine the level of amputation about the elbow (Fig. 2, p. 18).

2. Amputation at a level below the axilla and proximal to the biceps insertion is a 95% to 100% impairment of the upper extremity, depending on the location.

3. Use Table 3 (p. 20) to relate impairment of the upper extremity to impairment of the whole person.

Example: An amputation at the elbow joint level is a 96% impairment of the upper extremity (Fig. 2, p. 18) and a 58% impairment of the whole person (Table 3).

Abnormal Motion at the Elbow

The elbow functional unit represents 70% of upper extremity function. The elbow joint has two functional units of motion, each contributing a relative value to its function. Elbow motion impairments are converted to upper extremity impairments by multiplying their values by 70% as follows:

1. Flexion and extension: 60% of elbow function; 60% x 70% = 42% of upper extremity function.

2. Pronation and supination: 40% of elbow function; 40% x 70% = 28% of upper extremity function.

Impairment values for each of these units of motion have been derived according to the basic formula, A = E + F (p. 22), and expressed in graphs on a 100% scale (Figs. 31 and 34, at right, and p. 40). These graphs have been expressed in charts of upper extremity impairment by applying the relative value of each functional unit as a conversion factor (Figs. 32 and 35, pp. 40 and 41).

Elbow: Flexion and Extension

1. Measure the maximum flexion and extension and record the goniometer readings (Fig. 30, below). Round the figures to the nearest 10°. The normal range of motion is considered to be from 140° flexion to 0° extension. The position of function is 80° flexion.

Figure 30. Flexion and Extension of Elbow.

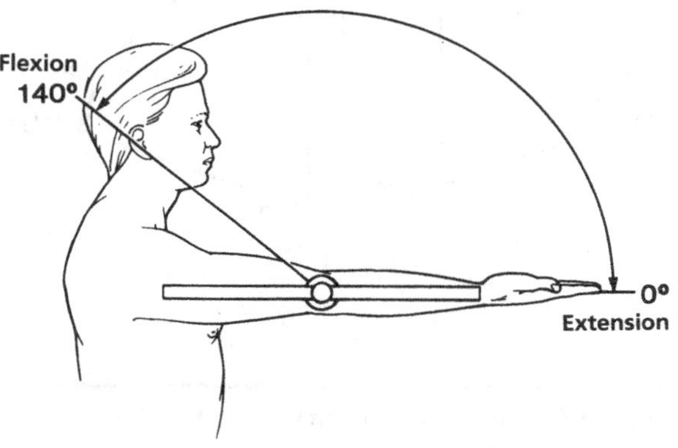

2. From Fig. 32, p. 40, match the measured flexion and extension angles (V) to their corresponding impairments of flexion (row headed $I_F\%$) and extension (row headed $I_E\%$).

3. *Add* the impairment values for flexion and extension loss to obtain the upper extremity impairment percent.

4. If the elbow is ankylosed, measure the position and match the angle (V) to the corresponding ankylosis impairment (row headed $I_A\%$) in Fig. 32. Ankylosis in the functional position (80° flexion) is given the lowest $I_A\%$, 21% impairment of the upper extremity.

Ankylosis in either 0° extension or 140° flexion represents a 100% loss of elbow flexion and extension function. This is equivalent to a 60% impairment of elbow function and a 42% (60% x 70%) impairment of the upper extremity (Fig. 32, p. 40).

Example: A patient has elbow extension lag of –40° and flexion to 70°:
$I_E\%$ = 4% impairment of the upper extremity (Fig. 32, p. 40);
$I_F\%$ = 15% impairment of the upper extremity;
4% + 15% = 19% impairment of the upper extremity.

Example: A patient's elbow has ankylosis in 140° flexion: $I_A\%$ is 42% impairment of the upper extremity (Fig. 32).

Figure 31. Impairment Curves for Ankylosis ($I_A\%$), Loss of Flexion ($I_F\%$), and Loss of Extension ($I_E\%$) of elbow joint. Ankylosis in functional position (80° flexion) is given the lowest $I_A\%$ (50%).*

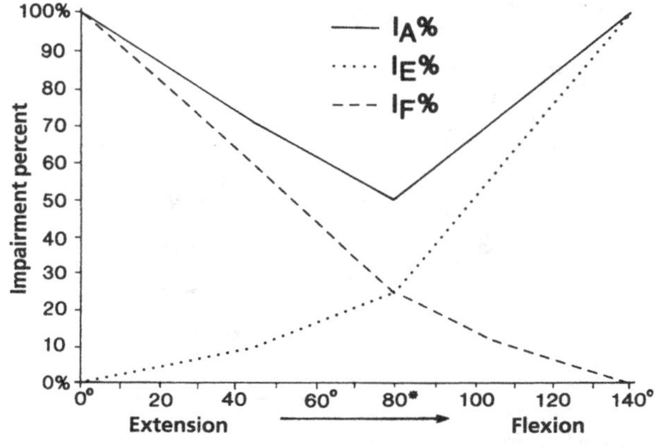

*Redrawn with permission from Swanson, AB, Goran-Hagert, C, de Groot Swanson, G[51], p. 64, Fig. 4-25.

Figure 32. Upper Extremity Impairments Due to Lack of Flexion and Extension of the Elbow Joint. Relative value of this functional unit to upper extremity impairment is 42%.†

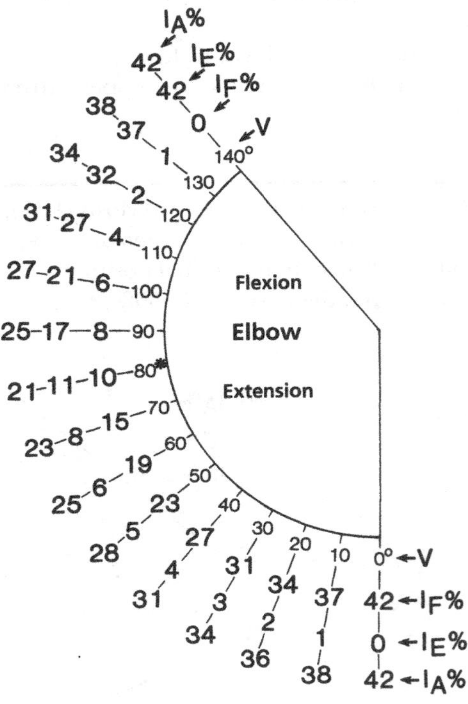

$I_A\%$ = Impairment due to ankylosis
$I_E\%$ = Impairment due to loss of extension
$I_F\%$ = Impairment due to loss of flexion
V = Measured angles of motion
* = Position of function

†Data from Swanson, AB, Goran-Hagert, C, de Groot Swanson, G[31], p. 64, Fig. 4-25.

Pronation and Supination at Elbow

1. Measure the maximum pronation and supination and record the goniometer readings (Fig. 33, at right). Round the figures to the nearest 10°. The normal range of motion is from 80° supination to 80° pronation. The position of function is 20° pronation.

2. From Fig. 35, p. 41, match the measured supination and pronation angles (V) to their corresponding impairments of pronation (row headed $I_P\%$) and supination (row headed $I_S\%$).

3. *Add* the pronation and supination impairment percents to obtain the upper extremity impairment percent.

4. If the elbow is ankylosed, measure the position and match the angle (V) to the corresponding ankylosis impairment (row headed $I_A\%$) in Fig. 35 (p. 41). Ankylosis in the functional position (20° pronation) is given the lowest $I_A\%$, or 8% impairment of the upper extremity.

Figure 33. Pronation and Supination of Forearm.

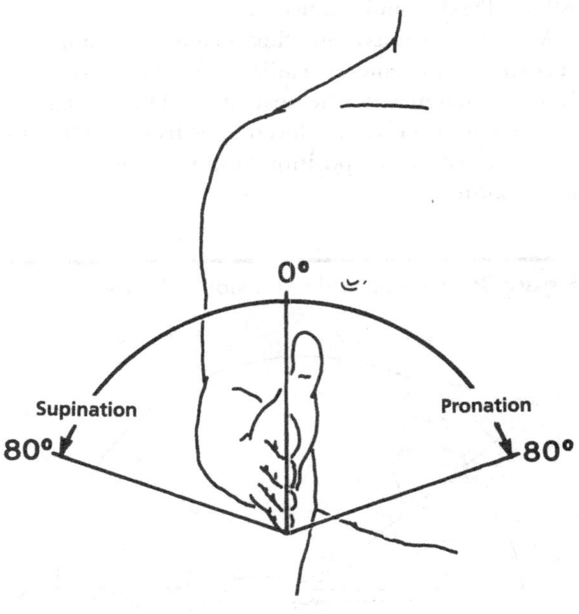

Figure 34. Impairment Curves for Ankylosis ($I_A\%$), Loss of Supination ($I_S\%$), and Loss of Pronation ($I_P\%$) of Elbow Joint. Ankylosis in functional position (20° pronation) is given the lowest $I_A\%$ (30%).*

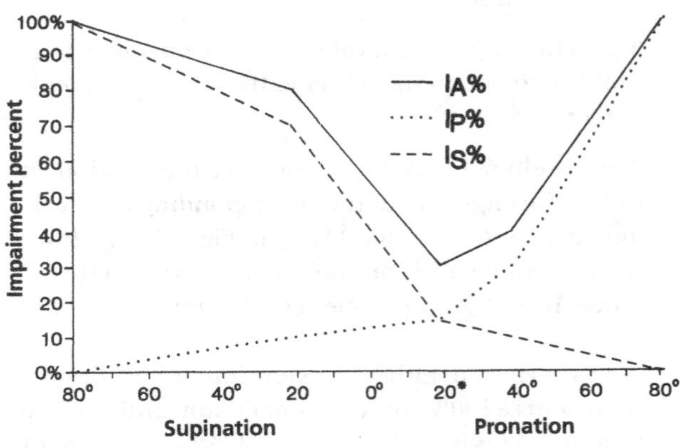

*Modified from Swanson, AB, Goran-Hagert, C, de Groot Swanson, G[31], p. 65, Fig. 4-26.

Ankylosis in 80° of pronation or supination represents a 100% impairment of forearm rotation. This is equivalent to 40% impairment of elbow function and 28% (40% x 70%) impairment of the upper extremity (Fig. 35 below).

Example: A patient can pronate the forearm to 30° and supinate to 10°:
I_P% = 3% impairment of the upper extremity (Fig. 35, below);
I_S% = 3% impairment of the upper extremity;
3% + 3% = 6% upper extremity impairment.

Example: A patient has elbow ankylosis in 80° supination:
I_A% = 28% impairment of the upper extremity (Fig. 35).

Figure 35. Upper Extremity Impairments Due to Lack of Pronation and Supination. Relative value of this functional unit to upper extremity impairment is 28%.†

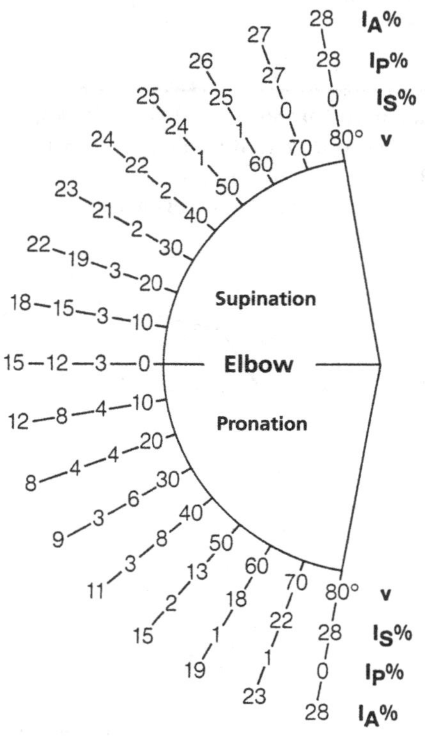

I_A% = Impairment due to ankylosis
I_P% = Impairment due to loss of pronation
I_S% = Impairment due to loss of supination
V = Measured angles of motion
* = Position of function

†Data from Swanson, AB, Goran-Hagert, C, de Groot Swanson, G[31], p. 65, Fig. 4-26.

Determining Impairments Due to Abnormal Motion of the Elbow Joint

1. Determine the impairment of the upper extremity contributed by abnormal elbow motions (flexion and extension, pronation and supination) as described in preceding parts.

2. Because the relative value of each elbow functional unit has been taken into consideration in the impairment figures, impairment values for the loss of each type of motion are *added* to determine the impairment of the upper extremity.

3. Use Table 3 (p. 20) to relate impairment of the upper extremity to impairment of the whole person.

Example: A patient has an upper extremity impairment of 19% due to loss of elbow flexion and extension, and one of 6% due to loss of pronation and supination:
19% + 6% = 25% impairment of the upper extremity, or 15% impairment of the whole person (Table 3, p. 20).

Example: An elbow has ankylosis in 140° flexion and 80° supination:
flexion I_A% = 42% (Fig. 32, p. 40);
supination I_A% = 28% (Fig. 35, at left);
42% + 28% = 70% impairment of the upper extremity, or 42% impairment of the whole person (Table 3, p. 20).

3.1j Shoulder

Amputation at Shoulder Level

An amputation at the shoulder level is considered to be a 100% impairment of the upper extremity (Fig. 2, p. 18) and a 60% impairment of the whole person (Table 3, p. 20).

Abnormal Motion of Shoulder

The shoulder functional unit represents 60% of upper extremity function. The shoulder has three functional units of motion, each contributing a relative value to shoulder function. The shoulder motion impairments are converted to upper extremity impairments by multiplying their values by 60% as follows:

1. Flexion: 40% of shoulder function.
Extension: 10% of shoulder function.
Flexion and extension: 50% of shoulder function, or 30% (50% x 60%) of upper extremity function.

2. Abduction: 20% of shoulder function.
Adduction: 10% of shoulder function.
Abduction and adduction: 30% of shoulder function, or 18% (30% x 60%) of upper extremity function.

3. Internal rotation: 10% of shoulder function.
External rotation: 10% of shoulder function.
Internal and external rotation: 20% of shoulder function, or 12% (20% x 60%) of upper extremity function.

Impairments for each of these units of motion have been derived according to the basic formula, A = E + F (p. 22), and expressed in graphs on a 100% scale (Figs. 37, 40, and 43, pp. 42, 44, and 45). These graphs were expressed in terms of upper extremity impairments by applying the relative value of each functional unit as a conversion factor (Figs. 38, 41, and 44, pp. 43 through 45).

Shoulder: Flexion and Extension

1. Measure the maximum flexion and extension and record the goniometer readings (Fig. 36, below). Round the figures to the nearest 10°. The normal range of motion is considered to be from 180° flexion to 50° extension. The position of function is considered to be from 40° flexion to 20° flexion.

2. From Fig. 38 (p. 43), match the measured flexion and extension angles (V) to their corresponding impairments of flexion (row headed $I_F\%$) and extension (row headed $I_E\%$).

Figure 36. Shoulder Extension and Flexion.

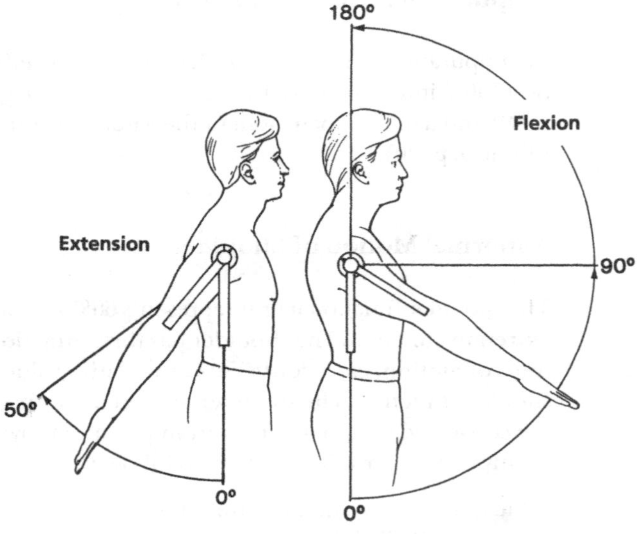

3. *Add* the impairment percents for loss of flexion and extension to obtain the percent of upper extremity impairment.

4. If the shoulder is ankylosed, measure the position and match the angle (V) to the corresponding ankylosis impairment (row headed $I_A\%$) in Fig. 38 (p. 43). Ankyloses in functional positions (40° flexion to 20° flexion) are given the lowest $I_A\%$, 15% impairment of the upper extremity.

Ankylosis in 50° extension or 180° flexion represents a 100% loss of shoulder flexion and extension function. This is equivalent to a 50% loss of shoulder function and a 30% (50% x 60%) impairment of the upper extremity (Fig. 38).

Example: A patient has shoulder flexion of 90° and extension of 0°:
$I_F\%$ = 6% impairment of the upper extremity (Fig. 38, p. 43);
$I_E\%$ = 3% impairment of the upper extremity;
6% + 3% = 9% impairment of the upper extremity.

Example: A patient's shoulder is ankylosed in 50° extension: $I_A\%$ = 30% impairment of the upper extremity (Fig. 38).

Figure 37. Impairment Curves for Ankylosis ($I_A\%$), Loss of Flexion ($I_F\%$), and Loss of Extension ($I_E\%$) of Shoulder. Ankyloses in functional positions (40° to 20° flexion) are given the lowest $I_A\%$ (50%).*

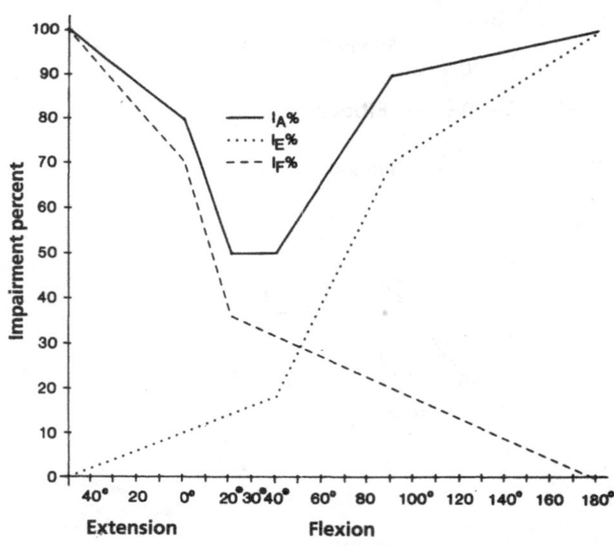

*Modified from Swanson, AB, Goran-Hagert, C, de Groot Swanson, G[31], p. 66, Fig. 4-27.

Figure 38. Upper Extremity Impairments Due to Lack of Flexion and Extension of Shoulder. Relative value of this functional unit to upper extremity impairment is 30%.†

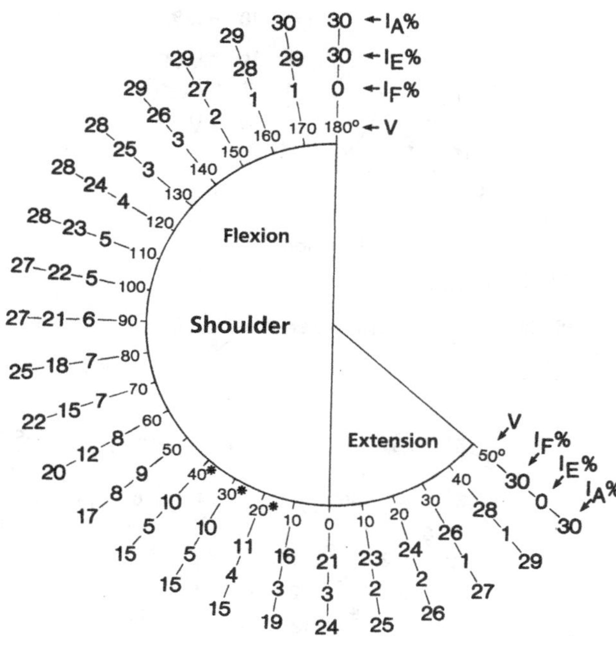

$I_A\%$ = Impairment due to ankylosis
$I_E\%$ = Impairment due to loss of extension
$I_F\%$ = Impairment due to loss of flexion
V = Measured angles of motion
* = Positions of function

†Data from Swanson, AB, Goran-Hagert, C, de Groot Swanson, G[31], p. 66, Fig. 4-28.

Abduction and Adduction of Shoulder

1. Measure the maximum abduction and adduction and record the goniometer readings (Fig. 39, at right). Round the figures to the nearest 10°. The normal range of motion is considered to be from 180° abduction to 50° adduction. The position of function is from 50° abduction to 20° abduction.

2. Using Fig. 41 (p. 44), match the measured abduction and adduction angles (V) to their corresponding impairments of abduction (row headed $I_{ABD}\%$) and adduction (row headed $I_{ADD}\%$).

3. *Add* the impairments for loss of abduction and adduction to obtain the upper extremity impairment.

4. If the shoulder is ankylosed, measure the position and match the angle (V) to the corresponding ankylosis impairment (row headed $I_A\%$) in Fig. 41. Ankyloses in functional positions (50° abduction to 20° abduction) are given the lowest impairment percent, 9% impairment of the upper extremity.

Ankylosis in either 50° adduction or 180° abduction represents a 100% loss of abduction or adduction function, respectively. This is equivalent to a 30% loss of shoulder function or an 18% (30% x 60%) impairment of the upper extremity (Fig. 41).

Example: A patient has shoulder abduction to 100° and adduction to 0°:
$I_{ABD}\%$ = 4% impairment of the upper extremity (Fig. 41, p. 44);
$I_{ADD}\%$ = 2% impairment of the upper extremity;
4% + 2% = 6% impairment of the upper extremity.

Example: Shoulder ankylosis in 180° abduction is an 18% impairment of the upper extremity (Fig. 41).

Figure 39. Shoulder Abduction and Adduction.

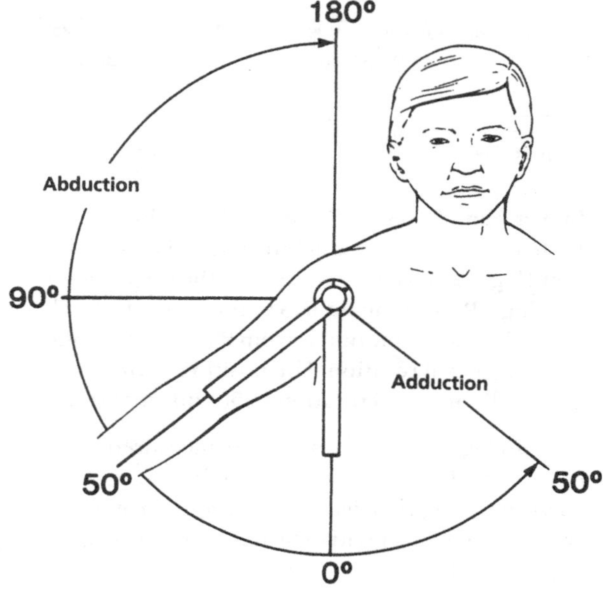

Figure 40. Impairment Curves for Ankylosis ($I_A\%$), Loss of Abduction ($I_{ABD}\%$), and Loss of Adduction ($I_{ADD}\%$) of Shoulder. Ankyloses in functional positions (50° to 20° abduction) are given the lowest $I_A\%$ (50%).*

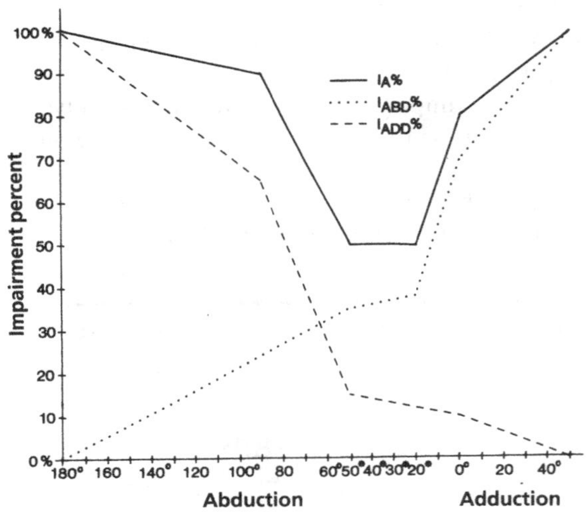

*Adapted from Swanson, AB, Goran-Hagert, C, de Groot Swanson, G[31], p. 66, Fig. 4-27.

Figure 41. Upper Extremity Impairments Due to Lack of Abduction and Adduction of Shoulder. Relative value of this functional unit to upper extremity impairment is 18%.†

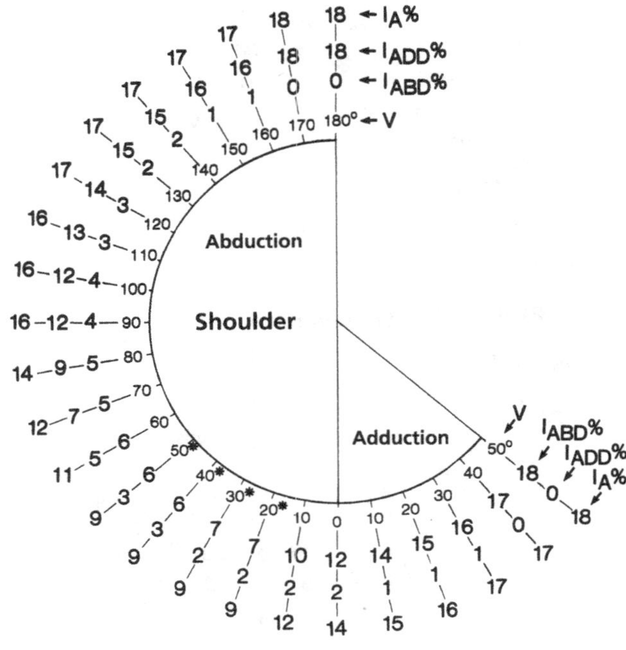

$I_A\%$ = Impairment due to ankylosis
$I_{ABD}\%$ = Impairment due to loss of abduction
$I_{ADD}\%$ = Impairment due to loss of adduction
V = Measured angles of motion
* = Positions of function

†Data from Swanson, AB, Goran-Hagert, C, de Groot Swanson, G[31], p. 66, Fig. 4-27.

Internal and External Rotation of Shoulder

1. Measure the maximum internal and external rotation (Fig. 42, at right) and record the goniometer readings. Round the figures to the nearest 10°. The normal range of motion is from 90° internal rotation to 90° external rotation. The position of function is from 30° internal rotation to 50° internal rotation.

2. From Fig. 44 (p. 45), match the measured internal and external rotation angles (V) to their corresponding impairments of internal rotation (row headed $I_{IR}\%$) and external rotation (row headed $I_{ER}\%$).

3. *Add* the impairment values for internal and external rotation loss to obtain the value for upper extremity impairment.

4. If the shoulder is ankylosed, measure the position and match the angle (V) to the corresponding ankylosis impairment (row headed $I_A\%$) in Fig. 44. Ankyloses in functional positions (30° to 50° internal rotation) are given the lowest $I_A\%$, 6% impairment of the upper extremity.

Ankylosis in either 90° internal or external rotation represents a 100% loss of shoulder rotation function. This is equivalent to a 20% impairment of shoulder function and a 12% (20% x 60%) impairment of the upper extremity (Fig. 44).

Figure 42. Shoulder External Rotation and Internal Rotation.

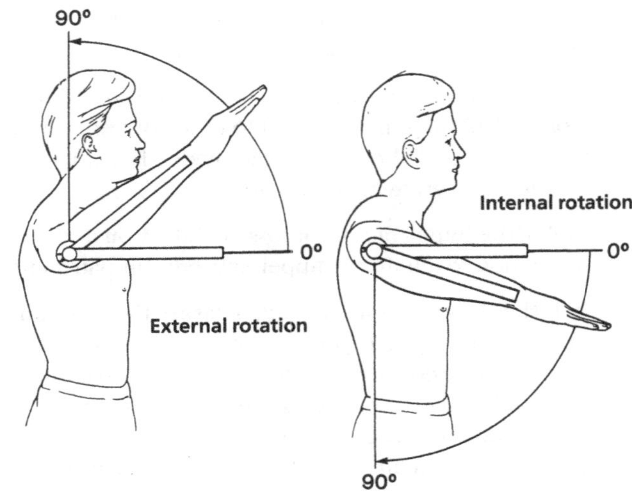

Example: A patient has shoulder internal rotation of 40° and external rotation of 50°:
$I_{IR}\%$ = 3% impairment of upper extremity (Fig. 44, at right);
$I_{ER}\%$ = 1% impairment of upper extremity;
3% + 1% = 4% impairment of upper extremity.

Example: Shoulder ankylosis in 90° external rotation:
$I_A\%$ = 12% impairment of the upper extremity (Fig. 44).

Determining Impairments Due to Abnormal Motions of the Shoulder Joint

1. Determine the impairments of the upper extremity that are contributed by abnormal shoulder motions (flexion and extension, abduction and adduction, internal and external rotation), using the methods described in preceding sections.

2. Because the relative value of each shoulder functional unit has been taken into consideration in the impairment charts, the impairment values for loss of each shoulder motion are *added* to determine the impairment of the upper extremity.

3. Use Table 3 (p. 20) to relate impairment of the upper extremity to impairment of the whole person.

Example: A patient has a shoulder flexion and extension impairment of 9%, an abduction and adduction impairment of 5%, and an internal and external rotation impairment of 2%:
9% + 5% + 2% = 16% impairment of the upper extremity or 10% impairment of the whole person (Table 3, p. 20).

Example: A patient has shoulder ankylosis in 0° extension, 0° adduction, and 0° rotation:
extension $I_A\%$ = 24% (Fig. 38, p. 43);
adduction $I_A\%$ = 14% (Fig. 41, p. 44);
rotation $I_A\%$ = 7% (Fig. 44, at right);
24% + 14% + 7% = 45% impairment of the upper extremity, or 27% impairment of the whole person (Table 3, p. 20).

Figure 43. Impairment Curves for Ankylosis ($I_A\%$), Loss of Internal Rotation ($I_{IR}\%$), and Loss of External Rotation ($I_E\%$) of the Shoulder. Ankyloses in functional positions (30° internal rotation to 50° internal rotation) are given the lowest $I_A\%$ (50%).

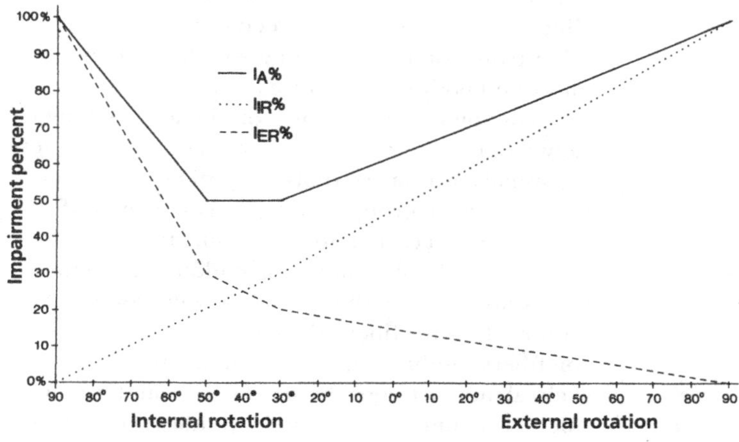

Figure 44. Upper Extremity Impairments Due to Lack of Internal and External Rotation of Shoulder. Relative value of this functional unit to upper extremity impairment is 12%.

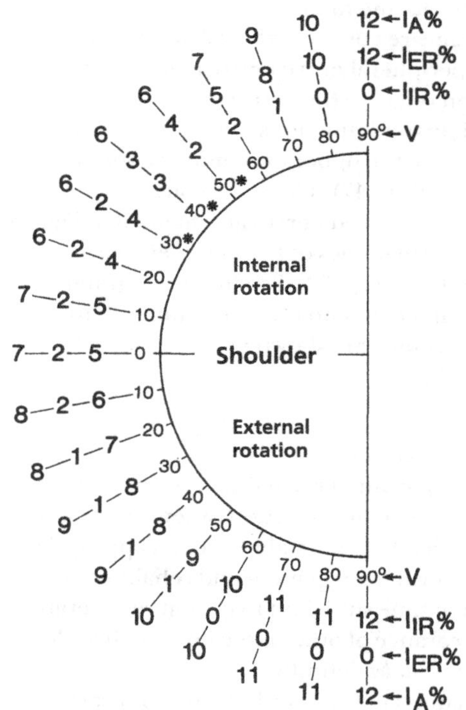

$I_A\%$ = Impairment due to ankylosis
$I_{IR}\%$ = Impairment due to loss of internal rotation
$I_{ER}\%$ = Impairment due to loss of external rotation
V = Measured angles of motion
* = Positions of function

3.1k Impairment of the Upper Extremity Due to Peripheral Nerve Disorders

The peripheral nerves constitute an intricate system that serves as the conductor of neural impulses traveling in both directions between the spinal cord and other tissues of the body and through which many important body functions are regulated.

The spinal nerves consist of 31 pairs of symmetrically arranged nerves, each of which leaves and enters the spinal cord via two roots. The spinal nerves contain three main groups of fibers: (1) sensory (afferent) fibers that carry impulses arising from various receptors in the skin, muscles, tendons, ligaments, bones, and joints to the central nervous system; (2) motor (efferent) fibers: the large *alpha* motor neuron fibers conduct impulses from the spinal cord to skeletal muscle fibers; the small *gamma* motor neuron fibers carry impulses to muscle spindles for feedback control; and (3) autonomic system fibers, which are efferent and are concerned with the control of smooth muscles and glands.

This section presents a method of evaluating upper extremity impairments related to disorders of the spinal nerves (C5 to T1), the brachial plexus, and the peripheral nerves of the upper extremity. Impairments relating to the spinal cord and central nervous system are considered in Chapter 4 of the *Guides.* The peripheral nerve impairments considered in this section relate to the entire upper extremity.

The origins and functions of the peripheral nerves that serve the upper extremity are summarized in Table 10 (p. 47). The cutaneous innervation and related nerves are mapped in Fig. 45 (p. 50). The dermatomes of the upper extremity are shown in Fig. 46 (p. 52). Schematic diagrams of the brachial plexus and the motor innervation of the upper extremity are shown in Figs. 47 and 48 (pp. 53 and 55).

Method of Evaluation

Permanent impairment related to a peripheral nerve may be described as an alteration of sensory or motor function that has become stable after an appropriate course of medical management and rehabilitation for a period of time sufficient to permit regeneration and the appearance of other indicators of physiologic recovery. The *Guides* definition of permanent impairment is explained in Chapter 1 and the Glossary.

To evaluate impairment resulting from the effects of peripheral nerve lesions, it is necessary to determine the extent of loss of function due to (1) sensory deficits or pain (Table 11, p. 48); and (2) motor deficits (Table 12, p. 49). Characteristic deformities and manifestations resulting from peripheral nerve lesions, such as restricted motion, atrophy, and vasomotor, trophic, and reflex changes, have been taken into consideration in preparing the estimated impairment percents shown in this section.

If an impairment results strictly from a peripheral nerve lesion, the physician should not *apply impairment percents from Sections 3.1f through 3.1j (pp. 24 through 45) of this chapter,* and *this section, because a duplication and an unwarranted increase in the impairment percent would result.*

If restricted motion cannot be attributed to a peripheral nerve lesion, the motion impairment should be evaluated according to Sections 3.1f through 3.1j and the nerve impairment according to this section. Then the motion impairment percent should be *combined* (Combined Values Chart, p. 322) with the peripheral nerve system impairment percent.

The severity of loss of function due to a sensory deficit (Table 11, p. 48) or a motor deficit (Table 12, p. 49) is graded with the appropriate table and related to the anatomic structure(s) involved. Maximum percentages of impairment due to motor and sensory deficits have been estimated for the spinal nerves (Table 13, p. 51), brachial plexus (Table 14, p. 52), and major peripheral nerves (Table 15, p. 54).

For each structure involved, impairment percents are calculated by multiplying the maximum impairment value of the nerve structure due to motor or sensory deficit (Tables 13, 14, and 15, pp. 51, 52, and 54) by the estimated grade of severity of the sensory or motor loss (Tables 11 and 12, pp. 48 and 49). When both functions are involved, the impairment percents are *combined* using the Combined Values Chart (p. 322).

Sensory Deficits and Pain

A wide range of abnormal sensations may be associated with peripheral nerve lesions, including anesthesia, dysesthesia, paresthesia, hyperesthesia, cold intolerance, and an intense, burning pain. Pain and sensory deficits associated with peripheral nerve disorders are evaluated according to the following criteria: (1) How does the pain or sensory deficit interfere with the individual's performance of daily activities? (2) To what extent does the pain or sensory deficit follow the defined anatomic pathways of the root, plexus, or peripheral nerve? (3) To what extent does the description of the pain or sensory deficit indicate that it is caused by a peripheral nerve abnormality? (4) To what extent does the pain or sensory deficit correspond to other disturbances of the involved nerve structure?

Table 10. Origins and Functions of the Peripheral Nerves of the Upper Extremity Emanating from the Brachial Plexus.

Nerves of plexus	Primary branches	Secondary branches	Function
Muscular branches	Unnamed		Motor to Longus colli, Scalenes, and Subclavius
Dorsal scapular (C5)			Motor to Rhomboideus major and minor, Levator scapulae
Long thoracic (C5, 6, 7)			Motor to Serratus anterior
Suprascapular (C5, 6)			Motor to Supraspinatus and Infraspinatus
Lateral pectoral (C5, 6, 7)			Motor to Pectoralis major
Medial pectoral (C8, T1)			Motor to Pectoralis major and minor
Upper subscapular (C5, 6)			Motor to Subscapularis
Lower subscapular (C5, 6)			Motor to Teres major and Subscapularis
Thoracodorsal (∓C6, C7, 8)			Motor to Latissimus dorsi
Medial brachial cutaneous (T1)			Sensory to anteromedial surface of arm (with intercostobrachial)
Medial antebrachial cutaneous (C8, T1)			Sensory to anteromedial surface of arm and ulnar surface of forearm
Musculocutaneous (C5, 6, 7)	Unnamed		Motor to Coracobrachialis, Biceps brachii, Brachialis
	Lateral antebrachial cutaneous		Sensory to radial surface of forearm
Axillary (C5, C6)	Posterior	Teres minor br	Motor to Teres minor Motor to posterior part of Deltoid
		Upper lateral brachial-cutaneous	Sensory to skin over lower two-thirds of Deltoid
	Anterior		Motor to central and anterior parts of Deltoid
Radial (C5, 6, 7, 8, ∓T1)	Unnamed		Motor to Triceps, Brachil, Anconeus, Brachioradialis, Extensor carpi radialis longus, Brachialis (Lateral part only)
	Ulnar collateral		Motor to medial head of Triceps brachii
	Posterior brachial cutaneous		Sensory to posteromedial surface of arm (with intercostobrachial) as far as olecranon
	Inferior lateral brachial cutaneous		Sensory to distal posterolateral surface of arm
	Posterior antebrachial cutaneous		Sensory to dorsal surface of arm and forearm and distal posterolateral one-third of arm
	Superficial and dorsal digitals		Sensory to dorsum of radial one-half of wrist and hand; thumb, index, middle and radial one-half of ring finger to middle phalanx
	Posterior interosseous		Motor to Extensor carpi radialis brevis, Supinator
		Superficial br	Motor to Extensor digitorum communis, Extensor digiti quinti proprius, Extensor carpi ulnaris
		Deep br	Motor to Extensor pollicis longus, Extensor pollicis brevis, Abductor pollicis longus, Extensor indicis proprius
		Terminal br	Sensory to wrist joint capsule
Median (∓C5, C6, 7, 8, T1)	Unnamed	Cubital fossa and forearm branches	Motor to Pronator teres, Flexor carpi radialis, Palmaris longus, Flexor digitorum superficialis
	Anterior interosseus		Motor to radial half of Flexor digitorum profundus of the index and middle fingers, Flexor pollicis longus, Pronator quadratus
	Palmar cutaneous		Sensory to radial surface of palm
	Common palmar radial digital	Thenar muscular branch	Motor to Abductor pollicis brevis, Flexor pollicis brevis and opponens pollicis
		Proper palmar digitals (1st, 2nd, 3rd)	Motor to first Lumbrical; sensory to first web space, to palmar and distal dorsal surfaces of thumb, and to index palmar surface and distal dorsal surface on radial side
	Common palmar central digital	Proper palmar digital (4th)	Motor to second Lumbrical; sensory to 2nd web space and to palmar surfaces and distal dorsal surfaces of continguous sides of index and middle fingers
	Common palmar ulnar digital	Proper palmar digital (5th)	Sensory to 3rd web space and to palmar surfaces and distal dorsal surfaces of contiguous sides of middle and ring fingers
Ulnar (∓C7, C8, T1)	Unnamed		Motor to Flexor carpi ulnaris, ulnar half of Flexor digitorum profundus of ring and little fingers
	Palmar and dorsal cutaneous		Sensory to ulnar half of hand, little finger and ulnar half of ring finger
	Superficial palmar		Motor to Palmaris brevis
	Deep palmar		Motor to Abductor pollicis, deep head of Flexor pollicis brevis, Abductor digiti quinti, Flexor digiti quinti brevis, Opponens digiti quinti, third and fourth Lumbricals, all Interossei

Only persistent pain or discomfort that leads to permanent loss of function, in spite of maximum effort toward medical rehabilitation and allowing an optimal period of time for physiologic adjustment, should be evaluated as a permanent impairment. Pain that does not meet one or more of the above criteria is not considered to be within the scope of this section.

Pain may be defined as "a disagreeable sensation that has as its basis a highly variable complex made up of afferent nerve stimuli interacting with the emotional state of the individual and modified by past experience, motivation, and state of mind."[34] Pain is a subjective symptom and is difficult to evaluate, but its presence, anatomic background, and intensity may be verified with a thorough examination. The subject of chronic pain is considered further in Chapter 15 (p. 303).

Motivation and malingering as they may relate to the presence or absence of an impairment or a supposed impairment are considered in the *Guides* chapter on mental and behavioral disorders (p. 291).

Table 11 (at right) provides a classification and procedure for determining impairment of the upper extremity due to a sensory deficit or pain resulting from a peripheral nerve disorder. Impairments relating to sensory losses of the hand are discussed in Sections 3.1c (p. 20), 3.1f (p. 24), and 3.1g (p. 30) of this chapter.

Example: After an injury to his elbow, a man continued to have pain and abnormal sensations (minor causalgia) in the medial aspect of his right forearm that prevented activity.

1. Area of involvement is the medial aspect of right forearm (Fig. 45, p. 50).

2. Nerve involved is the medial antebrachial cutaneous (Table 10, p. 47).

3. Maximum loss of function due to sensory deficit is 5% (Table 15, p. 54).

4. Grade of sensory deficit or pain is 61% to 80% (Table 11a right); use maximum value.

5. Impairment of the upper extremity is calculated to be 80% x 5%, or 4%. This is equivalent to a 2% whole-person impairment (Table 3, p. 20).

Table 11. Determining Impairment of the Upper Extremity Due to Pain or Sensory Deficit Resulting from Peripheral Nerve Disorders.

a. Classification

Grade	Description of sensory deficit or pain	% Sensory deficit
1	No loss of sensibility, abnormal sensation, or pain	0
2	Decreased sensibility with or without abnormal sensation or pain, which is forgotten during activity	1-25
3	Decreased sensibility with or without abnormal sensation or pain, which interferes with activity	26-60
4	Decreased sensibility with or without abnormal sensation or pain, which may prevent activity, and/or minor causalgia	61-80
5	Decreased sensibility with abnormal sensations and severe pain, which prevents activity, and/or major causalgia	81-100

b. Procedure

1. Identify the area of involvement using the dermatome charts (Figs. 45 and 46, pp. 50 and 52).
2. Identify the nerve(s) that innervate the area(s) (Table 10, Figs. 45 through 47, pp. 47, 50, 52, and 53).
3. Grade the severity of the sensory deficit or pain according to the classification given above.
4. Find the maximum impairment of the upper extremity due to sensory deficit or pain for each structure involved: spinal nerves (Table 13, p. 51), brachial plexus (Table 14, p. 52), and major peripheral nerves (Table 15, p. 54).
5. Multiply the severity of the sensory deficit by the maximum impairment value to obtain the upper extremity impairment for each structure involved.

Motor Deficits and Loss of Power

Involvement of peripheral or spinal nerves may lead to paralysis or weakness of the muscles they supply and to characteristic sensory changes. In the case of weakness, the patient often will attempt to substitute stronger muscles to accomplish the desired motion. Thus, the physician must understand which muscles help carry out the various movements of the body.

Muscle testing, including tests for strength, duration and repetition of contraction, and function, helps evaluate the motor function of specific nerves. Muscle testing rates one's ability to move a segment of the body through its full range of motion against gravity and hold the part against resistance. The motor function of individual muscles is tested and graded according to Table 12a (p. 49).

A classification and procedure for determining impairment of the upper extremity due to motor deficits resulting from peripheral nerve disorders are shown in Table 12 (p. 49). Loss of strength relating to other conditions is discussed in Section 3.1m (p. 64). *The evaluator should not apply impairment values from both sections to the same condition.*

Example: A patient sustained a subluxation of the right shoulder, which was reduced to its anatomic position as seen on roentgenograms. However, after an appropriate course of rehabilitation, a permanent impairment of function was present. The patient, while in a standing position, could abduct the shoulder fully against gravity and some resistance, starting with the arm placed alongside the body. There was some hypesthesia of the skin over the lower two thirds of the deltoid muscle that did not interfere with activity. The estimated impairment should take into consideration the motor and sensory deficits.

Table 12. Determining Impairment of the Upper Extremity Due to Loss of Power and Motor Deficits Resulting from Peripheral Nerve Disorders Based on Individual Muscle Rating*

a. Classification

Grade	Description of muscle function	% Motor deficit
5	Active movement against gravity with full resistance	0
4	Active movement against gravity with some resistance	1-25
3	Active movement against gravity only, without resistance	26-50
2	Active movement with gravity eliminated	51-75
1	Slight contraction and no movement	76-99
0	No contraction	100

b. Procedure

1. Identify the motion involved, such as flexion, extension, etc.
2. Identify the muscle(s) performing the motion and the motor nerve(s) involved.
3. Grade the severity of motor deficit of individual muscles according to the classification given above.
4. Find the maximum impairment of the upper extremity due to motor deficit for each nerve structure involved: spinal nerves (Table 13, p. 51), brachial plexus (Table 14, p. 52), and major peripheral nerves (Table 15, p. 54).
5. Multiply the severity of the motor deficit by the maximum impairment value to obtain the upper extremity impairment for each structure involved.

*Adapted from Medical Research Council[16]

Motor deficit calculation:

1. Muscle involved is the deltoid, which is innervated by the axillary nerve (Table 10, p. 47).

2. Maximum upper extremity impairment due to motor deficit of the axillary nerve is 35% (Table 15, p. 54).

3. Grade of loss of muscle strength is 25% (Table 12a above). Use maximum value.

4. Impairment of the upper extremity due to motor deficit of the axillary nerve is 25% x 35%, or 9%.

Sensory deficit calculation:

1. Cutaneous dermatome involved is innervated by the axillary nerve (Fig. 45, p. 50).

2. Maximum upper extremity impairment due to sensory deficit of the axillary nerve is estimated to be 5% (Table 15, p. 54).

3. Grade of severity of sensory deficit is 25% (Table 11a, p. 48).

4. Impairment of the upper extremity due to sensory deficit of the axillary nerve is 25% x 5%, or 1%.

The motor and sensory deficit of the upper extremity caused by axillary nerve dysfunction was 9% *combined* with 1%, or 10% (Combined Values Chart, p. 322); this is a 6% whole-person impairment (Table 3, p. 20).

Combining Multiple Deficits Due to Peripheral Nerve Disorders

The impairment percents due to pain or sensory deficits and those due to loss of power or motor deficits are determined for each peripheral nerve structure involved (spinal nerves, brachial plexus, and peripheral nerves).

The impairment for a structure with mixed motor and sensory fibers is calculated by *combining* the sensory and motor deficit impairments using the Combined Values Chart (p. 322).

When more than one structure is involved, the respective upper extremity impairments are *combined* using the Combined Values Chart to obtain the total upper extremity impairment due to peripheral nerve disorders.

When multiple impairments of the extremity are present, such as amputation, loss of motion, or vascular disorders, the peripheral nerve impairment is *combined* with the other impairments using the Combined Values Chart (p. 322) to obtain the total upper extremity impairment. The total upper extremity impairment is converted to a whole-person impairment using Table 3 (p. 20).

If there is bilateral upper extremity involvement, the unilateral impairments are determined separately, and each is converted to a whole-person impairment. The unilateral values then are *combined* using the Combined Values Chart.

Figure 45. Cutaneous Innervation of Upper Extremity and Related Peripheral Nerves and Roots.*

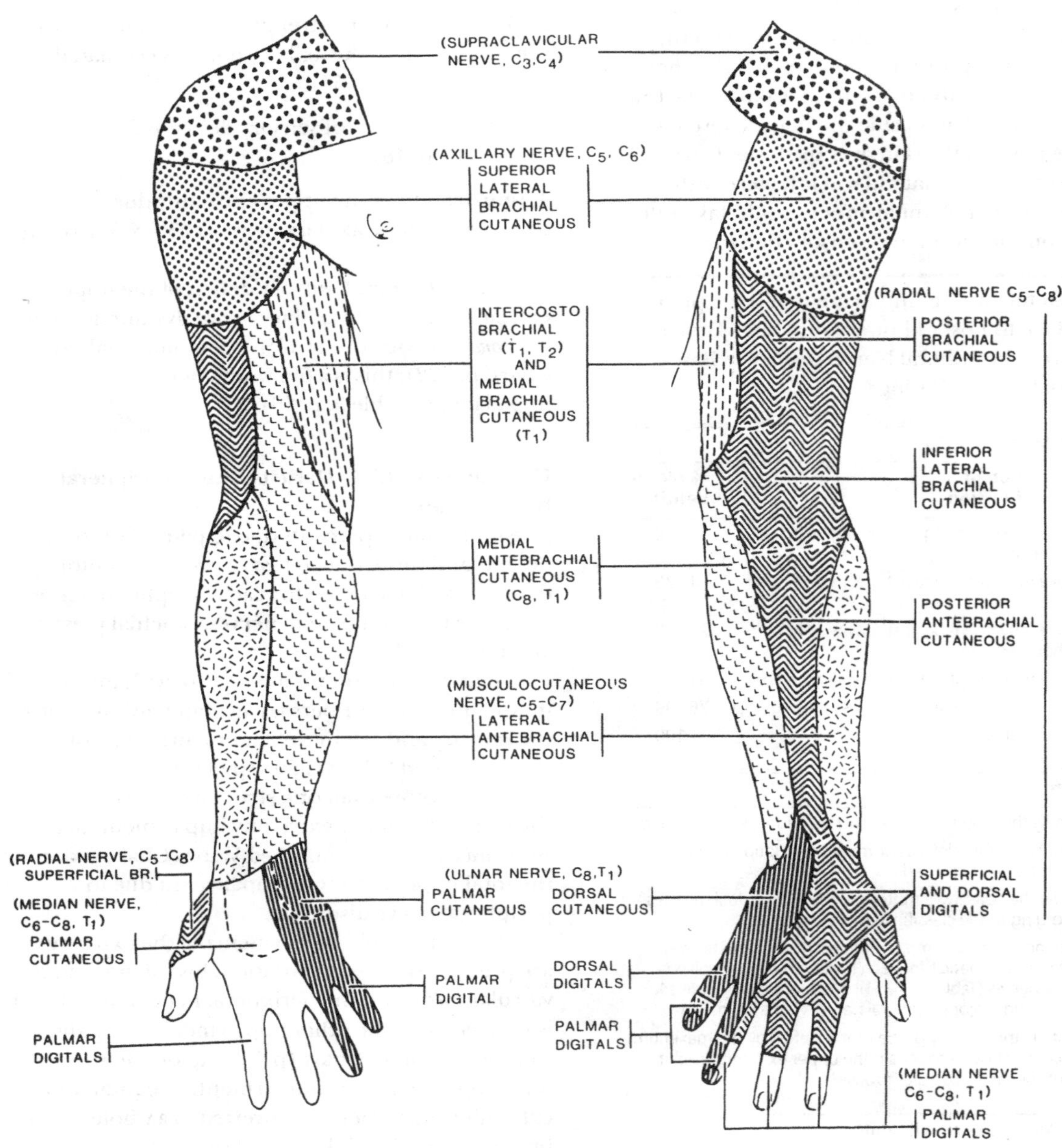

*Adapted with permission from an original painting by F. H. Netter from *The Atlas of Human Anatomy.* Copyright 1989, CIBA-GEIGY Corp., Summit, NJ.

Determination of Impairment

Impairment of the peripheral nerve system may involve the following structures:

1. Spinal nerves C5 to C8 and T1 (see below).
2. Brachial plexus (p. 52).
3. Major peripheral nerves (p. 54).
4. Entrapment neuropathies (p. 56).
5. Causalgia and reflex sympathetic dystrophy (p. 56).

Spinal Nerves

Evaluating impairment of the spinal nerves due to injuries or disease is based on the severity of loss of function of the peripheral nerves receiving fibers from specific spinal nerves. Because peripheral nerves receive fibers from more than one spinal nerve, the involvement of two or more spinal nerves giving fibers to the same peripheral nerve produces a greater loss of function than does the involvement of one spinal nerve; therefore, the impairment is evaluated according to brachial plexus impairment percents (Table 14, p. 52) rather than by *combining* individual spinal nerve root impairment percents, which are shown in Table 13 (below).

For example, the maximum upper extremity impairment due to *combined* motor and sensory deficits resulting from a lesion of the upper trunk (C5 and C6) is 81% (Table 14, p. 52); but *combining* the impairment percents for the individual nerves, C5 (34%) and C6 (40%) (Table 13, below), gives a 60% upper extremity impairment (Combined Values Chart, p. 322) and does not reflect the full severity of loss of function.

Table 13. Maximum Upper Extremity Impairment Due to Unilateral Sensory or Motor Deficits of Individual Spinal Nerves or to *Combined* Deficits.

Maximum % upper extremity impairment*			
Spinal nerve	**Due to sensory deficit or pain†**	**Due to motor deficit‡**	**Due to *combined* motor and sensory deficits**
C5	5	30	34
C6	8	35	40
C7	5	35	38
C8	5	45	48
T1	5	20	24

*See Table 3 (p. 20) to convert upper extremity impairments to whole-person impairments.
†See Table 11a (p. 48) to grade impairment from loss of function due to sensory deficit or pain.
‡See Table 12a (p. 49) to grade impairment from loss of function due to motor deficit.

Table 13 provides impairment percents for the spinal nerves that are most frequently involved in upper extremity permanent impairments. The percents are for unilateral upper extremity involvement only. If there is bilateral involvement, the impairment on each side is determined separately and converted to a whole-person impairment percent. Then the unilateral percents are *combined* using the Combined Values Chart (p. 322).

Impairment of a specific spinal nerve that is not mentioned in this section should be estimated by considering the percents suggested for a nerve that has fibers from the specific spinal nerve.

Spinal nerve impairment is derived as follows:

1. Estimate the severity of sensory deficit or pain according to Table 11a (p. 47) and that of motor deficit according to Table 12a (p. 48).
2. Find the values for maximum impairment of the upper extremity due to sensory and/or motor deficits of individual spinal nerves (Table 13, at left).
3. Multiply the severity of the sensory and/or motor deficit by the appropriate percent from Table 13 to determine the upper extremity impairment percent for each function.
4. *Combine* the sensory and motor impairment percents (Combined Values Chart, p. 322) to obtain the total upper extremity impairment.
5. Convert the upper extremity impairment to whole-person impairment (Table 3, p. 20).

Example: A 42-year-old man fell 30 feet and landed on his upper back. He complained of neck pain radiating down his right arm. Sixteen months later, after a maximum medical rehabilitation program and an optimal period for physiologic recovery, an examination disclosed a 20% sensory loss in the C5 area and 50% loss of power of the muscles innervated by C5. These losses were stable and were determined to be permanent impairments.

1. 20% of 5% (see Table 13, at left) equals 1% loss of function due to sensory deficit or pain.
2. 50% of 30% (Table 13) equals 15% loss of function due to loss of power.
3. 1% *combined* with 15% equals 16% impairment of the upper extremity (Combined Values Chart, p. 322).
4. A 16% impairment of the upper extremity is a 10% impairment of the whole person (Table 3, p. 20).

Brachial Plexus

The brachial plexus is formed by the anterior primary divisions of the C5 through C8 and T1 roots, which anastomose to form three primary trunks: upper trunk (C5 and C6), middle trunk (C7), and lower trunk (C8 and T1) (Fig. 47, p. 53). Specific findings result from the involvement of these structures.

Total brachial plexus paralysis causes a flail arm, paralysis of all muscles of the hand, and absence of sensation. Sudorific function is intact when the lesion is preganglionic.

Upper trunk (C5, C6) paralysis of the Erb-Duchenne type is responsible for paralysis of the biceps, deltoid, brachialis, supraspinatus, infraspinatus, and rhomboid muscles; weakness of the triceps, pectoralis major, and extensor carpi radialis brevis and longus; absent biceps reflex; and sensory deficit of C5 and C6 dermatomes (Fig. 46, at right). Most finger movements are intact.

Lower trunk (C8, T1) paralysis of the Dejerine-Klumpke type involves paralysis of all intrinsic muscles of the hand; weakness of flexor carpi ulnaris and flexor digitorum profundus of the little finger; and Horner syndrome (ptosis, mitosis, and enophthalmos). If the T1 root is avulsed from the spinal cord, a sensory deficit of C8 and T1 dermatomes is present (Fig. 46, at right).

Table 14. Maximum Upper Extremity Impairments Due to Unilateral Sensory or Motor Deficits of Brachial Plexus, or to *Combined* Deficits.

Maximum % upper extremity impairment*			
	Due to sensory deficit or pain†	**Due to motor deficit‡**	**Due to *combined* motor and sensory deficits**
Brachial plexus (C5 through C8, T1)	100	100	100
Upper trunk (C5, C6), Erb-Duchenne	25	75	81
Middle trunk (C7)	5	35	38
Lower trunk (C8, T1) Dejerine-Klumpke	20	70	76

*See Table 3 (p. 20) for converting upper extremity impairments to whole-person impairments.
†See Table 11a (p. 48) to grade impairment from loss of function due to sensory deficit or pain.
‡See Table 12a (p. 49) to grade impairment from loss of function due to motor deficit.

Figure 46. Dermatomes of the Upper Limb.*

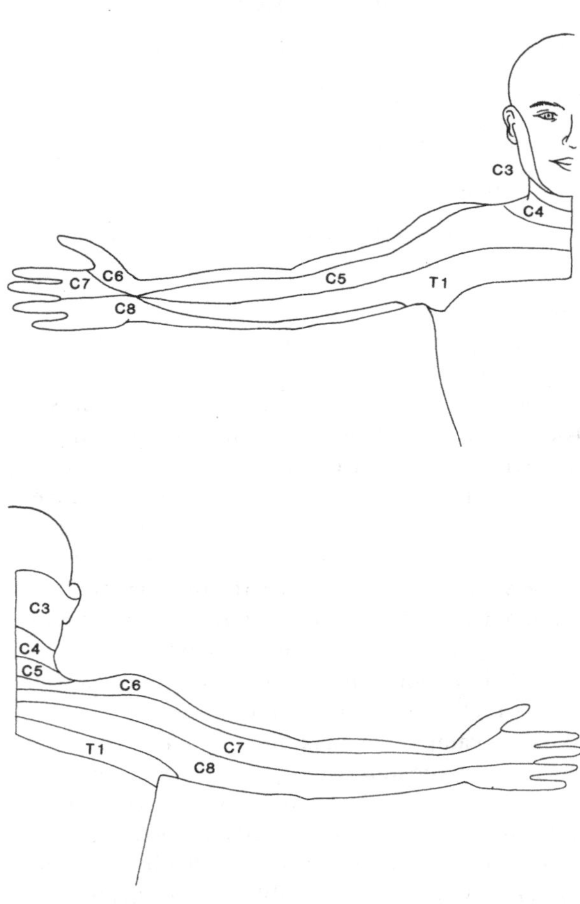

*Source: Netter FH: *The Atlas of Human Anatomy.* Summit, NJ, CIBA-GEIGY Corp., 1989.

Figure 47. The Brachial Plexus.

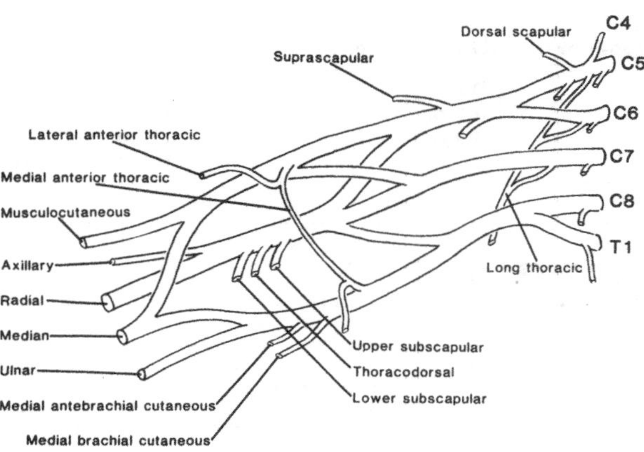

A brachial plexus-related impairment percent is derived as follows:

1. Rate the severity of sensory deficit or pain according to Table 11a (p. 48) and that of motor deficit according to Table 12a (p. 49).

2. Find the percents for maximum impairment of the upper extremity due to sensory and motor deficits of the brachial plexus and its trunks (Table 14, p. 52).

3. Multiply the severity of the sensory (Table 11a, p. 48) and/or motor (Table 12a, p. 49) deficits by the appropriate values from Table 14 to obtain upper extremity impairment percents for each function.

4. *Combine* the sensory and motor impairments to determine the impairment of the upper extremity (Combined Values Chart, p. 322).

5. Convert the upper extremity impairment to a whole-person impairment (Table 3, p. 20).

Example: A 22-year-old man was driving a pickup truck that flipped over during a crash. Days after the crash the man could not move his left arm. After a period of months, he had recovery of hand and forearm function but total paralysis along the C5 and C6 nerve distributions. As a result of grafts from C5 and C6 to truncal divisions, he had partial recovery within 4 years.

In the C5 and C6 distributions, the motor function of individual muscles was graded as follows (Table 12a, p. 49): supraspinatus, 4; infraspinatus, 3; deltoid, 3; biceps-brachialis, 4; brachioradialis, 3; and supinator, 3.

1. Supraspinatus muscle: a motor function grade of 4 was estimated to be a 25% motor deficit (Table 12a, p. 49). The maximum upper extremity impairment for involvement of the suprascapular nerve is 16% (Tables 10 and 15, pp. 47 and 54). The upper extremity impairment was estimated to be 25% x 16% or 4%.

2. Infraspinatus muscle: a motor function grade of 3 was estimated to be a 50% motor deficit (Table 12a). The maximum upper extremity impairment for suprascapular nerve involvement is 16% (Tables 10 and 15). The upper extremity impairment was calculated to be 50% x 16% or 8%.

3. Deltoid muscle: a motor function grade of 3 was estimated to be a 50% motor deficit (Table 12a). The maximum upper extremity impairment for involvement of the axillary nerve is 35% (Tables 10 and 15). The upper extremity impairment was estimated to be 50% x 35% or, rounding off, 18%.

4. Biceps brachialis muscle: a motor function grade of 4 represented a 25% motor deficit (Table 12a, p. 49). The maximum upper extremity impairment for involvement of the musculocutaneous nerve is 25% (Tables 10 and 15, pp. 47 and 54). The upper extremity impairment was estimated to be 25% x 25% or 6%.

5. Brachioradialis muscle: a motor function grade of 3 was estimated to be a 40% motor deficit (Table 12a). The maximum upper extremity impairment for involvement of the radial nerve with sparing of the triceps is 35% (Tables 10 and 15). The upper extremity impairment was estimated to be 40% x 35% or 14%.

6. Supinator muscle: a motor function grade of 3 was estimated to be a 40% motor deficit (Table 12a, p. 49). The maximum upper extremity impairment for involvement of the radial nerve with sparing of the triceps is 35% (Tables 10 and 15, pp. 47 and 54). The upper extremity impairment was 40% x 35% or 14%.

7. The impairments are *combined* using the Combined Values Chart (p. 322): 4% *combined* with 8% is 12%; 12% *combined* with 18% is 28%; 28% *combined* with 6% is 32%; 32% *combined* with 14% is 42%; 42% *combined* with 14% is 50%; the impairment of the upper extremity is 50%.

8. From Table 3 (p. 20), a 50% impairment of the upper extremity is seen to represent a 30% whole-person impairment.

Table 15. Maximum Upper Extremity Impairments Due to Unilateral Sensory or Motor Deficits or Combined Deficits of the Major Peripheral Nerves

Nerve	Maximum % upper extremity impairment*		
	Due to sensory deficit or pain †	Due to motor deficit ‡	Due to *combined* motor and sensory deficits
Pectorals (medial and lateral)	0	5	5
Axillary	5	35	38
Dorsal scapular	0	5	5
Long thoracic	0	15	15
Medial antebrachial cutaneous	5	0	5
Medial brachial cutaneous	5	0	5
Median (above midforearm)	38	44	65
Median (anterior interosseous branch)	0	15	15
Median (below midforearm)	38	10	44
Radial palmar digital of thumb	7	0	7
Ulnar palmar digital of thumb	11	0	11
Radial palmar digital of index finger	5	0	5
Ulnar palmar digital of index finger	4	0	4
Radial palmar digital of middle finger	5	0	5
Ulnar palmar digital of middle finger	4	0	4
Radial palmar digital of ring finger	2	0	2
Musculocutaneous	5	25	29
Radial (upper arm with loss of triceps)	5	42	45
Radial (elbow with sparing of triceps)	5	35	38
Subscapulars (upper and lower)	0	5	5
Suprascapular	5	16	20
Thoracodorsal	0	10	10
Ulnar (above midforearm)	7	46	50
Ulnar (below midforearm)	7	35	40
Ulnar palmar digital of ring finger	2	0	2
Radial palmar digital of little finger	2	0	2
Ulnar palmar digital of little finger	3	0	3

*See Table 3 (p. 20) to convert upper extremity impairments to whole-person impairments.
†See Table 11a (p. 48) to grade impairment from loss of function due to sensory deficit or pain.
‡See Table 12a (p. 49) to grade impairment from loss of function due to motor deficit.

Major Peripheral Nerves

Table 15 (above) lists the major peripheral nerves most frequently associated with impairments of the upper extremity. The percents are for unilateral involvement. When there is bilateral involvement, the impairment on each side is determined separately and converted to a whole-person impairment. Then the whole-person impairments are *combined* using the Combined Values Chart (p. 322).

The sensory and motor innervation of the upper extremity is shown in Figs. 45 and 48 (pp. 50 and 55) and Table 10 (p. 47).

Impairment of major peripheral nerves is derived as shown in steps 1 through 7 (p. 56). An example of a mixed peripheral nerve impairment is that given on p. 51, of the 42-year-old man who fell and landed on his back.

Figure 48. Motor Innervation of the Upper Extremity.

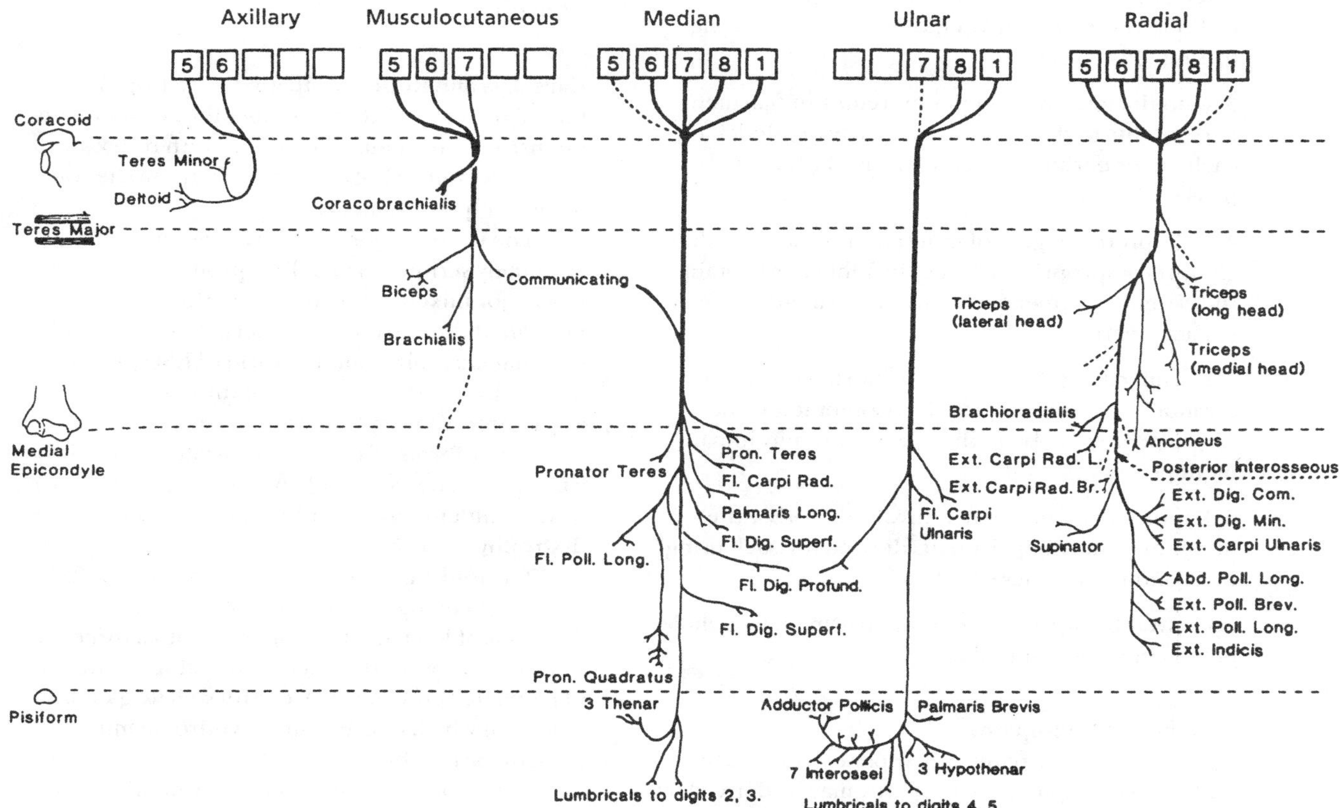

1. Identify the nerve(s) involved and determine the level of the lesion using Table 10 (p. 47) and Figs. 45 and 48 (pp. 50 and 55).

2. Rate the severity of sensory deficit or pain according to Table 11a (p. 48) and of motor deficit according to Table 12a (p. 49).

3. Find the maximum upper extremity impairment percent due to the motor and/or sensory deficit for each major peripheral nerve involved (Table 15, p. 54).

4. Multiply the degree of motor and/or sensory deficit by the appropriate percent in Table 15 to obtain the estimated upper extremity impairment related to each nerve.

5. For mixed nerves, *combine* the impairment estimates for motor and sensory deficits (Combined Values Chart, p. 322) to obtain the upper extremity impairment percent.

6. If more than one nerve is involved, *combine* the upper extremity impairments derived for each using the Combined Values Chart.

7. Convert the upper extremity impairment to a whole-person impairment (Table 3, p. 20).

Entrapment Neuropathy

Impairment of the hand and upper extremity secondary to entrapment neuropathy may be derived by measuring the sensory and motor deficits as described in preceding parts of this section.

An alternative method is provided in Table 16 (p. 57). The evaluator *should not* use both methods. Impairment of the upper extremity secondary to an entrapment neuropathy is estimated according to the severity of involvement of each major nerve at each entrapment site.

Example: A 35-year-old forklift mechanic had a 2-year history of median nerve compression in the right hand with abnormal results of median nerve conduction studies and an abnormal electromyogram. Seven months after surgical decompression of the median nerve in the right carpal tunnel, followed by a change of occupation to salesman, the man's only symptoms were infrequent, transient episodes of numbness in the thumb and index finger after 40 minutes of driving.

Examination showed a full range of movement of all joints and normal two-point discrimination sensory testing. Compared to the left hand, the right hand had a 60% strength loss index (Table 34, p. 65).

The upper extremity impairment due to a mild residual carpal tunnel syndrome is 10% (Table 16, p. 57) or 6% of the whole person (Table 3, p. 20). No additional impairment is allotted for loss of grip strength.

Causalgia and Reflex Sympathetic Dystrophy

Causalgia is a term that describes the constant and intense burning pain usually seen with reflex sympathetic dystrophy (RSD) when the causative lesion involves injury to a nerve.

The term "major causalgia" designates an extremely serious form of RSD produced by an injury to a major mixed nerve, usually in the proximal portion of the extremity. The term "minor causalgia" designates a more common form of RSD produced by an injury to the distal part of the extremity involving a purely sensory branch of a nerve.

Other forms of RSD not associated with injury of a peripheral nerve include minor traumatic dystrophy, shoulder-hand syndrome, and major traumatic dystrophy.

The four cardinal signs and symptoms of RSD are pain, swelling, stiffness, and discoloration. The diagnosis of RSD may be supported with a three-phase nucleotide flow study, cold stress testing, recurrence of pain after previously successful stellate ganglion blocks, in which case Horner's syndrome must be present, or Bier blocks.

The impairment secondary to causalgia and RSD is derived as follows:

1. Rate the upper extremity impairment due to loss of motion of each joint involved (Sections 3.1f through 3.1j).

2. Rate the sensory deficit or pain impairment according to instructions in this section and Table 11a (p. 48).

3. Rate the motor deficit impairment of the injured peripheral nerve, if it applies (Table 12a, p. 49).

4. The appropriate impairment percents for loss of motion, pain or sensory deficits, and motor deficits if present are *combined* using the Combined Values Chart (p. 322) to determine the upper extremity impairment. Major causalgia may result in a complete loss of function and an impairment of the extremity as great as 100%.

Table 16. Upper Extremity Impairment Due to Entrapment Neuropathy

Entrapped nerve	Entrapment site	Degree of severity and % upper extremity impairment: Mild	Moderate	Severe
Suprascapular		5	10	20
Axillary		10	20	38
Radial	Upper arm	15	25	45
Posterior interosseous	Forearm	10	20	35
Median	Elbow	15	35	55
Anterior interosseous	Proximal forearm	5	10	15
Median	Wrist	10	20	40
Ulnar	Elbow	10	30	50
Ulnar	Wrist	10	30	40

3.11 Impairment Due to Vascular Disorders of the Upper Extremity

Table 17 (below) provides a classification of impairments due to peripheral vascular disease. When amputation due to peripheral vascular disease is involved, the impairment due to amputation should be evaluated according to Sections 3.1f through 3.1j and *combined* with the appropriate value in Table 17 using the Combined Values Chart (p. 322).

Table 17. Impairment of Upper Extremity Due to Peripheral Vascular Disease

Symptoms	Upper Extremity impairment %: Class 1 (0%-9%)	Class 2 (10%-39%)	Class 3 (40%-69%)	Class 4 (70%-89%)	Class 5 (90%-100%)
Claudication	None	Intermittent with severe use	Intermittent with moderate use	Intermittent with mild use	
Pain at rest	None	None	None	Intermittent	Severe and constant
Edema	Transient	Persistent and moderate	Marked	Marked	Marked
Elastic support control		Incomplete	Partial	None	None
Signs of vascular damage	Loss of pulses; minimal loss of subcutaneous tissue of fingertips; arterial calcifi-cations on roentgenogram; asymptomatic dilation of veins or arteries not requiring surgery; no decreased activity	Healed painless amputation stump of one digit with persistent vascular disease or healed ulcer	Healed amputation stump of two or more digits with persistent vascular disease or super-ficial ulceration	Amputation of two or more digits of each extremity, or amputation at or above wrist of one extremity, with persistent widespread or deep ulceration of one extremity	Amputation of all digits or amputation at or above the wrist of each extremity, with persistent vascular disease or wide-spread or deep ulcerations of both extremities
Raynaud's phenomenon	At less than 0°C (32°F)	At less than 4°C (39°F)	At less than 10°C (50°F)	At less than 15°C (59°F)	At less than 20°C (68°F)
Medication control	Good	Good	Partial	Partial	Poor

3.1m Impairment Due to Other Disorders of the Upper Extremity

Derangements not previously described can contribute to impairments of the hand and upper extremity, and, if present, these should be considered in the final impairment determination. They include bone and joint disorders, presence of resection or implant arthroplasty, musculotendinous disorders, and loss of strength. The impairments are evaluated separately; appropriate impairment percents from Tables 19 through 30 are multiplied by percents from Table 18 (at right) representing the impaired parts. Appropriate impairment percents are *combined* with other impairment percents using the Combined Values Chart (p. 322). Skin disorders, including disfigurement, scars, and skin grafts, are evaluated with criteria in Chapter 13.

It is emphasized that impairments from the disorders considered in this section are usually estimated by using other criteria. The criteria described in this section should be used only when the other criteria have not adequately encompassed the extent of the impairments.

Table 18 (at right) shows impairment percents for loss of function of the digits, hand, wrist, elbow, and shoulder due to the conditions described in this section and relates the percents to larger units and the whole person. Table 18 differs from Figs. 2 and 3 (p. 18), which show impairment percents for amputation at the different levels.

Bone and Joint Deformities

Joint Crepitation with Motion

Joint crepitation with motion may reflect synovitis or cartilage degeneration. The impairment percent according to Table 19 (p. 59) is multiplied by the relative value of the joint (Table 18, at right).

The evaluator must take care to avoid duplication of impairments when other findings, such as synovial hypertrophy, carpal collapse with arthritic changes, or limited motion, are present. Those findings might indicate a greater severity of the same pathologic process and take precedence over evaluation of joint crepitation, which should not be rated in that instance.

Table 18. Impairment Values for Digits, Hand, Upper Extremity, and the Whole Person for Disorders of Specific Joints.

	% Impairment of			
Units and joints	**Unit**	**Hand**	**Upper extremity**	**Whole person**
Shoulder				
Glenohumeral	—	—	60	36
Acromioclavicular	—	—	25	15
Elbow				
Entire elbow	—	—	70	42
Ulnohumeral	—	—	50	30
Proximal radioulnar	—	—	20	12
Wrist				
Entire wrist	—	—	60	36
Radiocarpal	—	—	40	24
Distal radioulnar	—	—	20	12
Proximal carpal row	—	—	30	18
Entire hand	—	100	90	54
Thumb				
Entire thumb	100	40	36	22
Carpometacarpal	75	30	27	16
Metacarpo-phalangeal	10	4	4	2
Interphalangeal	15	6	5	3
Index and middle				
Entire finger	100	20	18	11
Metacarpo-phalangeal	100	20	18	11
Proximal interphalangeal	80	16	14	8
Distal interphalangeal	45	9	8	5
Ring or little				
Entire finger	100	10	9	5
Metacarpo-phalangeal	100	10	9	5
Proximal interphalangeal	80	8	7	4
Distal interphalangeal	45	4	4	2

Example: Mild joint crepitation of the carpometacarpal joint of the thumb would result in 10% x 75% = 8% impairment of the thumb (Table 18, above, and Table 19, p. 59), 3% impairment of the hand (Table 1, p. 18), 3% impairment of the upper extremity (Table 2, p. 19), and 2% impairment of the whole person (Table 3, p. 20).

Table 19. Impairment from Joint Crepitation.*

Crepitation severity	% Joint impairment†
Mild: inconstant during active range of motion	10
Moderate: constant during active range of motion	20
Severe: constant during passive range of motion	30

*Modified from Swanson, AB, Mays, JD, Yamauchi, Y[33], p. 1011, Fig. 9.
†Multiply by the relative value of the joint (Table 18, p. 58) to determine the joint crepitation impairment percent.

Joint Swelling Due to Synovial Hypertrophy

Impairment due to this condition usually is estimated through loss of motion. *Table 20 is used to estimate impairment only when there is full range of motion of the joint.* The percent of impairment from synovial hypertrophy according to Table 20 is multiplied by the relative value of the joint (Table 18, p. 58).

Table 20. Impairment from Synovial Hypertrophy.*

Description of joint swelling	% joint impairment†
Mild: visibly apparent	10
Moderate: palpably apparent	20
Severe: greater than 10% increase in size	30

*Modified from Swanson, AB, Mays, JD, Yamauchi, Y[33], p. 1011, Fig. 9.
†Multiply by the relative value for the joint (Table 18, p. 58) to determine the joint impairment.

Digit Lateral Deviation

The deviation from longitudinal alignment of each of the finger joints is measured in degrees during maximum active extension. Since lateral deviation at any level affects the longitudinal arch of the digit, deviation affects the entire digit. If lateral deviation is the *only impairment,* the degree of deviation (Table 21, at right) is multiplied by the relative value of the digit to the hand (Table 18, p. 58) to determine the hand impairment. If the digit has *other impairments, the lateral deviation impairment percent is* combined *with them* (Combined Values Chart, p. 322).

Example: A patient has 35° ulnar deviation at the proximal interphalangeal joint of the little finger after a ligamentous injury. Range of motion at that joint is –20° extension through 30° flexion.

1. Ulnar deviation impairment of the little finger is "severe," 30% (Table 21, at right).

Table 21. Impairment from Digit Ulnar or Radial Deviation.*

Deviation	% Digit impairment†
Mild: less than 10°	10
Moderate: 10° through 30°	20
Severe: Greater than 30°	30

*Modified from Swanson, AB, Mays, JD, Yamauchi, Y[33], p. 1011, Fig. 9.
†Multiply by the relative value of the digit (Table 18, p. 58) to determine the digit impairment.

2. Motion impairment of the little finger PIP joint:

$I_E\% = 7\%$; $I_F\% = 42\%$ (Fig. 21, p. 33);
$7\% + 42\% = 49\%$ motion impairment.

3. From the Combined Values Chart (p. 322), 30% *combined* with 49% is 64% impairment of the little finger, which is considered to be a 6% impairment of the hand and a 5% impairment of the upper extremity (Tables 1 and 2, pp. 18 and 19).

Digit Rotational Deformity

Rotational deformity of the distal, middle, or proximal phalanx is measured during maximum active flexion of the finger and expresses a malrotation of the normal axial alignment of the phalanx. Rotational deformity at any level affects the function of the entire digit, and the impairment percent is applied to the entire digit.

The impairment percent due to rotational deformity (Table 22, below) is multiplied by the relative value of the digit (Table 18, p. 58) to obtain the digit impairment. *If other impairments of the same digit are present, the rotational deformity impairment percent is* combined *with the other impairment percents using the Combined Values Chart* (p. 322).

Table 22. Impairment from Digit Rotational Deformity.*

Digit rotational deformity	% Digit impairment†
Mild: less than 15°	20
Moderate: 15° through 30°	40
Severe: greater than 30°	60

*Adapted from Swanson, AB[33], p. 1011, Fig. 9.
†Multiply the percent of impairment by the relative value of the digit (Table 18, p. 58) to determine the digit rotation deformity impairment percent.

Example: A 20° pronation deformity of the index finger is present following a healed fracture of the second metacarpal. This is a "moderate" deformity (Table 22, p. 59).

1. Rotational impairment of the index finger is 40%.

2. Relative value of the entire index finger to the hand is 20% (Table 18, p. 58).

3. Hand impairment is 40% x 20% = 8%; this is equivalent to 7% impairment of the upper extremity (Table 2, p. 19).

Persistent Joint Subluxation or Dislocation

When persistent joint subluxation or dislocation results in restricted motion, impairment percents are given only for lack of motion (Sections 3.1f through 3.1j). If there is *no* restricted motion, the values shown in Table 23 are multiplied by the relative value of the joint (Table 18, p. 58), to determine the joint impairment.

Table 23. Impairment from Persistent Joint Subluxation or Dislocation.*

Severity of joint subluxation or dislocation	% Joint impairment †
Mild: can be completely reduced manually	20
Moderate: cannot be completely reduced manually	40
Severe: cannot be reduced	60

*Modified from Swanson, AB, Mays, JD, Yamauchi, Y[33], p. 1011, Fig. 9.
†Multiply by the relative value of the joint (Table 18, p. 58) to determine the joint impairment.

Joint Instability

Excessive passive mediolateral motion is evaluated by comparing it with normal joint stability and is graded according to its degree of severity (Table 24, at right). Then the percentage of impairment is multiplied by the relative value of the joint (Table 18, p. 58) to obtain the joint impairment. *If other impairments of the same joint are present, they are* combined *using the Combined Values Chart (p. 322).*

Example: A patient has 15° passive radial deviation of the thumb IP joint due to collateral ligament injury, and surgery should be avoided.

1. 15° radial instability is a 40% joint impairment (Table 24).

2. Relative value of the IP joint to thumb motion is 15% (Table 18, p. 58).

Table 24. Impairment from Joint Mediolateral Instability.*

Amount of excessive passive mediolateral joint motion	% Joint impairment †
Mild: less than 10°	20
Moderate: 10° through 20°	40
Severe: greater than 20°	60

*Modified from Swanson, AB, Mays, JD, Yamauchi, Y[33], p. 1011, Fig. 9.
†Multiply by the relative value of the joint (Table 18, p. 58) to determine the joint impairment.

3. Thumb impairment is 40% x 15% or 6%; since the thumb value relative to the hand is 40%, this represents a 6% x 40%, or, rounding off, a 2% hand impairment and a 2% x 90% or, rounding to the nearest whole number, a 2% upper extremity impairment (Tables 1 and 2, pp. 18 and 19).

Wrist and Elbow Joint Radial and Ulnar Deviations

These angles are measured with the wrist or elbow in maximum active extension. The degree of severity of lateral deviation (Table 25, below) is multiplied by the relative value of the joint to the upper extremity (Table 18, p. 58) to obtain the upper extremity impairment. *If other impairments of the same joint are present, all the impairment percents are* combined *using the Combined Values Chart (p. 322).*

Table 25. Impairment from Wrist and Elbow Joint Radial and Ulnar Deviations.*

Deviation and severity	% Joint impairment †
Mild: less than 20°	10
Moderate: 20° through 30°	20
Severe: greater than 30°	30

*Modified from Swanson, AB, Mays, JD, Yamauchi, Y[33], p. 1011, Fig. 9.
†Multiply by the relative value of the joint (Table 18, p. 58) to determine the upper extremity impairment.

Example: An elbow injury with medial collateral ligament damage and radial head fracture is treated with simple radial head resection. One year later, the patient has a 25° lateral deviation of the elbow.

1. 25° lateral deviation of the elbow is a "moderate" or 20% impairment of the elbow (Table 25). The elbow joint's relative value is 70% of upper extremity (Table 18, p. 58). Impairment of the upper extremity is 20% x 70% or 14%.

2. Radial head resection is an 8% impairment of upper extremity (Table 27, at right).

3. Total elbow impairment is 14% *combined* with 8%, or 21% impairment of the upper extremity (Combined Values Chart, p. 322)

Carpal Instability

Carpal instability patterns resulting from lunate or scaphoid abnormalities are classified as mild, moderate, or severe, based on the severity of the roentgenographic findings (Table 26, below). The proximal carpal row represents half of the value of the wrist, or 30% of the upper extremity (Table 18, p. 58). Therefore, the grades of mild (20%), moderate (40%), and severe (60%) impairment represent upper extremity impairments of 6%, 12%, and 18%, respectively. These values may be *combined* with other upper extremity impairments due to wrist abnormalities using the Combined Values Chart (p. 322).

Only one category of severity of carpal instability impairment should be selected. The selection should be based on the greatest severity of the roentgenographic findings. The severity category percents for the various roentgenographic findings listed in Table 26 should not be added or combined.

To avoid duplicate impairment ratings, these roentgenographic criteria are used only when all other wrist factors are normal, except in instances after carpal bone resection or implant arthroplasty. In the latter situations, a carpal instability impairment (Table 26, below) is *combined* with an arthroplasty impairment (Table 27, at right) using the Combined Values Chart (p. 322).

Certain patients may have wrist pain and loss of strength related to a dynamic or nondissociative carpal instability that cannot be measured by changes of angles on roentgenograms. The examiner should assess the severity of this type of instability and estimate the resulting upper extremity impairment as mild (6%), moderate (12%), or severe (18%). Pain and loss of strength are *not* rated separately.

Table 26. Upper Extremity Impairment Due to Carpal Instability Patterns.

	Upper extremity impairment (%)		
Roentgenographic findings	**Mild (6%)**	**Moderate (12%)**	**Severe (18%)**
Radioscaphoid angle	45°-59°	60°-70°	>70°
Radiolunate angle	<10°	10°-30°	>30°
Carpal height collapse	<5%	5%-10%	>10%
Carpal translation	Mild	Moderate	Severe
Arthritic changes	Mild	Moderate	Severe

Example: A patient has roentgenographic evidence of a radioscaphoid angle of 60°, a radiolunate angle of 5°, and moderate arthritic changes. The greatest impairment is "moderate" (12%) for either the radioscaphoid angle or the arthritic changes. Therefore, the upper extremity impairment for carpal instability is 12%.

Arthroplasty

Arthroplasty of a joint may be carried out with or without an implant. Simple resection arthroplasty is given 40% impairment of the joint value; implant arthroplasty is given 50% impairment of the joint value. Table 27 provides impairment ratings for the upper extremity for arthroplasty of specific joints, based on these values.

Table 27. Impairment of the Upper Extremity After Arthroplasty of Specific Bones or Joints.

	% Impairment of upper extremity	
Level of arthroplasty*	**Resection arthroplasty (40%)**	**Implant arthroplasty (50%)**
Total shoulder	24	30
Distal clavicle (isolated)	10	—
Total elbow	28	35
Radial head (isolated)	8	10
Total wrist	24	30
Ulnar head (isolated)	8	10
Proximal carpal row	12	15
Carpal bones	12	15
Thumb†		
Carpometarcarpal	11	13
Metacarpophalangeal	1	2
Interphalangeal	2	3
Index or middle finger‡		
Metacarpophalangeal	7	9
Proximal interphalangeal	6	7
Distal interphalangeal	3	4
Ring or little fingers‡		
Metacarpophalangeal	3	4
Proximal interphalangeal	3	3
Distal interphalangeal	2	2

*If more than one level is involved, *combine* the levels from distal to proximal.

†If more than one thumb joint is involved, *add* the impairments.

‡If more than one joint is involved in the same finger, *combine* impairments. If multiple digits are involved, *add* the digit impairments.

In the presence of decreased motion, motion impairments are derived separately (Sections 3.1f through 3.1j) and *combined* with arthroplasty impairments using the Combined Values Chart (p. 322).

After arthrodesis procedures, impairment is rated only according to the guidelines for ankylosis impairment (I_A%) presented in Sections 3.1f through 3.1j, and is related to the measured joint angle (V).

Impairments involving the resection of malignant tumors with reconstructive surgery including arthroplasty should receive special consideration.

Example: A patient with rheumatoid arthritis presents the following findings: implant resection arthroplasty of the metacarpophalangeal (MP) joint of the index finger with a range of motion of –10° extension to 70° flexion; fusion of the index proximal interphalangeal (PIP) joint at 40° flexion; implant resection arthroplasty of the PIP joint of the middle finger with a range of motion of –10° extension to 60° flexion; fusion of the thumb MP joint in 20° flexion; and simple resection arthroplasty of the thumb carpometacarpal (CMC) joint with adduction to 1 cm, radial abduction to 40°, and opposition to 7 cm.

1. Index Finger: MP joint implant arthroplasty = 50% impairment of the MP joint. The MP joint value relative to the finger is 100% (Table 18, p. 58); 50% x 100% = 50% impairment of the finger.

MP joint –10° extension: I_E% = 7% impairment of the finger (Fig. 23, p. 34);
MP joint 70° flexion: I_F% = 11% impairment of the finger;
7% + 11% = 18% impairment of the index finger due to loss of MP joint motion.

The index finger impairment due to MP joint involvement is found by *combining* the impairment percent due to implant arthroplasty (50%) with that due to loss of motion (18%) using the Combined Values Chart (p. 322): 50% *combined* with 18% = 59% finger impairment due to MP joint involvement.

PIP joint fusion at 40° flexion: I_A% = 50% impairment of the finger (Fig. 21, p. 33).

The total index finger impairment is found by *combining* the impairment at the MP joint (59%) with the impairment at the PIP joint (50%); these *combine* to an 80% impairment of the index finger.

The index finger represents 20% of the hand (Table 18, p. 58); 80% x 20% = 16% impairment of the hand (Table 1, p. 18).

2. Middle Finger: PIP joint implant arthroplasty = 50% impairment of the finger PIP joint. The PIP joint's relative value to the finger is 80% (Table 18); 50% x 80% = 40% impairment of the finger.

PIP joint –10° extension: I_E% = 3% impairment of the finger;
PIP joint 60° flexion: I_F% = 24% impairment of the finger (Fig. 21, p. 33).
3% + 24% = 27% impairment of the middle finger due to loss of motion at the PIP joint.

The middle finger impairment is found by *combining* the impairment due to implant arthroplasty (40%) with the impairment due to loss of motion (27%) using the Combined Values Chart (p. 322); 40% *combined* with 27% is 56% impairment of the finger due to PIP joint involvement.

The middle finger represents 20% of the hand (Table 18, p. 58); 56% x 20% = 11% impairment of the hand related to the middle finger (Table 1, p. 18).

3. Thumb: CMC joint resection arthroplasty = 40% impairment of the CMC joint. The CMC joint's relative value to the thumb is 75% (Table 18, p. 58); 40% x 75% = 30% thumb impairment.

CMC joint range of motion impairment: adduction at 1 cm = 0% thumb impairment (Table 5, p. 28); radial abduction to 40° = 1% thumb impairment (Table 6, p. 28); opposition to 7 cm = 1% thumb impairment (Table 7, p. 29)

Fusion of the thumb MP joint at 20° flexion: I_A% = 5% thumb impairment (Fig. 13, p. 27).

Thumb motion impairments are *added* together: 0% + 1% + 1% + 5% = 7% thumb impairment due to loss of motion.

The thumb impairment due to resection arthroplasty of the CMC joint (30%) is *combined* with the thumb impairment due to loss of motion (7%) using the Combined Values Chart (p. 322); 30% *combined* with 7% is a 35% thumb impairment.

The thumb represents 40% of the hand (Table 18, p. 58); 35% x 40% = 14% hand impairment related to the thumb.

4. Total Hand and Upper Extremity Impairment: The total hand impairment is calculated by *adding* the hand impairments derived for each digit: 16% (index) + 11% (middle) + 14% (thumb) = 41% impairment of the hand.

The hand represents 90% of the upper extremity (Table 18); 41% x 90% = 37% upper extremity impairment related to the finger and thumb impairments.

Example: A patient with a total wrist replacement has flexion to 30° and extension to 20°:

1. Wrist implant arthroplasty = 30% impairment of upper extremity (Table 27, p. 61).

2. $I_F\%$ = 5% impairment of upper extremity;
$I_E\%$ = 7% impairment of upper extremity;
5% + 7% = 12% impairment of upper extremity due to loss of motion at the wrist (Fig. 26, p. 36).

3. 30% *combined* with 12% = 38% impairment of the upper extremity (Combined Values Chart, p. 322).

Musculotendinous Impairments

Intrinsic Tightness

Intrinsic tightness in the hand may be demonstrated by a test described by Bunnell. Hyperextension of the metacarpophalangeal (MP) joint in a normal hand still allows passive flexion of the proximal interphalangeal (PIP) joint. If the intrinsic muscles are tight or contracted, the available stretch of these muscles is taken up by the hyperextended position of the MP joint, and passive flexion of the PIP joint will be difficult.

If the active range of motion at the MP or PIP joint is already restricted, no additional impairment rating is given for intrinsic tightness.

The intrinsic tightness impairment (Table 28, below) is multiplied by the relative value of the digit (Table 18, p. 58) to derive the digit impairment percent, which should be *combined* with other impairments of the same digit using the Combined Values Chart (p. 322). The resulting finger impairment is converted to hand impairment using Table 1 (p. 18).

Table 28. Impairment from Intrinsic Tightness.‡

Intrinsic tightness severity (Passive flexion of PIP joint with MP joint hyperextended)	% Digit Impairment*
Mild: PIP flexion 80° to 60°	20
Moderate: PIP flexion 59° to 20°	40
Severe: PIP flexion ≤20°	60

*Multiply by the relative value of the digit (Table 18, p. 58) to determine the digit impairment.

‡Modified from Swanson, AB, Mays, JD, Yamauchi, Y[33], p. 1011, Fig. 9.

Constrictive Tenosynovitis

The impairment percent due to constrictive tenosynovitis (Table 29, at right) is multiplied by the relative value of the digit (Table 18, p. 58) to obtain the digit impairment. This value may be *combined* with other impairments of the digit using the Combined Values Chart (p. 322). The digit impairment is converted to hand impairment with Table 1 (p. 18). *If there already is restriction in the digit's active range of motion, no additional impairment percent is allowed for constrictive tenosynovitis.*

Table 29. Impairment Due to Constrictive Tenosynovitis.*

Constrictive tenosynovitis severity	% Digit impairment †
Mild: inconstant triggering during active range of motion	20
Moderate: constant triggering during active range of motion	40
Severe: constant triggering during passive range of motion	60

*Modified from Swanson, AB, Mays, JD, Yamauchi, Y[33], p. 1011, Fig. 9.

†Multiply by the relative value of the digit (Table 18, p. 58) to determine the digit impairment.

Extensor Tendon Subluxation at the MP Joint

The impairment estimate for extensor tendon subluxation at the metacarpophalangeal (MP) joint (Table 30) is multiplied by the relative value of the digit (Table 18, p. 58) to obtain the digit impairment. That percent may be *combined* with other impairments of the same digit using the Combined Values Chart (p. 322). The finger impairment is converted to hand impairment with Table 1 (p. 18).

If persistent extensor tendon subluxation results in a restricted range of motion, an impairment percent should be given only for the lack of motion (Sections 3.1f and 3.1g).

Table 30. Impairment Due to Extensor Tendon Subluxation.*

Extensor tendon subluxation severity	% Digit impairment †
Mild: ulnar tendon subluxation on MP joint flexion only	10
Moderate: reducible tendon subluxation in the intermetacarpal groove	20
Severe: nonreducible tendon subluxation in the intermetacarpal groove	30

*Modified from Swanson, AB, Mays, JD, Yamauchi, Y[33], p. 1011, Fig. 9.

†Multiply by the relative value of the digit (Table 18, p. 58) to determine the digit impairment.

Other Musculoskeletal System Defects

In a rare case, the severity of the clinical findings may not correspond to the extent of a musculoskeletal defect, as demonstrated with a variety of imaging techniques. This might occur in a patient in whom the loss of shoulder motion does not reflect the severity of an irreparable rotator cuff tear as demonstrated by MRI or visualization during surgery.

If the examiner determines that the estimate for the anatomic impairment does not sufficiently reflect the severity of the patient's condition, the examiner may increase the impairment percent, explaining the reason for the increase in writing.

Strength Evaluation

Because strength measurements are functional tests influenced by subjective factors that are difficult to control, and the *Guides* for the most part is based on *anatomic* impairment, the *Guides* does not assign a large role to such measurements. Those who have contributed to the *Guides* believe further research is needed before loss of grip and pinch strength is given a larger role in impairment evaluation.

In a rare case, if the examiner believes the patient's loss of strength represents an impairing factor that has not been considered adequately, the loss of strength may be rated separately. The loss of strength impairment would be *combined* (Combined Values Chart, p. 322) with other upper extremity impairments.

Impairments due to motor deficits secondary to disorders of the peripheral nerve system and various degenerative neuromuscular conditions are evaluated according to guidelines described in Section 3.1k of this chapter and the *Guides* chapter on the nervous system (p. 139). It should be understood that weakness or loss of strength can occur without muscle atrophy.

Grip and Pinch Strength

When evaluating strength, the examiner must have good reason to believe the patient has reached maximal improvement and that the condition is a "permanent" one as defined in Chapter 1 and the Glossary. This determination is best made with measurements taken over a period of time. Many factors, including fatigue, handedness, time of day, age, nutritional state, pain, and the patient's cooperation, influence strength measurements.

Tests repeated at intervals during an examination are considered to be reliable if there is less than 20% variation in the readings. If there is more than 20% variation, one may assume the patient is not exerting full effort. The test is usually repeated three times with each hand at different times during the examination, and the values are recorded and later compared.

Grip strength measurements are taken with a Jamar dynamometer. The second (4 cm) or third (6 cm) position, according to the size of the hand, usually allows the patient to apply maximal force comfortably. In weaker hands, strength can be recorded with a sphygmomanometer rolled to 5 cm in diameter and inflated to 50 mm Hg; as the cuff is squeezed, the increase in millimeters of mercury from 50 mm Hg represents the power of grip.

Two techniques have been reported to help detect individuals who exert less than maximal effort on grip strength testing. Stokes pointed out that the plotting of grip strength measurements from each of the five handle settings of the Jamar dynamometer would produce a bell-shaped curve. Those individuals not exerting maximal effort will produce results yielding a straight line or a flat curve.

An alternate method is the rapid exchange grip technique. The grip strength first is determined by standard techniques. The patient then is instructed to grip the dynamometer with *maximal* effort, first with one hand, then quickly with the other hand for at least five exchanges. Individuals who did not exert maximal effort with the standard technique will record significantly higher strength readings; if they become aware of this, the strength of both hands will drop dramatically.

Pinch strength measurements are done with a pinch gauge and may include chuck or three-digit pinch, key or lateral pinch, and tip pinch with separate digits. Key pinch measurements usually are sufficient. Measurements are repeated three times.

The three readings each for grip and pinch strength are averaged and compared to those of the opposite extremity, which usually is normal. If both extremities are involved, the strength measurements are compared to the average normal strengths listed in Tables 31 through 33 (pp. 64 and 65), which are from studies in 1970 by Swanson, Matev, and de Groot.[32]

Table 31. Average Strength of Unsupported Grip by Occupation in 100 Subjects*

	Grip Strength (kg)			
	Males		Females	
Occupation	Major hand	Minor hand	Major hand	Minor hand
Skilled	47.0	45.4	26.8	24.4
Sedentary	47.2	44.1	23.1	21.1
Manual	48.5	44.6	24.2	22.0
Average	47.6	45.0	24.6	22.4

*Adapted with permission from Swanson, AB, Matev IB, de Groot Swanson, G[32], p. 147, Table 1.

Table 32. Average Strength of Grip by Age in 100 Subjects.*

	Grip strength (kg)			
	Males		Females	
Age group	Major hand	Minor hand	Major hand	Minor hand
<20	45.2	42.6	23.8	22.8
20-29	48.5	46.2	24.6	22.7
30-39	49.2	44.5	30.8	28.0
40-49	49.0	47.3	23.4	21.5
50-59	45.9	43.5	22.3	18.2

*Adapted with permission from Swanson, AB, Matev, IB, de Groot Swanson, G[32], p. 147, Table 2.

Table 33. Average Strength of Lateral Pinch by Occupation in 100 Subjects.*

	Lateral pinch (kg)			
	Males		Females	
Occupation	Major hand	Minor hand	Major hand	Minor hand
Skilled	6.6	6.4	4.4	4.3
Sedentary	6.3	6.1	4.1	3.9
Manual	8.5	7.7	6.0	5.5
Average	7.5	7.1	4.9	4.7

*Adapted with permission from Swanson, AB, Matev, IB, de Groot Swanson, G[32], p. 151, Table 5.

If there is suspicion or evidence that the subject is exerting less than maximal effort, the grip strength measurements are invalid for estimating impairment. If both grip and pinch strength are decreased, the function with the greater loss or Strength Loss Index determines the extent of the upper extremity impairment. Both measures are *not* used.

It is acknowledged that wide variations exist in strength, even among persons doing the same kind of work. Little evidence exists that there is a significant difference in grip strength between the dominant and nondominant hand. The *Guides* does not recognize such a difference.

An index of loss of strength uses the following formula:

$$\frac{\text{Normal Strength} - \text{Abnormal Strength}}{\text{Normal Strength}} = \text{\% Strength Loss Index}$$

Impairments of the upper extremity due to loss of strength are based on the Strength Loss Index ranges shown in Table 34 (at right).

Table 34. Upper Extremity Impairment for Loss of Strength.

% Strength Loss Index	% Upper extremity impairment
10 - 30	10
31 - 60	20
61 - 100	30

Example: Grip strength of a patient's involved right hand is 20 kg and that of his left hand, which is normal, is 45 kg.

$$\frac{45\text{ kg} - 20\text{ kg}}{45\text{ kg}} = \frac{25}{45} = 56\% \text{ Strength Loss Index}$$

A 56% Strength Loss Index is considered to be a 20% impairment of the upper extremity (Table 34).

3.1n Combining Regional Impairments to Obtain Impairment of the Whole Person

1. Determine the impairments of each region (hand, wrist, elbow, and shoulder joints) as described in preceding sections.

2. Use the Combined Values Chart (p. 322) to *combine* impairments of the upper extremity contributed by each region.

Note: Digit and hand impairments must be converted to impairments of the upper extremity before regional impairments can be combined.

3. Use Table 3 (p. 20) to convert impairment of the upper extremity to impairment of the whole person.

Example: A patient sustained multiple injuries of the upper extremity and had the following regional impairments: 50% of the thumb, 10% of the index finger, 5% of the upper extremity due to the wrist, and 2% of the upper extremity due to the elbow.

According to Table 1 (p. 18), a 50% thumb impairment and a 10% index finger impairment convert to a 20% and a 2% impairment of the hand, respectively. These are *added* to obtain a 22% impairment of the hand.

According to Table 2 (p. 19), a 22% impairment of the hand is equivalent to a 20% impairment of the upper extremity. From the Combined Values Chart (p. 322), 20% *combined* with 5% is 24%; 24% *combined* with 2% is 26% impairment of the upper extremity, which according to Table 3 (p. 20) is a 16% whole-person impairment.

3.1o Summary of Steps for Evaluating Impairments of the Upper Extremity

I. Hand Region
Use Upper Extremity Evaluation Record Part 1 (p. 16).
A. Determine and record *amputation* impairments for each digit (thumb, p. 24; fingers, p. 30).

B. Determine and record *sensory* impairments for each digit (thumb, p. 24; fingers, p. 30).

C. Measure and record *motion* impairment for each digital joint (thumb IP, p. 25; MP, p. 26; CMC, pp. 28 and 29: finger DIP, p. 31; PIP, p. 33; MP, p. 34). The motion impairments are rounded to the nearest 10°.

The thumb motion impairments at the IP, MP, and basal joints are *added*. The motion impairments at the DIP, PIP, and MP joints of the fingers are *combined* (Combined Values Chart, p. 322).

D. Record digit impairments due to *other disorders* for each joint or digit (Section 3.1m, p. 58).

E. Individual digit impairment: *combine* impairments due to amputation, sensory loss, loss of motion, and other disorders (Combined Values Chart, p. 322).

F. *Convert* digit impairments to hand impairments (Table 1, p. 18).

G. Total hand impairment: *add* the hand impairment values related to the involved digits.

H. Convert hand impairment to upper extremity impairment (Table 2, p. 19).

I. If applicable, determine the upper extremity impairment percent due to loss of strength and *combine* this with other upper extremity impairments evaluated according to Section 3.1m, p. 64.

J. If other upper extremity impairments exist, such as those listed in steps II through VIII below, enter the upper extremity impairment due to involvement of the hand on line II of Part 2 (p. 17) of the Record.

K. If no other upper extremity impairment exists, convert the upper extremity impairment related to the hand region to whole-person impairment (Table 3, p. 20).

For steps II through XI, use the Upper Extremity Evaluation Record Part 2 (p. 17).

II. Wrist Region
Determine upper extremity impairments due to *loss of motion* (Section 3.1h, p. 35) and *other disorders* (Section 3.1m, p. 58) and *combine* the values to determine the upper extremity impairment related to the wrist region.

III. Elbow Region
Determine upper extremity impairments due to *loss of motion* (Section 3.1i, p. 38) and *other disorders* (Section 3.1m, p. 58) and *combine* the values to determine the upper extremity impairment related to the elbow region.

IV. Shoulder Region
Determine upper extremity impairments due to *loss of motion* (Section 3.1j, p. 41) and *other disorders* (Section 3.1m, p. 58) and *combine* the values to determine the upper extremity impairment involving the shoulder region.

V.
Determine the upper extremity impairment due to *amputation through arm or forearm* (pp. 35, 38, and 41).

VI.
Determine the upper extremity impairment due to *peripheral nerve disorders* (Section 3.1k, p. 46), *entrapment neuropathy* (p. 56), *causalgia, and RSD* (p. 56).

VII.
Determine the upper extremity impairment due to *peripheral vascular disorders* (Section 3.1l, p. 57).

VIII.
Determine the upper extremity impairments due to *other disorders not included in regional impairment* (Section 3.1m, p. 58).

IX.
Combine the upper extremity impairments due to *amputation* (other than hand), *regional disorders* (hand, wrist, elbow, shoulder), *peripheral vascular disorders, peripheral nerve disorders,* and *other disorders not included in regional impairment* (Combined Values Chart, p. 322).

X.
Convert the upper extremity impairment to a whole-person impairment (Table 3, p. 20).

XI.
When *both upper extremities* are involved, derive the whole-person impairment percent for each and then *combine* both values using the Combined Values Chart (p. 322).

Example 1: Fingertip Amputation and Neuroma
While cutting meat with a band saw, a butcher cut off the tip of his left index finger through the middle of the nail. Twelve months later he had good skin coverage, but a painful neuroma on the radial side of the stump kept him from using the finger. He refused surgery because there was no guarantee the sensitivity would be restored. His complaints included loss of the fingertip, painful neuroma, stiffness of the finger, and weakness of grip.

1. *Amputation* of the index finger through the midportion of the distal phalanx: 20% impairment of the finger (Fig. 17, p. 30).

2. *Motion impairment* of the index finger:

	Extension	Flexion	$I_E\% + I_F\%$	= Finger impairment %
DIP	−10°	20°	2% + 26%	= 28% (Fig. 19, p. 32)
PIP	0°	60°	0% + 24%	= 24% (Fig. 21, p. 33)
MP	+20°	70°	0% + 11%	= 11% (Fig. 23, p. 34)

The finger impairment due to loss of motion is obtained by *combining* the impairment of the three joints using the Combined Values Chart (p. 322). This equals 51% finger impairment.

3. The *total finger impairment* is found by *combining* the amputation impairment with the loss of motion impairment using the Combined Values Chart. This equals 61% finger impairment and converts to 12% hand impairment (Table 1, p. 18) and 11% upper extremity impairment (Table 2, p. 19).

4. *Painful neuroma* on the radial digital nerve of index finger: maximum loss of function due to pain is 5% (Table 15, p. 54). Gradation of pain is 61% to 80% (Table 11a, p. 48). Impairment of the upper extremity secondary to painful neuroma is 80% x 5% = 4%.

5. *Total impairment of the upper extremity* is derived by *combining* the upper extremity impairment of the digit (11%) with the upper extremity impairment secondary to the neuroma (4%) using the Combined Values Chart (p. 322). This equals a 15% upper extremity impairment or a 9% whole-person impairment (Table 3, p. 20). The 9% whole-person impairment adequately considers the patient's grip weakness.

Example 2 : Crushed Hand

A 36-year-old, right-handed construction worker sustained a closed crushing injury to his left hand, 1½ years before evaluation. The fractures healed with neither rotational nor angular deformity. Reconstructive surgery was completed 6 months before evaluation. The patient's impairment was considered permanent.

Factors relating to impairment included amputation through the PIP joint of the ring finger; sensory loss in the ring and little fingers; normal left wrist and proximal upper extremity; and reduced grip and pinch strength. Because of the extensive soft-tissue injury and subsequent fibrosis commonly seen in crushing injuries, it was believed that both the latter factors should be considered in assessing impairment. The right upper extremity was normal in all respects.

The impairment evaluation was calculated using the Upper Extremity Impairment Evaluation Record (Fig. 49, pp. 68 and 69).

Example 3 : Flexor Tendon and Digital Nerve Laceration

A 35-year-old machine operator sustained a deep laceration of the right middle finger, volar aspect, at the level of the PIP joint without joint involvement. This resulted in a complete laceration of the flexor digitorum profundus (FDP) and flexor digitorum superficialis (FDS) tendons and of the radial digital nerve. A primary flexor tenorrhaphy of the FDP and FDS tendons and a microneurorrhaphy of the radial digital nerve were done, and these were followed by a 3-month hand rehabilitation program.

One year after injury, the patient was examined for impairment. His complaints included numbness of the radial side of the middle finger; pain on flexion; and weakness of the right hand. Based on the anatomic examination, the impairment evaluation was as follows:

1. *Sensory impairment* of the middle finger: 9 mm of two-point discrimination on the radial side of the distal and middle phalanges of the middle finger corresponds to a partial sensory loss of 80% (PIP level) of the digit length. This is rated as a 12% impairment of the finger (Table 9, p. 31).

2. *Motion impairment* of the middle finger:

	Extension	Flexion	$I_E\% + I_F\%$	= Finger impairment %
DIP	0°	50°	0% + 10%	= 10% (Fig. 19, p. 32)
PIP	−20°	60°	7% + 24%	= 31% (Fig. 21, p. 33)
MP	+20°	90°	0% + 0 %	= 0% (Fig. 23, p. 34)

The finger impairment due to loss of motion is found by *combining* the impairment of the DIP and PIP joints (Combined Values Chart, p. 322), which gives a 38% finger impairment.

3. The *total finger impairment* is found by *combining* the sensory impairment (12%) with the motion impairment (38%) using the Combined Values Chart. This equals 45% finger impairment and converts to 9% hand impairment (Table 1, p. 18), 8% upper extremity impairment (Table 2, p. 19), and 5% impairment of the whole person (Table 3, p. 20).

Additional estimates are not given for pain and loss of strength.

Figure 49A. Upper Extremity Impairment Evaluation Record–**Part 1 (Hand)**** Side ☐ R ☒ L

Name A.B. EXAMPLE 2 Age 36 Sex ☒ M ☐ F Dominant hand ☒ R ☐ L Date ______

Occupation CONSTRUCTION WORKER Diagnosis CRUSH INJURY

Abnormal motion — Record motion, ankylosis, and impairment %

Digit	Joint		Flexion	Extension	Ankylosis	IMP%
Thumb	IP	Angle°	30	−10		6
		IMP%	4	2		
	MP	Angle°	30	−15		4
		IMP%	3	1		
			Motion		Ankylosis	IMP%
	CMC Radial abduction	Angle°	30			3
		IMP%	3			
	CMC Adduction	CMS	4			4
		IMP%	4			
	CMC Opposition	CMS	4			9
		IMP%	9			
	Add impairment % CMC + MP + IP = 26					[1]
			Flexion	Extension	Ankylosis	IMP%
Index	DIP	Angle°	30	−10		23
		IMP%	21	2		
	PIP	Angle°	70	−10		21
		IMP%	18	3		
	MP	Angle°	50	−10		29
		IMP%	22	7		
	• Combine impairment % MP + PIP + DIP = 56					[1]
Middle	DIP	Angle°	30	−10		23
		IMP%	21	2		
	PIP	Angle°	70	−10		21
		IMP%	18	3		
	MP	Angle°	50	−10		29
		IMP%	22	7		
	• Combine impairment % MP + PIP + DIP = 56					[1]
Ring	DIP	Angle°				
		IMP%				
	PIP	Angle°				
		IMP%				
	MP	Angle°	50	−20		32
		IMP%	22	10		
	• Combine impairment % MP + PIP + DIP =					[1]
Little	DIP	Angle°			10	33
		IMP%			33	
	PIP	Angle°			60	60
		IMP%			60	
	MP	Angle°	50	−20		32
		IMP%	22	10		
	• Combine impairment % MP + PIP + DIP = 84					[1]

Digit	Amputation (Mark level & impairment %)	Sensory loss (Mark type, level, & impairment %)	Other disorders (List type & impairment %)
Thumb	[2] IMP % =	[3] IMP % =	[4] IMP % =
Index	[2] IMP % =	[3] IMP % =	[4] IMP % =
Middle	[2] IMP % =	[3] IMP % =	[4] IMP % =
Ring	[2] IMP % = 80	U R; 12mm >15mm; [3] IMP % = 10+30=40	[4] IMP % =
Little	[2] IMP % =	U R; 8mm 10mm; [3] IMP % = 15+10=25	[4] IMP % =

Hand impairment% — • Combine digit IMP% *Convert to hand IMP%

	Thumb	Index	Middle	Ring	Little
Abnormal motion [1]	26	56	56	32	84
Amputation [2]				80	
Sensory loss [3]				40	25
Other disorders [4]					
Digit impairment % • Combine 1, 2, 3, 4	26	56	56	92	88
Hand impairment % *Convert above	10	11	11	9	9

Total hand impairment (Add hand impairment % for thumb + index + middle + ring + little finger) =	50 %
Upper extremity impairment (†Convert total hand impairment % to upper extremity impairment %) =	45 %; enter on Part 2, Line II
If hand region impairment is only impairment, convert upper extremity impairment to whole-person impairment:‡ =	%

• Combined Values Chart; (p. 322-324) *Use Table 1 (Digits to hand p. 18); †Use Table 2 (Hand to upper extremity p. 19) ‡Use Table 3 (p. 20)

**Courtesy of G. de Groot Swanson, MD

Figure 49B. Upper Extremity Impairment Evaluation Record–**Part 2 (Wrist, elbow, and shoulder)** Side ☐ R ☒ L

Name A.B. EXAMPLE 2 Age 36 Sex ☒ M ☐ F Dominant hand ☒ R ☐ L Date

Occupation CONSTRUCTION WORKER Diagnosis CRUSH INJURY

		Abnormal motion				Other disorders	Regional impairment %	Amputation
		Record motion, ankylosis and impairment %				List type & impairment %	• Combine [1] + [2]	Mark level & & impairment %
Wrist		Flexion	Extension	Ankylosis	IMP%			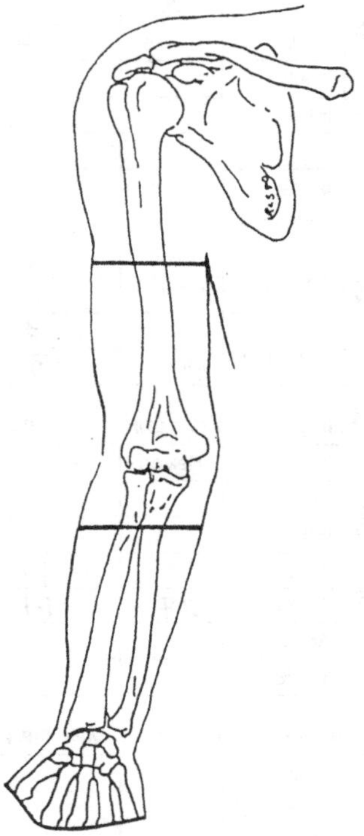
	Angle°							
	IMP%							
		RD	UD	Ankylosis	IMP%			
	Angle°							
	IMP%							
	Add IMP% F/E + RD/UD =				[1]	[2] **IMP% =**		
Elbow		Flexion	Extension	Ankylosis	IMP%			
	Angle°							
	IMP%							
		PRO	SUP	Ankylosis	IMP%			
	Angle°							
	IMP%							
	Add IMP% F/E + PRO/SUP =				[1]	[2] **IMP% =**		
Shoulder		Flexion	Extension	Ankylosis	IMP%			
	Angle°							
	IMP%							
		ADD	ABD	Ankylosis	IMP%			
	Angle°							
	IMP%							
		INT ROT	EXT ROT	Ankylosis	IMP%			
	Angle°							
	IMP%							
	Add IMP% F/E + ADD/ABD + IR/ER =				[1]	[2] **IMP% =**		**IMP %**

I. Amputation impairment (other than digitis)	=
II. Regional impairment of upper extremity • (Combine hand 45 % + wrist ____% + elbow ____% + shoulder ____%)	= 45 %
III. Peripheral nerve system impairment	=
IV. Peripheral vascular system impairment	=
V. Other disorders (not included in regional impairment) GRIP STRENGTH L = 24 Kg ; R = 52 Kg ; STRENGTH INDEX = 54 %	= 20%
Total upper extremity impairment (• Combine I + II + III + IV + V)	= 56 %
Impairment of the whole person (Use Table 3 p. 20)	= 34 %

If both limbs are involved, calculate the whole-person impairment for each on a separate chart and *combine* the percents (Combined Values Chart).

Figure 50A. Upper Extremity Impairment Evaluation Record**–**Part 1 (Hand)** Side ☐ R ☒ L

Name C.D. Example 5 Age 40 Sex ☒ M ☐ F Dominant hand ☒ R ☐ L Date

Occupation FIRE FIGHTER Diagnosis THERMAL BURN

			Abnormal motion				Amputation	Sensory loss	Other disorders	Hand impairment%	
			Record motion, ankylosis, and impairment %				Mark level & impairment %	Mark type, level, & impairment %	List type & impairment %	• Combine digit IMP% *Convert to hand IMP%	
			Flexion	Extension	Ankylosis	IMP%					
Thumb	IP	Angle°	40	-20		6		8mm			
		IMP%	3	3							
	MP	Angle°			10	6					
		IMP%			6						
				Motion	Ankylosis	IMP%					
	CMC	Radial abduction Angle°		10		9				Abnormal motion [1]	42
		Radial abduction IMP%		9						Amputation [2]	
		Adduction CMS		6		8				Sensory loss [3]	25
		Adduction IMP%		8						Other disorders [4]	
		Opposition CMS		3		13				Digit impairment % • Combine 1, 2, 3, 4	57
		Opposition IMP%		13							
Add impairment % CMC + MP + IP = 42 [1]							IMP % = [2]	IMP % = 25 [3]	IMP % = [4]	Hand impairment % *Convert above	23
			Flexion	Extension	Ankylosis	IMP%					
Index	DIP	Angle°			10	33		8mm		Abnormal motion [1]	81
		IMP%			33					Amputation [2]	
	PIP	Angle°	60	-40		38				Sensory loss [3]	25
		IMP%	24	14						Other disorders [4]	
	MP	Angle°			0	54				Digit impairment % • Combine 1, 2, 3, 4	86
		IMP%			54						
• Combine impairment % MP + PIP + DIP = 81 [1]							IMP % = [2]	IMP % = 25 [3]	IMP % = [4]	Hand impairment % *Convert above	17
Middle	DIP	Angle°			10	33		8mm		Abnormal motion [1]	81
		IMP%			33					Amputation [2]	
	PIP	Angle°	60	-40		38				Sensory loss [3]	25
		IMP%	24	14						Other disorders [4]	
	MP	Angle°			0	54				Digit impairment % • Combine 1, 2, 3, 4	86
		IMP%			54						
• Combine impairment % MP + PIP + DIP = 81 [1]							IMP % = [2]	IMP % = 25 [3]	IMP % = [4]	Hand impairment % *Convert above	17
Ring	DIP	Angle°			10	33		8mm		Abnormal motion [1]	81
		IMP%			33					Amputation [2]	
	PIP	Angle°	60	-40		38				Sensory loss [3]	25
		IMP%	24	14						Other disorders [4]	
	MP	Angle°			0	54				Digit impairment % • Combine 1, 2, 3, 4	86
		IMP%			54						
• Combine impairment % MP + PIP + DIP = 81 [1]							IMP % = [2]	IMP % = 25 [3]	IMP % = [4]	Hand impairment % *Convert above	9
Little	DIP	Angle°			10	33		8mm		Abnormal motion [1]	83
		IMP%			33					Amputation [2]	
	PIP	Angle°	70	-50		43				Sensory loss [3]	25
		IMP%	18	25						Other disorders [4]	
	MP	Angle°			0	54				Digit impairment % • Combine 1, 2, 3, 4	87
		IMP%			54						
• Combine impairment % MP + PIP + DIP = 83 [1]							IMP % = [2]	IMP % = 25 [3]	IMP % = [4]	Hand impairment % *Convert above	9

Total hand impairment (Add hand impairment % for thumb + index + middle + ring + little finger) = 75 %
Upper extremity impairment (†Convert total hand impairment % to upper extremity impairment %) = 68 %; enter on Part 2, Line II
If hand region impairment is only impairment, convert upper extremity impairment to whole-person impairment:‡ = %

• Combined Values Chart; (p. 322-324) *Use Table 1 (Digits to hand p. 18); †Use Table 2 (Hand to upper extremity p. 19) ‡Use Table 3 (p. 20)

** Courtesy of G. de Groot Swanson, MD

Figure 50B. Upper Extremity Impairment Evaluation Record–**Part 2 (Wrist, elbow, and shoulder)** Side ☐ R ☒ L

Name C. D. Age 40 Sex ☒ M ☐ F Dominant hand ☒ R ☐ L Date

Occupation FIRE FIGHTER Diagnosis THERMAL BURN

		Abnormal motion				Other disorders	Regional impairment %	Amputation
		Record motion, ankylosis and impairment %				List type & impairment %	• Combine [1] + [2]	Mark level & & impairment %
Wrist		Flexion	Extension	Ankylosis	IMP%			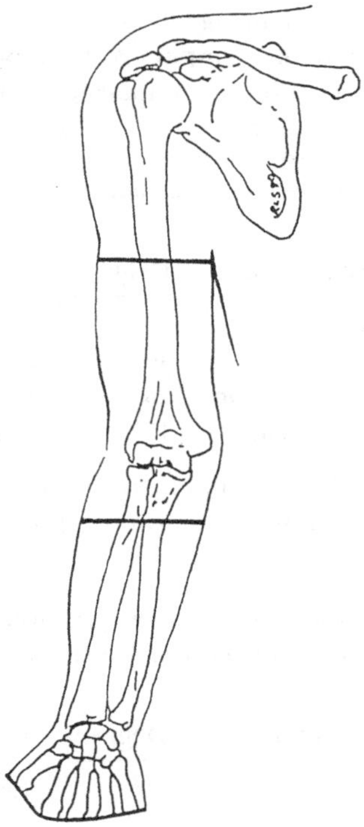
	Angle°	40	20		10			
	IMP%	3	7					
		RD	UD	Ankylosis	IMP%			
	Angle°	5	10		7			
	IMP%	3	4					
	Add IMP% F/E + RD/UD = 17				[1]	[2] **IMP% =**	17	
Elbow		Flexion	Extension	Ankylosis	IMP%			
	Angle°							
	IMP%							
		PRO	SUP	Ankylosis	IMP%			
	Angle°	50	40		4			
	IMP%	2	2					
	Add IMP% F/E + PRO/SUP = 4				[1]	[2] **IMP% =**	4	
Shoulder		Flexion	Extension	Ankylosis	IMP%			
	Angle°							
	IMP%							
		ADD	ABD	Ankylosis	IMP%			
	Angle°							
	IMP%							
		INT ROT	EXT ROT	Ankylosis	IMP%			
	Angle°							
	IMP%							
	Add IMP% F/E + ADD/ABD + IR/ER =				[1]	[2] **IMP% =**		**IMP %**

I. Amputation impairment (other than digitis)	=
II. Regional impairment of upper extremity • (Combine hand 68 % + wrist 17 % + elbow 4 % + shoulder ___ %)	= 74 %
III. Peripheral nerve system impairment	=
IV. Peripheral vascular system impairment	=
V. Other disorders (not included in regional impairment)	=

Total upper extremity impairment (• Combine I + II + III + IV + V)	= 74 %
Impairment of the whole person (Use Table 3 p. 20)	= 44 %

If both limbs are involved, calculate the whole-person impairment for each on a separate chart and *combine* the percents (Combined Values Chart).

Example 4: Colles' Fracture
A 45-year-old woman fell in a parking lot and sustained a Colles' fracture of the right distal radius. Fifteen months later she had full range of motion at the finger joints, some limitation of wrist motion, some deformity of the wrist, moderate pain with heavy activity, and a 40% Strength Loss Index.

The factors to be rated are the loss of motion of the wrist and forearm rotation. Strength loss should not be rated because it is not believed to be an additional impairing factor. No impairment estimate for deformity or pain is given. Based on the anatomic examination, the impairment evaluation is determined as follows.

1. *Wrist motion impairment:*

Wrist motion	Degrees	% Upper extremity impairment
Extension	30°	$I_E\% = 5\%$ (Fig. 26, p. 36)
Flexion	40°	$I_F\% = 3\%$ (Fig. 25, p. 36)
Radial deviation	20°	$I_{RD}\% = 0\%$ (Fig. 29, p. 38)
Ulnar deviation	10°	$I_{UD}\% = 4\%$ (Fig. 29, p. 38)

Add the upper extremity impairments contributed by wrist motion components: 5% + 3% + 4% = 12% impairment.

2. *Elbow motion impairment:* Forearm rotation is discussed in Section 3.1i (p. 38):

Elbow motion	Degrees	% Upper extremity impairment
Pronation	40°	$I_P\% = 3\%$ (Fig. 35, p. 41)
Supination	30°	$I_S\% = 2\%$ (Fig. 35, p. 41)

Add the upper extremity impairments contributed by elbow motion components. These equal a 5% upper extremity impairment.

3. *Combine* the upper extremity impairments contributed by the wrist (12%) and elbow (5%) (Combined Values Chart, p. 322). This yields a 16% upper extremity impairment and converts to a 10% impairment of the whole person (Table 3, p. 20).

Example 5: Severe Burn Contractures of the Hand
A firefighter sustained a severe thermal burn to his left hand in the line of duty. He underwent multiple skin grafting procedures and joint releases. Impairing factors included loss of motion of the finger joints and wrist and a sensory loss of the digits.

Sensory loss: static two-point discrimination measured between 7 and 12 mm in all digits. Partial sensory loss is rated at 50% of total sensory loss, or 25% of the amputation value (Fig. 5, Tables 8 and 9, pp. 22 and 31). A completed Upper Extremity Impairment Evaluation Record (Fig. 50, pp. 70 and 71) summarizes the impairment ratings.

Example 6: Multiple Finger Amputations
A 28-year-old punch press operator suffered multiple amputations of the right hand from a punch press injury. The stumps had good skin coverage, and there was no pain.

Factors to rate are the amputation level of each digit and the loss of motion of the proximal joints. The examination results and impairment calculations are shown in the Upper Extremity Impairment Evaluation Record (Fig. 51, p. 73).

Figure 51A. Upper Extremity Impairment Evaluation Record**–**Part 1 (Hand)**

Side ☒R ☐L

Name E.F. Example 6 Age 28 Sex ☒M ☐F Dominant hand ☒R ☐L Date

Occupation PUNCH PRESS OPERATOR Diagnosis MULTIPLE AMPUTATIONS

			Abnormal motion: Record motion, ankylosis, and impairment %				Amputation: Mark level & impairment %	Sensory loss: Mark type, level, & impairment %	Other disorders: List type & impairment %	Hand impairment%: • Combine digit IMP% *Convert to hand IMP%	
			Flexion	Extension	Ankylosis	IMP%					
Thumb	IP	Angle°	40	−10		5					
		IMP%	3	2							
	MP	Angle°	30	−10		4					
		IMP%	3	1							
				Motion	Ankylosis	IMP%					
	CMC	Radial abduction	Angle°							Abnormal motion [1]	9
			IMP%							Amputation [2]	30
		Adduction	CMS							Sensory loss [3]	
			IMP%							Other disorders [4]	
		Opposition	CMS							Digit impairment % • Combine 1, 2, 3, 4	36
			IMP%								
Add impairment % CMC + MP + IP = 9 [1]							[2] IMP % = 30	[3] IMP % =	[4] IMP % =	Hand impairment % *Convert above	14
			Flexion	Extension	Ankylosis	IMP%					
Index	DIP	Angle°								Abnormal motion [1]	17
		IMP%								Amputation [2]	80
	PIP	Angle°								Sensory loss [3]	
		IMP%								Other disorders [4]	
	MP	Angle°	60	+20		17				Digit impairment % • Combine 1, 2, 3, 4	83
		IMP%	17	0							
• Combine impairment % MP + PIP + DIP = 17 [1]							[2] IMP % = 80	[3] IMP % =	[4] IMP % =	Hand impairment % *Convert above	17
Middle	DIP	Angle°								Abnormal motion [1]	48
		IMP%								Amputation [2]	60
	PIP	Angle°	30	0		42				Sensory loss [3]	
		IMP%	42	0						Other disorders [4]	
	MP	Angle°	70	+20		11				Digit impairment % • Combine 1, 2, 3, 4	79
		IMP%	11	0							
• Combine impairment % MP + PIP + DIP = 48 [1]							[2] IMP % = 60	[3] IMP % =	[4] IMP % =	Hand impairment % *Convert above	16
Ring	DIP	Angle°	30	−10		23				Abnormal motion [1]	41
		IMP%	21	2						Amputation [2]	25
	PIP	Angle°	70	0		18				Sensory loss [3]	
		IMP%	18	0						Other disorders [4]	
	MP	Angle°	80	+20		6				Digit impairment % • Combine 1, 2, 3, 4	56
		IMP%	6	0							
• Combine impairment % MP + PIP + DIP = 41 [1]							[2] IMP % = 25	[3] IMP % =	[4] IMP % =	Hand impairment % *Convert above	6
Little	DIP	Angle°	30	0		21				Abnormal motion [1]	26
		IMP%	21	0						Amputation [2]	
	PIP	Angle°	90	0		6				Sensory loss [3]	
		IMP%	6	0						Other disorders [4]	
	MP	Angle°	90	+20		0				Digit impairment % • Combine 1, 2, 3, 4	26
		IMP%	0	0							
• Combine impairment % MP + PIP + DIP = 26 [1]							[2] IMP % =	[3] IMP % =	[4] IMP % =	Hand impairment % *Convert above	3

Total hand impairment (Add hand impairment % for thumb + index + middle + ring + little finger) = 56 %

Upper extremity impairment (†Convert total hand impairment % to upper extremity impairment %) = 50 %; enter on Part 2, Line II

If hand region impairment is only impairment, convert upper extremity impairment to whole-person impairment:‡ = 30 %

• Combined Values Chart; (p. 322-324) *Use Table 1 (Digits to hand p. 18); †Use Table 2 (Hand to upper extremity p. 19) ‡Use Table 3 (p. 20)

** Courtesy of G. de Groot Swanson, MD

Figure 51B. Upper Extremity Impairment Evaluation Record–**Part 2 (Wrist, elbow, and shoulder)** Side ☐ R ☐ L

Name__________ Age____ Sex ☐ M ☐ F Dominant hand ☐ R ☐ L Date__________

Occupation__________ Diagnosis__________

		Abnormal motion				**Other disorders**	**Regional impairment %**	**Amputation**
		Record motion, ankylosis and impairment %				List type & impairment %	• Combine [1] + [2]	Mark level & & impairment %
Wrist		Flexion	Extension	Ankylosis	IMP%			
	Angle°							
	IMP%							
		RD	UD	Ankylosis	IMP%			
	Angle°							
	IMP%							
	Add IMP% F/E + RD/UD =				[1]	**IMP% =** [2]		
Elbow		Flexion	Extension	Ankylosis	IMP%			
	Angle°							
	IMP%							
		PRO	SUP	Ankylosis	IMP%			
	Angle°							
	IMP%							
	Add IMP% F/E + PRO/SUP =				[1]	**IMP% =** [2]		
Shoulder		Flexion	Extension	Ankylosis	IMP%			
	Angle°							
	IMP%							
		ADD	ABD	Ankylosis	IMP%			
	Angle°							
	IMP%							
		INT ROT	EXT ROT	Ankylosis	IMP%			
	Angle°							
	IMP%							
	Add IMP% F/E + ADD/ABD + IR/ER =				[1]	**IMP% =** [2]		**IMP %**

I. Amputation impairment (other than digits)	=
II. Regional impairment of upper extremity • (Combine hand ____% + wrist ____% + elbow ____% + shoulder ____%)	=
III. Peripheral nerve system impairment	=
IV. Peripheral vascular system impairment	=
V. Other disorders (not included in regional impairment)	=

Total upper extremity impairment (• Combine I + II + III + IV + V)	=
Impairment of the whole person (Use Table 3 p. 20)	=

If both limbs are involved, calculate the whole-person impairment for each on a separate chart and *combine* the percents (Combined Values Chart).

3.2 The Lower Extremity

Anatomic, diagnostic, and functional methods are used in evaluating permanent impairments of the lower extremity. While some impairments may be evaluated appropriately by determining the range of motion of the extremity, others are better evaluated by the use of diagnostic categories or according to test criteria.

In general, only one evaluation method should be used to evaluate a specific impairment. In some instances, however, as with the example on p. 77, a combination of two or three methods may be required.

This section includes information on using some of the simpler, more reproducible methods of and tests for assessing function. It also includes examples illustrating how the physician selects the best approach to evaluate an impairment. Selecting the optimal approach or combining several methods requires judgment and experience. Also needed is careful testing that produces accurate and consistent results.

To make this section easier to use, the tables of the section show the impairment percents of the whole person, the lower extremity, and the specific part together. The whole-person impairments are *not* in parentheses, the lower-limb impairment percents are in parentheses ( ), and the specific part impairments are in brackets [ ]. Multiplying a lower extremity impairment percent by 0.4 yields the whole-person impairment percent. Multiplying the specific-part impairment percent by 0.7 yields the lower extremity impairment percent.

If the patient has several impairments of the same lower extremity part, such as the leg, or impairments of different parts, such as the ankle and a toe, the whole-person estimates for the impairments are *combined* (Combined Values Chart, p. 322). If both extremities are impaired, the impairment of each should be evaluated and expressed in terms of the whole person, and the two percents should be *combined* (Combined Values Chart, p. 322).

The figures for this section, which illustrate how to measure ranges of motion, the distribution of motor and sensory nerves, and the tibia-os calcis angle, are at the end of the section (pp. 90 through 93).

3.2a Limb Length Discrepancy

Measuring lower-extremity length by tape measure, or determining the iliac crest level when the subject is standing, has at least a 0.5- to 1-cm variance and is difficult in a patient with pelvic angulation, knee flexion contracture, or significant ankle edema. For this reason, teleroentgenography is recommended for estimating these impairments, which are classified in Table 35 (at right).

Table 35. Impairment from Limb Length Discrepancy.

Discrepancy (cm)	Whole-person (lower extremity) impairment (%)
0-1.9	0
2-2.9	2-3 (5-9)
3-3.9	4-5 (10-14)
4-4.9	6-7 (15-19)
5+	8 (20)

3.2b Gait Derangement

Gait derangement is a component of many different types of lower extremity impairments. Impairment estimates related to these conditions should be consistent with the pathologic findings, for instance, those seen by roentgenography. Except as otherwise noted, the percents given in Table 36 (p. 76) are for full-time derangements of persons who are dependent on assistive devices.

This part may serve as a general guide for estimating many lower extremity impairments. The lower limb impairment percents shown in Table 36 should stand alone and should *not* be combined with those given in other parts of Section 3.2. Whenever possible, the evaluator should use the more specific methods of those other parts in estimating impairments.

Section 3.2b does not apply to abnormalities based only on subjective factors, such as pain or sudden giving-way, as with, for example, a patient with low-back discomfort who chooses to use a cane to ease walking.

Example: A 61-year-old professor had symptoms of arthralgia in her left hip and difficulty with walking that required part-time use of a cane. On physical examination, the Trendelenburg test was mildly positive. The range of motion of the hip was normal. Roentgenography indicated moderately advanced hip arthritis.

Diagnosis: Antalgia (gait difficulty), moderately advanced arthritis requiring part-time use of a cane.

Impairment: 15% whole-person impairment.

Comment: The patient's impairment might be estimated by using the estimates for gait derangement, those for arthritic degeneration (p. 82), or those for hip abductor muscle weakness (p. 77).

In this case, the evaluator believed the patient's use of a cane best reflected the basic pathologic process and that using the estimates related to gait disturbance was proper.

Table 36. Lower Limb Impairment from Gait Derangement.

Severity	Patient's signs	Whole-person impairment (%)
Mild	a. Antalgic limp with shortened stance phase and documented moderate to advanced arthritic changes of hip, knee, or ankle	7
	b. Positive Trendelenberg sign and moderate to advanced osteoarthritis of hip	10
	c. Same as category **a** or **b** above, but patient requires part-time use of cane *or* crutch for distance walking but not usually at home or in workplace	15
	d. Requires routine use of short leg brace (ankle-foot orthosis [AFO])	15
Moderate	e. Requires routine use of cane, crutch, *or* long leg brace (knee-ankle-foot orthosis [KAFO])	20
	f. Requires routine use of cane *or* crutch *and* a short leg brace (AFO)	30
	g. Requires routine use of two canes *or* two crutches	40
Severe	h. Requires routine use of two canes *or* two crutches *and* a short leg brace (AFO)	50
	i. Requires routine use of two canes *or* two crutches *and* a long leg brace (KAFO)	60
	j. Requires routine use of two canes *or* two crutches *and* two lower-extremity braces (either AFOs or KAFOs)	70
	k. Wheelchair dependent	80

3.2c Muscle Atrophy (Unilateral)

In evaluating this condition, the corresponding part of the other limb should be normal and should be used for comparison. Neither limb should have swelling or varicosities that would invalidate the measurements. Diminished muscle function should be estimated under *only one* of several parts of this chapter, relating to gait derangement (p. 75), muscle atrophy (p. 76), manual muscle testing (p. 76), or peripheral nerve injury.

The evaluating physician should determine which method and approach best applies to the patient's impairment and use the most objective method that applies.

Example: A 49-year-old man fractured the right tibia in a fall while mountain climbing. Twelve months later, after the patient completed rehabilitation to a stable status of the injury, examination showed an undisplaced, healed tibial fracture with 2 cm of thigh muscle atrophy and 1 cm of calf muscle atrophy. Manual muscle testing showed normal strength.

The man was estimated to have a 3% whole-person thigh impairment and a 1% whole-person calf impairment (Table 37, p. 77), which are *combined* to give an estimated 4% whole-person impairment (Combined Values Chart, p. 322).

Comment: The healing times of fractured tibias are highly variable. Some patients require prolonged immobilization and inactivity, which may result in significant atrophy. A younger patient may be able to rebuild the leg muscle mass by following a rehabilitation program, but an older patient may not be able to do this.

Manual muscle testing gives an incomplete picture: even when results of muscle strength tests are normal, the injured extremity may fatigue more rapidly than usual. Evaluating the impairment in terms of atrophy gives an impairment estimate that more closely matches the patient's capabilities when results of manual muscle testing are normal.

3.2d Manual Muscle Testing

Manual muscle testing is performed by major groups, is dependent on the patient's cooperation, and is subject to the patient's conscious and unconscious control (Table 38, p. 77). The results should be concordant with observable pathologic signs and other medical evidence. Measurements should be consistent between two trained observers. If the measurements are made by one examiner, they should be consistent on different occasions. Even in a fully cooperative patient, strength may vary from one examination to another. Findings varying by more than one grade between observers, or such findings made by the same observer on separate occasions, are not valid. In those patients, impairment estimates should not be made with this section. Table 38 (p. 77) shows the criteria on which estimates and grades of the lower extremity's strength are based.

Patients whose weakness is based on a neurologic deficit would be expected to have positive electrodiagnostic findings. Patients whose performance is inhibited by pain or the fear of pain are not good candidates for manual muscle testing.

Example: A 30-year-old man had a healed tibial fracture without deformity but with residual signs of anterior compartment syndrome. When his condition was stable, he had grade 3 ankle extension power. The leg with the healed fracture appeared to have muscle atrophy.

Impairment: 10% impairment of the whole person.

Table 37. Impairments from Leg Muscle Atrophy.

Difference in circumference (cm)	Impairment degree	Whole-person (lower extremity) impairment (%)
a. Thigh: The circumference is measured 10 cm above the patella with the knee fully extended and the muscles relaxed.		
0-0.9	None	0
1-1.9	Mild	1-2 (3-8)
2-2.9	Moderate	3-4 (8-13)
3+	Severe	5 (13)
b. Calf: The maximum circumference on the normal side is compared with the circumference at the same level on the affected side.		
0-0.9	None	0
1-1.9	Mild	1-2 (3-8)
2-2.9	Moderate	3-4 (8-13)
3+	Severe	5 (13)

Table 38. Criteria for Grades of Muscle Function of the Lower Extremity.

Grade	Description of muscle function
5	Active movement against gravity with full resistance
4	Active movement against gravity with some resistance
3	Active movement against gravity only, without resistance
2	Active movement with gravity eliminated
1	Slight contraction and no movement
0	No contraction

Comment: The impairment from weakness is judged to be of greater significance to the patient than the atrophy impairment. Thus, manual muscle testing (Tables 38 and 39, below) is the better approach to estimating the patient's impairment.

3.2e Range of Motion

Evaluating permanent impairment of the lower extremity according to its range of motion is a suitable method. Principles similar to those for manual muscle testing apply because the patient's pain or motivation may affect the results. If it is clear to the evaluator that a restricted range of motion has an organic basis, multiple evaluations are unnecessary. If, however, multiple evaluations exist, inconsistency of a grade between the findings of two observers, or on separate occasions by the same observer, makes the results invalid. The arcs listed are examples of mild, moderate, and severe impairments and are to be used as guides.

Example: A 45-year-old woman sustained a fractured tibia in a crash. Months after the injury, when the residua were stable, she had lost half of the ankle flexion and extension motion, and she had severe, permanent stiffness of all toes.

Table 39. Impairments from Lower Extremity Muscle Weakness.

Muscle group		Whole-person (lower extremity) [foot] impairment (%)				
		Grade 0	Grade 1	Grade 2	Grade 3	Grade 4
Hip	Flexion	6 (15)	6 (15)	6 (15)	4 (10)	2 (5)
	Extension	15 (37)	15 (37)	15 (37)	15 (37)	7 (17)
	Abduction*	25 (62)	25 (62)	25 (62)	15 (27)	10 (25)
Knee	Flexion	10 (25)	10 (25)	10 (25)	7 (17)	5 (12)
	Extension	10 (25)	10 (25)	10 (25)	7 (17)	5 (12)
Ankle	Flexion (plantar flexion)	15 (37) [53]	15 (37) [53]	15 (37) [53]	10 (25) [35]	7 (17) [24]
	Extension (dorsiflexion)	10 (25) [35]	10 (25) [35]	10 (25) [35]	10 (25) [35]	5 (12) [17]
	Inversion	5 (12) [17]	5 (12) [17]	5 (12) [17]	5 (12) [17]	2 (5) [7]
	Eversion	5 (12) [17]	5 (12) [17]	5 (12) [17]	5 (12) [17]	2 (5) [7]
Great toe	Extension	3 (7) [10]	3 (7) [10]	3 (7) [10]	3 (7) [10]	1 (2) [3]
	Flexion	5 (12) [17]	5 (12) [17]	5 (12) [17]	5 (12) [17]	2 (5) [7]

*Hip adduction weakness is evaluated as an obturator nerve impairment (Table 68, p. 89).

Table 40. Hip Motion Impairments.

Motion	Whole-person (lower extremity) impairment (%)		
	Mild: 2% (5%)	**Moderate: 4% (10%)**	**Severe: 8% (20%)**
Flexion	Less than 100°	Less than 80°	Less than 50°
Extension	10°-19° flexion contracture	20°-29° flexion contracture	30° flexion contracture
Internal rotation	10°-20°	0°- 9°	
External rotation	20°-30°	0°-19°	
Abduction	15°-25°	5°-14°	Less than 5°
Adduction	0°-15°	—	—
Abduction contracture*	0°- 5°	6°-10°	11°-20°

*An abduction contracture of greater than 20° is a 15% whole-person impairment.

Table 41. Knee Impairments.

Motion	Whole-person (lower extremity) impairment (%)		
	Mild: 4% (10%)	**Moderate: 8% (20%)**	**Severe: 14% (35%)**
Flexion	Less than 110°	Less than 80°	Less than 60° +1% (2%) per 10° less than 60°
Flexion contracture	5°-9°	10°-19°	20°+
Deformity measured by femoral-tibial angle; 3° to 10° valgus is considered normal			
Varus	2° valgus-0° (neutral)	1°-7° varus	8°-12° varus; add 1% (2%) per 2° over 12°
Valgus	10°-12°	13°-15°	16°-20°; add 1% (2%) per 2° over 20°

Table 42. Ankle Motion Impairments.

Motion	Whole-person (lower extremity) [foot] impairment		
	Mild: 3% (7%) [10%]	**Moderate: 6% (15%)** [21%]	**Severe: 12% (30%)** [43%]
Plantar flexion capability	11°-20°	1°-10°	None
Flexion contracture	—	10°	20°
Extension	10°- 0° (neutral)	—	—

Table 43. Hindfoot Impairments.

Motion	Whole-person (lower extremity) [foot] impairment	
	Mild: 1% (2%) [3%]	**Moderate and severe: 2% (5%) [7%]**
Inversion	10°-20°	0°-9°
Eversion	0°-10°	—

Table 44. Ankle or Hindfoot Deformity Impairments.

Position	Whole-person (lower extremity) [foot] impairment		
	Mild: 5% (12%) [17%]	**Moderate: 10% (25%) [35%]**	**Severe: 20% (50%) [72%]**
Varus	10°-14°	15°-24°	25°+
Valgus	10°-20°	—	—

Table 45. Toe Impairments.

Type of impairment	Whole-person (lower extremity) [foot] impairment	
	Mild: 1% (2%) [3%]	**Moderate and severe: 2% (5%) [7%]**
Great toe		
Metatarsophalangeal, extension	15°-30°	Less than 15°
Interphalangeal, flexion	Less than 20°	—
Lesser toes		
Metatarsophalangeal, extension	Less than 10°	—

*The maximum whole-person impairment percent for impairments of 2 or more lesser toes of one foot is 2%.

Impairment: The woman's whole-person impairments were estimated to be moderate (6%) in terms of ankle motion (Table 42, at left) and severe (2%) (Table 45, above) in terms of toe impairment. The two impairments are *combined* by means of the Combined Values Chart (p. 322).

The whole-person impairment was 8%.

Comment: Comparing Tables 42 and 45 with Table 37 (p. 77), one can see that estimated impairment for loss of motion of the ankle and toes would exceed any estimated impairment for weakness or atrophy of the leg muscles. If the impairment is estimated on the basis of ankle and toe loss of motion, it should not be estimated on the basis of muscle atrophy also. Manual muscle testing is difficult to assess because of the lower leg muscles' limited range of motion of the ankle and toes.

3.2f Joint Ankylosis

Malposition in angulation or rotation of an arthrodesis or fused joint increases the magnitude of the impairment. Surgical correction usually is preferable to accepting a significant malposition. Impairment estimates for malposition are included for the infrequently encountered patient who is not a candidate for surgical correction.

The text and tables that follow indicate the optimal neutral positions for ankyloses of the lower extremity's parts and the impairment percents for ankyloses in the optimal positions. Any variation from the optimal neutral position of an ankylosed joint should be determined and the impairment percent increased by an appropriate percent according to the tables.

Table 46. Impairment* from Ankylosis in Hip Flexion.

Ankylosis in flexion (°)	Whole-person (lower extremity) impairment (%)	
0- 9	15	(37)
10-19	10	(25)
20-24	5	(12)
25-39	0	(0)
40-49	5	(12)
50-59	10	(25)
60-69	15	(37)
70+	20	(50)

*The appropriate ankylosis impairment percent is added to the impairment percent for ankylosis in the neutral position given in the text (at right).

Table 47. Impairment* from Ankylosis in Hip Internal Rotation.

Ankylosis in internal rotation (°)	Whole-person (lower extremity) impairment (%)	
5- 9	5	(12)
10-19	10	(25)
20-29	15	(37)
30+	20	(50)

*The appropriate ankylosis impairment percent is added to the impairment percent for ankylosis in the neutral position given in the text (at right).

Table 48. Impairment* from Ankylosis in Hip External Rotation.

Ankylosis in external rotation (°)	Whole-person (lower extremity) impairment (%)	
10-19	5	(12)
20-29	10	(25)
30-39	15	(37)
40+	20	(50)

*The appropriate ankylosis impairment percent is added to the impairment percent for ankylosis in the neutral position given in the text (below).

Table 49. Impairment* from Ankylosis in Hip Abduction.

Ankylosis in abduction (°)	Whole-person (lower extremity) impairment (%)	
5-14	10	(25)
15-24	15	(37)
25+	20	(50)

*The appropriate ankylosis impairment percent is added to the impairment percent for ankylosis in the neutral position given in the text (below).

Table 50. Impairment* from Ankylosis in Hip Adduction.

Ankylosis in abduction (°)	Whole-person (lower extremity) impairment (%)	
5- 9	10	(25)
10-14	15	(37)
15+	20	(50)

*The appropriate ankylosis impairment percent is added to the impairment percent for ankylosis in the neutral position given in the text (below).

Hip

The optimal position of ankylosis is 25° to 40° flexion and neutral rotation, adduction, and abduction. This position represents a 20% whole-person impairment and a 50% lower-extremity impairment.

Tables 46 through 50 (at left and above) provide impairment estimates for hip ankyloses in various positions. Figures 52 through 54 (pp. 90 and 91) illustrate the measurement of hip motion. Impairment estimates for extension, abduction, and adduction are combined (Combined Values Chart, p.322). The maximum hip impairment or lower limb impairment is 100%, which is a 40% whole-person impairment.

Table 51. Impairment* from Knee Ankylosis in Varus.

Ankylosis in Varus (°)	Whole-person (lower extremity) impairment (%)	
0 - 9	5	(12)
10 - 19	10	(25)
20+	13	(33)

*The appropriate ankylosis impairment percent is added to the impairment percent for ankylosis in the neutral position given in the text (below).

Table 52. Impairment* from Knee Ankylosis in Valgus.

Ankylosis in Valgus (°)	Whole-person (lower extremity) impairment (%)	
10 - 19	5	(12)
20 - 29	10	(25)
30+	13	(33)

*The appropriate ankylosis impairment percent is added to the impairment percent for ankylosis in the neutral position given in the text (below).

Table 53. Impairment* from Knee Ankylosis in Flexion.

Ankylosis in flexion (°)	Whole-person (lower extremity) impairment (%)	
20 - 29	5	(12)
30 - 39	10	(25)
40+	13	(33)

*The appropriate ankylosis impairment percent is added to the impairment percent for ankylosis in the neutral position given in the text (below).

Table 54. Knee Ankylosis Impairment* in Internal or External Malrotation.

Ankylosis in internal or external malrotation (°)	Whole-person (lower extremity) impairment (%)	
10 - 19	5	(12)
20 - 29	10	(25)
30+	13	(33)

*The appropriate ankylosis impairment percent is added to the impairment percent for ankylosis in the neutral position given in the text (below).

Knee

The optimal position is 10° to 15° flexion with good alignment. Figure 55 (p. 91) shows how the goniometer is used to measure knee flexion. Ankylosis in the optimal position is a 67% lower-extremity impairment or a 27% whole-person impairment.

Impairments beyond those of the neutral position are added according to Tables 51 through 54 (at left).

Malpositioning of the knee includes varus, excess valgus, and malrotation deformities, which can increase the impairment to 100% impairment of the lower extremity.

Ankle

The optimal ankylosis position is the neutral position without flexion, extension, varus, or valgus. Ankylosis in the neutral position is a 4% whole-person impairment, a 10% lower-extremity impairment, and a 14% foot impairment. A variation from the neutral position should be evaluated according to Tables 55 through 59 (pp. 80 and 81). The maximum impairments are 25% whole-person impairment, 62% lower-extremity impairment, and 88% ankle impairment.

Figure 56 (p. 91) illustrates the measurement of dorsiflexion and plantar flexion.

Table 55. Ankle Impairment* from Ankylosis in Plantar Flexion or Dorsiflexion.

Position	Whole-person (lower extremity) [foot] impairment (%)		
20°+ dorsiflexion	15	(37)	[53]
10° - 19° dorsiflexion	7	(17)	[24]
10° - 19° plantar flexion	7	(17)	[24]
20° - 29° plantar flexion	15	(37)	[53]
30°+ plantar flexion	21	(52)	[74]

*The appropriate ankylosis impairment percent is added to the impairment percent for ankylosis in the neutral position given in the text (above).

Table 56. Ankle Impairment* from Ankylosis in Varus Position.

Varus position (°)	Whole-person (lower extremity) [foot] impairment (%)		
5 - 9	10	(25)	[35]
10 - 19	15	(37)	[53]
20 - 29	18	(43)	[61]
30+	21	(52)	[74]

*The appropriate ankylosis impairment percent is added to the impairment percent for ankylosis in the neutral position given in the text (above).

Table 57. Ankle Impairment* from Ankylosis in Valgus Position.

Valgus Position (°)	Whole-person (lower extremity) [foot] impairment (%)		
10-19	10	(25)	[35]
20-30	15	(37)	[53]
30+	21	(52)	[74]

*The appropriate ankylosis impairment percent is added to the impairment percent for ankylosis in the neutral position given in the text (p. 80).

Table 58. Ankle Impairment* from Ankylosis in Internal Malrotation.

Internal malrotation (°)	Whole-person (lower extremity) [foot] impairment (%)		
0- 9	5	(12)	[17]
10-19	10	(25)	[35]
20-29	15	(37)	[53]
30+	21	(52)	[74]

*The appropriate ankylosis impairment percent is added to the impairment percent for ankylosis in the neutral position given in the text (p. 80).

Table 59. Ankle Impairment* from Ankylosis in External Malrotation.

External malrotation (°)	Whole-person (lower extremity) [foot] impairment (%)		
15-19	5	(12)	[17]
20-29	10	(25)	[35]
30-39	15	(37)	[53]
40+	21	(52)	[74]

*The appropriate ankylosis impairment percent is added to the impairment percent for ankylosis in the neutral position given in the text (p. 80).

Foot (Hindfoot, Midfoot, Forefoot)

For the subtalar part of the foot, the optimal ankylosis position is neutral, or 0°, without varus or valgus. The ankylosis impairment in the neutral position is 4% for the whole person, 10% for the lower extremity, and 14% for the foot.

Malpositioning may increase the whole-person impairment to as much as 25%, the lower-extremity impairment to 62%, and the foot impairment to 88%. Varus or valgus malpositioning is estimated in the same way as for the ankle (Tables 56 and 57, pp. 80 and 81).

Ankylosis impairment for loss of the tibia-os calcis angle is estimated according to Table 60 (below). The tibia-os calcis angle is made by the longitudinal axis of the os calcis and the longitudinal axis of the tibia with the ankle in neutral position (Fig. 57, p. 91).

For pantalar ankylosis, the optimal position is neutral; the impairment estimates for that position are 10% for the whole person, 25% for the lower extremity, and 35% for the foot. Further flexion, varus, and valgus impairments are estimated as shown in Tables 55 through 60 (pp. 80 and 81).

Toes

Table 61 (p. 82) indicates impairment estimates related to ankylosis of one or several toes. Figure 58 (p. 92) illustrates the use of a goniometer to measure a toe's range of motion.

Table 60. Impairments for Loss of the Tibia-Os Calcis Angle.*

Angle (°)	Whole-person (lower extremity) [foot] impairment (%)		
110-100	10	(25)	[35]
99- 90	15	(37)	[53]
Less than 90	21	(52)	[74]

*The tibia-os calcis angle is shown in Fig. 57 (p. 91).

Example: A 55-year-old diabetic man suffered a severe distal tibial and intra-articular ankle fracture that resulted in spontaneous bony ankylosis of his ankle in 15° dorsiflexion and 7° varus. Because of the diabetic condition and marginal circulation to the ankle region, corrective surgery was not recommended.

Impairment: 11% whole-person impairment related to ankle flexion (Table 55, p. 80) and 10% whole-person impairment related to the varus deformity (Table 56, p. 80). These ankle impairments are *combined,* giving a 20% impairment (Combined Values Chart, p. 322).

Comment: In this patient, considering the impairments for malpositioning and ankylosis is judged to be more appropriate than using the impairment for an intra-articular ankle fracture (Table 64, p. 86). Estimates for arthritic and range of motion impairments would not apply to an ankylosis impairment.

An impairment percent related to diabetes would be *combined* with the musculoskeletal system impairment percent.

Table 61. Impairment of the Foot Due to Impairments of Toes.

Digit(s) involved	Whole-person (lower extremity) [foot] impairment		
	Ankylosed in		
	Full Extension	Position of function	Full Flexion
Great	4 (10) [14]	4 (9) [13]	5 (13) [18]
Great, second	5 (12) [17]	4 (11) [15]	6 (15) [21]
Great, second, third	6 (14) [20]	5 (12) [17]	7 (17) [24]
Great, second, fourth	6 (14) [20]	5 (12) [17]	7 (17) [24]
Great, second, fifth	6 (14) [20]	5 (12) [17]	7 (17) [24]
Great, second, third, fourth	6 (16) [23]	5 (13) [19]	8 (19) [27]
Great, second, third, fifth	6 (16) [23]	5 (13) [19]	8 (19) [27]
Great, second, fourth, fifth	6 (16) [23]	5 (13) [19]	8 (19) [27]
Great, second, third, fourth, fifth	7 (18) [26]	6 (15) [21]	8 (21) [30]
Great, third	5 (12) [17]	4 (11) [15]	6 (15) [21]
Great, third, fourth	6 (14) [20]	5 (12) [17]	7 (17) [24]
Great, third, fifth	6 (14) [20]	5 (12) [17]	7 (17) [24]
Great, third, fourth, fifth	6 (16) [23]	5 (13) [19]	8 (19) [27]
Great, fourth	5 (12) [17]	4 (11) [15]	6 (15) [21]
Great, fourth, fifth	6 (14) [20]	5 (12) [17]	7 (17) [24]
Great, fifth	5 (12) [17]	4 (11) [15]	6 (15) [21]
Second	1 (2) [3]	0 (1) [2]	1 (2) [3]
Second, third	2 (4) [6]	1 (3) [4]	2 (4) [6]
Second, third, fourth	2 (6) [9]	1 (3) [4]	2 (6) [9]
Second, third, fifth	2 (6) [9]	2 (4) [6]	2 (6) [9]
Second, third, fourth, fifth	3 (8) [12]	2 (6) [8]	3 (8) [12]
Second, fourth	2 (4) [6]	1 (3) [4]	2 (4) [6]
Second, fourth, fifth	2 (6) [9]	2 (4) [6]	3 (8) [12]
Second, fifth	2 (4) [6]	1 (3) [4]	2 (4) [6]
Third	1 (2) [3]	0 (1) [2]	1 (2) [3]
Third, fourth	2 (4) [6]	1 (3) [4]	2 (4) [6]
Third, fourth, fifth	2 (6) [9]	2 (4) [6]	2 (6) [9]
Third, fifth	2 (4) [6]	1 (3) [4]	2 (4) [6]
Fourth	1 (2) [3]	0 (1) [2]	1 (2) [3]
Fourth, fifth	2 (4) [6]	1 (3) [4]	2 (4) [6]
Fifth	1 (2) [3]	0 (1) [2]	1 (2) [3]

3.2g Arthritis

Range of motion techniques are of limited value for estimating impairment secondary to arthritis. While there are some patients with arthritis for whom loss of motion is the principal impairment, most patients are impaired more by pain and weakness secondary to advanced joint surface degeneration but still can maintain functional ranges of motion.

Roentgenographic grading systems for inflammatory and degenerative arthritis are well established and widely used for treatment and scientific investigation. For most patients, roentgenographic grading is a more objective and valid method for assigning impairment estimates than physical findings, such as the range of motion or joint crepitation. Crepitation is an inconstant finding that depends on factors such as forces on joint surfaces and synovial fluid viscosity.

Certain roentgenographic findings that are of diagnostic importance, such as exostoses and reactive sclerosis, have no direct bearing on impairment. The best roentgenographic indicator of functional impairment for a patient with arthritis is the cartilage interval or joint space. The hallmark of all types of arthritis is thinning of the articular cartilage, and this correlates well with disease progression.

The need for joint replacement or major reconstruction usually corresponds with the complete loss of the articular surface. The impairments related to arthritis (Table 62, p. 83) are based on standard roentgenograms taken with the patient standing, if possible, and 36 inches from the machine, with the beam at the level of and parallel to the joint surface. The estimate for the patellofemoral joint is based on a "sunrise view" taken at 40° flexion or on a true lateral view.

In the case of the knee, the joint must be in neutral position (0°). Impairments of patients with flexion contractures should be estimated according to range of motion findings. Roentgenograms of the hip joint are taken in the neutral position. The cartilage interval of the hip is relatively constant in the various positions. The ankle roentgenogram must be taken in a mortise view, but 10° flexion or extension is permissible. Evaluation of the foot requires a lateral view for the hindfoot and an anteroposterior view for the forefoot. If there is doubt or controversy about the suitability of a specific patient for this rating method, range of motion techniques may be used.

A patient who has an intra-articular fracture and then rapid onset of arthritis should be evaluated with this section and with Section 3.2i (p. 84) on diagnosis-based estimates.

Table 62. Arthritis Impairments Based on Roentgenographically Determined Cartilage Intervals.

Joint	Whole-person (lower extremity) [foot] impairment (%)			
	Cartilage interval			
	3 mm	2 mm	1 mm	0 mm
Sacroiliac (3 mm)*	—	1 (2)	3 (7)	3 (7)
Hip (4 mm)	3 (7)	8 (20)	10 (25)	20 (50)
Knee (4 mm)	3 (7)	8 (20)	10 (25)	20 (50)
Patellofemoral†	—	4 (10)	6 (15)	8 (20)
Ankle (4 mm)	2 (5) [7]	6 (15) [21]	8 (20) [28]	12 (30) [43]
Subtalar (3 mm)	—	2 (5) [7]	6 (15) [21]	10 (25) [35]
Talonavicular (2 - 3 mm)	—	—	4 (10) [14]	8 (20) [28]
Calcaneocuboid	—	—	4 (10) [14]	8 (20) [28]
First metatarsophalangeal	—	—	2 (5) [7]	5 (12) [17]
Other metatarsophalangeal	—	—	1 (2) [3]	3 (7) [10]

*Normal cartilage intervals are given in parentheses.

†In a patient with a history of direct trauma, a complaint of patellofemoral pain, and crepitation on physical examination, but without joint space narrowing on roentgenograms, a 2% whole-person or 5% lower-extremity impairment is given.

Example: A 48-year-old dock worker had suffered a tibial fracture 23 years earlier. The fracture healed in 10° varus. The man complained now of knee pain toward the end of the day. An examination in the morning before work showed a nearly full range of motion of the injured knee, 0° through 125°, and mild crepitation. Standing roentgenograms showed the cartilage interval to be 2 mm on the medial side of the knee.

Impairment: 8% whole-person impairment and 20% impairment of the lower extremity (Table 62, above). The 8% whole-person impairment related to knee arthritis should be *combined* with an impairment percent reflecting the fracture malposition, 10° varus of the tibia, an 8% whole-person impairment (Table 64, p. 85). Combining two 8% whole-person impairments yields a 15% whole-person impairment (Combined Values Chart, p. 322).

Comment: The patient had moderate degenerative arthritis of the knee, and his symptoms worsened after a day's work. The cause of pain and impairment was the wearing away of the knee joint surfaces. Carefully taken, accurate roentgenograms are the most reliable method of estimating such an impairment.

3.2h Amputations

Impairments of the lower extremity due to amputations are estimated according to Table 63 (below).

Table 63. Impairment Estimates for Amputations.

Amputation	Whole-person (lower extremity) [foot] impairment (%)
Hemipelvectomy	50
Hip disarticulation	40 (100)
Above knee	
Proximal	40 (100)
Midthigh	36 (90)
Distal	32 (80)
Knee disarticulation	32 (80)
Below knee	
less than 3 inches	32 (80)
3 inches or more	28 (70)
Syme (foot)	25 (62) [100]
Midfoot	18 (45) [64]
Transmetatarsal	16 (40) [57]
First metatarsal	8 (20) [28]
Other metatarsals	2 (5) [7]
All toes at metatarso-phangeal (MTP) joint	9 (22) [31]
Great toe at MTP joint	5 (12) [17]
Great toe at interphalangeal joint	2 (5) [7]
Lesser toes at MTP joint	1 (2) [3] each

3.2i Diagnosis-based Estimates

Some impairment estimates are assigned more appropriately on the basis of a diagnosis than on the basis of findings on physical examination. A good example is that of a patient impaired because of the replacement of a hip, which was successful. This patient may be able to function well but may require prophylactic restrictions, a further impairment. For most diagnosis-based estimates, the ranges of impairment are broad, and the estimate will depend on the clinical manifestations.

The evaluating physician must determine whether diagnostic or examination criteria best describe the impairment of a specific patient. *The physician, in general, should decide which estimate best describes the situation and should use only one approach for each anatomic part.* For instance, a patient with a femoral neck fracture with nonunion, who requires one crutch, should be rated either for use of the crutch or for the nonunion plus the range of motion restriction, whichever is greater.

There may be instances in which elements from both diagnostic and examination approaches will apply to a specific situation. A patient with an acetabular fracture and a sciatic nerve palsy should have estimates made for both the hip joint impairment and the nerve palsy. The estimates for the fracture and the nerve condition would be *combined* (Combined Values Chart, p. 322).

The final lower extremity impairment must not exceed the impairment estimate for amputation of the extremity, 100%, or 40% whole-person impairment.

Fractures in and about joints with degenerative changes should be rated either by using this section and combining (Combined Values Chart, p. 322) the rating for arthritic degeneration or by using the range of motion section. It is recommended that the section providing the greater impairment estimate be used.

Example: A 40-year-old woman had a comminuted midshaft tibial fracture that healed with 2.5 cm (1 inch) of shortening and 10° of varus angulation. The patient was advised of the risks of midshaft tibial osteotomy and lengthening, and she declined surgery.

Impairment: The lower-extremity impairment estimate for the varus angulation is 20% (Table 64, p. 85); the impairment estimate for 2.5 cm of shortening is 8% (Table 35, p. 75). The 25% and 8% lower extremity impairments are *combined* using the Combined Values Chart (p. 322). The lower extremity impairment is 31%, which is a 12% whole-person impairment.

Comment: Impairment due to malunion of a fracture should be estimated according to the diagnosis. The expected muscle weakness or atrophy is included in the diagnosis-related estimates, but shortening is a different impairment.

If there were an associated nerve palsy, which usually does not occur with a fracture, the fracture and nerve palsy impairment percents reflecting impairments of different organ systems, would be *combined* (Combined Values Chart, p. 322), because they involve different organ systems.

Table 64. Impairment Estimates for Certain Lower extremity Impairments.

Region and condition	Whole-person (lower extremity) impairment (%)
Pelvis**	
Pelvic fracture	
Undisplaced, nonarticular, healed, without neurologic deficit or other sign	0
Displaced nonarticular fracture estimate by evaluating shortening and weakness	—
Acetabular fracture: estimate according to range of motion and joint changes	—
Sacroiliac joint fracture	1-3 (2-7)
Ischial bursitis (weaver's bottom) requiring frequent unweighting and limiting of sitting time	3 (7)
Hip	
Total hip replacement; includes endoprosthesis, unipolar or bipolar	
Good result, 85-100 points*	15 (37)
Fair result, 50-84 points*	20 (50)
Poor result, less than 50 points*	30 (75)
Femoral neck fracture, healed in	
Good position	Evaluate according to examination findings
Malunion	12 (30) plus range of motion criteria
Nonunion	15 (37) plus range of motion criteria
Girdlestone arthroplasty Or estimate according to examination findings; use the greater estimate	20 (50)
Trochanteric bursitis (chronic) with abnormal gait	3 (7)
Femoral shaft fracture	
Healed with 10°-14° angulation or malrotation	10 (25)
15°-19°	18 (45)
20°+	+1 (2) per degree up to 25 (62)
Knee	
Patellar subluxation or dislocation with residual instability	3 (7)
Patellar fracture	
Undisplaced, healed	3 (7)
Articular surface displaced more than 3 mm	5 (12)
Displaced with nonunion	7 (17)
Patellectomy	
Partial	3 (7)
Total	9 (22)
Meniscectomy, medial *or* lateral	
Partial	1 (2)
Total	3 (7)
Meniscectomy, medial *and* lateral	
Partial	4 (10)
Total	9 (22)
Cruciate *or* collateral ligament laxity	
Mild	3 (7)
Moderate	7 (17)
Severe	10 (25)
Cruciate *and* collateral ligament laxity	
Moderate	10 (25)
Severe	15 (37)
Plateau fracture	
Undisplaced	2 (5)
Displaced	
5°-9° angulation	5 (12)
10°-19° angulation	10 (25)
20°+ angulation	+1 (2) per degree up to 20 (50)
Supracondylar or intercondylar fracture	
Undisplaced fracture	2 (5)
Displaced fracture	
5°-9° angulation	5 (12)
10°-19° angulation	10 (25)
20°+ angulation	+1 (2) per degree up to 20% (50%)
Total knee replacement including unicondylar replacement	
Good result, 85-100 points*	15 (37)
Fair result, 50-84 points*	20 (50)
Poor result, less than 50 points*	30 (75)
Proximal tibial osteotomy	
Good result	10 (25)
Poor result	Estimate impairment according to examination and arthritic degeneration
Tibial shaft fracture, malalignment of	
10°-14°	8 (20)
15°-19°	12 (30)
20°+	+1 (2) per degree up to 20 (50)

*See Table 65 (p. 87) or Table 66 (p. 88) for point rating system.

**Refer also to section 3.4, p. 131.

Table 64 continued.

Region and Condition	Whole-person (lower extremity) [foot] impairment (%)
Ankle	
Ligamentous instability (based on stress roentgenograms*)	
Mild (2 - 3 mm excess opening)	2 (5) [7]
Moderate (4 - 6 mm)	4 (10) [14]
Severe (>6 mm)	6 (15) [21]
Fracture	
Extra-articular with angulation	
10° - 14°	6 (15) [21]
15° - 19°	10 (25) [35]
20°+	+1 (2) [3] per degree up to 15 (37) [53]
Intra-articular with displacement	8 (20) [28]
Hindfoot	
Fracture	
Extra-articular (calcaneal)	
With varus angulation 10° - 19°	5 (12) [17]
With varus angulation 20°+	0.5 (1) [1] per degree up to 10 (25)
With valgus angulation 10° - 19°	3 (7) [11]
With valgus angulation 20°+	0.5 (2) [1] per degree up to 10 (25%) [35]
Loss of tibia-os calcis angle†	
Angle is 120° - 110°	5 (12) [17]
Angle is 100° - 90°	8 (20) [28]
Angle is less than 90°	+1 (2) [3] per degree up to 15 (37) [54]
Intra-articular fracture with displacement	
Subtalar bone	6 (15) [21]
Talonavicular bone	3 (7) [10]
Calcaneocuboid bone	3 (7) [10]
Midfoot deformity	
Cavus	
Mild	1 (2) [3]
Moderate	3 (7) [10]
"Rocker bottom"	
Mild	2 (5) [7]
Moderate	4 (10) [14]
Severe	8 (20) [28]
Avascular necrosis of the talus	
Without collapse	3 (7) [10]
With collapse	6 (15) [21]

Region and Condition	Whole-person (lower extremity) [foot] impairment (%)
Forefoot deformity	
Metatarsal fracture with loss of weight transfer**	
1st metatarsal	4 (10) [14]
5th metatarsal	2 (5) [7]
Other metatarsal	1 (2) [3]
Metatarsal fracture with plantar angulation and metatarsalgia	
1st metatarsal	4 (10) [14]
5th metatarsal	2 (5) [7]
Other metatarsal	1 (2) [3]

*A stress roentgenogram is an anterior-posterior view taken with a varus or valgus stress applied by a knowledgeable physician.

**Loss of weight transfer is dorsal displacement of a metatarsal head greater than 5mm according to a lateral roentgenogram taken while weight-bearing.

†Estimates in this instance are slightly higher than those for ankylosis, because some movement is preserved. The tibia-os calcis angle is shown in Fig. 57 (p. 91).

Table 65. Rating Hip Replacement Results:*

	No. of points
a. Pain	
None	44
Slight	40
Moderate, occasional	30
Moderate	20
Marked	10
b. Function	
Limp	
None	11
Slight	8
Moderate	5
Severe	0
Supportive device	
None	11
Cane for long walks	7
Cane	5
One crutch	3
Two canes	2
Two crutches	0
Distance walked	
Unlimited	11
Six blocks	8
Three blocks	5
Indoors	2
In bed or chair	0
c. Activities	
Stairs climbing	
Normal	4
Using railing	2
Cannot climb readily	1
Unable to climb	0
Putting on shoes and socks	
With ease	4
With difficulty	2
Unable to do	0
Sitting	
Any chair, 1 hour	4
High chair	2
Unable to sit comfortably	0
Public transportation	
Able to use	1
Unable to use	0
d. Deformity	
Fixed adduction	
<10°	1
≥10°	0
Fixed internal rotation	
<10°	1
≥10°	0
Fixed external rotation	
<10°	1
≥10°	0
Flexion contracture	
<15°	1
≥15°	0
Leg length discrepancy	
<1.5 cm	1
≥1.5 cm	0
e. Range of Motion	
Flexion	
>90°	1
≤90°	0
Abduction	
>15°	1
≤15°	0
Adduction	
>15°	1
≤15°	0
External rotation	
>30°	1
≤30°	0
Internal rotation	
>15°	1
≤15°	0

*Add the points from categories a, b, c, d, and e to determine the total and characterize the result of replacement. Source: modified from refs. 42 and 43.

Table 66. Rating Knee Replacement Results.*

	No. of points
a. Pain	
None	50
Mild or occasional	45
Stairs only	40
Walking and stairs	30
Moderate	
Occasional	20
Continual	10
Severe	0
b. Range of motion	
Add 1 point per 5°	25
c. Stability (maximum movement in any position)	
Anteroposterior	
<5 mm	10
5-9 mm	5
>9 mm	0
Mediolateral	
5°	15
6°-9°	10
10°-14°	5
≥15°	0
Subtotal	
d. Deductions (minus)	
Flexion contracture	
5°-9°	2
10°-15°	5
16°-20°	10
>20°	20
e. Extension lag	
<10°	5
10°-20°	10
>20°	15
f. Alignment	
0°-4°	0
5°-10°	3 points per degree
11°-15°	3 points per degree
>15°	20
Deductions subtotal	—

*The point total for estimating knee replacement results is the sum of the points in categories a, b, and c minus the sum of the points in categories d, e, and f. Modified from ref. 44.

3.2j Skin Loss

Full-thickness skin loss about certain areas in the lower extremity results in significant impairment, as shown in Table 67 (at right), even when the areas are successfully covered with an appropriate form of skin graft.

3.2k Peripheral Nerve Injuries

Peripheral nerve injuries are divided into three components: motor deficits, sensory deficits, and dysesthesia or disordered sensation. Figures 59 and 60 (p. 93) show the sensory and motor nerves of the lower extremity. All estimates listed in Table 68 (p. 89) are for complete motor or sensory loss for the named peripheral nerves. Motor, sensory, and dysesthesia estimates should be *combined*. An impairment estimate for multiple peripheral nerve injuries should not exceed the whole-person impairment estimate for complete loss of a lower extremity (40%). Partial motor loss should be estimated on the basis of strength testing (Section 3.2d, p. 76).

Sensory deficits and dysesthesias are subjective and must be carefully evaluated. Ideally, two examiners should agree. Estimates for peripheral nerve impairments may be combined with those for other types of lower extremity impairments, except those for muscle weakness and atrophy, using the Combined Values Chart (p. 322).

Table 67. Impairments for Skin Loss.

Description	Whole-person (lower extremity) [foot] impairment (%)
Ischial covering that requires frequent unweighting and limits sitting time	5 (12)
Tibial tuberosity covering that limits kneeling	2 (5)
Heel covering that limits standing and walking time	10 (25) [35]
Plantar surface, metatarsal head covering that limits standing and walking time	
First metatarsal	5 (12) [17]
Fifth metatarsal	5 (12) [17]
Chronic osteomyelitis with active drainage	
Of femur	3 (7) [10]
Of tibia	3 (7) [10]
Of foot, requiring periodic redressing and limiting time using footwear	10 (25) [35]

Table 68. Impairments from Nerve Deficits.

	Whole-person (lower extremity) [foot] impairment (%)		
Nerve	**Motor**	**Sensory**	**Dysesthesia**
Femoral	15 (37)	1 (2)	3 (7)
Obturator	3 (7)	0	0
Superior gluteal	25 (62)	0	0
Inferior gluteal	15 (37)	0	0
Lateral femoral cutaneous	0	1 (2)	3 (7)
Sciatic	30 (75)	7 (17)	5 (12)
Common peroneal	15 (42)	2 (5)	2 (5)
Superficial peroneal	0	2 (5)	2 (5)
Sural	0	1 (2)	2 (5)
Medial plantar	2 (5) [7]	2 (5) [7]	2 (5) [7]
Lateral plantar	2 (5) [7]	2 (5) [7]	2 (5) [7]

3.2l Causalgia and Reflex Sympathetic Dystrophy

Causalgia is a burning pain due to injury of a peripheral nerve. Reflex sympathetic dystrophy is a disturbance of the sympathetic nervous system characterized by pain, swelling, stiffness, and discoloration, which may follow a sprain, fracture, or nerve or blood vessel injury.

When these conditions occur in the lower extremity, they should be evaluated as for the upper extremity (Section 3.1k, p. 56).

3.2m Vascular Disorders

Table 69 (below) classifies and provides criteria for impairments due to peripheral vascular disease of the lower extremity. When amputation due to peripheral vascular disease is involved, the impairment due to amputation should be evaluated according to the criteria in this section, and the impairment percent should be *combined* (Combined Values Chart, p. 322), with an appropriate percent based on Table 69.

Table 69. Lower Extremity Impairment Due to Peripheral Vascular Disease.

Class 1: (0%-9% impairment)	**Class 2: (10%-39% impairment)**	**Class 3: (40%-69% impairment)**	**Class 4: (70%-89% impairment)**	**Class 5: (90%-100% impairment)**
The patient experiences neither claudication nor pain at rest;	The patient experiences intermittent claudication on walking at least 100 yards at an average pace;	The patient experiences intermittent claudication on walking as few as 25 yards and no more than 100 yards at average pace;	The patient experiences intermittent claudication on walking less than 25 yards, or the patient experiences intermittent pain at rest;	The patient experiences severe and constant pain at rest;
and	**or**	**or**	**or**	**or**
The patient experiences only transient edema;	There is persistent edema of a moderate degree, incompletely controlled by elastic supports;	There is marked edema that is only partially controlled by elastic supports;	The patient has marked edema that cannot be controlled by elastic supports;	There is vascular damage as evidenced by signs such as amputations at or above the ankles of two extremities, or amputation of all digits of two or more extremities, with evidence of persistent vascular disease or of persistent, widespread, or deep ulceration involving two or more extremities
and	**or**	**or**	**or**	
On physical examination, not more than the following findings are present: loss of pulses; minimal loss of subcutaneous tissue; calcification of arteries as detected by roentgenographic examination; asymptomatic dilation of arteries or of veins, not requiring surgery and not resulting in curtailment of activity	There is vascular damage as evidenced by a sign such as a healed, painless stump of an amputated digit showing evidence of persistent vascular disease, or a healed ulcer	There is vascular damage as evidenced by a sign such as healed amputation of two or more digits of one extremity, with evidence of persisting vascular disease or superficial ulceration	There is vascular damage as evidenced by signs such as an amputation at or above an ankle, or amputation of two or more digits of two extremities with evidence of persistent vascular disease, or persistent widespread or deep ulceration involving one extremity	

Figure 52. Using a Goniometer to Measure Flexion of the Right Hip.

(a) Goniometer is placed at the right hip, and the pelvis is locked in the neutral position by flexing the left hip until the lumbar spine is flat.

(b) Patient flexes the right hip until the anterior superior iliac spine begins to move, when the angle is recorded.

(c) To measure loss of extension of the right hip, the left hip is flexed until the lumbar spine is flat on the examining table, as determined by the examiner's hand, which is placed between the lumbar spine and table surface. The right thigh should rest flat on the table; any right hip flexion is recorded as a flexion contracture.

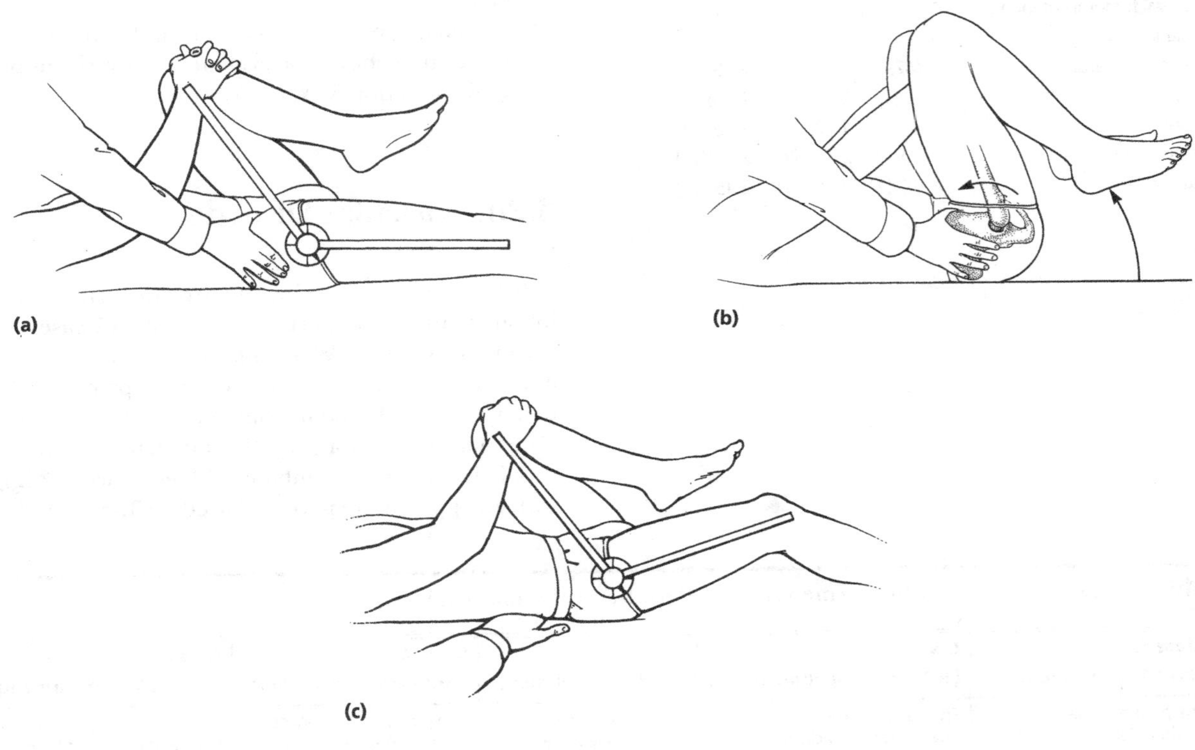

Figure 53. Neutral Position (a), Abduction (b), and Adduction (c) of Right Hip.
The patient is supine on a flat surface.

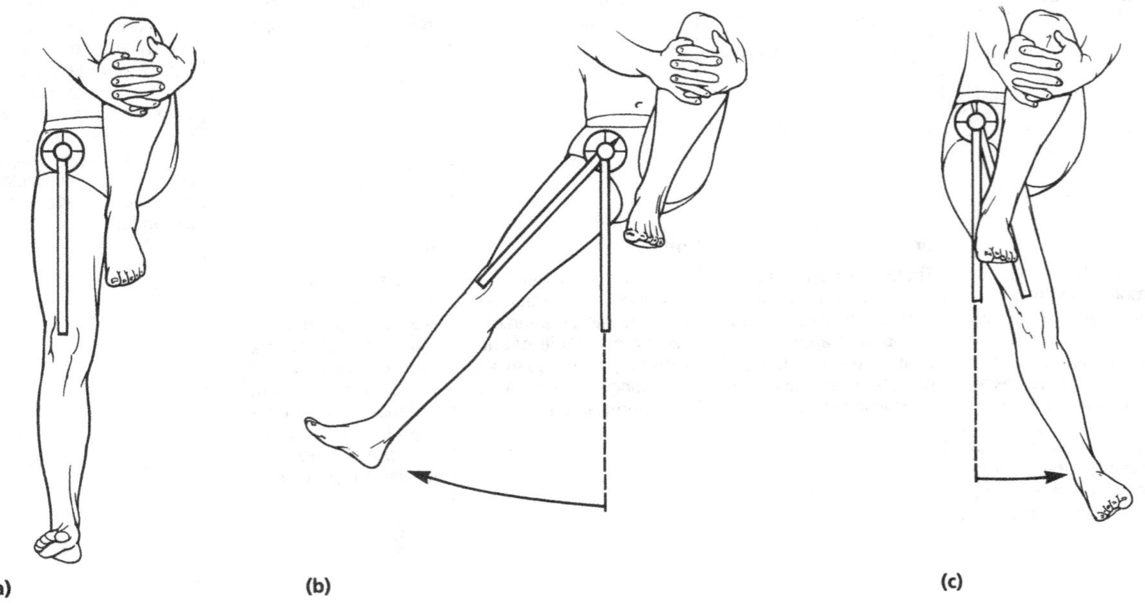

Figure 54. Measuring Internal and External Hip Rotation.*

The patient is prone on a flat surface, and the knee is flexed 90°. One part of the goniometer is parallel to the flat surface, and the other is along the tibia. The examiner while testing should place the hand on the knee to determine if there is significant laxity of the knee joint.

*Source: Adapted from American Orthopaedic Association. Manual of Orthopedic Surgery. Rosemont, Ill.; 1966.

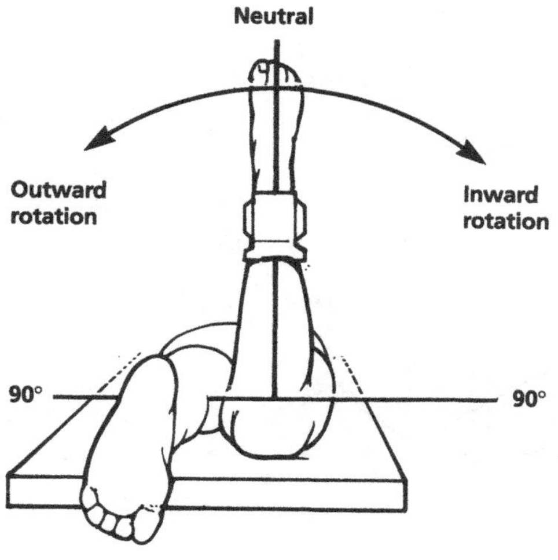

Figure 55. Measuring Knee Flexion.

(a) The patient is supine and the goniometer is next to the knee joint; one goniometer arm is parallel to the lower leg, and the other is parallel to the femur. Any deviation from 0° is recorded.

(b) Patient exerts maximum effort to flex the knee, and the angle subtended by the maximum arc of motion is read.

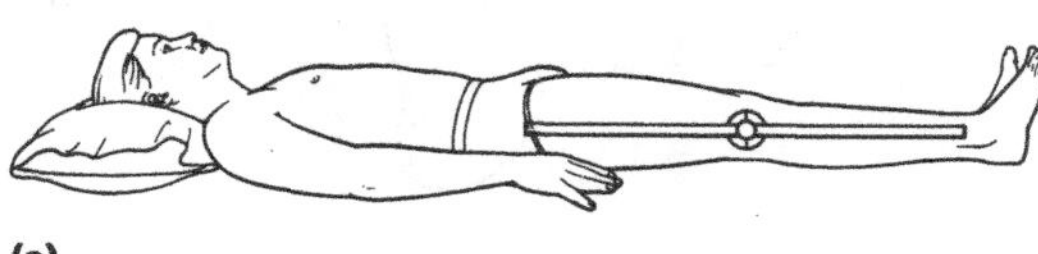

(a)

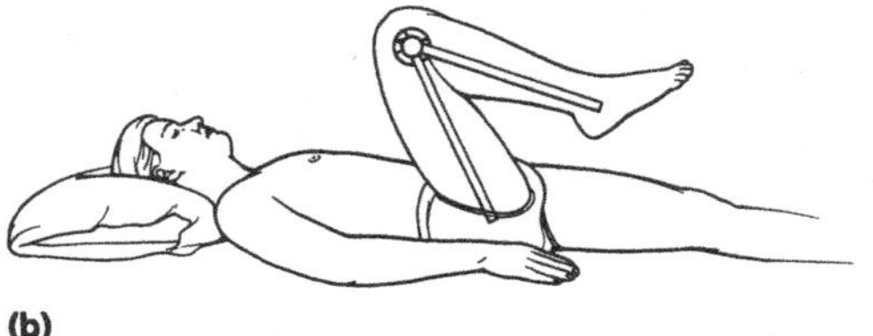

(b)

Figure 56. Measuring Foot Dorsiflexion and Plantar Flexion. The goniometer's pivot is centered over the ankle, and one arm parallels the tibia. The examiner reads the angles subtending the maximum arcs of motion for dorsiflexion and plantar flexion.

The test is repeated with the knee flexed to 45°. The averages of the maximum angles represent dorsiflexion and plantar flexion ranges of motion.

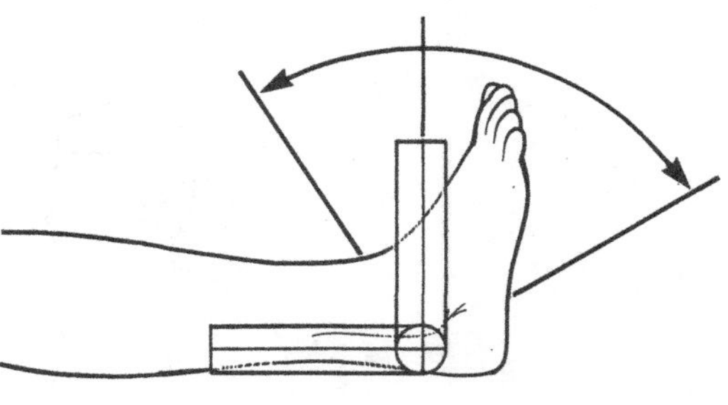

Figure 57. Tibia-Os Calcis Angle.*

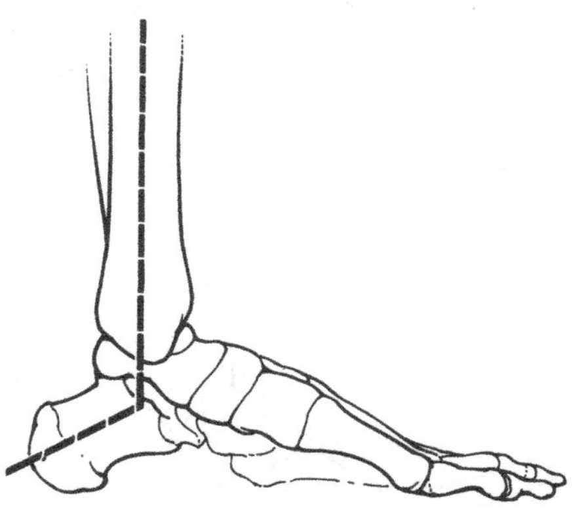

*The tibia-os calcis angle is the angle between the longitudinal axis of the os calcis and the vertical tibia, as shown by this drawing based on a lateral roentgenogram of the foot and ankle in the *neutral* position.

Figure 58. Evaluating the Range of Motion of a Toe, the Metatarsophalangeal (MTP) Joint of the Great Toe.

(a) The patient is seated in the position for evaluating the toes. The knee is flexed to 45° and the foot and MTP joint are in the neutral position.

(b) Extension: The goniometer is under the MTP joint, and its angle is read as a baseline. The patient extends (dorsiflexes) the toe maximally, and the angle subtending the maximum arc of motion is read; the baseline angle is subtracted.

(c) Flexion: The goniometer is placed over the MTP joint. The baseline angle is read. The patient plantar flexes the MTP joint maximally. The angle subtending the maximum arc of motion is read, and the baseline angle is subtracted.

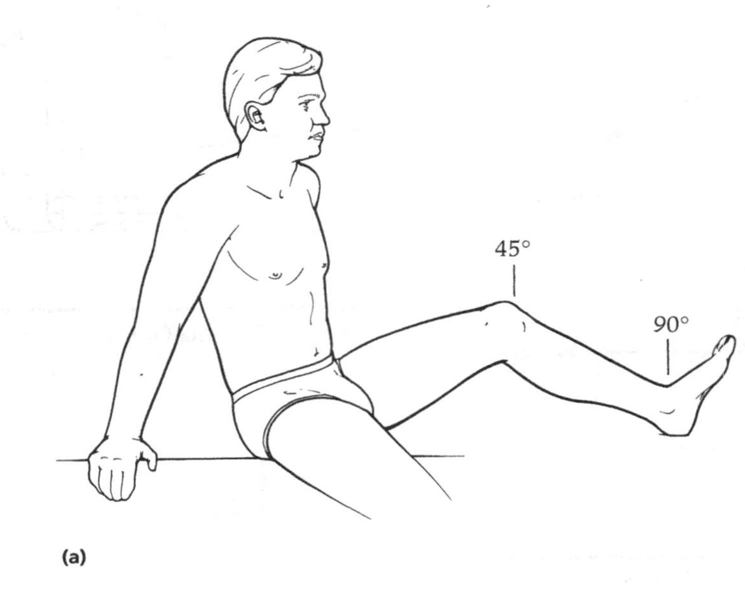

(a)

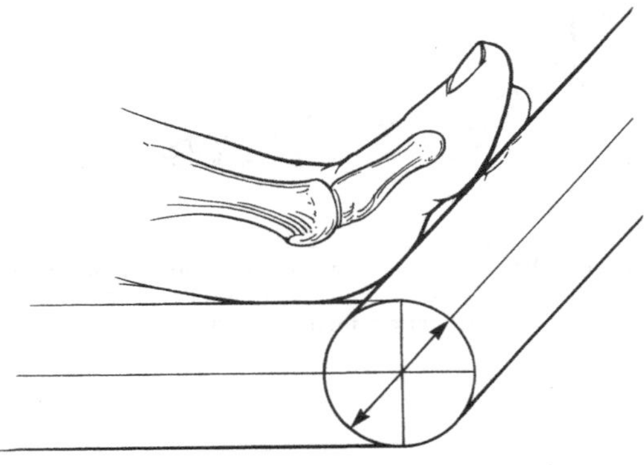

(b)

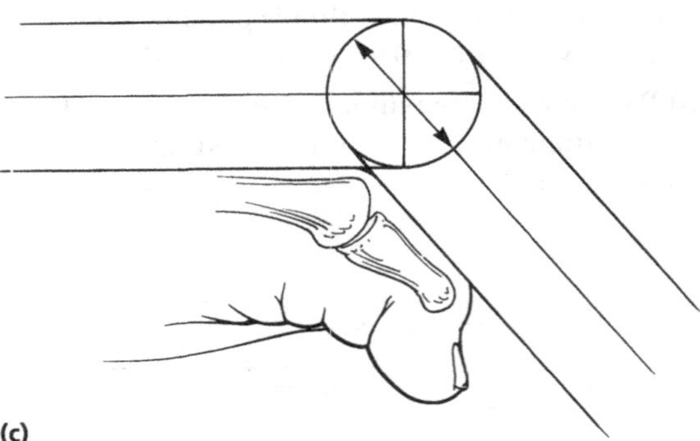

(c)

Figure 59. Sensory Nerves of the Lower Extremity and Their Roots of Origin.

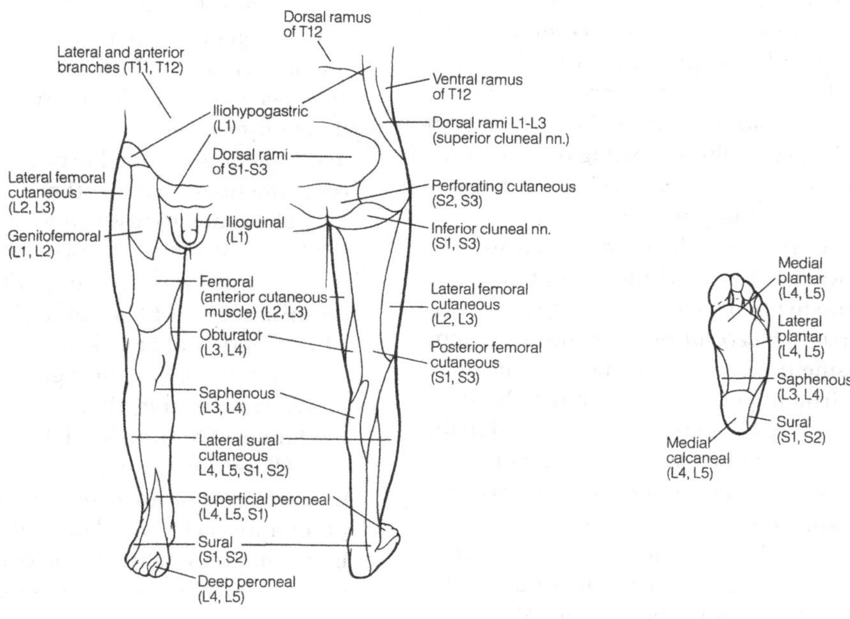

Figure 60. Motor Innervation of the Lower Extremity.

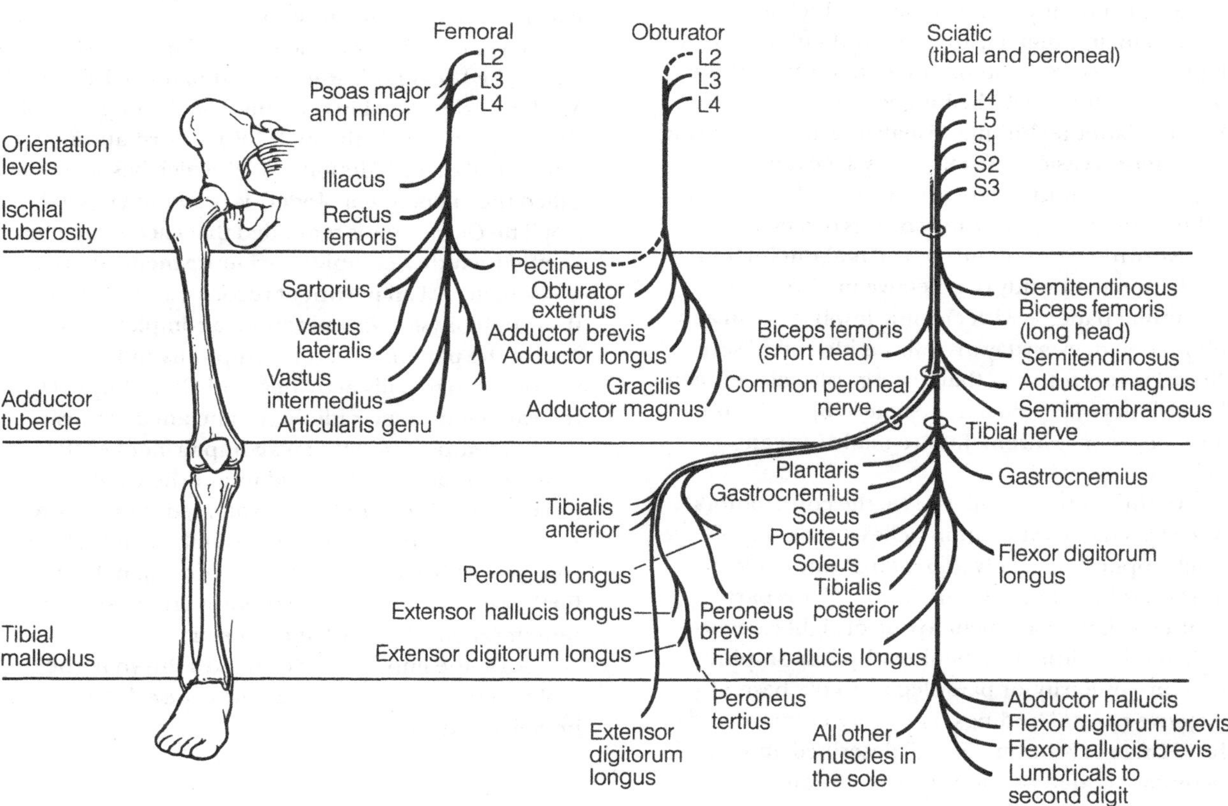

3.3 The Spine

Symptoms related to the back and spine are among the most common of adults' everyday complaints. In most instances, people accept and tolerate the symptoms as one of the consequences of growing older, making minor concessions in activity. When the symptoms follow an injury or illness, sorting out the injury or illness component from the age-related component may be difficult or impossible.

One of the purposes of the *Guides* is to lead to similar results when different clinicians evaluate illnesses and impairments. For evaluating spine impairments, past *Guides* editions have used a system based on assessing the degree of spine motion and assigning impairment percents according to limitations of motion. Impairment percents related to the range of motion were to be combined with percents based on diagnoses or therapeutic approaches and neurologic impairments.

One concern with the range of motion system has been that in applying it, other clinical data and diagnostic information tend to be ignored. Also, some physicians are concerned about the accuracy and reproducibility of mobility measurements, while others believe the system fails to account for the effects of aging.

Spine mobility measurements, which are carried out with inclinometers, are more difficult to perform than are measurements of ranges of motion of the extremities, for which the hinged goniometer is used. With the latter technique, visualizing and measuring movement is easier, one extremity's movement may be checked against that of the other, and the patient's willingness to cooperate may be less of a factor.

Notwithstanding the concerns about inclinometers, a recent study of objective methods for examining patients with chronic low-back pain and self-reported, everyday disabilities identified seven clinical measurements that distinguish well between the patients with pain and normal subjects.[68] Four of the seven measurements are made with an inclinometer.

In this edition of the *Guides*, the contributors have elected to use two approaches. One component, which applies especially to patients' traumatic injuries, is called the "Injury Model." This part involves assigning a patient to one of eight categories, such as minor injury, radiculopathy, loss of spine structure integrity, or paraplegia, on the basis of objective clinical findings. The other component is the "Range of Motion Model," described above and recommended in previous *Guides* editions.

This approach to the evaluation of spine impairments was developed with the advice of an ad hoc committee of authorities knowledgeable about the musculoskeletal system, orthopedic surgery, neurosurgery, internal medicine, rehabilitation, impairment evaluation, and medical science. It is acknowledged that the approach is different from that of previous *Guides* editions, and that future developments may lead to refinement or to a different recommendation altogether.

The evaluator assessing the spine should use the Injury Model, if the patient's condition is one of those listed in Table 70 (p. 108). That model, for instance, would be applicable to a patient with a herniated lumbar disk and evidence of nerve root irritation. If none of the eight categories of the Injury Model is applicable, then the evaluator should use the Range of Motion Model.

All persons evaluating impairments according to *Guides* criteria are cautioned that either one *or* the other approach should be used in making the final impairment estimate. If one component were used according to *Guides* recommendations, then a final impairment estimate using the other component usually would not be pertinent or germane. However, if disagreement exists about the category of the Injury Model in which a patient's impairment belongs, then the Range of Motion Model may be applied to provide evidence on the question.

The newer Injury Model, which may also be called the "Diagnosis-Related Estimates (DRE) Model," is described in sections 3.3a through 3.3i of this chapter (pp. 95 through 106). Information on using the Range of Motion Model, which has also been called the "Functional Model," is presented in section 3.3j. The *Guides* user is reminded that each evaluation should include a complete, accurate medical history and a review of all pertinent records, a careful and thorough physical examination, a complete description of the patient's current symptoms and their relationship to daily activities, and all findings of relevant laboratory, radiologic, and ancillary tests.

It is emphasized that if an impairment evaluation is to be accepted as valid under the *Guides* criteria, the impairment being evaluated should be a *permanent* one, that is, one that is stable, unlikely to change within the next year, and not amenable to further medical or surgical therapy (refer to definition in *Guides* Chapter 1 and Glossary).

All spine impairment estimates shown in the tables of this section are estimates of *whole-person* impairments.

3.3a The Spine History

Much of the historical part of the impairment evaluation should be based on the patient's own statements rather than on secondhand information. While the medical history that the physician gathers should consider objective data from others, the physician should be cautious about using *only* information from others, especially subjective information. It is not appropriate to question the patient's integrity. If information from the patient does not make sense, or there are inconsistencies in the history, the physician should note this and describe the discrepancies in the record.

The medical history of the patient's spine-related symptoms and complaints must describe the chief complaint and the pain, numbness, weakness, anatomic location, frequency, and duration, then describe specifically how the condition interferes with daily activities (Fig. 61, p. 96). The physician should elicit the facts about when the condition started, the circumstances, the relationship to any previous spine problems, any precipitating events or factors, and the impact of the problem on daily activities.

The history should use the patient's description in his or her own words as to how the symptoms developed, the cause, the response to treatment, and the results of special studies that have been performed. The physician should review the roentgenograms personally, or report the roentgenographic findings as being those of another reviewer. It is helpful to record the patient's future plans, should the present symptoms and limitations not improve. A review of systems and of the medical history are needed to provide potentially useful information and to identify any complicating problems and requirements for diagnosis or care.

3.3b The Spine Examination

Many aspects of the physical examination are covered in other parts of the *Guides*. Much of the information pertaining to the examination for spine injury and impairment is neurologic in nature; thus, the physician must have a good grasp of neurologic principles and understand the material covered in the *Guides* chapter on the nervous system (p. 139) and in Section 3.1k (p. 46) of this chapter. Guided by the history (Fig. 61, p. 96), the physician should focus attention on spine-related physical findings, such as motor abilities, reflexes, muscle atrophy, anal tone, and the need for assistive devices.

Findings of atrophy should be related to possible explanations for the abnormality other than spine impairment, for instance, previous joint surgery or hypertrophy of the contralateral side from overuse. Other objective findings may be present relating to the motor and sensory systems, ranges of motion, and sciatic nerve tension. Examination of the vascular system and a follow-up of any possibly significant information from the history and physical examination will prepare the physician to make reasonable recommendations.

The physician should note any physical findings that are not consistent with the medical history. The physician should identify any information based on the patient's verbal responses or interpretation and not confuse it with objective clinical findings.

It is difficult to separate the cervical, thoracic, lumbar, and sacral spine regions functionally, because the signs related to the different regions commonly overlap. Upper lumbar spine impairments tend to behave more like those of the thoracic region than those of the lower lumber region, and the involved nerve plexuses expand the effects from the different levels. For instance, the brachial plexus is made up of nerve trunks from both the cervical and the upper thoracic regions, and the sciatic nerve includes components from both the lower lumbar and the sacral regions.

With the Injury or DRE Model, the main spine regions are termed the cervicothoracic, thoracolumbar, and lumbosacral regions. With this model, the cervicothoracic spine is considered to comprise 35% of total body function, the thoracolumbar spine 20%, and the lumbosacral spine 75%. Under the Range of Motion or Functional Model, the main regions are called the cervical, thoracic, and lumbar regions. With that model, the cervical spine is considered to be involved with 80% of the individual's functioning, the thoracic spine is involved with 40%, and the lumbosacral spine is involved with 90%. However, the structural, neurologic, vascular, and other activities mediated by the spine regions overlap and are difficult to separate.

With both the Injury Model and the Range of Motion Model, the normal percent of function of the spine or the whole person is 100%.

For the purposes of this book, the cervical region may be considered to represent the cervicothoracic region, the thoracic region to represent the thoracolumbar region, and the lumbar region to represent the lumbosacral region.

Figure 61. History of Spine Complaint.

Name:____________________ Soc. Sec. No.: ________________ Date: __________

1. History of impairment or injury

Describe all symptoms, location, frequency of occurrence, duration, quality with particular attention to time and circumstances of onset, course of condition, treatment, treatment response; note presence of pain, numbness, weakness, stiffness:

2. Condition limits the patient or interferes with which daily activities?

List the activities. What activities has the patient reduced or given up? Describe them:

3. Patient's perceptions

a. How long at one time and over an 8-hour period can the patient do the following without serious discomfort? (Express in terms of half-hours or hours and note the unit used.)

Sit ________________ Walk ________________

Stand ________________

b. How many pounds can the patient lift at frequent intervals? ________________

Occasionally? ________________

4. Present symptoms

a. Starting date of present symptoms ________________.

b. How long have symptoms been the same? If they are changing, describe how.

c. Previous back or neck problems or surgeries (give dates):

1. ________________
2. ________________
3. ________________
4. ________________

d. Special tests or procedures:

Type	Date	Results

e. What exercises does the patient usually do to stay physically fit or "in shape?"

Type	Duration	To what heart rate minimum?	Freq./wk.

f. Usual daily activities and postures (check those that apply):

Sit __________ Walk __________

Stand __________ Lift __________ Max. no. lb. __________

Other (describe) __________

5. Patient's understanding of reason for this impairment evaluation:

History taken by: __________
(print name)

Evaluation of Sciatic Nerve Tension Signs

Sciatic nerve tension signs are important indicators of acute compression of the lumbosacral nerve roots. However, in chronic nerve root compression due to spinal stenosis, tension signs may be absent or not obvious. Though different methods of evaluating sciatic tension have been recommended, variations of the straight-leg-raising test are the most common.

Research indicates that maximum excursion of nerve roots in the region of the nerve root foramina occurs at an angle of the leg with the trunk in the range of 20° to 70°.[62] However, this may vary widely according to the patient's body position and duration of symptoms. Sciatic nerve tension signs are most reliable when pain elicited by the procedure is in a focal neurologic distribution.

With time, patients' spine-related symptoms usually improve, and their patterns of discomfort tend to migrate proximally and be elicited at the extremes of leg raising. The best means of verifying straight leg raising related to disk herniation is straight leg raising of the asymptomatic limb, which produces increased sciatic discomfort in the limb with symptoms. There are other means of validating straight leg raising, for instance, by comparing it with the patient's response to equivalent sciatic tension while sitting and extending the knee.[69]

Results of the straight-leg raising test can be further validated by recording the response of the supine patient to gentle dorsiflexion and plantar flexion of the ankle, and to internal and external rotation of the hip when the straightened leg is raised to the point where symptoms begin. Normally, ankle dorsiflexion and hip internal rotation increase the pain, and ankle plantar flexion and hip external rotation decrease the complaints.[62]

Loss of Motion Segment Integrity

A motion segment of the spine is defined as two adjacent vertebrae, an intercalated disk, and the vertebral facet joints. Loss of motion segment or structural integrity is defined as abnormal back-and-forth motion (translation) or abnormal angular motion of a motion segment with respect to an adjacent motion segment.

The loss of integrity is defined as an anteroposterior motion or slipping of one vertebra over another greater than 3.5 mm for a cervical vertebra or greater than 5 mm for a vertebra in the thoracic or lumbar spine (Fig. 62, at right); or a difference in the angular motion of two adjacent motion segments greater than 11° in response to spine flexion and extension (Fig. 63, at right). Motion of the spine segments is evaluated with flexion and extension roentgenograms. Loss of integrity of the lumbosacral joint is defined as an angular motion between L-5 and S-1 that is 15° greater than the motion at the L-4, L-5 level.

Abnormal motion or translation is depicted in Fig. 62 (below). In that figure, if line A + line B > 5 mm, there is more than 5 mm of translation, which meets the criterion of loss of segmental integrity. The criterion for the cervical spine is that the translation is greater than 3.5 mm.

Figure 62. Loss of Motion Segment Integrity: Translation.*

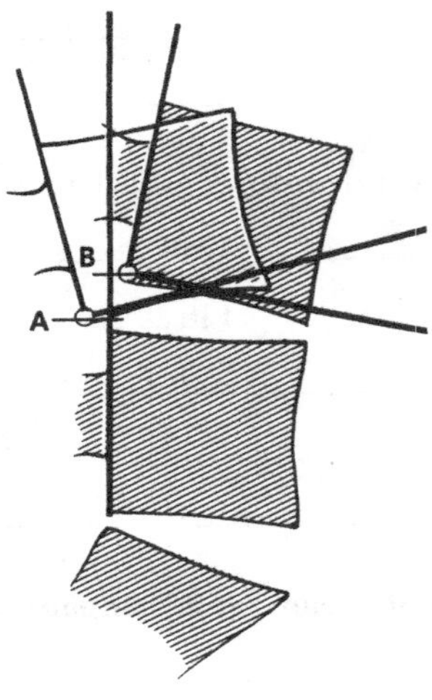

*Source: ref 64.

Figure 63. Loss of Motion Segment Integrity: Angular Motion.*

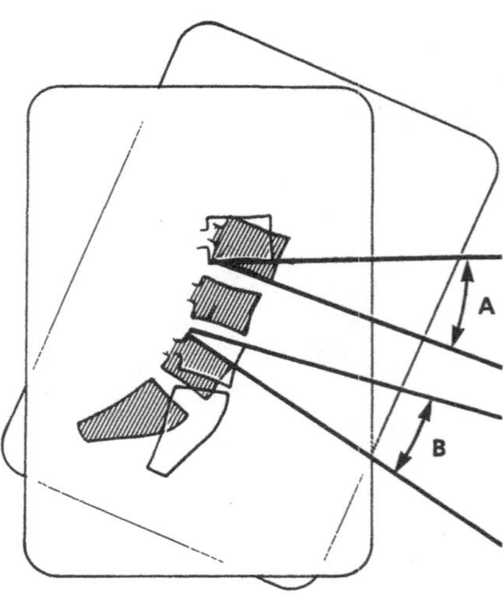

*Source: ref 64.

Figure 63 (p. 98) illustrates the measurements for angular motion. If the difference in motion, measured by flexion and extension films, between two angles (such as angles A and B in Fig. 63) is more than 15° at the lumbosacral joint or more than 11° at any other joint, there is loss of structural integrity.

The importance of careful and accurate roentgenographic studies cannot be overemphasized.

Special Studies

The patient may have undergone roentgenographic, dye, electromyographic or electrodiagnostic, cystometric, or other types of studies. The examining physician should determine when, where, and by whom the studies were made, the findings, and who interpreted them. These records should be summarized in the history form (Fig. 61, p. 96) and included with the Report of Medical Evaluation (p. 11).

Differentiators

In using the Injury Model, the physician or examiner may use certain clinical procedures or determinations in placing the patient's impairment in the proper category. These "differentiators" are described in Table 71 (p. 109) and are listed below.

No differentiator is required to place a patient in any impairment category. However, if a differentiator is present, it provides important evidence as to the category in which the patient belongs.

Impairment Category Differentiators

- Guarding
- Loss of reflex(es)
- Decreased muscle circumference
- Electrodiagnosis
- Lateral motion roentgenograms
- Loss of bowel or bladder control
- Bladder studies
- Range of Motion Model

If the physician cannot decide into which DRE category the patient belongs, the physician may refer to and use the Range of Motion Model, which is described in Section 3.3j (p. 113). Using the procedures of that model, the physician combines an impairment percent based on the patient's diagnosis with a percent based on the patient's spine motion impairment and a percent based on neurologic impairment, if it is present. The physician uses the estimate determined with the Range of Motion Model to decide placement within one of the DRE categories. The proper DRE category is the one having the impairment percent that is closest to the impairment percent determined with the Range of Motion Model.

Structural Inclusions

Certain spine fracture patterns may lead to significant impairment and yet not demonstrate any of the findings involving the differentiators. Therefore, with the Injury Model, "structural inclusions" are included in some of the DRE categories. If the patient has a condition that meets the definition of a category that includes a structural inclusion, the physician need not determine if the other criteria for that category are present.

If the patient demonstrates the structural inclusions of two categories, the physician should place the patient in the category with the higher impairment percent.

3.3c Impressions, Diagnoses, and Impairment Estimates

Impressions should be expressed in logical fashion, progressing from symptoms, such as "back and leg pain," to a documented diagnosis that may or may not be remediable, such as "L5 nerve root compression due to a herniated disk between L4 and L5."

Impairment estimates are based on the history, objective findings and data, impression, and any other information collected during the evaluation. The physician's report should describe and explain any qualifications or inconsistencies that may be present (Report of Medical Evaluation, p. 11). The impairment evaluation report may consider relevant factors, such as the patient's literacy, general capability, and overall health.

3.3d Evaluating Impairments: The Injury or Diagnosis-related Estimates Model

The Injury Model relies not only on the medical history and physical examination, but also on medical data other than those that relate to the range of motion.

What is called osteoarthritis of the spine is due more to increments of age than to injury or illness, while similar structural changes in the hip or glenohumeral joint are more likely to be injury related. For example, roentgenographic evidence of aging changes in the spine, called osteoarthritis, are found in 40% of people by age 35 years,[67] and there is a poor correlation with symptoms, while roentgenographic evidence of osteoarthritic changes of the hip are found in 5% to 7% of 70-year-olds, in whom the correlation with acute injury is greater.

The Injury Model attempts to document physiologic and structural impairments relating to insults other than common developmental findings, such as (1) spondylolysis, found normally in 7% of adults; (2) spondylolisthesis, found in 3%; (3) herniated disk without radiculopathy, found in more than 30% of individuals by age 40 years[53, 62, 71]; and (4) aging changes, common in 40% of adults after age 35 years.[67]

The Injury Model relies especially on evidence of neurologic deficits and uncommon, adverse structural changes, such as fractures, dislocations, and loss of motion segment integrity. Under this model, DREs are differentiated according to clinical findings that are verifiable using standard medical procedures.

With the Injury Model, surgery to treat an impairment does not modify the original impairment estimate, which remains the same in spite of any changes in signs or symptoms that may follow the surgery and irrespective of whether the patient has a favorable or unfavorable response to treatment.

3.3e General Approach and Directions

The medical history, physical examination, and clinical workup described in Sections 3.3a through 3.3c will guide the examiner to the appropriate impairment category. Is there radiculopathy of the lumbosacral spine? This impairment is in lumbosacral impairment category III (Table 72, p. 110). Loss of motion segment or structural integrity of the lumbosacral spine is in category IV. Impairment due to a vertebral body fracture with both radiculopathy and instability would be in category III, IV, or V (Table 70, p. 108), and a vertebral body fracture without either characteristic would be in category II, III, or IV. Categories and tables are provided for the cervicothoracic (Table 73, p. 110), thoracolumbar (Table 74, p. 111), and lumbosacral (Table 72, p. 110) regions.

The physician should start with Table 70 (p. 108) as a guide toward the appropriate category for the spine impairment. A series of differentiators (Table 71, p. 109) describes clinical criteria that correlate with serious physiologic dysfunction or structural change, which the physician should use to help define the patient's impairment. The dysfunctions include documentable neurologic compromise of the limbs (Table 71, p. 109, differentiators 2, 3, and 4) or of bowel or bladder function (Table 71, differentiators 6 and 7) and documentable loss of normal spine motion segment integrity (Table 71, differentiator 5; Figs. 62 and 63, p. 98). Adverse conditions are possible for each spine segment or region, and appropriate DREs are given for all of the regions.

In the Injury Model, the lumbosacral spine segment is considered to represent 75% of total body function; the cervicothoracic spine is considered to represent 35% of total body function; and the thoracolumbar spine is considered to represent 20% of total body function. Thus, the maximum whole-person spine impairments are 75% for the lumbosacral spine and, *without long-tract signs*, 35% for the cervicothoracic spine and 20% for the thoracolumbar spine.

Having a whole-person impairment estimate greater than 35% for the cervicothoracic spine (Table 73, p. 110) or an estimate greater than 20% for the thoracolumbar spine (Table 74, p. 111) depends on the existence of documentable long-tract nervous system signs of bowel and bladder or lower-extremity impairment. If these signs or differentiators, which are explained in Table 71 (p. 109), are present, the examiner may combine an appropriate long-tract impairment percent with the percent for the specific DRE category. Tables 73 and 74 (pp. 110 and 111) explain further the combining of DRE category percents with percents related to long-tract signs.

Long-tract-sign-related percents are combined only with cervicothoracic and thoracolumbar spine impairments.

To express a spine impairment and a bladder impairment, or any other combination of organ system impairments, as an impairment of the whole person, the whole-person impairment estimates for the respective organ systems should be *combined* using the Combined Values Chart (p. 322).

Spine-related complaints in category II involve mild to moderately impaired spine function but are considered to be minor impairments. Categories III through VIII relate to specific, documentable findings more serious than those that most people develop without injuries or illnesses and include radiculopathy, loss of motion segment integrity, potentially unstable vertebral body fractures, dislocations, multilevel neurologic dysfunction, and severe neurologic losses. In the last category are the cauda equina-like syndromes associated with loss of lower-limb function, bowel and bladder dysfunction, and paraplegia.

3.3f Specific Procedures and Directions

1. Take a careful history (Fig. 61, p. 96) from the patient, perform a thorough medical examination, and review all of the pertinent records. This will provide sufficient information for an initial impression about the presence of radiculopathy, fracture, loss of structural integrity, and severe loss of strength in the lower extremities with or without bowel and bladder derangement.

2. Review special studies. Doing so will raise or lower the suspicion of radiculopathy, help estimate the potential for meeting criteria for loss of motion segment integrity, and help estimate the possibility spine impairment is affecting the extremities, bowel, and bladder. Table 71 (p. 109) lists and explains the clinical findings that differentiate the impairment categories.

3. Select the region that is primarily involved, that is, the lumbosacral, thoracolumbar, or cervicothoracic spine region (Tables 72, 73, and 74, pp. 110 and 111), and identify the patient's most serious objective findings. Refer to the clinical differentiators if necessary (Table 71), especially to differentiators 4, 5, and 7, which may provide objective clinical information.

If the criteria of one impairment category cannot be met, then compare the findings in the patient with the criteria of other categories. If the Injury Model is not applicable, refer to and use the Range of Motion Model (Section 3.3j, p. 113). If an organ system other than the spine and musculoskeletal system is seriously involved, consult the *Guides* chapter and the criteria in it referring to that system and determine the whole-person impairment.

4. Consider the permanency of the impairment, referring to *Guides* Chapter 1 and the Glossary as needed. If the impairment is resolving, changing, unstable, or expected to change significantly within 12 months, it is *not* a permanent impairment, and it should not be described as one under *Guides* criteria.

5. If one spine region is primarily involved, then determine the spine-related whole-person impairment using the impairment table referring to that region.

6. If the physician cannot place the patient into an impairment category, or if disagreement exists about which of two or three categories to use for the patient, the physician should use the Range of Motion Model as a differentiator, as explained in Section 3.3b (p. 99, "Differentiators").

If spine motion examinations under the Range of Motion Model do not meet validity standards, then only a percent in Table 75 (p. 113), which provides estimates based on diagnoses under the Range of Motion Model, should be used. If no diagnosis in Table 75 is applicable, the Range of Motion Model should not be used. Instead, the patient should be placed in the lowest of the DRE categories in question.

When the Range of Motion Model is used as a differentiator, the impairment percent assigned to the patient under the Injury Model should not be lower than that of the lowest category of the Injury Model in question nor higher than that of the highest category in question.

7. If there is impairment of the cervicothoracic or thoracolumbar region and if long-tract signs are present, consider combining another impairment percent from the involved region that reflects the long-tract signs.

8. If more than one spine region is impaired, determine the impairment of the other region(s). *Combine* the regional impairments using the Combined Values Chart (p. 322) to express the patient's total spine impairment.

9. From historical information and previously compiled medical data, determine if there was a preexisting impairment. If the previously compiled data can be verified as being accurate, they may be used in apportionment (see Glossary). The percent based on the previous findings would be subtracted from the percent based on the current findings.

10. Use the report form on spine impairment (Fig. 80, p. 135) and the standard *Guides* Report of Medical Evaluation (p. 11) to describe the evaluation findings and indicate the patient's whole-person impairment.

3.3g Lumbosacral Spine Impairment

Tables 70 and 72 (pp. 108 and 110) list commonly encountered impairments of the lumbosacral spine, and the paragraphs below describe their characteristics. The impairments are described as diagnosis-related estimates (DREs) and are in categories. The whole-person impairment percents based on the categories designated I through VIII may be used in conjunction with impairment estimates for other organ systems.

DRE Lumbosacral Category I: Complaints or Symptoms

Description and Verification: The patient has no significant clinical findings, no muscle guarding or history of guarding, no documentable neurologic impairment, no significant loss of structural integrity on lateral flexion and extension roentgenograms, and no indication of impairment related to injury or illness.

Structural Inclusions: None.

Impairment: 0% whole-person impairment.

DRE Lumbosacral Category II: Minor Impairment

Description and Verification: The clinical history and examination findings are compatible with a specific injury or illness. The findings may include significant intermittent or continuous muscle guarding that has been observed and documented by a physician, nonuniform loss of range of motion (dysmetria, differentiator 1, Table 71, p. 109), or nonverifiable radicular complaints. There is *no* objective sign of radiculopathy and *no* loss of structural integrity. See Table 71, differentiator 1 (p. 109).

Structural Inclusions: (1) Less than 25% compression of one vertebral body; (2) posterior element fracture *without* dislocation (not developmental spondylolysis); the fracture is healed, and there is no loss of motion segment integrity.

A spinous or transverse process fracture with displacement without a vertebral body fracture is a category II impairment because it does not disrupt the spinal canal.

Impairment: 5% whole-person impairment.

DRE Lumbosacral Category III: Radiculopathy

Description and Verification: The patient has significant signs of radiculopathy, such as loss of relevant reflex(es), or measured unilateral atrophy of greater than 2 cm above or below the knee, compared to measurements on the contralateral side at the same location. The impairment may be verified by electrodiagnostic findings. See Table 71, p. 109, differentiators 2, 3, and 4.

Structural Inclusions: (1) 25% to 50% compression of one vertebral body; (2) posterior element fracture, but *not* fracture of transverse or spinous process, *with* displacement disrupting the spinal canal, healed without loss of structural integrity. Radiculopathy may or may not be present.

Differentiation from congenital and developmental conditions may be accomplished by examining preinjury roentgenograms or a bone scan performed after onset of the condition.

Impairment: 10% whole-person impairment.

DRE Lumbosacral Category IV: Loss of Motion Segment Integrity

Description and Verification: The patient has loss of motion segment integrity (differentiator 5, Table 71, p. 109). Loss of motion segment or structural integrity is defined as at least 5 mm of translation of one vertebra on another, or angular motion at the involved motion segment that is 11° more than that at an adjacent motion segment (Figs. 62 and 63, p. 98). Loss of structural integrity at the lumbosacral joint is defined as at least 15° more angular motion than at the L4 and L5 motion segment.

A documented history of muscle guarding and pain is present. Neurologic abnormalities need not be present. If they are present, the examiner should consider using category V.

Structural Inclusions: (1) Greater than 50% compression of one vertebral body without residual neurologic compromise; (2) multilevel spine segment structural compromise, as with fractures or dislocations, without residual neurologic motor compromise.

Impairment: 20% whole-person impairment.

DRE Lumbosacral Category V: Radiculopathy and Loss of Motion Segment Integrity

Description and Verification: The patient meets the criteria of DRE lumbosacral category III and DRE lumbosacral category IV, that is, both radiculopathy and loss of motion segment integrity are present (Table 71, differentiators 2, 3, 4, and 5, p. 109). Significant lower-extremity impairment is indicated by atrophy or loss of reflex(es), numbness with an anatomic basis, or electromyographic findings as in lumbosacral category III *and* loss of spine motion segment integrity as in lumbosacral category IV.

Structural Inclusions: Structural compromise is present, as is documented neurologic or motor compromise.

Impairment: 25% whole-person impairment.

DRE Lumbosacral Category VI: Cauda Equina-like Syndrome Without Bowel or Bladder Signs

Description and Verification: Patients in this category have a cauda equina-like syndrome with objectively demonstrated, permanent, partial loss of lower-extremity function bilaterally. They may or may not have loss of motion segment integrity. They do *not* have objectively demonstrated bowel or bladder impairment.

Structural Inclusion: None.

Impairment: 40% whole-person impairment.

DRE Lumbosacral Category VII: Cauda Equina Syndrome with Bowel or Bladder Impairment

Description and Verification: Cauda equina-like syndrome as defined in category VI is present, *and* the patient has bowel and bladder involvement requiring an assistive device. Evidence from electromyography or other neurologic test or cystometrogram may be present, indicating spinal nerve compression.

Structural Inclusions: None.

Impairment: 60% whole-person impairment.

DRE Lumbosacral Category VIII: Paraplegia, Total Loss of Lumbosacral Spinal Cord Function

Description and Verification: The patient has complete or nearly complete paraplegia because of neural compression in the lumbar spine region.

Structural Inclusions: None.

Impairment: 75% whole-person impairment.

Example 1: A 24-year-old man hurt his back while lifting a large, heavy box. He described the pain as being in the lumbosacral area. The physician's examination disclosed no positive findings. The man was treated with an analgesic.

Five months later, the physician was asked to evaluate the man's clinical status. The man had no symptoms. A physical examination disclosed numbness of an area of one leg not along the distribution of a nerve. A straight-leg-raising test was normal. No other positive finding was present.

Impairment: Lumbosacral category I, 0% whole-person impairment.

Example 2: A 45-year-old woman had onset of back and right-leg pain immediately after being in a crash. She had a history of mild intermittent back pain but denied ever having had leg pain. Roentgenograms taken in the emergency room on the day of the crash and repeated at a later clinic visit showed significant slipping of L4 on L5 that was measured at 7 mm. Examination of roentgenograms taken years earlier in an orthopedist's office demonstrated significant spondylolisthesis between L4 and L5.

Conservative treatment of the woman's symptoms was ineffective, and she developed signs of a radiculopathy on the right side, with diminished reflexes and a positive straight-leg-raising test. A magnetic resonance image showed a herniated nucleus pulposus at L4.

The woman underwent an operation for disk removal and one-level spine fusion. She did well after the operation, her signs and symptoms receded, and she resumed full daily activities. Ten months after the injury, when her condition was stable, the physician evaluated her condition.

Impairment: Lumbosacral category III (Table 72, p. 110); 10% whole-person impairment.

Comment: The woman had a ruptured disk as a result of the crash. The resolution of her symptoms after a surgical procedure does not reduce the impairment estimate. The slipping of L4 on L5 shown after the crash does not enter into the estimate, because the responsible condition was present years earlier, according to roentgenographic evidence.

3.3h Cervicothoracic Spine Impairment

A DRE cervicothoracic category II, III, IV, or V percent may be supplemented with a cervicothoracic category VI, VII, or VIII percent, if the appropriate long-tract signs are present (Table 73, p. 110).

DRE Cervicothoracic Category I: Complaints or Symptoms

Description and Verification: The patient has no significant clinical findings, no muscular guarding or history of guarding, no documentable neurologic impairment, no significant loss of integrity on lateral flexion and extension roentgenograms, and no indication of impairment related to injury or illness.

Structural Inclusions: None.

Impairment: 0% whole-person impairment.

DRE Cervicothoracic Category II: Minor Impairment

Description and Verification: The history and findings are compatible with a specific injury and include intermittent or continuous muscle guarding observed by a physician, nonuniform loss of range of motion (dysmetria, differentiator 1, Table 71, p. 109), or nonverifiable radicular complaints. There is *no* objective evidence of radiculopathy or loss of structural integrity.

Structural Inclusions: (1) Less than 25% compression of one vertebral body; (2) posterior element fracture without dislocation (not developmental spondylolysis) is present and healing has occurred without loss of structural integrity or radiculopathy. A patient with a spinous or transverse process fracture with displacement should be placed in this category, because the fracture does not disrupt the spinal canal.

Impairment: 5% whole-person impairment.

If the patient qualifies for cervicothoracic category II and also has long-tract signs, the evaluator should refer to cervicothoracic categories VI, VII, and VIII (Table 73, p. 110).

DRE Cervicothoracic Category III: Radiculopathy

Description and Verification: The patient has significant signs of radiculopathy, such as (1) loss of relevant reflexes or (2) unilateral atrophy with greater than a 2-cm decrease in circumference compared with the unaffected side, measured at the same distance above or below the elbow. The neurologic impairment may be verified by electrodiagnostic or other criteria (differentiators 2, 3, and 4, Table 71, p. 109).

Structural Inclusions: (1) 25% to 50% compression of one vertebral body; (2) posterior element fracture, but *not* fracture of transverse or spinous process; a mild displacement disrupts the spinal canal, but the fracture is healed without loss of structural integrity. Radiculopathy may or may not be present. Differentiation from congenital and developmental conditions may be accomplished by examining preinjury roentgenograms or bone scans performed after onset of the condition.

Impairment: 15% whole-person impairment.

If the patient qualifies for cervicothoracic category III and also has long-tract signs, the evaluator should refer to cervicothoracic categories VI, VII, and VIII (Table 73, p. 110).

DRE Cervicothoracic Category IV: Loss of Motion Segment Integrity or Multilevel Neurologic Compromise

Description and Verification: The patient has loss of motion segment or structural integrity or bilateral or multilevel radiculopathy (Table 71, differentiators 2, 3, 4, 5, p. 109). Loss of structural integrity is defined as more than 3.5 mm of translation of one vertebra on another, or angular motion at one motion segment that is more than 11° greater than the angular motion at an adjacent motion segment (Table 71, differentiator 5, and Figs. 62 and 63, p. 98). Radiculopathy as defined in category III, if present, should be bilateral or involve several levels. A documented history of muscle guarding and pain should be present.

Structural Inclusions: (1) Greater than 50% compression of one vertebral body without residual neurologic compromise; (2) multilevel motion segment structural compromise without residual neurologic motor compromise, for example, multilevel fracture or dislocation.

Impairment: 25% whole-person impairment.

If the patient qualifies for cervicothoracic category IV and also has long-tract signs, the evaluator should refer to cervicothoracic categories VI, VII, and VIII (Table 73, p. 110).

DRE Cervicothoracic Category V: Severe Upper Extremity Neurologic Compromise

Description and Verification: The patient has objectively demonstrated a significant upper-extremity impairment requiring the use of upper-extremity external functional or adaptive device(s). There may be total neurologic loss at a single level or severe, multilevel neurologic loss.

Structural Inclusions: Structural compromise is present with severe upper extremity motor compromise but without severe lower extremity involvement.

Impairment: 35% whole-person impairment.

If the patient qualifies for cervicothoracic category V based on cervical region signs and also has long-tract signs, the evaluator should refer to cervicothoracic categories VI, VII, and VIII (Table 73, p. 110).

Supplementary Cervicothoracic Impairments for Severe Long-tract Impairment or Paraplegia

In patients with severe cervicothoracic injuries, there may be long-tract signs in the lower extremities or bowel and bladder compromise. In these cases, estimates for impairments of the spine and upper extremities for categories II, III, IV, and V should be *combined* (Combined Values Chart, p. 322) with estimates from cervicothoracic categories VI through VIII for lower extremity and long-tract involvement.

If a patient has cervical injury-related bowel or bladder symptoms *without* verifiable lower extremity symptoms, the physician should estimate the bladder and bowel impairment according to criteria in the *Guides* chapters on the urinary and reproductive and digestive systems and *combine* the bladder and bowel impairment percents with an impairment percent from one of the cervicothoracic impairment categories II through V.

If there is lower extremity neurologic compromise without involvement of the bowel or bladder the physician should place the patient in category V or VI.

DRE Cervicothoracic Category VI: Cauda Equina Syndrome Without Bowel or Bladder Signs

Description and Verification: The patient has a cauda equina-like syndrome with objectively documented, permanent, severe, partial loss of function of one or both lower extremities that requires use of an external ambulation device. The impairment may be verified by electromyographic or other evidence (differentiators 4, 6, and 7, Table 71, p. 109). There is no bowel or bladder impairment. If the patient does not require an ambulatory assistive device, the physician should place the patient in cervicothoracic category V.

Structural Inclusions: None except those of DRE categories II through V.

Impairment: 40% whole-person impairment.

An impairment estimate in cervicothoracic category VI should be combined with an appropriate estimate from cervicothoracic category II, III, IV, or V using the Combined Values Chart (p. 322).

DRE Cervicothoracic Category VII: Cauda Equina Syndrome with Bowel or Bladder Compromise

Verification and Description: The patient has severe lower extremity impairment as defined in cervicothoracic category VI, with permanent bowel or bladder involvement requiring an assistive device.

Structural Inclusions: None except for those of cervicothoracic categories II through V.

Impairment: 60% whole-person impairment.

An impairment estimate in cervicothoracic category VII should be combined with the most appropriate impairment estimate from cervicothoracic category II, III, IV, or V using the Combined Values Chart (p. 322).

DRE Cervicothoracic Category VIII: Paraplegia, Total Loss of Lower-Extremity Function

Description and Verification: A patient in this category has total or near-total lower-extremity paralysis with or without loss of bowel or bladder function.

Structural Inclusions: None except for those included in cervicothoracic categories II, III, IV, and V.

Impairment: 75% whole-person impairment.

A cervicothoracic category VIII impairment estimate should be combined with an appropriate impairment estimate from cervicothoracic category II, III, IV, or V using the Combined Values Chart (p. 322).

Example 1: A 37-year-old woman had onset of right-arm pain, and the medical workup and clinical tests showed a large herniated nucleus pulposus between C5 and C6 and C6 radiculopathy. Excision of the herniated disk with fusion surgery was performed because of the patient's radiculopathy, and the symptoms resolved. The woman later was classified as having had a category III impairment.

Impairment: Cervicothoracic category III, 15% whole-person impairment.

Example 2: A 28-year-old athlete had a C5 vertebral body fracture with almost 50% compression and had radicular pain in the left arm, which was verified as a C6 level radiculopathy by positive sharp waves in three arm muscles. The man underwent a three-level posterior fusion. After his condition became stable, he had no bladder symptoms, but he was unable to walk without leg braces.

The patient's impairment was in cervicothoracic category III and also in category VI because of the lower extremity weakness. The category III impairment of 15% would be *combined* with a 40% category IV impairment representing lower extremity weakness.

Impairment: 49% whole-person impairment; this represents 15% combined with 40% (Combined Values Chart, p. 322).

Example 3: A 60-year-old woman, after a motor vehicle crash, had bilateral facet dislocation at the C4 and C5 levels and had loss of C5 and C6 function in the upper extremity, no bowel or bladder symptoms, some remaining motor function of the lower extremities, and inability to walk. The cervicothoracic category V impairment of 35% is *combined* with 75%, which represents the category VIII long-tract signs, that is, the inability to walk.

Impairment: 84% whole-person impairment; this represents 35% combined with 75% (Combined Values Chart, p. 322).

3.3i Thoracolumbar Spine

DRE Thoracolumbar Category I: Complaints or Symptoms

Description and Verification: The patient has no significant clinical findings, no documented or observed muscle guarding, no documentable neurologic impairment, no significant loss of structural integrity on lateral flexion and extension roentgenograms, and no indication of impairment related to injury or illness.

Structural Inclusions: None.

Impairment: 0% whole-person impairment.

DRE Thoracolumbar Category II: Minor Impairment

Description and Verification: The patient's history and findings are compatible with injury or illness and may include significant, intermittent or continuous, muscle guarding observed by a physician, nonuniform loss of range of motion (dysmetria, differentiator 1, Table 71, p. 109), or nonverifiable radicular complaints. There is no objective sign of neurologic impairment and no loss of structural integrity.

Structural Inclusions: (1) Less than 25% compression of one vertebral body; (2) posterior element fracture without dislocation and not due to developmental spondylolysis is present and healing is occurring without loss of structural integrity or radiculopathy. Spinous or transverse process fracture or displacement is a thoracolumbar category II impairment, because it does not disrupt the spinal canal.

Impairment: 5% whole-person impairment.

If a patient qualifies for thoracolumbar category II based on the presence of a structural inclusion *and* has long-tract signs, the evaluator should refer to thoracolumbar category VI, VII, or VIII (Table 74, p. 111).

If a patient in thoracolumbar category II has bowel or bladder symptoms but does not have long-tract signs, then appropriate impairment estimates based on the *Guides* chapters on the digestive and urinary and reproductive systems should be combined with the category II estimate.

DRE Thoracolumbar Category III: Radiculopathy

Description and Verification: The patient has ongoing minor neurologic impairment of the lower extremity related to thoracolumbar injury. This is documented through examination of reflexes and findings of unilateral atrophy above or below the knee related to no other condition, and it may be verified by electrodiagnostic testing. These differentiating signs 2, 3, and 4 are described in Table 71 (p. 109).

Structural Inclusions: (1) 25% to 50% compression fracture of one vertebral body; (2) posterior element fracture other than fracture of transverse or spinous process, with mild displacement disrupting the canal, healed without loss of structural integrity. Radiculopathy may or may not be present.

Differentiation from a congenital or developmental condition should be accomplished, if possible, by examining preinjury roentgenograms or a bone scan performed after onset of the condition.

Impairment: 15% whole-person impairment.

If the patient qualifies for thoracolumbar category III based on the presence of a structural inclusion *and* has long-tract signs, the evaluator should refer to thoracolumbar category VI, VII, or VIII (Table 74, p. 111).

If a patient in thoracolumbar category III has bowel or bladder symptoms but does not have long-tract signs, then appropriate impairment estimates based on criteria in the *Guides* chapters on the digestive and urinary and reproductive systems should be combined with the category III estimate.

DRE Thoracolumbar Category IV: Loss of Motion Segment Integrity or Multilevel Neurologic Compromise

Description and Verification: The patient has loss of motion segment or structural integrity *or* bilateral or multilevel radiculopathy. Loss of structural integrity is defined as translation of one vertebra on another of more than 5 mm, or angular motion at one motion segment that is 11° more than the angular motion at an adjacent motion segment (Figs. 62 and 63, p. 98). There is a documented history of muscle guarding and pain.

Radiculopathy as defined in thoracolumbar category III need not be present, if there is loss of motion segment integrity. If a patient is to be placed in thoracolumbar category IV because of radiculopathy, the latter must be bilateral or involve several levels. The category differentiators are numbers 2, 3, 4, and 5 (Table 71, p. 109).

Structural Inclusions: (1) More than 50% compression of one vertebral body without residual neural compromise; (2) multilevel motion segment compromise as with multilevel fractures or dislocations.

Impairment: 20% whole-person impairment.

If the patient qualifies for thoracolumbar category IV based on the presence of thoracic signs *and* has long-tract signs, the evaluator should refer to thoracolumbar categories VI, VII, or VIII (Table 74, p. 111).

If a patient in thoracolumbar category IV has bowel or bladder symptoms but does not have long-tract signs, then appropriate impairment estimates based on the *Guides* chapters on the digestive and urinary and reproductive systems should be *combined* with the estimate from thoracolumbar category IV (Combined Values Chart, p. 322).

DRE Thoracolumbar Category V: Radiculopathy and Loss of Motion Segment Integrity

Description and Verification: The patient has impairment of the lower extremities, as defined in thoracolumbar category III and indicated by differentiators 2, 3, and 4 (Table 71, p. 109), *and* loss of structural integrity (Table 71, differentiator 5), as defined in thoracolumbar category IV.

Structural Inclusions: Structural compromise causing neural motor compromise but *not* a cauda equina syndrome.

Impairment: 25% whole-person impairment.

Caution: An impairment estimate from thoracolumbar category V, which involves impairments of both the musculoskeletal and nervous systems, should *not* be combined with one from thoracolumbar categories VI through VIII, because this would magnify the estimated impairment.

If the examiner believes it is appropriate to supplement a thoracolumbar category V impairment with a thoracolumbar category VI, VII, or VIII impairment relating to long-tract signs, the examiner should *combine* either the 20% estimate from category IV (Loss of Motion Segment Integrity) or the 15% estimate from category III (Radiculopathy) with the appropriate percent representing the thoracolumbar category VI, VII, or VIII long-tract signs. The Combined Values Chart (p. 322) should be used.

Severe Long-Tract Impairment or Paraplegia

Patients with severe thoracolumbar injuries may have long-tract signs in the lower extremities and bowel and bladder compromise. In these cases, impairment estimates for thoracolumbar categories II, III, or IV should be combined with impairment estimates for involvement of the lower extremities from thoracolumbar categories VI, VII, or VIII (Table 74, p. 111).

If thoracolumbar injury-related bowel or bladder symptoms exist without verifiable lower-extremity involvement, then appropriate estimates for bowel and bladder impairments from the *Guides* chapters on the urinary and reproductive and digestive systems should be combined (Combined Values Chart, p. 322) with an impairment percent from one of the thoracolumbar categories II through IV.

If the patient has lower-extremity neurologic compromise without involvement of the bowel or bladder, the patient should be placed in category V or VI.

DRE Thoracolumbar Category VI: Cauda Equina Syndrome Without Bowel or Bladder Impairment

Description and Verification: Patients in this category have a cauda equina-like syndrome with objectively verified, severe impairment, with partial loss of use of one or both lower extremities that requires the use of an external ambulation device. The impairment may be verified by electromyographic or other neurologic evidence (Table 71, p. 109, differentiators 2, 3, and 4). There is no bowel or bladder impairment. If an external ambulation device is not required, the patient is placed in category V.

Structural Inclusions: None except for those included in thoracolumbar categories II, III, and IV.

Impairment: 35% whole-person impairment.

An impairment estimate from thoracolumbar category VI should be combined with an appropriate estimate from thoracolumbar categories II, III, or IV using the Combined Values Chart (p. 322).

DRE Thoracolumbar Category VII: Cauda Equina Syndrome with Severe Bowel or Bladder Impairment

Description and Verification: A patient in this category has a severe lower extremity impairment as defined in category VI and has permanent bowel or bladder involvement that requires internal or external assistive devices.

Structural Inclusions: None except those included in cervicothoracic categories II, III, and IV.

Impairment: 55% whole-person impairment.

An impairment estimate in thoracolumbar category VII should be combined with an appropriate estimate from thoracolumbar categories II, III, or IV, using the Combined Values Chart (p. 322).

DRE Thoracolumbar Category VIII: Paraplegia

Description and Verification: The patient has total or near-total loss of lower extremity function with or without loss of bowel or bladder function (Table 71, p. 109, differentiators 4, 6, and 7).

Structural Inclusions: None except for those of thoracolumbar categories II, III, and IV.

Impairment: 70% whole-person impairment.

Table 70. Spine Impairment Categories for Cervicothoracic, Thoracolumbar, and Lumbosacral Regions.

	Category					Category *		
Patient's condition	**I**	**II**	**III**	**IV**	**V**	**VI**	**VII**	**VIII**
Complaints or symptoms	I							
Vertebral body compression, less than 25%		II						
Posterior element fracture, healed, stable, no dislocation or radiculopathy		II						
Transverse or spinous process fracture with dislocation of fragment, healed, stable		II						
Vertebral body compression fracture 25%–50%			III					
Posterior element fracture with spinal canal displacement or radiculopathy, healed, stable			III					
Radiculopathy			III					
Loss of motion segment integrity				IV				
Vertebral body compression, greater than 50%				IV	V			
Multilevel structural compromise				IV	V			
Cauda equina syndrome *without* bowel or bladder impairment						VI		
Cauda equina syndrome *with* bowel or bladder impairment							VII	
Paraplegia								VIII
Spondylolysis *without* loss of motion segment integrity or radiculopathy	I	II						
Spondylolysis *with* loss of motion segment integrity or radiculopathy			III	IV	V			
Spondylolisthesis *without* loss of motion segment integrity or radiculopathy	I	II						
Spondylolisthesis *with* loss of motion segment integrity or radiculopathy			III	IV	V			
Spondylolisthesis *with* cauda equina syndrome						VI	VII	VIII
Vertebral body fracture *without* loss of motion segment integrity or radiculopathy		II	III	IV				
Vertebral body fracture *with* loss of motion segment integrity or radiculopathy			III	IV	V			
Vertebral body fracture *with* cauda equina syndrome						VI	VII	VIII
Vertebral body dislocation *without* loss of motion segment integrity or radiculopathy		II	III	IV				
Vertebral body dislocation *with* loss of motion segment integrity or radiculopathy			III	IV	V			
Vertebral body dislocation *with* cauda equina syndrome						VI	VII	VIII
Previous spine operation *without* loss of motion segment integrity or radiculopathy		II	III	IV				
Previous spine operation *with* loss of motion segment integrity or radiculopathy			III	IV	V			
Previous spine operation *with* cauda equina syndrome						VI	VII	VIII
Stenosis, or facet arthrosis or disease, or disk arthrosis	I	II						

*Long-tract categories VI, VII, and VIII for long-tract signs may be combined (Combined Values Chart, p. 322) with impairment percents of cervicothoracic categories II–V or thoracolumbar categories II–IV (see Tables 73 and 74, pp. 110 and 111).

An impairment estimate in thoracolumbar category VIII should be combined with an appropriate estimate from thoracolumbar category II, III, or IV using the Combined Values Chart (p. 322).

Example: An 18-year-old man fell from a roof and suffered a TI2 burst fracture. Examination when the man's signs and symptoms were stable indicated he had neurologic impairment of the lower legs meeting thoracolumbar category III criteria and bladder and bowel impairment meeting thoracolumbar category VII criteria. To determine the whole-person impairment, the impairment percent for the radicular signs would be combined with that for the cauda equina syndrome.

Impairment: 15% (thoracolumbar category III or IIIB, Table 74, p. 111) combined with 55% (thoracolumbar category VII, Table 74) is 62% (Combined Values Chart, p. 322). Thus, the patient has a 62% whole-person impairment.

Table 71. DRE Impairment Category Differentiators.

In many cases, as with patients who have localized, severe pressure on spinal nerve roots, physicians can differentiate one type of impairment from another. But it may be difficult to reach agreement when the clinical findings are not obvious. The criteria below will help differentiate spine impairments and place them in impairment categories for the cervicothoracic, thoracolumbar, and lumbosacral regions.

The more objective and important differentiators are marked with an asterisk; the physician should use these to determine the highest impairment category. If the physician cannot place a patient's impairment in one of the categories, or if there is disagreement about the most appropriate category, he or she should use the Range of Motion Model (Section 3.3j, p. 113) to evaluate the magnitude of the impairment and identify the most appropriate category (see Sections 3.3b, p. 95, and 3.3f, p. 101).

1. Guarding
Paravertebral muscle guarding or spasm or nonuniform loss of range of motion, dysmetria, is present or has been documented by a physician. Radicular complaints that follow anatomic pathways but cannot be verified by neurologic findings belong with this type of differentiator.

2. Loss of reflexes
Spine-injury-related loss of arm or leg reflexes is present; this may be verified by differentiator 4 below.

3. Decreased circumference, atrophy
Spine-injury-related circumferential measurements show loss of girth of 2 cm or more above or below the elbow or knee. The atrophy cannot be explained by non-spine-related problems or contralateral hypertrophy, as might occur with a dominant limb or greatly increased use of a limb. The neurologic impairment may be verified by differentiator 4 below.

4.* Electrodiagnostic evidence
Unequivocal electrodiagnostic evidence exists of acute nerve root compromise, such as multiple positive sharp waves or fibrillation potentials; or H-wave absence or delay greater than 3 mm/sec; or chronic changes such as polyphasic waves in peripheral muscles.

5.* Loss of motion segment integrity
Flexion and extension comparison roentgenograms show significant injury-related anterior-to-posterior translation of two adjacent vertebral bodies of 5 mm or more in the lumbar or thoracic spine, or of 3.5 mm or more in the cervical spine; or the roentgenograms show 15° more angular motion in the sagittal plane of L5 and S1 than at L4 and L5, or 11° more angular motion in the sagittal plane of a motion segment above L5 than in the adjacent motion segment. See Figs. 62 and 63 (p. 98).

6. Loss of bowel or bladder control
Rectal examination indicates loss of sphincter tone, or there is loss of bladder control requiring the use of an assistive device such as a catheter.

7.* Bladder studies
Cystometrograms show unequivocal neurologic compromise of the bladder with resulting incontinence.

*More objective and important differentiators.

Table 72. DRE Lumbosacral Spine Impairment Categories.

DRE impairment category	Description	% Impairment of the whole person
I	Complaints or symptoms	0
II	Minor impairment: clinical signs of lumbar injury are present without radiculopathy or loss of motion segment integrity	5
III	Radiculopathy: evidence of radiculopathy is present	10
IV	Loss of motion segment integrity: criteria for this condition are described in Section 3.3b, p. 95	20
V	Radiculopathy and loss of motion segment integrity	25
VI	Cauda equina-like syndrome *without* bowel or bladder impairment	40
VII	Cauda equina syndrome *with* bowel or bladder impairment	60
VIII	Paraplegia	75

Table 73. DRE Cervicothoracic Spine Impairment Categories.*

DRE impairment category	Description	% Impairment of the whole person	Impairment (%) with long-tract signs* combined		
			VI (40)	VII (60)	VIII (75)
I	Complaints or symptoms	0			
II	Minor impairment: clinical signs of neck injury are present without radiculopathy or loss of motion segment integrity	5	43	62	76
III	Radiculopathy: evidence of radiculopathy is present	15	49	66	79
IV	Loss of motion segment integrity or multilevel neurologic compromise	25	55	70	81
V	Severe upper extremity neurologic compromise: single-level or multilevel loss of function	35	61	74	84
VI	Cauda equina syndrome *without* bowel or bladder impairment	40	The 40% impairment for category VI must be combined with the impairment percent from the most appropriate cervicothoracic impairment category, II, III, IV, or V.		
VII	*Cauda equina* syndrome *with* bowel or bladder impairment	60	The 60% impairment for category VII must be combined with the impairment percent from the most appropriate cervicothoracic impairment category, II, III, IV, or V.		
VIII	Paraplegia	75	The 75% impairment for category VIII must be combined with the impairment percent from the most appropriate cervicothoracic impairment category, II, III, IV, or V.		

*If a patient has an impairment in cervicothoracic spine impairment category VI, VII, or VIII, the appropriate impairment percent should be *combined* (Combined Values Chart, p. 322) with the percent in cervicothoracic impairment category II, III, IV, or V that best reflects the patient's condition.

If the patient's bowel or bladder function is impaired and there is no cervicothoracic or lower-limb impairment that meets the criteria of categories VI, VII, or VIII, the impairment should be evaluated according to criteria in the *Guides* chapters on the digestive or urinary and reproductive systems.

Table 74. DRE Thoracolumbar Spine Impairments.

DRE impairment category	Description	% Impairment of the whole person	Impairment (%) with long-tract signs* combined		
			VI (35)	VII (55)	VIII (70)
I	Complaints or symptoms	0			
II	Minor impairment				
	A. Clinical signs of thoracolumbar injury are present without radiculopathy or loss of motion segment integrity	5			
	B. Structural inclusions are present, ie, less than 25% compression of vertebral body or posterior element fracture without dislocation	5	38	57	72
III	Radiculopathy				
	A. Neurologic evidence of limb impairment is present	15			
	B. Structural inclusions are present, ie, 25% to 50% compression fracture of 1 vertebral body or posterior element fracture disrupting spinal canal	15	45	62	75
IV	Loss of motion segment integrity or multilevel neurologic compromise	20	48	64	76
V	Radiculopathy and loss of motion segment integrity	25	Impairment percents in thoracolumbar category V are *not* combined with impairment percents representing long-tract signs for the thoracolumbar spine.		
VI	Cauda equina syndrome *without* bowel or bladder impairment	35	The 35% thoracolumbar category VI impairment must be combined with the impairment percent from the most appropriate thoracolumbar impairment category, II, III, or IV.		
VII	Cauda equina syndrome *with* bowel or bladder impairment	55	The 55% thoracolumbar category VII impairment must be combined with the impairment percent from the most appropriate thoracolumbar impairment category, II, III, or IV.		
VIII	Paraplegia	70	The 70% thoracolumbar category VIII impairment must be combined with the impairment percent from the most appropriate thoracolumbar impairment category, II, III, or IV.		

**Note:* If a patient has an impairment in thoracolumbar spine impairment category VI, VII, or VIII, the impairment percent for that category should be *combined* (Combined Values Chart, p. 322) with the percent in thoracolumbar category II, III, or IV (*not* V) that bests reflects the patient's condition.

Combining a thoracolumbar category II or category III impairment percent with an impairment percent representing long-tract signs (thoracolumbar categories VI, VII, VIII) is appropriate only if the patient qualifies for category IIB or category IIIB because of the presence of structural inclusions.

A thoracolumbar category V impairment should *not* be combined with a category VI, VII, or VIII impairment representing presence of long-tract signs.

If the patient's bowel or bladder function is impaired but the patient does not have thoracolumbar or lower extremity impairment that meets the criteria of categories VI, VII, or VIII, the bowel or bladder impairment should be evaluated according to criteria in the *Guides* chapters on the digestive or urinary and reproductive systems.

3.3j The Range of Motion Model

Determining the range of motion of a patient's spine is a clinically useful procedure,[68] and it is the second of the two methods recommended in the *Guides* for evaluating spine impairment. This approach uses a diagnosis-based component, based on Table 75 (p. 113), a method for determining the range of motion of the impaired spine region described in this section, and a component based on any spinal nerve deficit (Section 3.1k, p. 46).

The Range of Motion Model should be used only if the Injury Model is not applicable, or if more clinical data on the spine are needed to categorize the individual's spine impairment.

The spine consists of three major regions: cervical, thoracic, and lumbar (Fig. 64, below). Under the *Guides* approach to impairment evaluation, the spine is considered to be equivalent to the whole person. As described in Section 3.3b (p. 95), with the Range of Motion Model, the cervical spine is considered to be involved with 80% of the individual's functioning, the thoracic spine involved with 40%, and the lumbosacral spine involved with 90%.

Figure 64. The Whole Spine Divided Into Regions Indicating the Maximum Whole-person Impairment Represented by Total Impairment of One Region (Range of Motion Model).

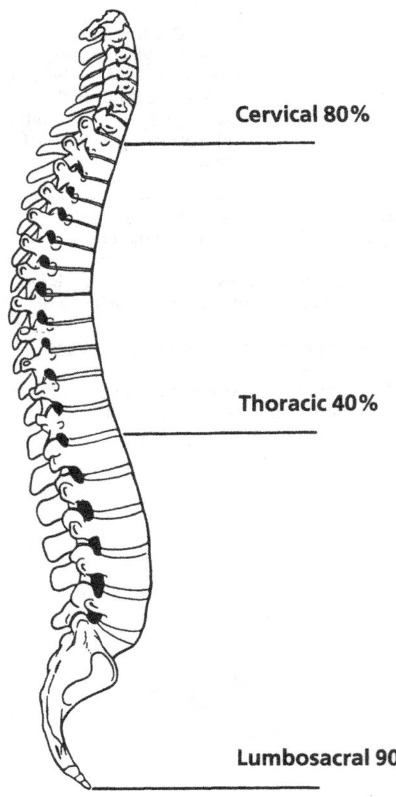

All impairment estimates shown in the tables of this section are expressed as whole-person impairments. Section 3.3k (p. 135) explains how to express a whole-person spine impairment as a regional spine impairment. The tables in this section provide estimates for judging ankylosis as well as range of motion impairments.

Regional spine motion is a compound motion, and it is essential to measure simultaneously the motion of both the upper and lower extremes of the spine region being examined. Because the small joints of the spine do not lend themselves readily to goniometer measurements, and the difficulty of measuring a spine segment's mobility is compounded by motion above and below the measurement points, using an inclinometer is a better way of obtaining accurate, reproducible measurements in a simple, practical, and inexpensive way.

The data on standards and normal functioning described in this section are based both on medical studies and consensus judgments. The impairment measurements and estimates involving the three major regions should be recorded in Figs. 77-80 (pp. 132-134).

General Measurement Principles

An individual's impairment should be evaluated when the impairment has become stable after the completion of all necessary medical, surgical, and rehabilitative treatment. This principle precludes performing the evaluation when acute illness is present. If acute muscle spasm is present, this should be noted in the examiner's report; however, the mobility measurements would *not* be valid for estimating permanent impairment, because by definition the evaluation must be carried out when the acute condition has resolved.

Pain, fear of injury, or neuromuscular inhibition may limit mobility by diminishing the patient's effort, leading to inaccurately low and inconsistent measurements and inflated impairment estimates. The reproducibility of a patient's performance is one indicator of an optimum effort.

In measuring a range of motion, the examiner should select at least three consecutive measurements and calculate the mean or average of the three. If the average is less than 50°, three of the measurements must fall within 5° of it; if the average is greater than 50°, three measurements must fall within 10% of it. Measurements may be repeated up to six times to obtain three *consecutive* measurements that meet these criteria. If inconsistency persists, all measurements of that part of the examination are invalid.

An impairment based on loss of mobility is valid only if there is medical evidence of a documented injury or illness with a physiologic residual.

Table 75. Whole-person Impairment Percents Due to Specific Spine Disorders:*

Disorder	% Impairment of the whole person		
	Cervical	Thoracic	Lumbar
I. Fractures:			
A. Compression of one vertebral body			
0%-25%	4	2	5
26%-50%	6	3	7
>50%	10	5	12
B. Fracture of posterior element (pedicle, lamina, articular process, transverse process)	4	2	5
Note: An impairment due to compression of a vertebra and one due to fracture of a posterior element are *combined* using the Combined Values Chart (p. 322). Fractures or compressions of several vertebrae are *combined* using the Combined Values Chart.			
C. Reduced dislocation of one vertebra.	5	3	6
If two or more vertebrae are dislocated and reduced, *combine* the estimates using the Combined Values Chart (p. 322). An unreduced dislocation causes impairment until it is reduced; the physician should then evaluate the impairment on the basis of the subject's condition with the dislocation reduced. If no reduction is possible, the physician should evaluate the impairment on the basis of the range of motion and the neurologic findings according to criteria in this chapter and the nervous system chapter.			
II. Intervertebral disk or other soft-tissue lesion			
A. Unoperated on, with no residual signs or symptoms	0	0	0
B. Unoperated on, stable, with medically documented injury, pain, and rigidity† associated with *none to minimal* degenerative changes on structural tests, such as those involving roentgenography or magnetic resonance imaging.	4	2	5
C. Unoperated on, stable, with medically documented injury, pain, and rigidity† associated with *moderate to severe* degenerative changes on structural tests; includes unoperated on herniated nucleus pulposus with or without radiculopathy	6	3	7
D. Surgically treated disk lesion without residual signs or symptoms; includes disk injection	7	4	8
E. Surgically treated disk lesion with residual, medically documented pain and rigidity	9	5	10
F. Multiple levels, with or without operations and with or without residual signs or symptoms	Add 1% per level		
G. Multiple operations *with* or without residual symptoms:			
1. Second operation	Add 2%		
2. Third or subsequent operation	Add 1% per operation		
III. Spondylolysis and spondylolisthesis, not operated on			
A. Spondylolysis or grade I (1%-25% slippage); or grade II (26%-50% slippage) spondylolisthesis, accompanied by medically documented injury that is stable, and medically documented pain and rigidity with or without muscle spasm	6	3	7
B. Grade III (51%-75% slippage) or grade IV (76%-100% slippage) spondylolisthesis, accompanied by medically documented injury that is stable and medically documented pain and rigidity with or without muscle spasm	8	4	9
IV. Spinal stenosis, segmental instability, spondylolisthesis, fracture, or dislocation, operated on			
A. Single-level decompression *without* spinal fusion and *without* residual signs or symptoms	7	4	8
B. Single-level decompression *with* residual signs or symptoms	9	5	10
C. Single-level spinal fusion with or without decompression *without* residual signs or symptoms	8	4	9
D. Single-level spinal fusion with or without decompression *with* residual signs or symptoms	10	5	12
E. Multiple levels, operated on, with residual, medically documented pain and rigidity with or without muscle spasm	Add 1% per level		
1. Second operation	Add 2%		
2. Third or subsequent operation	Add 1% per operation		

***Instructions:**

1. Identify the most significant impairment of the primarily involved region.
2. The diagnosis-based impairment estimates and percents shown above should be combined with range of motion impairment estimates and with whole-person impairment estimates involving sensation, weakness, and conditions of the musculoskeletal, nervous, or other organ systems.
3. List the diagnosis-based, range of motion, and other whole-person impairment estimates on the Spine Impairment Summary Form (Fig. 80, p. 134).

†The words "with medically documented injury, pain, and rigidity" imply not only that an injury or illness has occurred, but also that the condition is stable, as shown by the evaluator's history, examination, and other data, and that a permanent impairment exists, which is at least partly due to the condition being evaluated and not only due to preexisting disease.

Principles of Inclinometry

Spinal inclinometry is a feasible and potentially accurate method of measuring spine mobility, because the subcutaneous bony structures that mark the upper and lower ends of the three spine regions can be palpated readily.

Inclinometers are small, reasonably priced angle-measuring instruments that operate on the principle of gravity. A mechanical inclinometer has a starting or zero position that usually is indicated by a fluid level or a weighted needle or pendulum (Fig. 65, below). An electronic inclinometer uses a form of gravity sensor to determine an angle and then indicates the angle. Most fluid-filled inclinometers allow for rotation of the inclinometer face, so any number on the face can be set as the initial position.

Figure 65. A Mechanical Inclinometer.

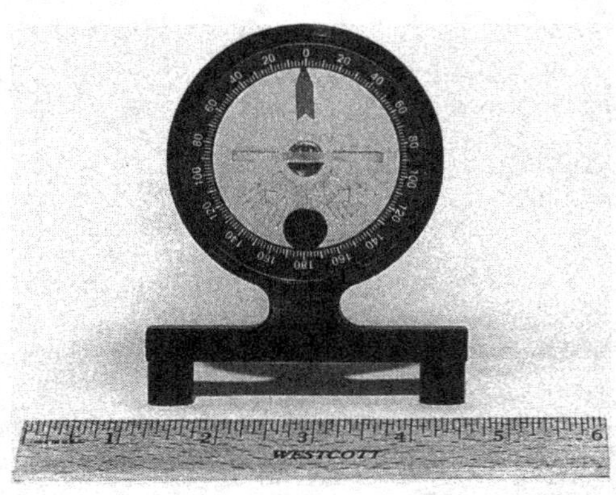

Electronic inclinometers must be calibrated to 0° for each measurement, but they display angles automatically and may be more precise than mechanical inclinometers. An electronic inclinometer may contain a microprocessor and a memory that store two readings and determine the difference. Electronic inclinometers are more expensive than mechanical inclinometers.

At the end of this section (p. 130) is a list of companies that produce or distribute inclinometers. *The American Medical Association does not endorse or recommend the use of any type or brand of inclinometer.*

The following principles apply to the use of inclinometers; observing the principles is mandatory for obtaining accurate measurements. A recent publication describes in detail the applicable principles and methods for using the inclinometer and measuring ranges of motion.[52]

Gravitational plane: An inclinometer works only in the vertical position or plane, which enables the pointer or sensor to move freely in response to gravity. An inclinometer will not operate properly in a tilted position and will not operate at all when laid down. Therefore, the subject being tested must be placed in a position that permits motion of the part being tested in a vertical plane. For measurements of the spine made in the standing or sitting position, the sagittal and coronal planes should be vertical (Fig. 66, below). Measurements in the transverse or axial plane must be made with the patient in the supine, prone, or flexed hip position.

Figure 66. Body Planes for Measuring Motion.*

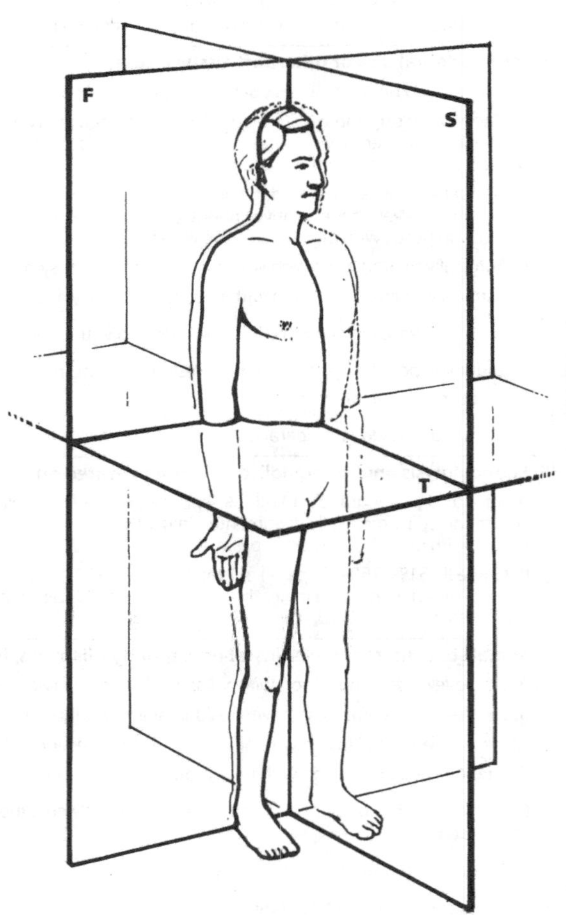

S: sagittal plane; a vertical plane that divides the body into right and left parts

T: transverse plane; a crosswise plane that divides the body into upper and lower parts and is perpendicular to the sagittal and frontal planes

F: frontal (coronal) plane; a vertical plane that divides the body into anterior and posterior parts

*Source: adapted from Gerhardt JJ.[52]

Stabilization: If the caudad or bottom part of a spine region can be stabilized so that it does not move when the top or cephalad component is moved, a single mechanical inclinometer may be used, as in measuring rotation of the cervical spine (Fig. 67, p. 116). In most circumstances involving the use of manual inclinometers, however, two inclinometers are needed to measure the movements of the extreme portions of the spine region.

Manual Pressure During Use: The inclinometer should be held so that it remains firmly applied to the subcutaneous skeletal structure while the structure is moving through the entire range of motion. The inclinometer must not deviate from the original position because of skin movement or uneven pressure on the skin overlying the bone structure, which might occur with an obese patient. The inclinometer design is important; a good design allows proper application of the inclinometer to bone structures. In measuring the range of motion, firm contact of two points of the instrument with the structure is essential, especially if a convex surface such as the sacrum or calvarium is involved.

Ankylosis and Motion with Ankylosis

Ankylosis is defined as the complete absence of joint motion or as a fixed position. In the spine, which has multiple motion segments in each region with vertebrae moving together and separately, complete absence of regional motion is rare. For the purposes of spine impairment evaluation, in instances in which the subject cannot reach the neutral 0° position, *the position or angle of restriction closest to the neutral position is considered to be the position of ankylosis.*

Considering a position of ankylosis as an impairment excludes using abnormal motion as an impairment. If the motion of the tested joint or member crosses the neutral 0° position in any plane, the examiner should use the abnormal motion section of the appropriate table to determine the impairment.

In determining ankylosis impairments, the examiner should *add* all ankylosis impairments occurring in a single plane of motion of a spine region and *combine* the ankylosis impairments in several planes of a single region or the ankylosis impairments of two or more regions (Combined Values Chart, p. 322). If a region has several range of motion impairments and an ankylosis impairment, the range of motion impairments are added and the total is *combined* with the ankylosis impairment. Under either the Injury Model or the Range of Motion Model, impairments of two or more regions are always *combined* (Combined Values Chart, p. 322).

Example: An individual who can flex the cervical region from 30° to 60° and who lacks 30° of motion in reaching the neutral 0° position has the same estimated impairment as if he or she had ankylosis at 30° of cervical flexion. According to Table 76 (p. 118), the patient's impairment is 30% of the whole person.

Estimating Whole-person Impairment

1. Select the primarily impaired region, cervical, thoracic, or lumbar. Only the most important diagnosis relevant to the patient's signs and symptoms should be considered.

2. Using Table 75 (p. 112), determine the estimated diagnosis-related impairment percent for the primarily involved region. This percent will be combined with those representing the impaired range(s) of motion and the neurologic deficit (steps 7 and 8 below).

3. Test the range of motion in the sagittal, frontal (coronal), and transverse planes (Fig. 66, p. 114) as appropriate, and determine any angle of ankylosis or restricted motion that is present.

4. Determine whether the impairment is stable and unlikely to change during coming months. If it is changing, unstable, or likely to change substantially in the future, it is not a "permanent impairment" according to *Guides* criteria.

5. Carry out at least three sets of measurements of the types of motion measured, that is, flexion, extension, and movement in the sagittal, coronal, and axial planes. Determine which measurements meet the accuracy criteria described above under General Measurement Principles (p. 112). Calculate the average of each set of three measurements and determine whether the three measurements in each set fall within 5° or 10%, whichever is larger.

6. If the measurements do not meet the consistency requirements described in step 5 above, perform additional tests up to a maximum of six until the reproducibility criteria are satisfied. If the test results remain inconsistent after six measurements, consider that part invalid and repeat the tests at a later date or disallow impairment related to that motion.

7. Use the maximum angle of a valid set of measurements of the range of motion to determine the impairment percent from the appropriate table. Refer to the Ankylosis and Motion with Ankylosis section (at left) if there are several range of motion or ankylosis impairments in a region.

8. Determine any impairments due to neurologic deficits, such as radiculopathy or nerve injury. Refer to Section 3.1k (p. 46) and to Table 83 (p. 130) on lumbar nerve root impairment as needed. Express the neurologic impairments as a whole-person impairment.

9. Combine the diagnosis-based and range of motion impairment percents using the Combined Values Chart (p. 322).

10. Repeat steps 1 through 7 above for either of the other two regions with significant involvement related to the primary diagnosis.

11. Combine the regional impairments into a single whole-person impairment using the Combined Values Chart (p. 322).

12. Combine the whole-person spine impairment with the whole-person neurologic or nervous system impairment using the Combined Values Chart.

13. Record the results of the evaluation on the Spine Impairment Summary Form (Fig. 80, p. 134).

Example: A 35-year-old woman had months of moderately severe pain after a motor vehicle crash injury, but at the time of examination her condition was medically stable and showed severe C6 and C7 degenerative changes on roentgenograms. Three consecutive occipital flexion angles obtained with the inclinometer held on the skull were 60°, 40°, and 50° (Fig. 67, below). The T1 flexion angles were 20°, 5°, and 5°, respectively, making the true regional cervical flexion angles 40°, 35°, and 45°, respectively.

The mean of the cervical flexion angles was 40°, and all three measurements were within 5° of the mean. Thus, measurement validity criteria were met. The maximum flexion angle of the valid set, 45°, was used. The woman's whole-person spine impairment was estimated to be 0.5% or, rounding off, 1% (Table 76, p. 118). The diagnosis-based component of the impairment (Table 75, p. 112, diagnosis II-C) was 6%. There was no weakness or loss of sensation. The whole-person impairment is 7% (Combined Values Chart, p. 322).

Figure 67. Two-inclinometer Measurement Technique for Cervical Flexion and Extension.

(a) The subject is sitting with the head in the neutral position, and the inclinometers are held over the occiput and T1.

(b) With the subject flexing the neck fully, determine the lower inclinometer angle. Then subtract the lower angle from the upper angle.

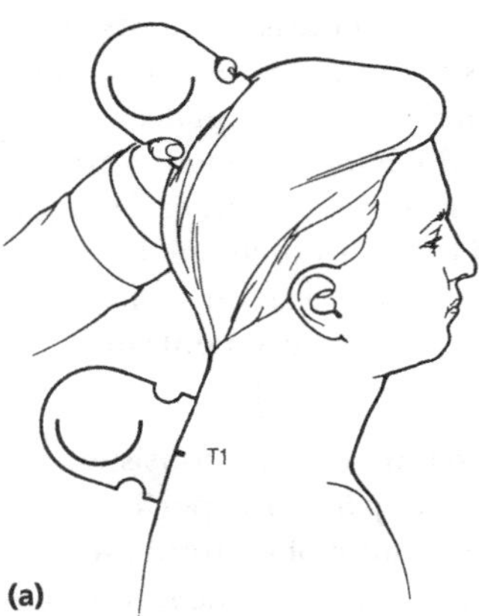

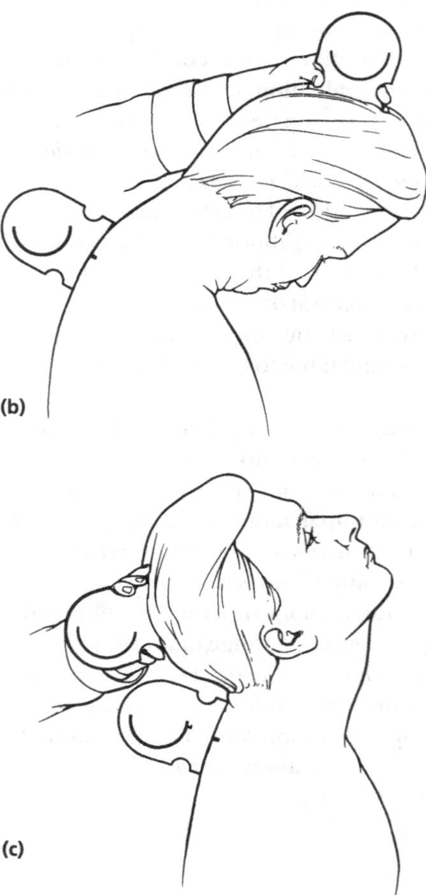

(c) With the patient extending the neck, read the two angles and subtract the T1 angle to determine the extension angle.

Figure 68. Single-inclinometer Measurement Technique for Cervical Flexion.

(a) Obtain 0° readings first at T1 (position 1) and then over the occiput (position 2).

(b) Flex the spine, first measuring the occipital angle (position 3) and then the T1 angle (position 4).

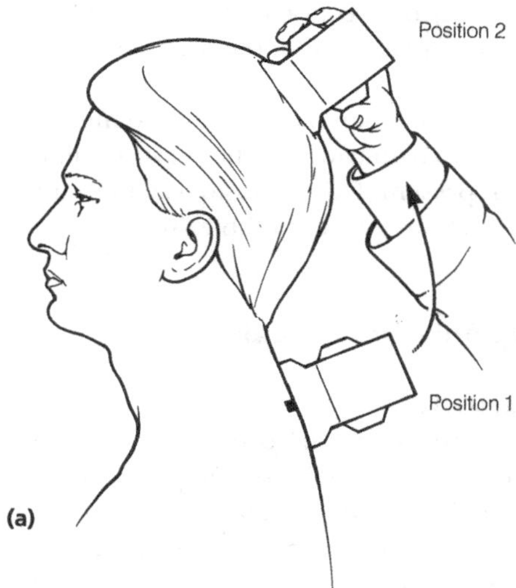

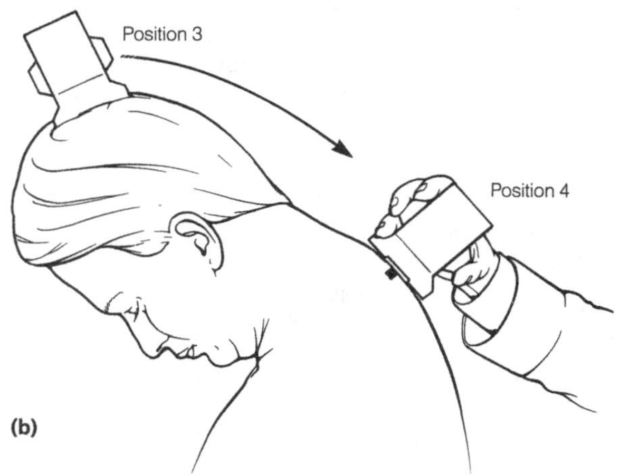

(c) Calculate the cervical flexion angle and estimate the whole-person impairment as indicated in the text (below).

Cervical Region: Range of Motion Impairments

Flexion and Extension: Two-inclinometer Technique

1. Locate and place a skin mark over the T1 spinous process. With the patient seated, place the first inclinometer aligned in the sagittal plane over the T1 spinous process while holding the second inclinometer over the occiput (Fig. 67, p. 116). The head should be in the neutral position while the inclinometers are set at 0°.

2. Ask the subject to flex maximally and record both angles. Subtract the T1 angle from the occipital angle to obtain the cervical flexion angle (Fig. 67). Return the head to the neutral position so that both inclinometers read 0° again.

3. Instruct the subject to extend the neck as far as possible, again recording both inclinometer angles. Subtract the T1 angle from the occipital angle to obtain the cervical extension angle (Fig. 67[c]). Ask the subject to return the head to the neutral position.

4. Repeat the procedure three times. The cervical flexion angle and the cervical extension angle should be consistently measured within ± 10% or 5°, whichever is greater. The final impairment is that for the greatest angle measured of a valid set of three consecutive measurements.

5. Consult the Abnormal Motion section of Table 76 (p. 118) to determine the whole-person impairment.

Flexion and Extension: One-inclinometer Technique

Use an automated device that can calculate and show compound joint motions.

1. Locate and place a skin mark over the T1 spinous process. With the subject in the seated position, place the inclinometer aligned in the sagittal plane over the skin mark and set the first 0° reading (Fig. 68, position 1). Move the inclinometer to the occiput and set the second 0 reading (Fig. 68, position 2).

2. Ask the subject to flex the head maximally and record the occipital flexion angle (Fig. 68[b], position 3). Move the inclinometer to the T1 skin mark and record the angle while the subject maintains the head in the flexed position (Fig. 68[b], position 4). Then ask the subject to move the head back to the neutral position. Subtract the first T1 reading from the second, then calculate the cervical flexion angle.

3. After recording the 0° readings first at T1, and then over the occiput, ask the subject to carry out full cervical extension and rerecord the angles at the occiput and T1 to obtain the cervical extension angle.

4. Repeat the procedure three times. The cervical flexion angle and extension angle each should be measured consistently within 10% or 5° of the mean, whichever is greater. The final impairment is that for the greatest angle measured of a valid set.

5. Consult the Abnormal Motion part of Table 76 (p. 118) to determine the impairment of the whole person.

Table 76. Cervical Region Impairment from Abnormal Flexion or Extension or Ankylosis.

Abnormal Motion **Average range of flexion and extension is 110°; the proportion of all cervical motions is 40%.**				
a.	**Flexion** from neutral position (0°) to:	Degrees of cervical motion		% Impairment of the whole person
		Lost	Retained	
	0°	50	0	5
	15°	30	15	4
	30°	15	30	2
	50°	0	50	0
b.	**Extension** from neutral position (0°) to:			
	0°	60	0	6
	20°	40	20	4
	40°	20	40	2
	60°	0	60+	0
c.	**Ankylosis** Region ankylosed at:			
	0° (neutral position)			12
	15°			20
	30°			30
	50° (full flexion)			40
	Region ankylosed at:			
	0° (neutral position)			12
	20°			20
	40°			30
	60° (full extension)			40

Example: A patient has occipital flexion measurements of 60°, 40°, and 45°, which are matched with T1 flexion measurements of 20°, 5°, and 5°, respectively. This provides cervical flexion angle measurements of 40°, 35°, and 40°. Measurement validity is satisfactory. The largest flexion angle is 40°, and the impairment due to abnormal motion is 1% (Table 76, above).

Cervical Region: Ankylosis

1. Note whether there is motion of the cervical spine in the sagittal plane, or whether the spine is not able either to flex or to extend beyond the neutral point. Determine if the ankylosis or restricted motion is in flexion or extension. If some motion is possible in the sagittal plane, ask the subject to hold the position closest to the neutral point.

2. Place the inclinometer's base against a vertical surface to measure the neutral 0° position. Place the inclinometer in the sagittal plane at the upper aspect of the cervical spine along the long axis of the cervical spine with the head in the position as described for evaluating flexion and extension (Fig. 67, p. 116).

3. Place the inclinometer at T1 and record the T1 angle. Subtract the T1 angle from the upper cervical spine angle to obtain the ankylosis angle or angle of restriction in either flexion or extension.

4. Consult the Ankylosis section of Table 76 (at left) to determine the impairment of the whole person.

Example: A 55-year-old man has a set of valid measurements indicating that ankylosis of the cervical spine at 20° extension is present. This is considered to be a 20% whole-person impairment (Table 76).

Cervical Region: Lateral Flexion

Two-inclinometer Technique

1. Locate and place a skin mark over the T1 spinous process. With the subject in the seated position, place the first inclinometer aligned in the coronal plane over the T1 spinous process while holding the second inclinometer over the occiput, the back part of the head (Fig. 69[a], p. 119). The head should be in the neutral position while the inclinometers are set at 0°.

2. Ask the subject to incline the head maximally to the right and record both angles (Fig. 69[b]). Subtract the T1 angle from the occipital angle to determine the degrees of right lateral flexion. Return the head to the neutral position.

3. Instruct the subject to incline the head maximally to the left as far as possible, recording both inclinometer angles and subtracting the T1 angle from the occipital angle to determine cervical left lateral flexion (Fig. 69[c]).

4. Repeat the above procedure at least three times. The left and right lateral flexion angles should be measured within ± 10% or 5°, whichever is greater, of the mean of the three measurements. The selected measurement for impairment evaluation is the greatest angle measured of a valid set of three consecutive measurements.

5. Consult the Abnormal Motion section of Table 76 (at left) to determine the whole-person impairment.

One-inclinometer Technique

Use an automated device that can calculate and show compound joint motions.

1. With the subject in the seated position, locate and place a skin mark over the T1 spinous process (position 1, Fig. 70, p. 120). Place the inclinometer

Figure 69. Two-inclinometer Measurement Technique for Cervical Lateral Flexion.

(a) The subject is sitting with his head in the neutral position, and the inclinometers are over the occiput and T1.

(b) Full right lateral flexion position. Subtract the bottom from the top angle to determine the lateral flexion.

(c) Repeat the process with the patient flexing the neck laterally to the left.

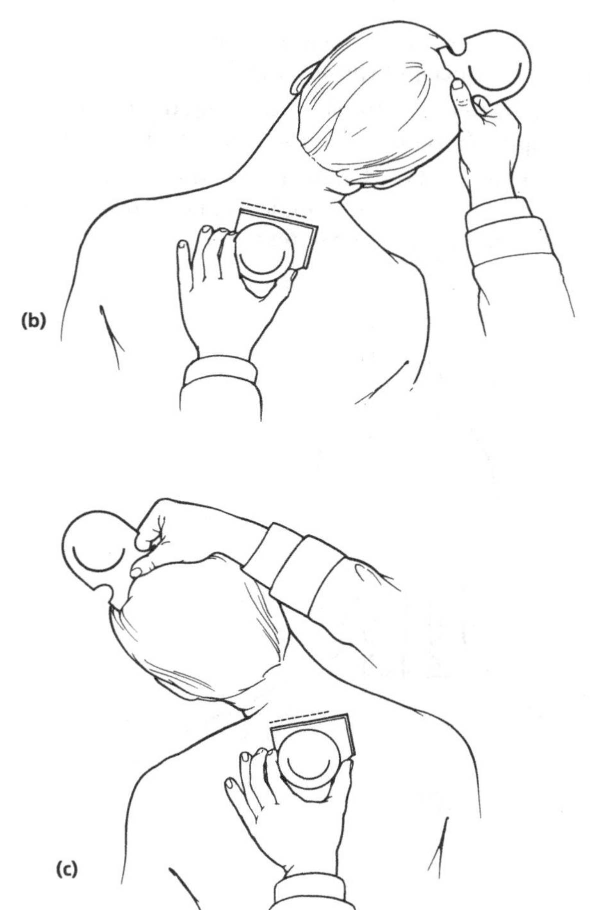

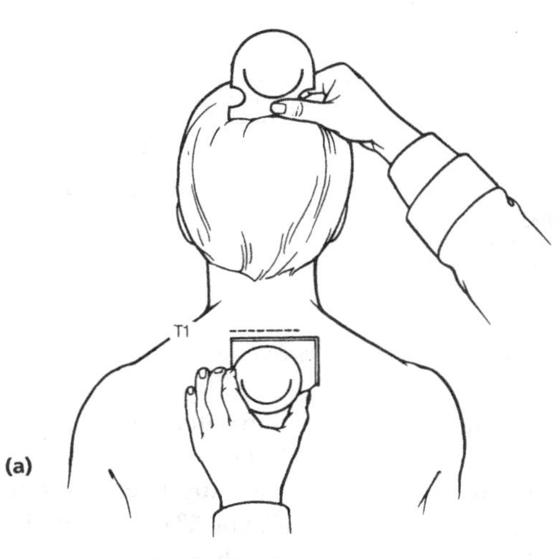

aligned in the coronal plane over the skin mark and set the first 0° reading. Move the inclinometer to the occiput and set the second 0° reading (position 2, Fig. 70, p. 120).

2. Ask the subject to incline the head maximally to the right and record the occipital flexion angle (position 3, Fig. 70, p. 120). Move the inclinometer to the T1 skin mark, duplicating the original inclinometer position and record the angle (position 4, Fig. 70).

Repeat the procedure three to six times to obtain a valid measurement set. Ask the subject to resume the neutral head position, and calculate the cervical right lateral flexion angle by subtracting (position 4 angle–position 1 angle) from (position 3 angle–position 2 angle).

3. Record the 0° readings at T1, then over the occiput, and ask the subject to incline the head maximally to the left. Rerecord the angles at the occiput and at T1 and calculate the cervical left lateral flexion angle.

4. Repeat the procedure three times to six times to obtain three valid measurements. The left and right lateral flexion angles should be consistently measured within ± 10% or 5° of the average, whichever is greater. The angle used to estimate impairment is the greatest angle measured of a valid set.

5. Consult the Abnormal Motion part of Table 76 (p. 118) to determine the impairment of the whole person.

6. *Add* the impairment percents from left lateral flexion and right lateral flexion. Their sum represents the whole-person impairment related to abnormal lateral flexion of the cervical region.

Figure 70. Single-inclinometer Technique for Cervical Lateral Flexion.

(a) Obtain 0° readings first at T1 (position 1) and then over the occiput (position 2).

(b) Have patient flex the spine laterally, then note the occipital (position 3) and T1 (position 4) angles.

(c) Calculate total flexion degrees by subtracting the (position 4–position 1) angle from the (position 3–position 2) angle. See text.

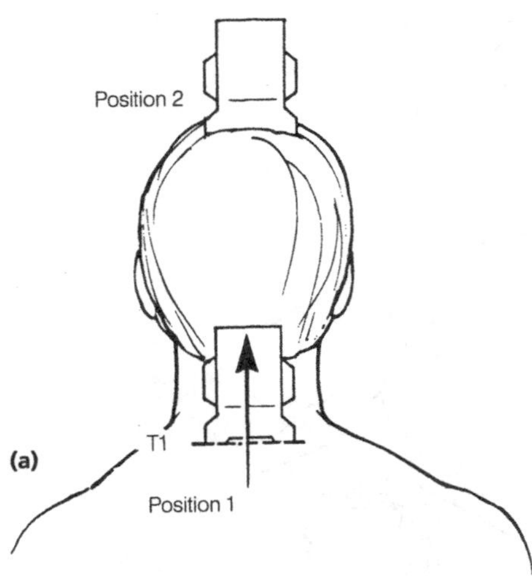

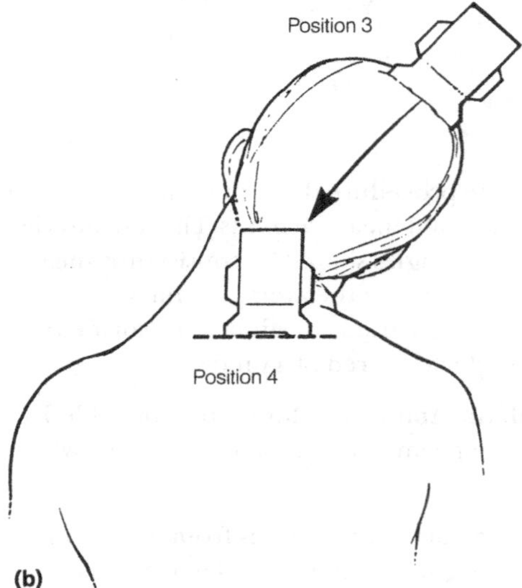

Table 77. Impairment Due to Abnormal Motion and Ankylosis of the Cervical Region: Lateral Flexion.

Abnormal Motion **The average range of lateral flexion is 90°; the proportion of all cervical motions is 25%.**				
a.	**Right lateral flexion** from neutral position (0°) to:	Degrees of cervical motion Lost	Retained	% Impairment of the whole person
	0°	45	0	4
	15°	30	15	2
	30°	15	30	1
	45°	0	45	0
b.	**Left lateral flexion** from neutral position (0°) to:			
	0°	45	0	4
	15°	30	15	2
	30°	15	30	1
	45°	0	45+	0
c.	**Ankylosis** Region ankylosed at:			
	0° (neutral position)			8
	15°			20
	30°			30
	45° (full right or left lateral flexion)			40

Example: A patient's occipital right lateral flexion angle measures 20°, 35°, 35°, and 40°. The matching T1 measurements are 15°, 5°, 10°, and 10°. The degrees of flexion are 5°, 30°, 25°, and 30°. The 5° determination is discarded, and the succeeding three measurements fulfill the validation criteria. The greatest lateral flexion angle of the three trials is 30°, and the impairment is 1% (Table 77, above).

Cervical Region: Lateral Flexion, Ankylosis

One-inclinometer Technique

1. Determine whether the subject has cervical lateral motion or is unable to attain the neutral position. If there is motion, ask the patient to maintain the position closest to neutral.

2. Place the inclinometer base against a desk or tabletop to obtain the neutral 0° coronal plane position. Place the inclinometer at the upper edge of the cervical spine in the coronal plane (T1 position, Fig. 70, at left) aligned at a right angle to the long axis of the cervical spine; record any deviation from 0°.

3. With the cervical region at the position of ankylosis, again place the inclinometer at the T1 position. Subtract the first T1 angle from the second T1 angle and determine the difference.

4. With the patient maintaining the ankylotic position, place the inclinometer at the occiput (position 3, Fig. 70, p. 120). Subtract the baseline angle or difference from step 3 above to determine the degrees of ankylosis.

5. Consult the Ankylosis part of Table 77 (p. 120) to determine the whole-person impairment.

6. Repeat on the contralateral side if indicated.

Example: A patient's cervical region has an ankylosis angle to the right of 35°, and the baseline angle is 5°. Thus, the ankylosis in right lateral flexion is 30°. This is equivalent to a 30% impairment of the whole person (Table 77, p. 120).

Cervical Region: Rotation

Because the technique for evaluation stabilizes the shoulders in the supine position, only one inclinometer is required for measurement of rotation.

Measurement of Cervical Rotation

1. Have the subject lie supine on a flat examination table with shoulders exposed to permit observation of shoulder rotation. Stand at the head of the table and place the inclinometer in the coronal plane with the base applied to the forehead (Fig. 71, at right). Record the neutral 0° position with the subject's nose pointing to the ceiling (Fig. 71[a]).

2. Ask the subject to rotate the head maximally to the right, and record the cervical right rotation angle (Fig. 71).

3. Ask the subject to rotate the head maximally to the left, and record the cervical left rotation angle.

4. Repeat the procedure three to six times to get a valid set of three measurements. The right and left cervical rotation angles should be within 5° or 10%, whichever is greater, of the mean of a valid set. The final impairment is that for the greatest impairment angle of a valid set.

Figure 71. Measurement of Cervical Rotation.

(a) The subject is in the supine position with the inclinometer held in the coronal plane in the neutral position.

(b) The head is rotated to the right with the inclinometer indicating the right rotation angle. The shoulders must remain flat on the table and the spine straight.

(c) Subtract the first angle from the second, refer to Table 78 (p. 122), and determine the impairment.

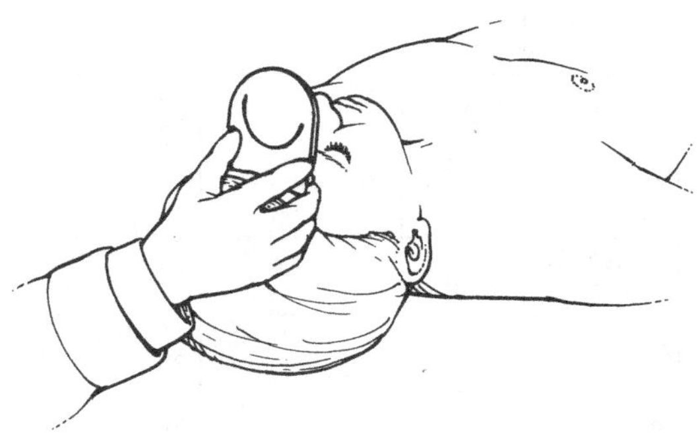

(a)

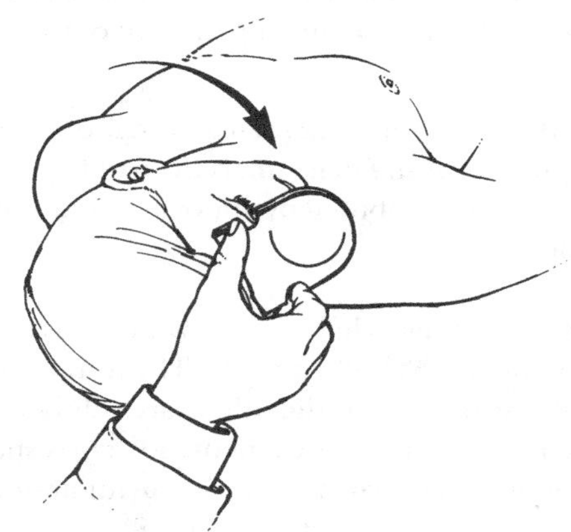

(b)

Table 78. Impairment Due to Abnormal Motion and Ankylosis of the Cervical Region: Rotation.

	Abnormal Motion **Average range of rotation is 160°; the proportion of all cervical motion is 35%.**			
a.	**Right rotation** from neutral position (0°) to:	Degrees of cervical motion		% Impairment of the whole person
		Lost	Retained	
	0°	80	0	6
	20°	60	20	4
	40°	40	40	2
	60°	20	60	1
	80°	0	80+	0
b.	**Left rotation** from neutral position (0°) to:			
	0°	80	0	6
	20°	60	20	4
	40°	40	40	2
	60°	20	60	1
	80°	0	80+	0
c.	**Ankylosis** Region ankylosed at:			
	0° (neutral position)			12
	20°			20
	40°			30
	60°			40
	80° (full right or left rotation)			50

5. Consult the Abnormal Motion part of Table 78 (above) to determine the impairment of the whole person.

6. *Add* the impairment percents for left rotation and right rotation. Their sum is the whole-person impairment contributed by abnormal rotation of the cervical region.

Example: A woman's left cervical rotation is measured to be 15°, 35°, 40°, and 35°. The initial measurement is discarded, and the others are valid measurements. The largest measurement, 40°, corresponds to a whole-person impairment estimate for abnormal left cervical rotation of 2% (Table 78).

Ankylosis

1. Determine whether the subject has cervical axial motion and is unable to attain the neutral position. If the patient has some motion, ask him or her to maintain the position closest to neutral.

2. Place the base of the inclinometer on a horizontal flat surface such as a desktop, to obtain the neutral 0° position. With the subject supine, place the inclinometer on the patient's forehead in line with the nose to obtain the baseline reading (Fig. 71, p. 121).

3. With the cervical region in the ankylosis position, record the ankylosis angle.

4. Subtract the first angle from the second. Repeat steps 1 through 3 to obtain three valid measurements.

5. Consult the Ankylosis part of Table 78 (at left) to determine the impairment of the whole person.

Example: A patient's three readings for ankylosis in right cervical rotation are consistent at 25° and 5°. Thus, ankylosis in right rotation is 20°, and the whole-person ankylosis impairment is 20% (Table 78, at left).

Thoracic Region: Range of Motion Impairments

Flexion and Extension

Thoracic flexion and extension are relatively limited motions, with the degree of extension determined mainly by the subject's posture and the degree of fixed kyphosis or curvature of the thoracic spine. To determine the ranges of motion of this region, the subject is measured in the "military brace" posture to obtain the angle of minimum kyphosis. Then, with the patient fully flexing the thoracic spine, the flexion angle is determined. The angle of minimum kyphosis is actually a measure of ankylosis, and impairment resulting from this angle is found in the Ankylosis part of Table 79.

Table 79. Impairment Due to Abnormal Motion (Flexion) and Ankylosis of the Thoracic Region.

Average range of flexion and extension is 50°; the proportion of all thoracic motion is 60%.			
Abnormal Motion			
Flexion from erect position (angle of thoracic flexion) to:	Degrees of thoracic motion		% Impairment of the whole person
	Lost	Retained	
0°	50	0	4
15°	35	15	2
30°	20	30	1
60°	0	50	0
Ankylosis Angle of minimum kyphosis			
−30° (Extension thoracic lordosis)			20
0° (neutral)			0
60°			5
80°			20
100°			40

Two-inclinometer Technique

The technique is illustrated on p. 123, Fig. 72.

1. Locate and place skin marks over the T1 and T12 spinous processes. Place both inclinometers against a true vertical surface, such as a wall, and set the neutral 0° positions. Place the inclinometers over the T1

Figure 72. Two-inclinometer Measurement Technique for Obtaining Angles of Minimum Kyphosis and Measuring Thoracic Flexion.

(a) Standing technique.

(b) Sitting technique; the inclinometers are at T1 and T12, and the subject is in the erect, "military brace" posture to determine the angle of minimum kyphosis.

(c and d) Standing and sitting techniques. The inclinometers are over T1 and T12. The thoracic spine is flexed maximally to obtain the angle of thoracic flexion.

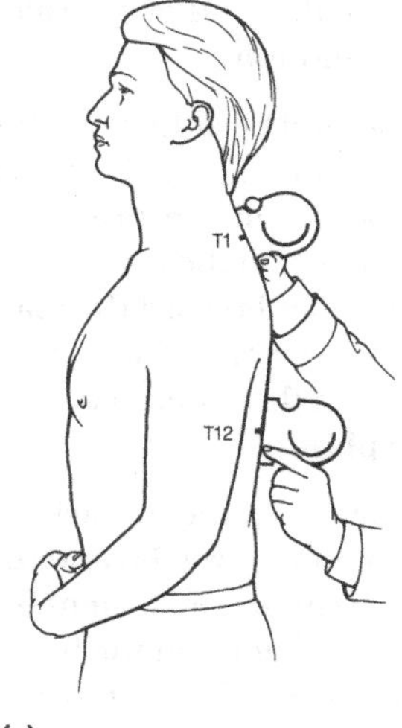

(a)

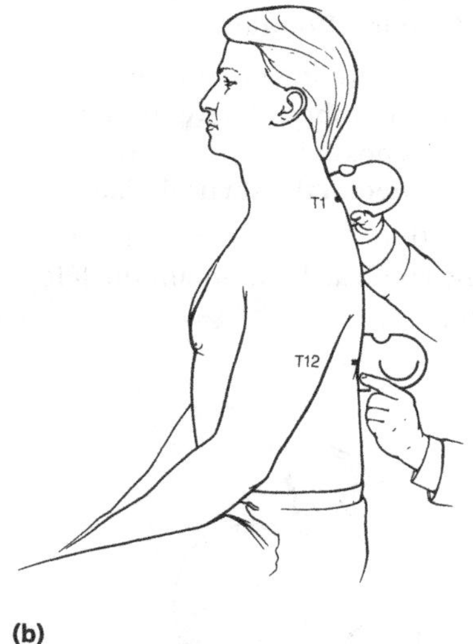

(b)

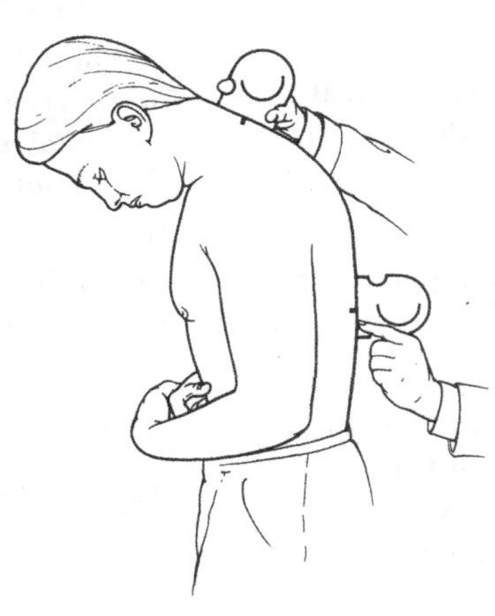

(c)

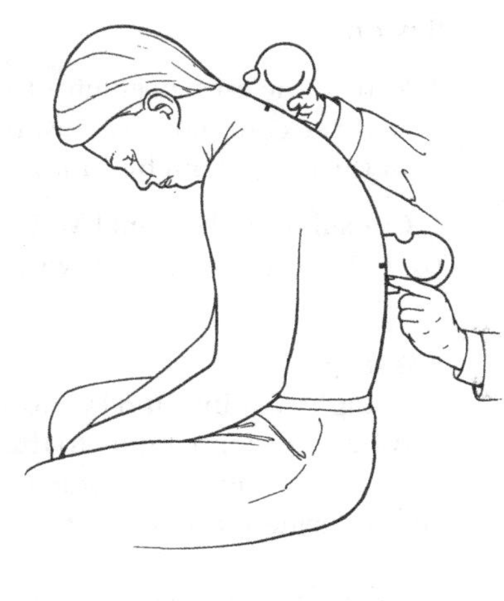

(d)

and T12 spinous processes while instructing the subject to maintain the maximally extended "military brace" straight posture position (Figs. 72[a] and [b], above). Subtract the T12 inclinometer reading from the T1 inclinometer reading to obtain the angle of minimum kyphosis. Find the impairment percent in the Ankylosis part of Table 79 (p. 122).

2. Set the inclinometers to 0° with the subject in the erect "military brace" posture. Then ask the subject to flex fully by curving the thoracic spine. Bending at the hips is permitted. Subtract the T12 inclinometer reading from the T1 reading obtained in step 1 above to obtain the angle of thoracic flexion (Figs. 72[c] and [d], above).

3. A reproducibility test is done in the sitting position. Seat the subject on a stool and ask the subject to flex the thoracic spine maximally from the "military brace" position after the neutral 0° position is recorded. The angle of thoracic flexion while the patient sits should be identical to the flexion angle obtained in the erect position.

4. Repeat either the sitting or standing test up to six times to obtain three measurements that are within 10% or 5° of the mean, whichever is greater.

5. Consult the Abnormal Motion part of Table 79 (p. 122) to determine the whole-person impairment.

Thoracic Region: Flexion and Extension

One-inclinometer Technique

Use an automated device that can calculate and show compound joint motions.

1. The patient should be either standing or sitting, as with the two-inclinometer method (p. 122). Set the neutral or 0° reading on a vertical surface, such as a wall. With the subject in the erect position, place the inclinometer at T1 and record the reading, then obtain an inclinometer reading at T12. Subtract one measurement from the other to determine the angle of minimum kyphosis.

2. Ask the subject to flex the thoracic spine maximally, place the inclinometer over T1, and record the reading. Facilitate maximum movement by asking the subject to place the hands on the hips if in the standing position or to lower the head between the knees if sitting. Then move the inclinometer and record the reading at the T12 skin mark; subtract the T12 reading from the T1 reading to determine the degrees of flexion.

3. Repeat the measurements to obtain a valid set, at least three consecutive measurements within 10% or 5° of the mean, whichever is greater.

4. Consult the Abnormal Motion part of Table 79 (p. 122) to determine the whole-person impairment.

Ankylosis

The angle of minimum kyphosis of the thoracic spine may be considered equal to the angle of ankylosis. Excessive kyphosis or thoracic lordosis is evaluated as an impairment according to Table 79 (p. 122).

Example: A subject with ankylosing spondylitis attempts to extend his thoracic spine fully but demonstrates an angle of minimum kyphosis of 60°. With maximum flexion, T1 readings of 35°, 45°, and 55° are recorded, which are matched with T12 flexion angles of 25°, 30°, and 40°, respectively.

The angles of thoracic flexion, which are derived by subtracting the T1 angles from the T12 angles, are 10°, 15°, and 15°. These meet validity criteria. According to Table 79 (p. 122), the impairment due to ankylosis (angle of minimum kyphosis) of 60° is 5% of the whole person, and considering maximum flexion, the impairment due to abnormal motion of 15° is 2%. The total impairment is the *greater* of the ankylosis and abnormal motion percentages, in this instance, 5%.

Thoracic Region: Rotation

Two-inclinometer Technique

1. The subject should be seated or standing, whichever is more comfortable, in a forward flexed position, with the thoracic spine in as horizontal a position as can be achieved (Fig. 73, below). Locate and place a skin mark over the T1 and T12 spinous processes. Place the first inclinometer aligned in the axial and vertical planes over the T1 spinous process while holding the second over the T12 spinous process. The trunk should be in the neutral position for rotation while the inclinometers are set at 0°.

2. Ask the subject to rotate the trunk maximally to the right and record both angles. Subtract the T12 angle from the T1 angle to obtain the thoracic right rotation angle (Fig. 73, below). Return the trunk to the neutral position.

Figure 73. Two-inclinometer Measurement Technique for Left Thoracic Rotation.

(a) The subject may be standing or sitting in a forward flexed position and should have the spine as parallel to the floor as possible to permit the inclinometers to be aligned in the vertical plane.

(b) In the full left rotation position, subtract the angle to T12 from the angle at T1 to obtain the left thoracic rotation angle.

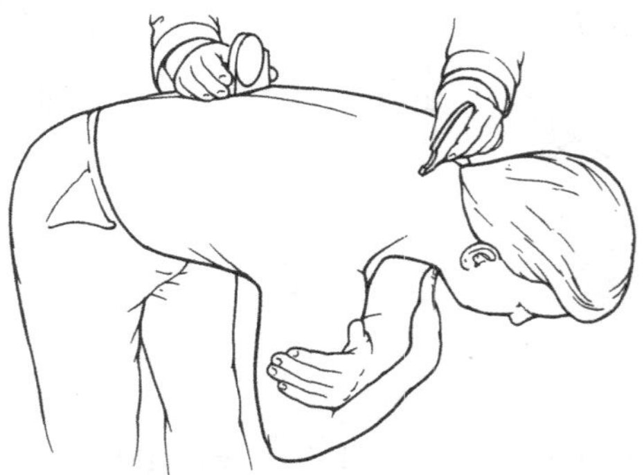

(a) Neutral position

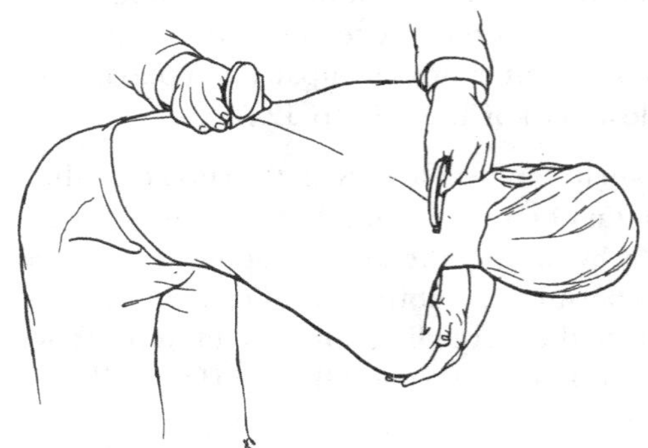

(b) Left rotation

3. Instruct the subject to rotate the trunk maximally to the left, again recording both inclinometer angles; subtract the T12 angle from the T1 angle to obtain the thoracic left rotation angle.

4. Repeat the procedure three to six times per side to obtain a valid set of three measurements. The angles of a valid set should be within ± 10% or 5°, whichever is greater, of the mean of the set. The final impairment percent is based on the best (least impairing) angle measured.

5. Consult the Abnormal Motion part of Table 80 (p. 126) to determine the whole-person impairment.

One-inclinometer Technique
Use an automated device that can calculate and show compound motion.

1. The subject should be seated or standing, whichever is more comfortable, in a forward flexed position with the thoracic spine in as *horizontal* a position as can be achieved. Locate and place a skin mark over the T1 and T12 spinous processes. Place the inclinometer aligned in the axial and vertical planes over the T12 spinous process and set the first 0° reading. Move the inclinometer to T1 and set the second 0° reading.

2. Ask the subject to rotate the trunk maximally to the right and record the T1 rotation angle. Move the inclinometer to the T12 skin mark, duplicating the original inclinometer position, and record the angle. Subtract the corrected T12 angle from the corrected T1 angle to determine the right rotation angle.

3. Again record the 0° readings at T12 and then at T1; ask the subject to produce full thoracic left rotation and rerecord the angles at T1 and T12 to obtain the calculated thoracic left rotation angle.

4. Repeat the procedure three to six times per side. Each of a valid set of three rotation angles should be within ± 5° or 10% of the mean, whichever is greater.

5. Consult the Abnormal Motion part of Table 80 (p. 126) to determine the whole-person impairment.

Example: A patient's T1 rotation to the right measures 15°, 20°, and 15°. Matching T12 rotation angles measure 5°, 10°, and 5°. The measurements are valid, and the right rotation angle is 10°. The whole-person impairment is 2% (Table 80, p. 126).

Alternative Single-inclinometer Technique
1. The subject lies supine on the examining table. Locate the manubrium sterni, and place the inclinometer across the upper sternum just below the notch. The trunk should be in the neutral position and the inclinometer should be set at 0° (Fig. 74, at right).

2. Ask the subject to rotate the trunk maximally to the left and record the angle of the sternum inclinometer, making certain that an assistant holds the pelvis to the table without permitting rotation. Read the angle, which measures the left thoracolumbar rotation. Subtract 5°, which represents lumbar rotation during the test, to obtain the estimated left thoracic rotation angle.

3. Instruct the subject to rotate the trunk maximally to the right (Fig. 74[b]), again maintaining pelvic stabilization. Read the sternum inclinometer angle and subtract 5° to obtain the right thoracic rotation angle.

Figure 74. Alternative Single-inclinometer Technique for Thoracic Spine Rotation.

(a) Patient is supine on the examining table. The manubrium and pelvis are in the neutral (0°) position. The inclinometer is on the upper part of the sternum below the sternal notch. An assistant stabilizes the pelvis.

(b) Patient's shoulders are rotated maximally to the right or left; 5° is subtracted from the inclinometer reading to account for lumbar spine rotation during the test.

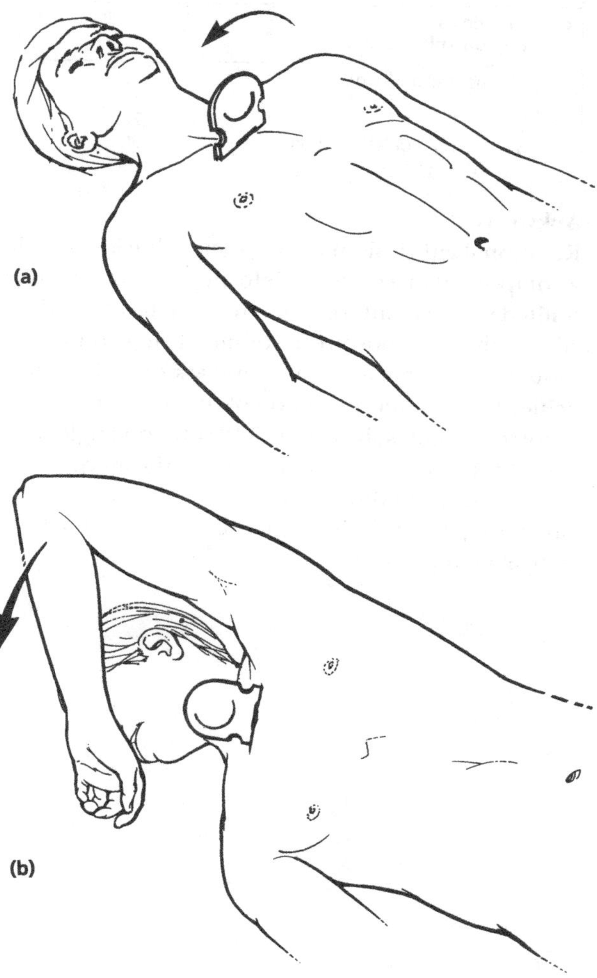

4. Repeat the procedure three to six times to obtain a valid set of measurements. The impairment estimate is based on the best (least impairing) of the three measurements of a valid set.

5. Consult the Abnormal Motion part of Table 80 (below) to determine the whole-person impairment.

Table 80. Impairment Due to Abnormal Motion and Ankylosis of the Thoracic Region: Rotation.

	Abnormal Motion **Average range of flexion and extension is 60°; the proportion of all thoracic spine motion is 40%.**			
a.	**Right rotation** from neutral position (0°) to:	Degrees of thoracic motion		% Impairment of the whole person
		Lost	Retained	
	0°	30	0	3
	10°	20	10	2
	20°	10	20	1
	30°	0	30	0
b.	**Left rotation from neutral position (0°) to:**			
	0°	30	0	3
	10°	20	10	2
	20°	10	20	1
	30°	0	30	0
c.	**Ankylosis** **Region ankylosed at:**			
	0° (neutral position)			6
	5°			10
	25°			20
	35° (full right or left rotation)			30

Ankylosis

Rotational ankylosis in the thoracic spine is generally a component of a scoliosis deformity and creates only limited impairment. To evaluate this type of ankylosis, use the same posture as for measuring abnormal motion in the thoracic spine, and ask the subject to achieve maximum correction of the rotation deformity. Then subtract the T12 rotation angle from the T1 rotation angle and determine the ankylosis angle or angle of restricted motion. Refer to the Ankylosis part of Table 80 (above) to determine the impairment percent.

Lumbosacral Region: Range of Motion Abnormalities

Flexion and Extension

A useful validity test is available to check lumbar spine flexion. Lumbar flexion is a compound movement of both the lumbar spine and the hips, measured at the sacrum, in which sacral or hip flexion normally accounts for at least 50% of total flexion and lumbar spine flexion accounts for the remainder. Comparing hip flexion to straight leg raising on the tightest side provides the validity test.

A lumbar spine flexion test is invalid and should be repeated at a later date if the following criterion is *not* met, unless the test shows that sacral hip flexion plus extension exceeds 65° for the female patient or 55° for the male patient: tightest straight-leg-raising angle —(hip flexion angle + hip extension angle) ≤ 15°.

Two-inclinometer Technique

1. Locate and place skin marks over the T12 spinous process and the sacrum. Place the first inclinometer aligned in the sagittal plane over the T12 spinous process while holding the second over the sacrum. It is generally convenient to place the sacral mark at or near the sacral midpoint, because if the mark is placed too high on the sacral convexity, the inclinometer may be displaced when measuring extension.

The subject should be in the standing position with knees straight and weight balanced on both feet, ideally with hands on hips for support to permit greater motion. The trunk should be in the neutral position while the inclinometers are set at 0° (Fig. 75, p. 127).

2. Ask the subject to flex maximally and record both angles (Fig. 75[b]). Subtract the sacral (hip) inclination from the T12 inclinometer angle to obtain the true lumbar flexion angle. Return the trunk to the neutral position.

3. Instruct the subject to extend the trunk as far as possible (Fig. 75[c]), again recording both inclinometer angles and subtracting the sacral (hip) angle from the T12 inclinometer angle to obtain the true lumbar extension angle. Ask the subject to return the trunk to the neutral position.

4. Repeat the procedure at least three times for flexion or extension, and six times at most in each case, to obtain a valid measurement set. Only the true lumbar spine flexion and extension angles need to be consistently measured within ± 10% or 5°, whichever is greater. The impairment is based on the maximum true flexion or extension angle.

Figure 75. Two-inclinometer Measurement Technique for Lumbosacral Flexion and Extension.

(a and b) Neutral position and flexion are shown with the inclinometers at T12 and over the sacrum.

(c) True lumbar extension is the T12 inclination angle minus the sacral inclination angle (hip motion).

(d) Straight-leg-raising angle on the tightest side should be within 15° of the total hip motion (hip flexion + hip extension); see text.

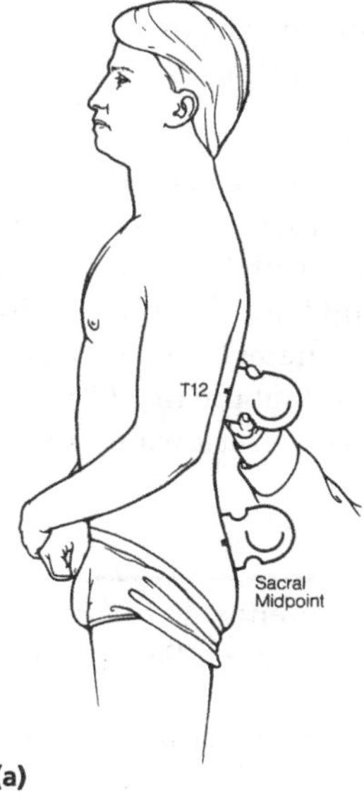

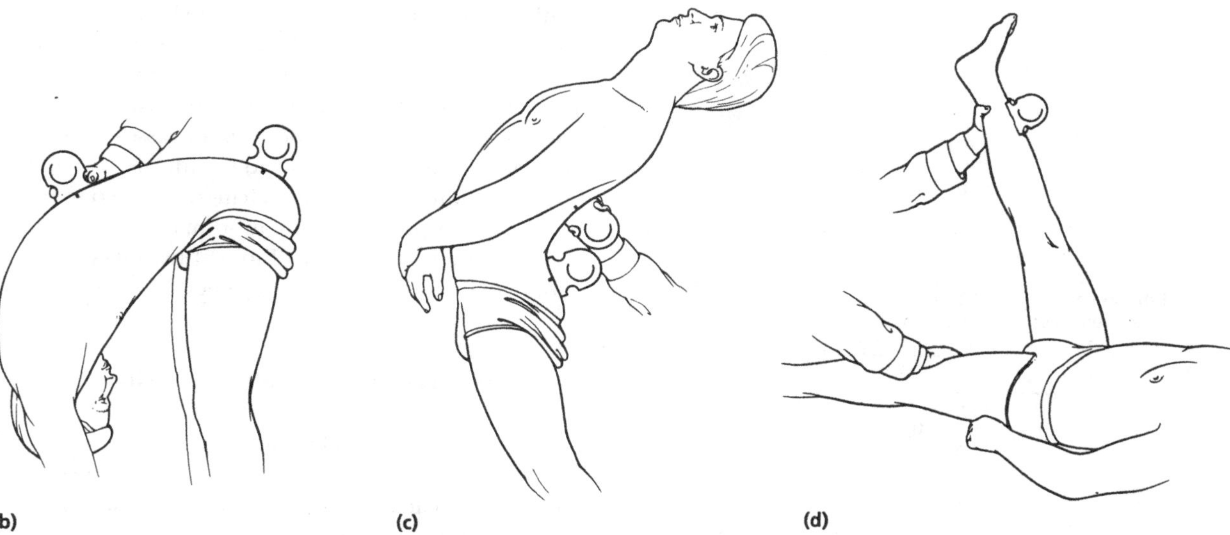

5. *Validity test* for lumbosacral flexion and extension: Record the straight-leg-raising angle of the supine patient by placing an inclinometer on each tibial tuberosity with the knees extended. Compare the tighter straight-leg-raising angle to the sum of the sacral flexion and extension (sacral or hip motion) angles. If the tighter SLR angle exceeds the sum of the sacral flexion and extension angles by more than 15°, the lumbosacral flexion test is invalid. The examiner should either repeat the test or disallow impairment for lumbosacral spine flexion and extension.

This validity test should *not* be used if the total sacral (hip) motion (flexion plus extension) exceeds 55° for men or 65° for women.

6. Consult the Abnormal Motion part of Table 81 (p. 126) to determine the impairment of the whole person.

Lumbosacral Region: Flexion and Extension

One-inclinometer Technique

Use an automated device that can calculate and show compound joint motions.

1. Locate and place skin marks over the T12 spinous process and the sacrum. Place the mark on the sacrum at or near the midpoint. The subject should be in the standing position, with knees straight, weight balanced on both feet, and hands on the hips for support. Place the inclinometer in the sagittal plane over the T12 skin mark and set the first 0° reading. Move the inclinometer to the sacrum and set the second 0° reading.

Table 81. Impairment Due to Abnormal Motion of the Lumbosacral Region: Flexion and Extension*

The proportion of flexion and extension of total lumbosacral motion is 75%.			
Sacral (hip) flexion angle	**True lumbar spine flexion angle (°)**		% Impairment of the whole person
45°+	60°+		0
	45°		2
	30°		4
	15°		7
	0°		10
30-45	40+		4
	20		7
	0		10
0-29	30+		5
	15		8
	0		11
True lumbar spine extension from neutral position (0°) to:	Degrees of lumbosacral spine motion		
	Lost	Retained	
0°	25	0	7
10°	15	10	5
15°	10	15	3
20°	5	20	2
25°	0	25	0

*Use this table only if the sum of sacral (hip) flexion and sacral (hip) extension is within 15° of the straight-leg-raising test on the tighter side; see text below.

2. Ask the subject to flex the trunk maximally and record the sacral (hip) flexion angle. Then move the inclinometer to the T12 skin mark and record the lumbar flexion angle. Ask the subject to resume the neutral position and calculate the true lumbar flexion angle.

3. Again set the 0° readings, first at T12, then over the sacrum; ask the subject to produce full lumbosacral extension, record the angles at the sacrum and T12, and calculate the true lumbar extension angle.

4. Repeat the procedure three to six times to obtain a valid set of measurements and follow instructions for the validity test described on p. 127.

5. Consult the Abnormal Motion part of Table 81 (at left) to determine the impairment of the whole person.

Example: A 40-year-old male truck driver has a T12 flexion measurement of 60° that is matched with sacral (hip) flexion measurement of 20° and a sacral (hip) extension angle of 10°. The measured left straight-leg-raising angle is the tighter one, 70°. Thus, the man has total sacral (hip) motion of 20° + 10°, or 30°, compared to a straight-leg-raising angle of 70°. The difference between 70° and 30° is greater than 15°; the validity test is applicable, because the patient's total sacral motion, 30°, is less than 55°.

The examiner knows that true lumbar flexion is good (60° –20° = 40°). The examiner has the choice of either encouraging the patient to repeat the test with greater effort or invalidating any finding of lumbosacral spine range of motion impairment in the sagittal plane.

Ankylosis

Ankylosis in the lumbosacral spine has significance only if immobility occurs in *both* the hips and the lumbar spine region, so the neutral position cannot be attained in the sagittal plane. This is a rare event.

Isolated fusions of either a hip or two or three nearby vertebrae place additional stresses on adjacent segments but do not lead to failure of the lumbosacral unit. Ankylosis impairments related to fusion of the hip or part of the hip motion complex should be evaluated according to Table 81 (at left) on abnormal motion of the lumbosacral region.

Lumbosacral Region: Lateral Flexion

Two-inclinometer Technique

1. With the subject standing erect with knees straight, locate and place skin marks over the T12 spinous process and the sacrum. Place the first inclinometer aligned in the frontal (coronal) plane over the T12 spinous process while holding the second over the sacrum (Fig. 76[a], p. 129). The trunk should be in the neutral position while the inclinometers are set at 0.

2. Instruct the subject to bend the trunk maximally to the right and record both angles. Subtract the sacral (hip) inclination angle from the T12 inclination angle to determine the lumbar right lateral flexion angle (Fig. 76[b]). Return the trunk to the neutral position.

3. Instruct the subject to bend the trunk to the left as far as possible, again recording both inclinometer angles and subtracting the sacral (hip) angle from the T12 inclinometer angle to obtain the lumbar left lateral flexion angle. Ask the subject to return to the neutral position.

4. Repeat the procedure at least three times per side. To be valid, three of six consecutive measurements must lie within ±10% or 5° of the mean, whichever is greater. The impairment estimate is based on the best (least impairing) angle of a valid set.

5. Consult the Abnormal Motion part of Table 82 (p. 130) to determine the whole-person impairment.

Figure 76. Two-inclinometer Measurement Technique for Lumbosacral Lateral Bend.

(a) Set the inclinometers at T12 and over the sacrum in the frontal (coronal) plane with the inclinometers set at 0° in the erect position.

(b) With the subject bending maximally to the right, subtract the sacral inclinometer reading from the T12 reading to obtain the right lumbar lateral bending angle.

(c) Carry out the procedure on the left side.

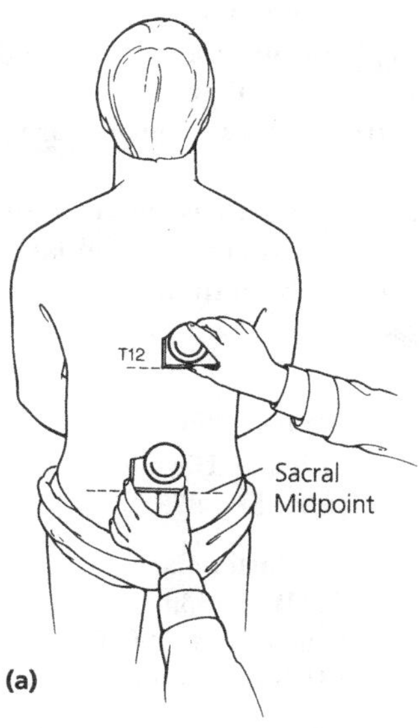

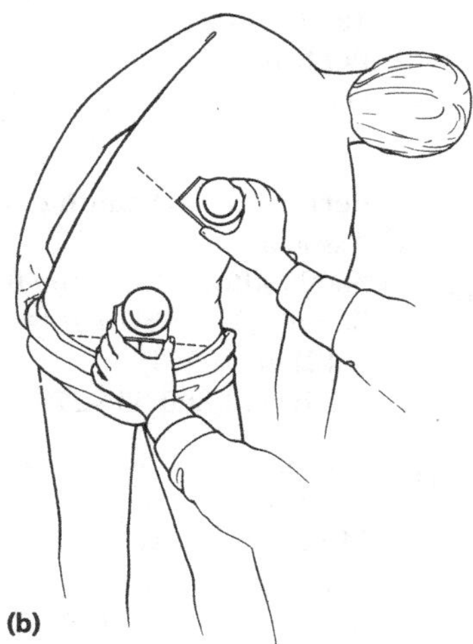

Lumbosacral Region: Lateral Flexion

One-inclinometer Technique

Use an automated device that can determine compound joint motions and indicate the involved angles.

1. With the subject standing erect with the knees straight, locate and place skin marks over the T12 spinous process and the sacrum. Place the inclinometer aligned in the coronal plane over the T12 skin mark and set the first 0° reading. Move the inclinometer to the sacrum and set the second 0° reading.

2. Ask the subject to bend the trunk maximally to the right, and record the sacral (hip) flexion angle. Move the inclinometer to the T12 skin mark and record the angle. Then ask the subject to resume the neutral position, and calculate the lumbar right lateral flexion angle.

3. Set the 0° readings first at T12, then over the sacrum. Ask the subject to flex fully to the left, and determine the angles at the sacrum and T12. Calculate the lumbar left lateral flexion angle.

4. Repeat the procedure three to six times. To be a valid set, three of six measurements should lie within ± 5° or 10% of the mean, whichever is greater. The final impairment estimate is based on the best (least impairing) angle of a valid set.

5. Consult the Abnormal Motion part of Table 82 (p. 130) to determine the whole-person impairment.

Example: In a 55-year-old man who complains of persisting back pain, T12 angles for right flexion are 20°, 20°, 30°, and 25°. Matching sacral (hip) lateral flexion measurements to the right are 15°, 5°, 10°, and 10°. Subtracting, the lumbosacral right lateral flexion angles are 5°, 15°, 20°, and 15°, respectively. The first measurement is discarded, and the next three measurements fulfill validation criteria. The best right lateral flexion angle is 20°, and the impairment is 1% (Table 82).

Ankylosis

Ankylosis in lumbosacral spine lateral flexion generally represents a scoliosis and usually produces only limited impairment. Mark the T12 and sacral spinous processes and ask the subject to stand in the most erect position possible that corrects the deformity. Using the simple measurements made in the coronal plane, subtract the sacral (hip) inclination from the T12 inclination and record the ankylosis angle or the angle of restriction. Consult Table 82 (p. 130).

Table 82. Impairment Due to Abnormal Motion and Ankylosis of the Lumbosacral Region: Lateral Flexion.

Abnormal Motion **Average range of lateral flexion is 50°; the proportion of total lumbosacral motion is 40%.**				
a.	**Right lateral flexion** from neutral position (°) to:	Degrees of lumbosacral motion		% Impairment of the whole person
		Lost	Retained	
	0°	25	0	5
	10°	15	10	3
	15°	10	15	2
	20°	5	20	1
	25°	0	25	0
b.	**Left lateral flexion** from neutral position (0°) to:			
	0°	25	0	5
	10°	15	10	3
	15°	10	15	2
	20°	5	20	1
	25°	0	25	0
c.	**Ankylosis** Region ankylosed at:			
	0° (neutral position)			10
	30°			20
	45°			30
	60°			40
	75° (full flexion)			50

Lumbar Nerve Root Impairment

The nerve roots most frequently associated with lower-extremity impairments are listed in Table 83 (at right), which provides impairment estimates for unilateral sensory or motor loss. The evaluator should follow the procedures described in Tables 11 and 12, Section 3.1k (pp. 47 and 48). In brief, the sensory or motor impairment percent for the impaired nerve root is multiplied by a percent from Table 11 or Table 12 that represents the degree of sensory or motor impairment.

If there is both sensory and motor impairment of a nerve root, the impairment percents are determined for both modalities and the percents are *combined* (Combined Values Chart, p. 322) to determine the lower-extremity impairment. If both lower extremities are impaired, the impairment percent for each is determined and the two percents are *combined* (Combined Values Chart).

The *whole-person* impairment percent corresponding to a lower-extremity impairment percent is determined by multiplying the lower-extremity impairment percent by 0.4. If there is bilateral lower-extremity impairment, the whole-person impairment percent related to each extremity should be determined and the two whole-person impairment percents *combined* (Combined Values Chart).

Table 83. Unilateral Spinal Nerve Root Impairment Affecting the Lower Extremity.*

Nerve root impaired	Maximum % loss of function due to sensory deficit or pain	Maximum % loss of function due to strength deficit	Range of lower extremity impairment (%)
L3	5	20	0-24
L4	5	34	0-37
L5	5	37	0-40
S1	5	20	0-24

*For description of the process of determining impairment percent, see text at left.

Inclinometers and Inclinometer Sources

Inclinometers, called "angle finders" by some, are small angle-measuring devices that are used by carpenters and mechanics and are useful to physicians also. The inclinometer works like a plumb bob. A satisfactory inclinometer can be purchased in the hand tool section of a well-stocked hardware store. An inclinometer used by a physician should be marked off in 5° increments or less and should be in good operating condition. Electronic types of devices are also available.

Each of the following companies has informed the AMA that it distributes an inclinometer or a similar device. To receive information about their products, *Guides* users should contact the companies.

Biokinetics
5413 W. Cedar Ln.,
Unit 103C
Bethesda, MD 20814
(301) 530-2224;
toll free, 1-800-289-4664.

BTE,
Baltimore Therapeutic Equipment Co.
7455-L New Ridge Rd.,
Hanover, MD 21076-3105
(410) 850-0333.

Cybex
2100 Smithtown Ave.
Ronkonkoma, NY 11779-0903
(516) 585-9000;
toll free, 1-800-645-5392.

Faro Medical Technologies Inc.
125 Technology Park
Lake Mary, FL 32746-6204
toll free, 1-800-736-6063.

Isomed, Inc.
PO Box 22248
Portland, OR 97269-2248
(503) 653-2008.

J Tech
PO Box 720
Midvale, UT 84047
(801) 565-8737.

McMaster Carr
PO Box 4335
Chicago, IL 60680
(312) 834-9600.

MI Tech Inc., Medical Instruments Technology
4239 S. Atlantic Ave.,
PO Box 7471
Daytona Beach, FL 32016
(904) 788-6399.

Performance Attainment Associates
3600 LaBore Rd., Suite 6
St. Paul, MN 55110-4144
(612) 484-0004;
toll free, 1-800-835-2766.

The Saunders Group, Inc.
7750 W. 78th St.
Minneapolis, MN 55439
(612) 944-1656;
toll free, 1-800-654-8357.

3.3k Determining Regional Spine Impairment

In some instances the evaluator may be asked to express an impairment in terms of the involved spine region rather than in terms of the whole person. This is done by dividing the whole-person impairment estimate by the percent of spine function that has been assigned to that region (see Sections 3.3b, p. 95, and 3.3j, p. 113).

Under the Injury Model, a whole-person estimate being converted to a regional estimate should be divided by 0.35 for the cervicothoracic spine, 0.20 for the thoracolumbar spine, or 0.75 for the lumbosacral spine. Under the Range of Motion Model, a whole-person estimate being converted to a regional estimate should be divided by 0.80 for the cervical spine, 0.40 for the thoracic spine, or 0.90 for the lumbosacral spine.

Example: A 24-year-old office worker sustained a cervical injury that, after it was healed and stable, was estimated to be a whole-person impairment of 20%. Her cervicothoracic spine impairment, estimated by using the Injury Model, was 20% ÷ 0.35, or 57%.

Example: A 55-year-old man had a permanent whole-person impairment of the cervical spine, an ankylosis impairment estimated under Range of Motion Model criteria to be 20%. The estimated impairment of the cervical spine was 20% ÷ 0.80, or 25%.

3.4 The Pelvis

The following shows impairment values associated with selected disorders of the pelvis:

Disorder	% Impairment of the whole person
1. Healed fracture *without* displacement or residual sign(s)	0
2. Healed fracture *with* displacement and *without* residual sign(s) involving:	
a. Single ramus	0
b. Rami, bilateral	0
c. Ilium	0
d. Ischium	0
e. Symphysis pubis, without separation	5
f. Sacrum	5
g. Coccyx	0
3. Healed fracture(s) *with* displacement, deformity, and residuals sign(s) involving:	
a. Single ramus	0
b. Rami, bilateral	5
c. Ilium	2
d. Ischium, displaced 1 inch or more	10
e. Symphysis pubis, displaced or separated	15
f. Sacrum, into sacroiliac joint	10
g. Coccyx, nonunion or excision	5
h. Fracture into acetabulum	Evaluate on basis of restricted motion of hip joint

The impairment estimate for hemipelvectomy is 50% of the whole person (Table 63, p. 83, lower extremity).

Figure 77. Cervical Range of Motion (ROM)*

Name ______________________ Soc. Sec. No. ______________ Date ______________

Movement	Description	Range					
Cervical Flexion	Occipital ROM						
	T1 ROM						
	Cervical flexion angle						
	±10% or 5°?	Yes	No				
	Maximum cervical flexion angle						
	% Impairment						
Cervical Extension	Occipital ROM						
	T1 ROM						
	Cervical extension angle						
	±10% or 5°?	Yes	No				
	Maximum cervical extension angle						
	% Impairment						
Cervical Ankylosis in Flexion/Extension	Position		(Excludes any impairment for abnormal flexion or extension motion)				
	% Impairment						
Cervical Right Lateral Flexion	Occipital ROM						
	T1 ROM						
	Cervical right lat flexion angle						
	±10% or 5°?	Yes	No				
	Maximum cervical right lat flexion angle						
	% Impairment						
Cervical Left Lateral Flexion	Occipital ROM						
	T1 ROM						
	Cervical left lat flexion angle						
	±10% or 5°?	Yes	No				
	Maximum cervical left lat flexion angle						
	% Impairment						
Cervical Ankylosis in Lateral Flexion and Extension	Position		(Excludes any impairment for abnormal lateral flexion or extension motion)				
	% Impairment						
Cervical Right Rotation	Cervical right rotation angle						
	±10% or 5°?	Yes	No				
	Maximum cervical right rotation angle						
	% Impairment						
Cervical Left Rotation	Cervical left rotation angle						
	±10% or 5°?	Yes	No				
	Maximum cervical left rotation angle						
	% Impairment						
Cervical Ankylosis in Rotation	Position		(Excludes any impairment for abnormal rotation)				
	% Impairment						

Total cervical range of motion and ankylosis* impairment ________ %

*If ankylosis is present, combine the ankylosis impairment with the range of motion impairment (Combined Values Chart, p. 322). If ankyloses in several planes are present, combine the estimates (Combined Values Chart), then combine the result with the range of motion impairment.

Figure 78. Thoracic Range of Motion (ROM)*

Name ______________________ Soc. Sec. No. ______________ Date ______________

Movement	Description	Range					
Angle of Minimum Kyphosis (Thoracic Ankylosis in Extension)	T1 reading		XXXX	XXXX	XXXX	XXXX	XXXX
	T12 reading		XXXX	XXXX	XXXX	XXXX	XXXX
	Angle of minimum kyphosis		XXXX	XXXX	XXXX	XXXX	XXXX
	% Impairment due to thoracic ankylosis		(Use larger of either ankylosis or flexion impairment)				
Thoracic Flexion	T1 ROM						
	T12 ROM						
	Thoracic flexion angle						
	± 10% or 5°?	Yes	No				
	Maximum thoracic flexion angle						
	% Impairment						
Thoracic Right Rotation	T1 ROM						
	T12 ROM						
	Thoracic right rotation angle						
	± 10% or 5°?	Yes	No				
	Maximum thoracic right rotation angle						
	% Impairment						
Thoracic Left Rotation	T1 ROM						
	T12 ROM						
	Thoracic left rotation angle						
	± 10% or 5°?	Yes	No				
	Maximum thoracic left rotation angle						
	% Impairment						
Thoracic Ankylosis in Rotation	Position		(Excludes any impairment for abnormal flexion or extension motion)				
	% Impairment						

Total thoracic range of motion and ankylosis* impairment ______ %

*If ankylosis is present, combine the ankylosis impairment with the range of motion impairment (Combined Values Chart, p. 322). If ankyloses in several planes are present, combine the ankylosis estimates (Combined Values Chart), then combine the result with the range of motion impairment.

Figure 79. Lumbar Range of Motion (ROM)*

Name ____________ Soc. Sec. No. ____________ Date ____________

Movement	Description	Range						Notes
Lumbar Flexion	T12 ROM							
	Sacral ROM							
	True lumbar flexion angle							
	±10% or 5°?	Yes	No					
	Maximum true lumbar flexion angle							
	% Impairment							
Lumbar Extension	T12 ROM							
	Sacral ROM							
	True lumbar extension angle							
	±10% or 5°?	Yes	No					
	Maximum true lumbar extension angle							(Add sacral flexion and extension ROM and compare to tightest straight-leg-raising angle)
	% Impairment							
Straight Leg Raising (SLR), Right	Right SLR							
	±10% or 5°?	Yes	No					(If tightest SLR ROM exceeds sum of sacral flexion and extension by more than 15°, lumbar ROM test is invalid)
	Maximum SLR right							
Straight Leg Raising, Left	Left SLR							
	±10% or 5°?	Yes	No					(If tightest SLR ROM exceeds sum of sacral flexion and extension by more than 15°, lumbar ROM test is invalid)
	Maximum SLR Left							
Lumbar Right Lateral Flexion	T12 ROM							
	Sacral ROM							
	Lumbar right lateral flexion angle							
	±10% or 5°?	Yes	No					
	Maximum lumbar right lateral flexion angle							
	% Impairment							
Lumbar Left Lateral Flexion	T12 ROM							
	Sacral ROM							
	Lumbar left lateral flexion angle							
	±10% or 5°?	Yes	No					
	Maximum lumbar left lateral flexion angle							
	% Impairment							
Lumbar Ankylosis in Lateral Flexion	Position							(Excludes any impairment for abnormal flexion or extension motion)
	% Impairment							

Total lumbar range of motion and ankylosis* impairment ________ %

*If ankylosis is present, combine the ankylosis impairment with the range of motion impairment (Combined Values Chart, p. 322). If ankyloses in several planes are present, combine the ankylosis estimates (Combined Values Chart), then combine the result with the range of motion impairment.

Figure 80. Spine Impairment Summary.

Name:__________ Soc. Sec. No.:__________ Date:__________

Impairment	**Cervical *or* Cervicothoracic**	**Thoracic *or* Thoracolumbar**	**Lumbar *or* Lumbosacral**
1. Injury Model impairment			
2. Range of Motion Model impairment a. Based on diagnosis (Table 64, pp. 85-86) b. Based on range of motion c. Neurologic system 1. Loss of sensation 2. Loss of strength			
3. Regional impairment totals *Combine* impairments in each column using the Combined Values Chart (p. 322).			
4. Total spine impairment (*Combine* regional impairments)			

References

Upper Extremity

1. American Board of Electrodiagnostic Medicine; American Association of Electrodiagnostic Medicine; 21 Second St SW, Rochester, MN 55902.

2. Bechtol CO. Grip test, the use of a dynamometer with adjustable handle spacings. *J Bone Joint Surg Am.* 1954;36A:820-824.

3. Boyes JH, ed. *Bunnell's Surgery of the Hand.* 5th ed. Philadelphia, Pa: JB Lippincott Co; 1970.

4. Bunnell S. The management of the nonfunctional hand: reconstruction vs prosthesis. *Artif Limbs.* 1957;4:76-102.

5. Crenshaw AH, ed. *Campbell's Operative Orthopaedics.* 5th ed. St. Louis, Mo: CV Mosby Co; 1971.

6. Culver J. Personal written and oral communication. The Cleveland Clinic, Cleveland, Ohio, 1990-1992.

7. De Palma A. *Surgery of the Shoulder.* 2nd ed. Philadelphia, Pa: JB Lippincott Co; 1973.

8. Dellon AL, Kallman CH. Evaluation of functional sensation in the hand. *J Hand Surg.* 1983;8:865-870.

9. Goldner JL. Pain: extremities and spine: evaluation and differential diagnosis. In: Omer GE Jr, Spinner M, eds. *Management of Peripheral Nerve Problems.* Philadelphia, Pa: WB Saunders Co; 1980; chap 8.

10. Kline DG. Caution in the evaluation of results of peripheral nerve surgery. In Samiit M, ed. *Peripheral Nerve Lesions.* Berlin, Germany: Springer-Verlag; 1990.

11. Lankford LL. Reflex sympathetic dystrophy. In: Omer GE Jr, Spinner M, eds. *Management of Peripheral Nerve Problems.* Philadelphia, Pa: WB Saunders Co; 1980; chap 12.

12. Litchman HM, Paslay PR. Determination of finger-motion impairment by linear measurement: description of method and comparison with angular measurement. *J Bone Joint Surg Am.* 1974;56A:85-91.

13. Luck JV Jr, Florence DW. A brief history and comparative analysis of disability systems and impairment rating guides. *Orthop Clin North Am.* 1988;19:839-844.

14. Mannerfelt L. Motor function testing. In: Omer GE, Spinner M, eds. *Management of Peripheral Nerve Problems.* Philadelphia, Pa: WB Saunders Co; 1980:16-29.

15. McBride ED. *Disability Evaluation.* 6th ed. Philadelphia, Pa: JB Lippincott Co; 1963.

16. Medical Research Council. *Aids to the Examination of the Peripheral Nervous System.* Memorandum No. 45. London, England: Her Majesty's Stationery Office; 1976.

17. Moberg E. Objective methods for determining the functional value of sensibility in the hand. *J Bone Joint Surg Br.* 1958;40B:454-476.

18. Omer GE Jr. Nerve compression syndromes. *Hand Clin.* 1992;8:317-324.

19. Omer GE Jr. Management techniques for the painful upper extremity. In: Murray JA, ed. *Instructional Course Lectures, American Academy of Orthopaedic Surgeons.* St. Louis, Mo: CV Mosby Co; 1984;33:513-528.

20. Omer GE Jr. Report of the committee for evaluation of the clinical result in peripheral nerve injury. *J Hand Surg.* 1983;8(part 2):754-758.

21. Omer GE Jr. Physical diagnosis of peripheral nerve injuries. *Orthop Clin North Am.* 1981;12:207-228.

22. Omer GE Jr. Methods of assessment of injury and recovery of peripheral nerves. *Surg Clin North Am.* 1981;61:303-319.

23. Omer GE Jr. Sensibility testing. In: Omer GE, Spinner M, eds. *Management of Peripheral Nerve Problems.* Philadelphia, Pa: WB Saunders Co; 1980:3-15.

24. Slocum DB, Pratt DR. Disability evaluation for the hand. *J Bone Joint Surg.* 1946;28:491-450.

25. Smith WC. *Principles of Disability Evaluation.* Philadelphia, Pa: JB Lippincott Co; 1959.

26. Stokes HM. The seriously injured hand: weakness of grip. *J Occup Med.* 1983;25:683-684.

27. Swanson AB, de Groot Swanson G, Blair SJ. Evaluation of impairment of hand and upper extremity function. In: Barr JS Jr, ed. *Instructional Course Lectures, American Academy of Orthopaedic Surgery.* St. Louis, Mo: CV Mosby Co; 1989;38(part B):77-102.

28. Swanson AB, Goran-Hagert C, de Groot Swanson G. Evaluation of impairment of hand function. In: Hunter JM, Schneider LH, Mackin E, Callahan A. *Rehabilitation in the Hand.* 1st ed. St. Louis, Mo: CV Mosby Co; 1978:31-69.

29. Swanson AB, Hagert CG, de Groot Swanson G. Evaluation of impairment of hand function. *J Hand Surg.* 1983;8(part 2):709-722.

30. Swanson AB. Evaluation of disabilities and recordkeeping. In: Swanson AB. *Flexible Implant Resection Arthroplasty in the Hand and Extremities.* St. Louis, Mo: CV Mosby Co; 1973; chap 5.

31. Swanson AB, Goran-Hagert C, de Groot Swanson G. Evaluation of impairment of hand function. In: Hunter JM, Schneider LH, Mackin E, et al. *Rehabilitation of the Hand.* St. Louis, Mo: CV Mosby Co; 1978:31-69.

32. Swanson AB, Matev IB, de Groot Swanson G. The strength of the hand. *Bull Prosthet Res.* Fall 1970; 145-153.

33. Swanson AB, Mays JD, Yamauchi Y. A rheumatoid arthritis evaluation record for the upper extremity. *Surg Clin North Am.* 1968;48:1003-1013.

34. Swanson AB. Evaluation of impairment of function in the hand. *Surg Clin North Am.* 1964;44:925-940.

35. Taylor CL. Biomechanics of the normal and the amputated upper extremity. In: Klopsteg PE, Wilson PD, eds. *Human Limbs and Their Substitutes.* New York, NY: McGraw-Hill Book Co; 1954.

36. Tubiana R, Michon J, Thomime J. Scheme for assessment of deformities of Dupuytren's disease. *Surg Clin North Am.* 1968;48:979-984.

37. Tubiana R, Valentin P. Opposition of the thumb. *Surg Clin North Am.* 1968;48:967-977.

38. Van't Hof A, Heiple KG. Flexor-tendon injuries of the fingers and thumb: a comparative study: a report on sixty primary tendon repairs by the authors, to which reports of other series have been added to furnish statistics on 310 cases. *J Bone Joint Surg Am.* 1958;40A:256-262.

Lower Extremity

39. American Orthopaedic Association (AOA). *Manual of Orthopaedic Surgery.* Rosemont, Ill: American Orthopaedic Association; 1966.

40. Anderson G. Hip assessment: a comparison of nine different methods. *J Bone and Joint Surg Br.* 1972;54B:621-625.

41. Callaghan JJ, Dysart SH, Savory CF, Hopkinson WJ. Assessing the results of hip replacement: a comparison of five different rating systems. *J Bone Joint Surg Br.* 1990;72B:1008-1009.

42. Gross AE, McDermott AGP, Lavoie MV, et al. The use of allograft bone in revision hip arthroplasty. In: Brand R, ed. *Proceedings of the Fourteenth Open Scientific Meeting of the Hip Society.* St. Louis, Mo: CV Mosby Co; 1987:49.

43. Harris AH. Traumatic arthritis of the hip after dislocation and acetabular fractures: treatment by mold arthroplasty. *J Bone Joint Surg Am.* 1969;51A:741-742.

44. Insall JN, Dorr LD, Scott RD. Rationale of the Knee Society clinical rating system. *Clin Orthop.* 1989;248:14.

45. Luck JV, Beardmore TD, Kaufman R. Disability evaluation in arthritis. *Clin Orthop.* 1987;221:59-67.

46. Luck JV, Florence DW. Brief history and comparative analysis of disability systems and impairment rating guides. *Orthop Clin North Am.* 1988;19:839-844.

47. Ranawat C, Shine JJ. Duo-condylar total knee arthroplasty. *Clin Orthop.* 1973;94:188-189.

Spine

48. Adams M, Dolan P, Marks C, Hutton C. An electron-clinometer technique for measuring lumbar curvature. *Clin Biomech.* 1986;1:130-134.

49. Battie MC, Bigos SJ, Fisher LD, et al. The role of spinal flexibility in back pain complaints within industry: a prospective study. *Spine.* 1989;15:768-773.

50. Dvorak J, Antinnes J, Panjabi M, et al. Age and gender related normal motion of the cervical spine. *Spine.* 1992;17(S):393-398.

51. Fitzgerald G, Wynveen K, Rheauit W, Rothschild B. Objective assessment with establishment of normal values for lumbar spinal range of motion. *Phys Ther.* 1983;63:1776-1781.

52. Gerhardt JJ. *Documentation of Joint Motion.* rev. 3rd ed. Portland, Ore: Oregon Medical Association; 1992.

53. Hitselberger WE, Witten CWM. Abnormal myelograms in asymptomatic patients. *J Neurosurg.* 1968;28:204-206.

54. Keeley J, Mayer T, Cox R, et al. Quantification of lumbar function: reliability of range of motion measures in the sagittal plane and in vivo torso rotation measurement techniques. *Spine.* 1986;11:31-35.

55. Loebl W. Measurements of spinal posture and range in spinal movements. *Ann Phys Med.* 1967;9:103-110.

56. Lowery WD, Wiesel SW, Boden SD, Horn TTJ. Impairment evaluation based on spinal range of motion in normal subjects. Presented at the 59th Annual Meeting of American Academy of Orthopedic Surgeons; Washington, DC; February 20, 1992. Paper 15.

57. Mayer T, Tencer A, Kristoferson S, Mooney V. Use of noninvasive techniques for quantification of spinal range of motion in normal subjects and chronic low-back dysfunction patients. *Spine.* 1984;9:588-595.

58. Mellin G. Measurement of thoracolumbar posture and mobility with myrin inclinometer. *Spine.* 1986;11:759-776.

59. Mellin G. Method and instrument for non-invasive measurements of thoracolumbar rotation. *Spine.* 1987;12:28-31.

60. Moll J, Wright V. Measurements of spinal movement. In: Jayson M, ed. *The Lumbar Spine and Low Back Pain.* New York, NY: Grune & Stratton, Inc; 1976.

61. Nachemson AL. Lumbar spine instability, a critical update and symposium summary. *Spine.* 1985;10:290-291.

62. Nachemson AL, Bigos SJ. The low back. In: Cruess RL, Rennie WRJ, eds. *Adult Orthopedics.* New York, NY: Churchill Livingstone; 1984; chap 16.

63. Pearcy M, Portek I, Sheperd J. The effect of low back pain on lumbar spinal movements measured by three dimensional x-ray analysis. *Spine.* 1985;10:150-153.

64. Posner I, White AA, Edwards WT, Hayes WC. A biomechanical analysis of the clinical stability of the lumbar and lumbosacral spine. *Spine.* 1982;7:374-389.

65. Reynolds P. Measurement of spinal mobility: a comparison of three methods. *Rheum Rehabil.* 1975;14:180-185.

66. Symmons DPM, van Hemert AM, Vandenbroucke JP, Valkenburg HA. A longitudinal study of back pain and radiological changes in the lumbar spines of middle aged women, II: radiographic findings. *Ann Rheum Dis.* 1991;50:161-165.

67. Valkenburg HA, Haanen HCN. The epidemiology of low back pain. In: White AA, Gordon SL, eds. *Symposium on Idiopathic Low Back Pain.* St Louis, Mo: CV Mosby Co; 1982;9-22.

68. Waddell G, Somerville D, Henderson I, Newton M. Objective clinical evaluation of physical impairment in chronic low back pain. *Spine.* 1992;17:617-628.

69. Waddell G, McCulloch, JA, Kummel E, Venner RM. Non-organic physical signs in low back pain. *Spine.* 1980;5:117-125.

70. White AA, Johnson RM, Panjabi MM, Southwick WO. Biomechanical analysis of clinical stability in the cervical spine. *Clin Orthop.* 1975;109:85-96.

71. Wiesel SW, Feffer HL, Rothman RH. Industrial low back: a prospective evaluation of a standardized diagnostic and treatment protocol. *Spine.* 1984;9:199-203.

Chapter 4

The Nervous System

This chapter provides criteria for evaluating permanent impairments resulting from dysfunction of the brain, brain stem, cranial nerves, spinal cord, nerve roots, and peripheral nerves.

Before using the information in this chapter, the reader should peruse Chapters 1 and 2 and the Glossary, which discuss the general purposes of the *Guides*, the situations in which they are useful, and the basic definitions pertaining to impairments. Chapters 1 and 2 also discuss the methods and techniques of examining patients and preparing reports. A medical report on an impairment evaluation should include information such as that outlined below.

A. Medical Evaluation
- History of medical condition
- Results of most recent clinical evaluation
- Assessment of current clinical status and description of further medical plans
- Diagnosis

B. Analysis of Findings
- Impact of medical conditions on daily activities
- Explanation for concluding that the condition being evaluated is stable and is unlikely to change
- Explanation for concluding that the individual is or is not likely to suffer further impairment by engaging in usual activities
- Explanation for concluding that accommodations or restrictions related to the impairment are or are not warranted

C. Comparison of Analysis with Impairment Criteria
- Description of clinical findings and how these findings relate to specific criteria
- Explanation of each impairment estimate or rating
- Summary list of impairment estimates
- Overall estimate of whole-person impairment

This chapter is organized according to the approach to the neurologic examination of the patient. The chapter's sections and the subjects they consider are listed below.

The emphasis of this chapter is on deficits or impairments that may be identified during the neurologic evaluation and demonstrated by standard clinical techniques. The impairment criteria are defined in terms of the restrictions or limitations that the impairments impose on the patient's ability to carry out activities of daily living, rather than in terms of specific diagnoses. Nevertheless, before evaluating and estimating the extent of an impairment, the physician should attempt to establish an accurate diagnosis.

Neurologic impairment is intimately related to mental and emotional processes and their functioning. Thus, the examiner should refer to the *Guides*' chapters on behavioral and mental disorders and pain when evaluating neurologic impairments.

If the patient has impairments involving several parts of the nervous system, for instance, the brain, spinal cord, and peripheral nerves, separate evaluations of the impairments should be made and the whole-person impairment estimates should be combined by means of the Combined Values Chart (p. 322). In general, only the medical condition causing the greatest impairment should be evaluated.

4.1 The Central Nervous System—Cerebrum or Forebrain

The forebrain or cerebrum is that portion of the nervous system located within the skull and above the tentorium of the posterior fossa of the skull. The most complex cerebral processes and integrative functions are only partially understood.

The more common categories of impairment resulting from disorders of the forebrain are as follows: (1) disturbances of consciousness and awareness; (2) aphasia or communication disturbances; (3) mental status and integrative functioning abnormalities; (4) emotional or behavioral disturbances; (5) special types of preoccupation or obsession; (6) major motor or sensory abnormalities; (7) movement disorders; (8) episodic neurologic disorders; and (9) sleep and arousal disorders. Sleep and arousal disorders are considered in the *Guides*' chapter on the respiratory system (p. 153).

A patient may have more than one of the types of cerebral dysfunction listed above. *The most severe of the first five categories shown above* should be used to represent the cerebral impairment. Any impairments in the last four categories may be *combined* with the most severe of the first five by means of the Combined Values Chart (p. 322); the result would represent the estimate of total cerebral impairment.

In evaluating the forebrain, the physician first should determine the presence or absence of aphasia, because communication is paramount to the evaluation of the patient's mental status. Mood, including depression, can modify cerebral function. The patient's level of education, also a modifier, should be determined. When a mental status evaluation is performed, the patient must be awake, alert, and cooperative.

Example: A patient had a communication impairment estimated at 35%, a complex, integrated, cerebral functioning impairment estimated at 15%, an emotional state disturbance resulting in an estimated impairment of 30%, and a disturbance of consciousness impairment estimated at 5%. All of the impairments were thought to be caused by cerebral hemorrhage related to long-standing hypertension. The patient's impairment of cerebral function was designated as that of the greatest impairment, 35%.

The patient also had a monaural hearing or eighth cranial nerve impairment of 15%. To estimate the patient's total impairment, the whole-person impairment percents of the two organ systems would be *combined*. Combining the impairments resulted in an estimated impairment of 45% (Combined Values Chart, p. 322).

Sensory Disturbances

While patients' descriptions of sensory disturbances may be fairly typical, the evidence gathered during the medical examination may be of only limited value. Thalamic pain, phantom limb sensations, causalgia, and other disturbances of sensation may be of such duration and severity as to be classified as impairments. Judgment on the part of the physician is needed in deciding whether a sensory disturbance qualifies as a "permanent" impairment. Chapter 1 (p. 1) and the Glossary (p. 315) define permanent impairments.

Motor Disturbances

Motor disturbances without paresis or weakness may affect daily activities and result in permanent impairment. These include, but are not limited to, the following: (1) involuntary movements, such as tremors, chorea, athetosis, and hemiballismus; (2) disturbances of tone and posture; (3) various forms of limitation of voluntary movements, as in parkinsonism with or without bradykinesia; (4) impairment of associated and synergistic movements, as in abnormal conditions of the extrapyramidal system, cerebellum, and basal ganglia; (5) complex gait and manual dexterity disturbances, as in ataxia; and (6) convulsive or seizure disorders of simple or complex, focal or generalized cerebral involvement.

The evaluation of sensory and motor impairments due to central nervous system disorders should be documented in terms of how they affect the patient's ability to perform daily activities, such as dressing, eating, walking, using the upper extremity, communicating, controlling the functioning of bladder and bowel, and carrying out responsibilities at home and in the workplace.

If the condition being evaluated involves another organ system, such as the musculoskeletal or digestive system, the condition should be evaluated in terms of that system also. Then the whole-person impairment percents of both systems relating to the underlying condition should be *combined* by means of the Combined Values Chart (p. 322).

4.1a Aphasia and Communication Disturbances

Communication involves comprehension, understanding, language, and effective interactions between and among individuals. Aphasia involves the lack of ability to comprehend; deficits in vision, hearing, and understanding of spoken and written language; and the inability to implement discernible and appropriate language symbols by voice, action, writing, or pantomime. Understandable speaking and articulation, or their lack, involve the structure and function of the brain stem or medulla, which is evaluated according to a later part of this chapter (p. 145). Speech and communication are considered also in the *Guides* chapter on the ear, nose, throat, and related structures.

Aphasia should be differentiated from dysarthria, which is imperfect articulation of speech due to disordered muscle control, and dysphonia, which is voice impairment causing difficulty in speaking.

Impairment due to aphasia or dysphasia is based on a presumed hierarchy of severity of impairment and on the results of specific tests of communication (Table 1, at right). Some of the latter include (1) naming objects by sight or describing them after reading about them; (2) repeating speech; (3) following oral and written commands; (4) reading aloud and silently and understanding what was read; (5) writing from sight and dictation and copying; (6) spelling; and (7) pantomiming about the use of an object.

Example: A 64-year-old man was brought to a physician by family members because he appeared unable to speak with them, was unable to dress himself, and could not care for his body functions, especially excretion. These symptoms had been stable for 4 months.

The man was right-handed. His vital signs were normal, as were results of basic laboratory tests. Examination disclosed a flaccid paralysis and no deep tendon reflexes of the right arm and leg. He was unable to name a key, a pen, or a comb, could not read a simple newspaper paragraph, and could not describe the paragraph's contents. He could stand but not walk without help.

The man's impairment related to dysphasia was estimated to be 45% (Table 1, at right); the impairment related to the upper extremity was estimated to be 55%; and gait impairment was judged to be 65% (Table 13, p. 148). These estimates *combined* to give an estimated whole-person impairment of 91% (Combined Values Chart, p. 322).

Table 1. Impairments Related to Aphasia or Dysphasia.

Description	% Impairment of the whole person
Minimal disturbance in comprehension and production of language symbols of daily living	0 - 9
Moderate impairment in comprehension and production of language symbols of daily living	10 - 24
Inability to comprehend language symbols; production of unintelligible or inappropriate language for daily activities	25 - 39
Complete inability to communicate or comprehend language symbols	40 - 60

4.1b Disturbances of Mental Status and Integrative Functioning

Deficits in these functions include the general effects of organic brain syndrome, dementia, and some specific, focal, neurologic deficiencies. Documentation of mental status should include information about the following characteristics or capabilities of the patient: (1) orientation concerning time, person, and place; (2) recent recall; (3) ability to remember and repeat a series of digits and repeat them in reverse order; (4) ability to perform serial subtraction of 7s from 100 or 3s from 20; (5) ability to do other simple calculations; (6) ability to repeat three unrelated words; (7) ability to spell a word such as "world" forward and backward; (8) ability to repeat a short paragraph; (9) ability to understand and explain proverbs or abstract thoughts; and (10) judgment.

Before evaluating the patient's mental status, the physician should determine the presence or absence of aphasia. If there is no aphasia, tests of integrative functions and abilities such as those listed above may be performed. If the patient has a communication disturbance and a disturbance of the highest integrative functions, then the greater of the dysphasia and the integrative functioning impairments should be used as the impairment estimate. The criteria for evaluating mental status are shown in Table 2 (p. 142).

4.1c Emotional or Behavioral Disturbances

These types of disturbances illustrate the interrelationships between the fields of neurology and psychiatry. The disturbances may be the result of

Table 2. Mental Status Impairments.

Impairment description	% Impairment of the whole person
Impairment exists, but ability remains to perform satisfactorily most activities of daily living	1 - 14
Impairment requires direction and supervision of daily living activities	15 - 29
Impairment requires directed care under continued supervision and confinement in home or other facility	30 - 49
Individual is unable without supervision to care for self and be safe in any situation	50 - 70

neurologic impairments but may have psychiatric features as well, which may range from irritability to outbursts of rage or panic and from aggression to withdrawal. These illnesses may include depression, manic states, emotional fluctuations, socially unacceptable behavior, involuntary laughing or crying, and other kinds of central nervous system responses. The criteria for evaluating these disturbances (Table 3, below) relate to the criteria for mental and behavioral impairments (Chapter 14, p. 291).

Table 3. Emotional or Behavioral Impairments.

Impairment description	% Impairment of the whole person
Mild limitation of daily social and interpersonal functioning	0 - 14
Moderate limitation of *some* but not all social and interpersonal daily living functions	15 - 29
Severe limitation impeding useful action in *almost all* social and interpersonal daily functions	30 - 49
Severe limitation of all daily functions requiring total dependence on another person	50 - 70

4.1d Permanent Disturbances in Level of Consciousness and Awareness

These neurologic disturbances result in permanent loss of responsiveness, communication, and awareness and are seen in stupor, coma, and the persistent vegetative state. The criteria for these disturbances (Table 4, below) *do not* apply to sleep or seizure disorders or syncope.

Example: A 55-year-old man had a severe cerebrovascular hemorrhage, and 5 months later, when his condition was stable, he remained paralyzed on the right side and dependent on others for daily living activities and functions. He had to be fed, and the care of nurses or a family member was required for his bladder and bowel functioning.

A physical examination confirmed the presence of right hemiplegia and the patient's total dependence. The patient was unable to express himself clearly, and generalized weakness was present.

Impairment: The greater of the patient's impairment in consciousness and that related to aphasia was judged to be in his level of consciousness and awareness. The latter impairment was estimated to be 49% (Table 4, below). The upper-extremity impairment was estimated to be 60% (Table 14, p. 148). The impairments of the two organ systems were *combined* (Combined Values Chart, p. 322), and the estimated whole-person impairment was 80%.

Table 4. Impairment of Consciousness and Awareness.

Impairment description	% Impairment of the whole person
Brief repetitive or persisting alteration of state of consciousness, limiting ability to perform usual activities	0 - 14
Prolonged alteration of state of consciousness diminishing capabilities in personal care and other activities of daily living	15 - 29
State of semicoma with complete dependency and subsistence by artificial medical means	30 - 49
Persistent vegetative state, or irreversible coma requiring total medical support	50 - 90

4.1e Episodic Neurologic Disorders

Intermittent but persisting disorders of neurologic function may be grouped into conditions with syncope or loss of awareness, convulsive disorders, and arousal and sleep disorders. These conditions may involve other body systems, such as the cardiovascular, respiratory, and autonomic nervous systems. Many mechanisms, including behavioral factors, can precipitate convulsions.

Complete resolution and identification of the mechanism underlying the disorder may not be possible. The physician should attempt to identify the disorder as being in one of the three categories, syncope, seizure, or arousal or sleep disorder. In some cases the disorder may be static, but in others it may worsen. A disorder that is expected to change to a moderate or greater degree in the next year is not a "permanent impairment" (see Chapter 1 and Glossary).

In assessing permanent impairment due to episodic conditions, the physician must complete a thorough neurologic evaluation, allow sufficient time to establish the pattern of the disorder's occurrence by time, estimate its effects on daily activities, and evaluate the effects of appropriate treatment. If other organ systems are involved, any permanent impairments should be expressed as whole-person impairments, and the percentages should be *combined* with the neurologic system impairment percentage (Combined Values Chart, p. 322). As explained in Chapter 2, the control of an episodic disorder does not necessarily prevent its being properly considered a permanent impairment.

Transient loss of awareness or consciousness after a period of cerebral ischemia may be due to various mechanisms. These may include hypotension or decreased brain perfusion, inadequate cardiac output, periodic metabolic defects, or reflex actions. The autonomic nervous system (ANS) innervates the functioning of many organ systems. Failure of this system to respond appropriately may cause an individual's impairment (see section on the ANS, p. 151).

Focal failure of the ANS may result in causalgia, or the painful syndrome of reflex sympathetic dystrophy of an extremity. Some neurologic conditions have associated ANS involvement that is a part of the impairment. These include some polyneuropathies, familial dysautonomia, Guillain-Barre syndrome, syringomyelia, porphyria, brain and spinal cord tumors, and myelopathy.

Epilepsy, seizures and convulsive disorders, and related impairments should be described according to their onset, frequency, and duration and how they affect the patient's performance of daily activities. Attempts to control the seizures should be documented and the results described. Daytime episodes of loss of consciousness with tonic or clonic seizures, or nocturnal episodes with daytime residua, may interfere significantly with daily activities. The criteria for evaluating seizures and convulsive disorders are given in Table 5 (at right).

Table 5. Impairments Related to Epilepsy, Seizures, and Convulsive Disorders.

Impairment description	% Impairment of the whole person
Paroxysmal disorder with predictable characteristics and unpredictable occurrence that does not limit usual activities but is a *risk* to the patient or limits performance of daily activities	0 - 14
Paroxysmal disorder that interferes with *some* activities of daily living	15 - 29
Severe paroxysmal disorder of such frequency that it limits activities to those that are supervised, protected, or restricted	30 - 49
Uncontrolled paroxysmal disorder of such severity and constancy that it *totally limits* the individual's daily activities	50 - 70

Minor seizures with alterations of awareness or consciousness, transient manifestations of unconventional behavior, or interruptions of daytime activity may indicate impairment. The severity of major or minor seizures should be judged as they interrupt or affect daily activities.

Arousal and sleep disorders include disorders related to initiating and maintaining sleep or inability to sleep; disorders of excessive somnolence, including those associated with sleep-induced respiratory impairment; disorders of sleep-wake schedules; and dysfunctions associated with sleep, sleep stages, or parasomnias.

The categories of impairment that may arise from sleep disorders (Table 6, below) relate to (1) the nervous system, with reduced daytime attention, concentration, and other cognitive abilities; (2) mental and behavioral factors, including depression, irritability, interpersonal difficulties, and social problems; (3) the cardiovascular system, with systemic and pulmonary hypertension, cardiac enlargement,

Table 6. Impairment Criteria for Sleep and Arousal Disorders.

Description	% Impairment of the whole person
Reduced daytime alertness with sleep pattern such that patient can carry out most daily activities	1 - 9
Reduced daytime altertness requiring some supervision in carrying out daytime activities	10 - 19
Reduced daytime alertness that significantly limits daily activities and requires supervision by caretakers	20 - 39
Severe reduction of daytime alertness that causes the patient to be unable to care for self in any situation or manner	40 - 60

congestive heart failure, or arrhythmias; and (4) the hematopoietic system and polycythemia. Sleep disorders relating to these systems should be evaluated according to the *Guides* chapters that deal with the respective systems.

The subject of sleep disorders is considered also in the chapter on the respiratory system.

4.1f The Cranial Nerves

The olfactory nerve (cranial nerve I) is concerned with the sense of smell and the recognition of odors. Lack of the sense of smell may reduce the perception of taste, which is mediated by cranial nerves VII and IX. Partial or complete right or left anosmia may occur. A perversion of the sense of smell, parosmia, may occur. An impairment estimate for anosmia or parosmia, which should be given only if the anosmia interferes significantly with daily activities, would be *combined* with any other permanent impairment (Combined Values Chart, p. 322). The maximum impairment from anosmia is 5%.

The optic nerve (cranial nerve II) relates to vision, the eye, the optic chiasm, visual fields, and the visual cortex. Table 7 (at right) considers optic nerve impairments; the reader should refer to the *Guides* chapter on the visual system (p. 209) for detailed instructions on evaluating visual impairments. Visual loss related to the optic nerve may be partial or complete, unilateral or bilateral, hemianopic or quadrantanopic.

Loss of visual acuity due to nerve dysfunction is usually unilateral. For bilateral nerve involvement, reference to the chapter on the visual system is indicated. After estimating an optic nerve impairment, the physician should combine the estimate with any other visual system impairment estimate (Combined Values Chart, p. 322).

Testing for loss of visual fields is difficult, and the reader is referred to the *Guides* chapter on the visual system (p. 209) for detailed instructions. Consultation with and referral to an ophthalmologist is recommended. Table 8 (at right), which provides impairment estimates for some losses, may be used when central visual acuity is normal.

For noncongruous or partial defects, refer to the method of assessing visual field loss in the chapter on the visual system (p. 209). That method involves calculating the remaining degrees of visual fields in eight principal meridians.

Use Table 5 in the *Guides* chapter on the visual system (p. 214) to determine the percentage of visual field loss. If central visual acuities are normal and there is no diplopia, then the percentage of field loss equals the percentage of visual impairment of each eye. Use Table 7 of the visual system chapter to determine the percentage of impairment of the visual system. Use Table 6 of the same chapter to determine the whole-person impairment.

If there are permanent impairments of other organ systems, *combine* the percentages with the whole-person impairment percentage related to the visual system (Combined Values Chart, p. 322) to estimate the individual's total impairment.

Table 7. Selected Optic Nerve Impairment Criteria.*

1. Partial visual impairment with best-corrected visual acuity better than 20/200: refer to the Guides chapter on visual system (p. 209)
2. Best-corrected visual acuity in one eye is 20/200 to 20/400 for distance *and* near: this is an 89% to 94% impairment of central vision and approximately a 23% whole-person impairment, depending on the visual fields
3. Best-corrected visual acuity in one eye is poorer than 20/400 at distance and 20/200 at near: this is a 97% impairment of central vision and a 24% impairment of the whole person
4. Complete destruction of an optic nerve is a 25% impairment of the visual system and a 24% impairment of the whole person
5. Complete destruction of both optic nerves is a 100% impairment of the visual system and an 85% impairment of the whole person

*Refer to *Guides* chapter on visual system (p. 209).

Table 8. Visual Field Impairment.*

Visual field loss	Impairment (%)	
	Visual field	Whole person
Dense, congruous, complete, homonymous, hemianopia or bitemporal hemianopia	66	62
Dense, congruous, complete, superior quadrantanopia	25	24
Dense, congruous, complete, inferior quadrantanopia	30	28

*This table may be used when central visual acuity is normal. Refer to *Guides* chapter on visual system (p. 209)

Example: A 27-year-old woman, who previously was in good health and had normal vision, experienced a progressive loss of vision in the left eye during a 6 month period. During the next 6 months there was slight return of visual acuity, but she no longer could read with that eye or see television images.

Results of a physical examination were normal, as were results of basic laboratory tests. The woman's visual acuity was 20/200 at near and far with the left eye and 20/20 with the right eye. The findings on neurologic examination were otherwise normal.

Impairment: The woman's whole-person impairment was estimated to be 23% (Table 7, above). Because careful documentation of such an impairment requires an ophthalmologic evaluation, the woman was referred to an ophthalmologist.

4.2 The Brain Stem

The cranial nerves with origins within the brain stem may be grouped into those originating in the midbrain, pons-cerebellum, and posterior hindbrain or medulla. The spinal accessory nerve originates in the cervical cord but exits from the skull and is called cranial nerve XI. Its loss of function is indicated by the combination of cranial nerve dysfunction and dysfunction of the associated long tracts of the motor and sensory systems that pass near the nerve or its nucleus.

4.2a The Midbrain

This segment of the brain stem contains the nuclei of cranial nerve III, the oculomotor nerve, and cranial nerve IV, the trochlear nerve. It also contains the red nucleus of the cerebellum and its crossings or decussations, the crossed long sensory tracts, and the corticospinal or pyramidal tracts. Diplopia and loss of cerebellar or corticospinal function are the most common impairments related to the segment. Oscillopsia, a condition in which visualized objects seem to move back and forth or jerk, is an uncommon cause of impairment.

The oculomotor and trochlear nerves (cranial nerves III and IV) and cranial nerve VI, the abducens, innervate the muscles that move the eyeball and control the size of the pupil. If there is permanent impairment of one or more of these nerves, resulting in loss of ability to perceive a single image with both eyes, the whole-person impairment may be significant. Correction of double vision by occluding one eye does not preclude properly making an impairment estimate.

Unless a patient has diplopia within 30° of the center of vision, the diplopia rarely causes significant visual impairment. An exception is with looking downward. The steps for estimating visual system impairment are described in detail in the chapter on the visual system (p. 209). Abnormalities of other organ systems also can occur with neurologic system syndromes and illnesses. Such abnormalities should be expressed as whole-person impairments and *combined* with the estimated whole-person impairment of the nervous system (Combined Values Chart, p. 322).

4.2b The Pons-Cerebellum Segment

The upper portion of the pons contains cranial nerve V, the trigeminal nerve; cranial nerve VI, the abducens; cranial nerve VII, the facial; and cranial nerve VIII, the auditory nerve. Impairment syndromes involving this region may include cerebellar abnormalities, hemiparesis, hemisensory defects, or Horner's syndrome. Parts of the nerves may be involved as they lead to the final end organ. There may be dysfunction of a single cranial nerve, as in trigeminal neuralgia, Bell's palsy, Ramsey-Hunt syndrome, and Meniere's syndrome. The reader should consult the *Guides* chapters on the visual system and the ear, nose, throat, and related structures as necessary. Combined neurologic syndromes are considered in this chapter.

The trigeminal nerve (cranial nerve V) is a mixed nerve having sensory fibers to the face, cornea, anterior scalp, nasal and oral cavities, tongue, and the supratentorial dura mater. The nerve also transmits motor impulses to the muscles of mastication.

Sensation in the parts served by the three major divisions of the trigeminal nerve is tested with the usual techniques for evaluating sensation, that is, pain, temperature, and touch; the two sides of the face or body are compared. Bilateral loss of facial sensation is uncommon. An impairment percentage for loss of sensation involving the trigeminal nerve is *combined* with an estimated impairment percentage for pain or motor loss.

Trigeminal neuralgia may be severe and uncontrolled. Both atypical, episodic facial pain and typical neuralgic pain may be evaluated (Table 9, below) if they have occurred for a period of months and interfere with daily activities. Motor impairment of the trigeminal nerve may affect chewing, swallowing, and speech articulation and may be accompanied by pain or a tic. Bilateral impairment is rare and may be severe. Daily activities may precipitate the pain.

Impairments of speech, chewing, and swallowing are considered also in the *Guides* chapter on the ear, nose, throat, and related structures (p. 223).

Table 9. Cranial Nerve V (Trigeminal) Impairment Criteria.

Impairment description	% Impairment of the whole person
Mild impairment due to uncontrolled facial neuralgic pain	0 - 14
Moderately severe, uncontrolled, facial neuralgic pain	15 - 24
Severe, uncontrolled, neuralgic pain, unilateral or bilateral	25 - 35

The abducens nerve (cranial nerve VI) has as its major function the innervation of the lateral rectus muscle of the eye and abduction of the eye laterally. With its location in the medial section of the brain stem, the nerve is intimately positioned near the facial nerve, the motor and main sensory nuclei of the trigeminal nerve, and the auditory nerve. If there is impairment of these nerves and the parts they serve, the appropriate parts of this and other *Guides* chapters should be consulted.

Example: A 55-year-old man had onset of diplopia 4 months before examination and almost immediately his symptoms stabilized. The persistent condition interfered with his workplace responsibilities, recreational pursuits, and his hobby of stamp collecting.

Results of physical examination and laboratory tests were normal except for the neurologic system. There was diplopia on forward fixation of gaze, and the patient was unable to abduct the right eye.

Impairment: The diplopia impairment was estimated, by means of the criteria in Chapter 8, to be a 20% impairment of the visual system, or a 19% whole-person impairment (Table 6, Chapter 8).

The facial nerve (cranial nerve VII) is a mixed nerve of which the motor part innervates the facial muscles of expression and accessory muscles for chewing and swallowing. The sensory fibers carry tactile sensations from a part of the external auditory canal, ear, tympanic membrane, and soft palate and adjacent pharynx, and sensory fibers mediating taste to the anterior two thirds of the tongue. Special fibers innervate the lacrimal and salivary glands.

Sensory loss related to the facial nerve does not interfere with the patient's activities of daily living. Loss of taste usually is not considered to be a major impairment. Impairment criteria are given in Table 10 (below).

Unilateral motor impairment poses the risk of vision impairment because of loss of blinking and corneal injury. Eating and speaking also can be affected.

Table 10. Impairment Criteria for Cranial Nerve VII (Facial) and Adjoining Region.

Impairment description	% Impairment of the whole person
Complete loss of taste of anterior tongue	1 - 4
Mild unilateral facial weakness	1 - 4
Mild bilateral facial weakness	5 - 19
Severe *unilateral* facial paralysis with 75% or greater facial involvement	5 - 19
Severe *bilateral* facial paralysis with 75% or greater facial involvement	20 - 45

The auditory nerve (cranial nerve VIII) is composed of nerves from two adjacent nuclei. The cochlear portion of the nerve is concerned with hearing, and the vestibular portion of the nerve is concerned with vertigo and position and orientation in space. The reader should consult the *Guides* chapter on the ear, nose, throat, and related structures (p. 223) regarding the evaluation of hearing impairment without known nerve dysfunction.

Tinnitus in the presence of *unilateral* hearing loss may impair speech discrimination and adversely influence the ability to carry out daily activities. Therefore, up to 5% may be added because of tinnitus to an impairment estimate for severe *unilateral* hearing loss.

Dysfunction of the vestibular part of the eighth nerve may be unilateral or bilateral. The impaired person may or may not be able to compensate for a unilateral loss. With bilateral loss of vestibular function, equilibrium and station are dependent on other systems, such as those for visual cues and kinesthetic senses; however, those systems may be inadequate for normal movement or ambulation.

Vertigo is the most disturbing symptom of vestibular dysfunction. Associated symptoms include nausea, vomiting, headache, fear of movement, ataxia, and nystagmus. The patient's movement or movement of objects in the environment may worsen these uncomfortable symptoms. Vertigo as a single entity is evaluated in the *Guides* chapter on the ear, nose, throat, and related structures (p. 223). Impairment of equilibrium and balance (Table 11, below) assumes significance, if the patient undertakes daily activities such as bicycle riding or working in high places or other hazardous locations.

Table 11. Impairment Criteria for Cranial Nerve VIII (Auditory Nerve).

Impairment description	% Impairment of the whole person
Minimal impairment of equilibrium exists, with limitation required only of activities in hazardous surroundings	1 - 9
Minimal impairment of equilibrium exists, with limitation required of all daily activities except simple ones for self-care	10 - 29
Moderate impairment of equilibrium exists, with limitation required of all daily activities including those for self-care	30 - 49
Severe impairment of equilibrium exists, with such limitation of daily activities that assistance is required for self-care and ambulation, and confinement may be needed	50 - 70

Combinations of cranial nerve impairments with dysfunctioning of the long tracts passing nearby should be evaluated by means of appropriate parts of the *Guides*, including Chapter 3 on the musculoskeletal system. Effects on several systems would be expressed in whole-person impairment percents, and the percents would be *combined* by means of the Combined Values Chart (p. 322).

4.2c The Medulla or Posterior Hindbrain

This segment has been called the mouth segment, because it moderates functions involving the mouth and the digestive and respiratory systems. Mixed nerves from the segment supply the oropharynx, larynx, and trachea; the autonomic fibers supply the thoracic and upper abdominal viscera. Abnormalities of breathing, swallowing, and speaking and visceral functions may be related to impairments of the medulla. The reader should consult the *Guides* chapters that relate to these functions.

The glossopharyngeal and vagus nerves (cranial nerves IX and X) are mixed nerves that supply sensory fibers chiefly to the posterior one third of the tongue and to the pharynx, larynx, and trachea. Involvement of the glossopharyngeal nerve by neuralgia usually is self-limiting or treatable and not permanent; the nerve's involvement may cause a condition similar to trigeminal (V) nerve tic or neuralgia. If the neuralgia persists for a period of months and is stable, the physician may be justified in assigning a percentage of impairment that is consistent with other impairments. Reference may be made to Table 9 (p. 145) on trigeminal nerve impairment. Sensory impairments may contribute to difficulties with breathing, swallowing, speaking, and visceral functions.

The spinal accessory nerve (cranial nerve XI) assists the vagus nerve in supplying some of the muscles of the larynx and innervates the cervical parts of the sternocleidomastoid and trapezius muscles.

Impairment of this nerve would be judged according to the effects on swallowing and speech, which are considered in the chapter on the ear, nose, throat, and related structures (p. 223). The nerve also can affect head turning and shoulder motion; related impairments would be evaluated according to criteria in *Guides* Chapter 3.

Table 12. Impairment Criteria for Cranial Nerves IX and XII.

Impairment description	% Impairment of the whole person
Mild dysarthria, dystonia, or dysphagia with choking on liquids or semisolid food; or uncontrolled spasmodic torticollis	1 - 14
Moderately severe dysarthria or dysphagia with hoarseness, nasal regurgitation, and aspiration of liquids or semisolid foods	15 - 39
Severe inability to swallow or handle oral secretions without choking, with need for assistance and suctioning	40 - 60

The hypoglossal nerve (cranial nerve XII) is a motor nerve that innervates the musculature of the tongue. Unilateral loss of function is not considered to be an impairment. Bilateral loss may result in impaired swallowing, breathing, and speech articulation (Table 12, at left). Swallowing is considered in the chapter on the ear, nose, throat, and related structures.

4.3 The Spinal Cord

The spinal cord conveys nerve impulses for motor, sensory, and visceral functions. Disorders of impulse transmission can result in permanent impairment, and the magnitude of the impairment would be estimated according to the effects on daily activities and the results of neurologic examination and testing.

Impairments resulting from spinal cord injuries and other adverse conditions include those relating to station and gait; use of the upper extremities; respiration; urinary bladder function; anorectal function; sexual function; and gait.

Sensory disturbances, including the loss of touch, pain, temperature perception, and sense of vibration and joint position, and paresthesias, dysesthesias, and phantom limb sensations may indicate spinal cord dysfunction. Autonomic system disorders, including disturbances in sweating patterns, regulation of circulation, and temperature regulation, may occur. Impairment is determined according to the amount of functional impairment and the level of involvement.

If the patient has impairments of several functions or systems, for instance, those of station and gait, as with hemiparesis and ataxia, of dexterity in using the upper extremity, and of bladder, bowel, or sexual functioning, the Combined Values Chart (p. 322) should be used to *combine* the whole-person impairment estimates for the several functions.

Accompanying disorders, such as trophic lesions, urinary calculi, osteoporosis, nutritional disturbances, infections, and reactive psychological states may occur. The degree to which any of these conditions augments spinal cord impairment should be based on the criteria given in the *Guides* chapters dealing with those disorders.

4.3a Station and Gait

The ability to stand and walk safely and with dexterity provides the basis of criteria for evaluating various neurologic syndromes involving the forebrain, brain stem, spinal cord, and peripheral nervous system

(Table 13, below). These impairments may need to be combined with those of other organ systems by means of the Combined Values Chart (p. 322).

Example: A 60-year-old man was referred with complaints of difficulty in walking and loss of strength of the hands; these complaints had not changed in the preceding 4 months.

Physical examination and laboratory studies disclosed the following abnormalities: gait spasticity and paraparesis, atrophy of the intrinsic muscles of the left hand, loss of sensation at the lateral aspects of the hands, increased deep tendon reflexes in the legs, and extensor plantar responses.

The man's impairments were estimated to be 55% gait impairment (Table 13, below); 12% whole-person impairment related to weakness of hand muscles; and 4% whole-person impairment of hand sensation. These *combine* to give an estimated whole-person impairment of 62% (Combined Values Chart, p. 322).

Table 13. Station and Gait Impairment Criteria.

Impairment description	% Impairment of the whole person
Patient can rise to a standing position and can walk but has difficulty with elevations, grades, stairs, deep chairs, and walking long distances	1 - 9
Patient can rise to a standing position and can walk some distance with difficulty and without assistance but is limited to level surfaces	10 - 19
Patient can rise to a standing position and can maintain it with difficulty but cannot walk without assistance	20 - 39
Patient cannot stand without help of others, mechanical support, and a prosthesis	40 - 60

4.3b Use of Upper Extremities

The basic tasks of everyday living are dependent on the dexterous use of the preferred or dominant upper extremity. Loss of the use of that extremity results, in most instances, in greater impairment than with impairment of the limb on the nonpreferred side.

Impairment of the preferred extremity (Table 14, at right) should be evaluated periodically, because the nonpreferred extremity eventually may become as capable of functioning as the preferred extremity. When the spinal cord disorder affects both upper extremities, the individual's impairment is greater than a simple combination of impairments of the preferred and nonpreferred extremities. The criteria for spinal cord disorders affecting both upper extremities are given in Table 15 (at right).

Table 14. Criteria for One Impaired Upper Extremity.

Impairment description	% Impairment of the whole person	
	Preferred extremity	Nonpreferred extremity
Patient can use the involved extremity for self-care, daily activities, and holding, but has difficulty with digital dexterity	1 - 9	1 - 4
Patient can use the involved extremity for self-care, can grasp and hold objects with difficulty, but has *no* digital dexterity	10 - 24	5 - 14
Patient can use the involved extremity but has difficulty with self-care activities	25 - 39	15 - 29
Patient cannot use the involved extremity for self-care and daily activities	40 - 60	30 - 45

Table 15. Criteria for Two Impaired Upper Extremities.

Impairment description	% Impairment of the whole person
Patient can use both upper extremities for self-care, grasping, and holding, but has difficulty with digital dexterity	1 - 19
Patient can use both upper extremities for self-care, can grasp and hold objects with difficulty, but has *no* digital dexterity	20 - 39
Patient can use both upper extremities but has difficulty with self-care activities	40 - 79
Patient cannot use upper extremities	80+

Example: A 58-year-old man had sudden onset of weakness of the left arm associated with occurrence of a severe headache. Living by himself in a small home, he had difficulty with bathing and caring for himself after the episode; a few months later his symptoms were stable.

On physical examination the patient's vital signs were normal. Results of basic laboratory tests and an electrocardiogram were normal. The man was able to stand steady and walk on the level floor. Questioning indicated he was right-handed. There was a moderately pronounced sensory loss on the left side, affecting the face, arm, and leg, and a mild loss of strength with increased deep tendon reflexes on the left. Visual field tests indicated that he had a left, congruous, homonymous hemianopia.

Diagnosis: Hemorrhagic infarct, right basal ganglia.

Impairment: Whole-person impairments were estimated to be 35% of the upper extremity (Table 14, above); 24% related to sensation; and 60% related to visual loss. These impairments *combine* to an estimated whole-person impairment of 80% (Combined Values Chart, p. 322).

4.3c Respiration

Neurologic impairment of one's ability to breathe is considered in Table 16 (below) only in terms of neurologic limitations. Other aspects of respiratory function are covered in the *Guides* chapter on the respiratory system (p. 153).

Table 16. Neurologic Impairment of Respiration.

Impairment description	% Impairment of the whole person
Patient can breathe spontaneously but has difficulty in activities of daily living that require exertion	5 - 19
Patient is capable of spontaneous respiration but is restricted to sitting, standing, or limited ambulation	20 - 49
Patient is capable of spontaneous respiration but to such a limited degree that he or she is confined to bed	50 - 89
Patient has no capacity for spontaneous respiration	90+

4.3d Urinary Bladder Dysfunction

The ability to control bladder emptying provides the criterion for evaluating permanent bladder impairment resulting from spinal cord and central nervous system disorders (Table 17, below). Documentation by cystometric or other tests may be necessary.

When evaluating impairments of the bladder, the physician also must consider the status of the upper urinary tract. The reader should refer to the *Guides* chapter on the urinary and reproductive systems and apply the Combined Values Chart (p. 322) if whole-person impairments of several organ systems are present.

Table 17. Criteria for Neurologic Impairment of Bladder.

Impairment description	% Impairment of the whole person
Patient has some degree of voluntary control but is impaired by urgency or intermittent incontinence	1 - 9
Patient has good bladder reflex activity, limited capacity, and intermittent emptying without voluntary control	10 - 24
Patient has poor bladder reflex activity, intermittent dribbling, and no voluntary control	25 - 39
Patient has no reflex or voluntary control of bladder	40 - 60

4.3e Anorectal Dysfunction

The ability to control emptying provides the criterion for evaluating permanent impairment of the anus and rectum due to spinal cord or other neurologic dysfunction (Table 18, below).

Table 18. Criteria for Neurologic Anorectal Impairment.

Impairment description	% Impairment of the whole person
Anorectum has reflex regulation but only limited voluntary control	1 - 19
Anorectum has reflex regulation but no voluntary control	20 - 39
Anorectum has *no* reflex regulation or voluntary control	40 - 50

4.3f Sexual Functioning

Awareness and capability of having an orgasm are the criteria for evaluating permanent impairment of sexual functioning that may result from spinal cord or other neurologic system disorders (Table 19, below). The patient's previous sexual functioning should be considered by the physician. The patient's age is only one criterion for evaluating previous sexual functioning.

Table 19. Sexual Impairment Criteria.

Impairment description	% Impairment of the whole person
Sexual functioning is possible but with difficulty of erection or ejaculation in men or lack of awareness, excitement, or lubrication in either sex	1 - 9
Reflex sexual functioning is possible but there is no awareness	10 - 19
No sexual functioning or awareness is present	20

4.4 The Muscular and Peripheral Nervous Systems

The spinal roots, plexuses, and peripheral nerves constitute an intricate conduction system that conveys impulses to and from the spinal cord and the tissues of the body including the muscles. Impairments due to disorders of the peripheral nervous system affect three main groups of fibers: sensory (afferent) fibers; motor (efferent) fibers; and autonomic system peripheral nerve fibers. The characteristics and functions of these groups are described in Chapter 3, Section 3.1k (p. 46).

Chapter 3 considers the musculoskeletal system and impairments of the extremities, spine, and pelvis, including those that involve nerves and blood vessels. Some material from that chapter, including tables for evaluating pain, sensation, and strength, is included in this chapter.

In evaluating finger sensation, the physician should understand that finger impairments involving total sensory losses are considered to be 50% of those for finger amputation. The physician should refer to Sections 3.1b (p. 19) and 3.1k (p. 46) for further relevant information.

At present, an approach to evaluating muscles and nerves that considers physiologic functioning or anatomic changes, or a combination of those approaches, is the one recommended in this part and in Chapter 3 to evaluate permanent impairments of sensation or muscle functioning.

The physician or other person evaluating the adverse condition of the neurologic system must understand the fundamental definition of a permanent impairment, which is described in Chapter 1 and the Glossary of the *Guides.*

4.4a Method of Neurologic Evaluation

Evaluating the peripheral nervous system requires documentation of the extent of loss of function due to sensory deficit, pain, or discomfort; loss of muscular strength and control of specific muscles or groups of muscles; and alteration of ANS control. Documentation of these deficiencies should include, if possible, descriptions of the spinal root(s), portion of the plexus, and peripheral nerve(s) that are involved.

Neurologic evaluation of pain is based first on the patient's description of the character, location, intensity, duration, and persistence of the discomfort and on verification of the anatomic distribution of the neurologic defect. Appropriate laboratory, radiographic, electrophysiologic, or autonomic testing may be required. A description of the ways and the degrees to which the pain interferes with the individual's performance in daily activities and the factors that augment the discomfort should be included. Anatomic descriptions should be made according to the usual distributions of the roots, plexuses, and nerves of the nervous system, which are described in Section 3.1k (p. 46) of Chapter 3.

Grading procedures for sensory and motor impairments are found in Chapter 3 (pp. 48 and 49) and are reproduced in this chapter (Tables 20 and 21, p. 151). The muscle strength grading system (Table 21, p. 151) is similar to the system recommended by the Medical Research Council of the United Kingdom, except that the numbers representing the categories of loss of strength are in reverse order.

4.4b Motor Deficits and Loss of Power

Involvement of peripheral nerves or roots may lead to paralysis or weakness of the muscles supplied by them, as well as to characteristic sensory changes. The system of the Medical Research Council is the one recommended in the *Guides* for evaluating muscle function and testing impairments (Table 21, p. 151). In this system, movement of the part is tested against the examiner's resistance plus gravity, without the effect of gravity, against gravity, and for slight or no movement. The contralateral extremity is tested also, and the results are compared with those in the affected limb.

4.4c Combining Multiple Deficits Due to Peripheral Nervous System Disorders

The impairment estimates for each neurologic deficit are determined by *combining* the motor and sensory impairments by means of the Combined Values Chart (p. 322). Conversion of an extremity impairment to a whole-person impairment is made only after all impairments involving that extremity have been combined, for instance, those due to loss of motion, vascular disorders, and neurologic deficits.

If there is bilateral extremity involvement, one determines the unilateral extremity impairments separately and converts each to a whole-person impairment. Then the two impairment percents are combined (Combined Values Chart, p. 322).

Example: A 60-year-old woman with diabetes mellitus developed a persistent and painful numbness of the right lower extremity during a 6-month period. This sensation involved the lateral aspect of the lower leg and extended in a more severe fashion down to the dorsum of the foot.

A physical examination disclosed the following abnormalities: a decrease in perception of pinpoint, cold, and light touch on the dorsum of the foot extending to the upper lateral calf area; painful par-

Table 20. Classification and Procedure for Determining Impairment Due to Pain or Sensory Deficit Resulting from Peripheral Nerve Disorders.

a. Classification

Class	Description of sensory loss or pain	% Sensory impairment
1	No loss of sensation, abnormal sensation, or pain	0
2	Normal sensation except for pain, or decreased sensation with or without pain, forgotten during activity	1 - 25
3	Decreased sensation with or without pain, interfering with activity	26 - 60
4	Decreased sensation with or without pain or minor causalgia that may prevent activity	61 - 80
5	Decreased sensation with severe pain or major causalgia that prevents activity	81 - 95

b. Procedure

1. Identify the area of involvement, using the dermatome charts in Chapter 3 (pp. 50 and 52).

2. Identify the nerve, part of plexus, or root that innervates the area.

3. Find the value for maximum loss of function of the specific nerve or root due to pain or loss of sensation, using the appropriate table in the *Guides* chapter on the musculoskeletal system (Chapter 3, p. 13).
Use Table 13 (p. 51) for the cervical roots; Table 14 (p. 52) for the brachial plexus; Table 15 (p. 54) for upper extremity nerves; Table 83 (p. 130) for the lumbosacral roots; and Table 68 (p. 89) for the lower extremity nerves.

4. Grade the degree of decreased sensation or pain according to the classification given above.

5. Multiply the percentage associated with the nerve identified in procedure 3 (above) by the percentage associated with the decreased sensation.

6. Determine other nerve impairments by the same procedure; *combine* the impairments using the Combined Values Chart (p. 322) to determine the whole-person impairment of the nervous system.

esthesias and dysesthesias of the foot; and mild weakness of dorsiflexion of the foot with a mild foot drop, characteristic of a peroneal nerve neuropathy.

Impairment:

1. Loss of function due to motor involvement of the common peroneal nerve (strength): 25% strength deficit (Table 68, p. 89) x 15% representing motor strength of nerve (Table 21, above) = 6% whole-person impairment.

2. Loss of function due to sensory involvement of common peroneal nerve: 25% representing sensory loss (Table 20, above) x 2% representing sensory function of common peroneal nerve (Table 68, p. 89) = 0.5%, or rounding, 1% whole-person impairment.

3. A 6% whole-person impairment combined with a 1% whole-person impairment is a 7% whole-person impairment (Combined Values Chart, p. 322).

Table 21. Classification and Procedure for Determining Nervous System Impairment Due to Loss of Muscle Power and Motor Function Resulting from Peripheral Nerve Disorders.

a. Classification

Grade	Description of muscle function	% Motor deficit
5	Active movement against gravity with full resistance	0
4	Active movement against gravity with some resistance	1 - 25
3	Active movement against gravity only, without resistance	26 - 50
2	Active movement with gravity eliminated	51 - 75
1	Slight contraction and no movement	76 - 99
0	No contraction	100

b. Procedure

1. Identify the motion involved, such as flexion or extension.

2. Identify the muscle(s) performing the motion and the motor nerve(s) involved.

3. Grade the severity of motor deficit of the individual muscles according to the classification given above.

4. Find the maximum impairment due to the motor deficit for each nerve structure involved, as listed in Chapter 3: upper extremity (Table 15, p. 54), brachial plexus (Table 14, p. 52), lower extremity nerves (Table 68, p. 89); and lumbosacral nerves (Table 83, p. 130).

5. Multiply the severity of the motor deficit by the percentage associated with the nerve(s) identified in procedure 4 (above) to obtain the estimated impairment from strength deficit for each structure involved.

4.4d The Autonomic Nervous System

The ANS influences the functioning of many organ systems; thus, failure of the system can increase impairment. Neurologic conditions that have ANS involvement include polyneuropathy of various causes, familial dysautonomia, Guillain-Barré syndrome, syringomyelia, porphyria, cord and brain tumors, and myelopathy.

Lack of control of blood pressure, body thermal regulation, and bladder and bowel elimination are prominent signs of ANS failure. Impairments related to transient loss of awareness or consciousness after a period of cerebral ischemia may be due to various mechanisms, including orthostasis, reflex actions, or cardiopulmonary disorders, and may be estimated by means of Table 22 (p. 152). Referring to other *Guides* chapters also may be necessary to estimate the magnitudes of the impairments.

Causalgia or reflex sympathetic dystrophy may be moderate or severe. The physician should assign a percentage on the basis of the severity of the pain and the degree to which it interferes with the activities of daily living. The evaluator should refer to the *Guides* chapters on the Musculoskeletal System and pain (pp. 13 and 303).

Impairments of spinal nerves, roots, plexuses, or peripheral nerves by various diseases or injuries may be partial or complete, unilateral or bilateral, related to motor or sensory functions, with or without pain. Each of these attributes or characteristics should be evaluated. When there is bilateral involvement, the two unilateral impairments should be determined; then the Combined Values Chart (p. 322) should be used to estimate the whole-person impairment.

Table 22. Impairments Related to Syncope or Transient Loss of Awareness.*

Level	Description	% Impairment of the whole person
1	*Mild* loss of awareness with drop in blood pressure of 15 mm Hg/10 mm Hg without compensatory increase in pulse rate, lasting more than 2 minutes after precipitating event	1 - 9
2	*Moderate* loss of blood pressure of 25 mm Hg/15 mm Hg, with loss of awareness or consciousness lasting 1-2 minutes	10 - 29
3	Levels 1 and 2 are present with *repeated severe* losses of blood pressure of 30 mm Hg/20 mm Hg, and additional neurologic symptoms or signs of focal or generalized nature also are present	30 - 49
4	Level 3 is present with *uncontrolled loss of consciousness* and muscle control without recognized cause and with risk of body injury	50 - 70

*This table is applicable to patients receiving treatment.

4.4e Nerves of Head and Neck, Trunk, and Inguinal Region

Tables 23 and 24 provide estimates for sensory abnormalities or loss of strength related to certain nerves of the head and neck and perineal regions. Any sensory or motor abnormalities of the nerves should be documented with the standard techniques of neurological evaluation. Using the listed percents, whole-person impairment estimates may be made by applying the classification and procedure of Table 20 or 21 (p. 151).

If a nerve is impaired because of an abnormality involving both sensation and strength, the whole-person estimates for the two kinds of impairment should be *combined* (Combined Values Chart, p. 322). If there is bilateral involvement, the whole-person impairment estimates for the nerves on the two sides should be *combined.*

The maximum impairment percent for a sensory or motor abnormality of a *thoracic nerve* is 2%. The final whole-person impairment estimate depends on the severity of the abnormality, and the classification and procedure of Table 20 or 21 (p. 151) should be used to determine the estimate. If both a sensory and a motor abnormality exist, the whole-person impairment estimates for the two types of abnormality should be *combined* to estimate the nerve's impairment (Combined Values Chart). If two or more nerves are involved, the impairment percents for the nerves should be *combined.*

Table 23. Impairments of Spinal Nerves in the Head and Neck Region.

Nerve	% Impairment of the whole person	
	Due to sensory deficit, pain, or discomfort	Due to loss of strength
Greater occipital	5	0
Lesser occipital	3	0
Great auricular	3	0

Table 24. Impairments of Spinal Nerves Affecting the Inguinal and Perineal Regions.

Nerve	% Impairment of the whole person	
	Due to sensory deficit, pain, or discomfort	Due to loss of strength
Iliohypogastric	3	0
Ilioinguinal	5	0
Coccygeal	5	0

4.5 Pain

Impairment due primarily to intractable pain may greatly influence an individual's ability to function. Psychological factors can influence the degree and perception of pain: different individuals in similar circumstances may be impaired by pain to different degrees.

Pain may be related to conditions as diverse in their causes, characteristics, and outcomes as angina pectoris, periodic (migraine) headache, a bone spur on the os calcaneus, and trigeminal neuralgia.

In some instances, pain will affect the proper functioning of a specific organ system. In the *Guides,* impairment percents shown in the chapters considering the various organ systems make allowance for the pain that may accompany the impairing conditions. However, chronic pain, also termed the chronic pain syndrome, should be evaluated according to criteria in the chapter on pain.

References

1. Baker AB, Joynt RJ, eds. *Clinical Neurology.* Philadelphia, Pa: JB Lippincott Co; 1991.

2. Wyngaarden JB, Smith LH, Bennett JC, eds. *Cecil's Textbook of Medicine.* 19th ed. Philadelphia, Pa: WB Saunders Co; 1992.

3. Walton J, Gilliatt RW, Hutchinson M, et al, eds. *Aids to the Examination of the Peripheral Nervous System.* London, England: Bailliere Tindall; 1988.

4. Osterweis M, Kleinman A, Mechanic D, eds. *Pain and Disability: Clinical, Behavioral, and Public Policy Perspectives.* Washington, DC: National Academy Press; 1987.

5. Johnson RH, Lambie DG, Spalding JMK. The autonomic nervous system. In: Joynt RJ, ed. *Clinical Neurology.* Philadelphia, Pa: JB Lippincott Co; 1989.

6. Raskin NH. *Headache.* 2nd ed. New York, NY: Churchill Livingstone; 1988.

7. Dalessio DJ. *Wolff's Headache and Other Head Pain.* New York, NY: Oxford University Press; 1987.

8. Haber A, LaRocca N, eds. *Minimal Record of Disability for Multiple Sclerosis. Developed by International Federation of Multiple Sclerosis Societies.* New York, NY: National Multiple Sclerosis Society; 1985.

9. Scheinberg L. Quantitative techniques in the assessment of multiple sclerosis: the problem and current solutions. In: Munsat T, ed. *Quantification of Neurologic Deficit.* Boston, Mass: Butterworth Publishers; 1989.

Chapter 5

The Respiratory System

This chapter provides a framework for the recognition and assessment of respiratory abnormalities that affect the individual's ability to function in the everyday world. Such an assessment requires collecting several types of information, organizing it into an understandable whole, and integrating it with other pertinent information that concerns the individual.

Before using the information in this chapter, the reader should become familiar with Chapters 1 and 2 and the Glossary, which discuss the general purpose of the *Guides*, the situations in which they are useful, and basic definitions relating to impairments. Chapter 2 discusses methods for examining patients and preparing reports. An impairment evaluation report should include information such as that shown below.

A. Medical Evaluation
- History of medical condition(s)
- Results of most recent clinical evaluation
- Assessment of current medical status and statement of further plans
- Diagnoses

B. Analysis of Findings
- Impact of medical condition(s) on life activities
- Explanation for concluding that the condition has been present for several months and is stable and unlikely to change
- Explanation for concluding that the individual is or is not likely to suffer further impairment by engaging in usual activities
- Explanation for concluding that accommodations or restrictions are or are not warranted

C. Comparison of Analysis with Impairment Criteria
- Description of clinical findings and how these relate to pertinent criteria
- Explanation of each impairment estimate
- Summary of all impairment estimates
- Estimated whole-person impairment

5.1 Assessing the Respiratory System

Assessment of the respiratory system should begin with the patient's description of the specific complaints related to respiration. Then a review should follow of personal habits and workplace exposures to potentially toxic substances that might explain or contribute to the existence of the symptoms. During the physical examination, the physician evaluates structural or movement abnormalities of the chest and its contents. Radiologic techniques provide visual evidence of internal anatomic abnormalities that are not apparent by external inspection of the chest wall or auditory assessment of the lungs, heart, and pleural space.

While each of the techniques mentioned above provides a certain amount of information about the severity of any respiratory abnormality, their main objectives are diagnostic and qualitative rather than quantitative. Pulmonary function testing, on the other hand, provides an objective assessment of the severity of respiratory abnormality but only a small amount of diagnostic information. The appropriate techniques are discussed below, the major emphasis being on the quantitation of abnormalities in terms of pulmonary function testing.

Symptoms Associated with Respiratory Dysfunction

Symptoms associated with respiratory dysfunction include dyspnea, cough, sputum production, hemoptysis, wheezing, chest pain, and soaking night sweats. Although questions should be asked about each of these symptoms during history taking, quantification of the symptoms is difficult in view of their subjective nature.

Dyspnea

Dyspnea is the most common presenting symptom in patients with any type of pulmonary impairment. Its importance is matched only by its nonspecificity and resistance to quantification. Dyspnea can be caused by diseases of cardiac, hematologic, metabolic, or neurologic origin; anxiety also can play a major role in its genesis.

Various schemes have been used to grade dyspnea. The one proposed by the American Thoracic Society (ATS) and shown in Table 1 (below) has been used widely. It is important to remember that the proper function of the classification is to enable comparison of the individual's symptoms with objective measurements of the individual's respiratory function. If there is a great disparity between the subjective and the objective findings, a nonrespiratory component of the dyspnea should be suspected.

Table 1. Classification of Dyspnea.*

Severity	Definition and question
Mild	Do you have to walk more slowly on the level than people of your age because of breathlessness?
Moderate	Do you have to stop for breath when walking at your own pace on the level?
Severe	Do you ever have to stop for breath after walking about 100 yards or for a few minutes on the level?
Very severe	Are you too breathless to leave the house, or breathless after dressing or undressing?

*The patient's lowest level of physical activity and exertion that produces breathlessness denotes the severity of dyspnea.

Cough, Sputum Production, and Hemoptysis

Although cough is an important indicator of disease in the respiratory tract, there are few generally accepted measures of the severity of that symptom. For this reason, the presence of a cough should not be used as an objective determinant of pulmonary impairment. Nonetheless, it is incumbent on the physician to document its presence or absence, its productive or nonproductive nature, its duration, and its association with hemoptysis. The purpose of this documentation is to identify individuals who require further evaluation of the respiratory system.

An acute, self-limited cough most commonly is due to infection or irritation. A subacute or recurrent nonproductive cough may be a manifestation of asthma and should be investigated further with pulmonary function testing. A chronic, productive cough is often a marker of bronchitis; according to ATS criteria, the term "chronic bronchitis" may be used to describe a cough productive of sputum that occurs on most days of at least 3 consecutive months per year, for at least 2 years in succession.

Hemoptysis frequently accompanies bronchitis and pneumonia, usually in the form of blood-streaking of the sputum. The more serious causes of hemoptysis include bronchogenic carcinoma, pulmonary emboli, bronchiectasis, tuberculosis, aspergilloma, and arteriovenous malformations. The presence of hemoptysis requires radiologic evaluation, which may uncover a disease that might lead to a respiratory or other type of impairment.

Wheezing

High-pitched, musical sounds often are reported as wheezing by patients with partial airway obstruction. These sounds can be generated at any point along the respiratory tract from the glottis to the bronchioles. The symptomatic manifestations of wheezing are helpful clues to the anatomic site of abnormality. Inspiratory wheezing, known as stridor, suggests laryngeal disease, while expiratory wheezing indicates bronchospasm or localized bronchial narrowing. Information about the seasonal occurrence of wheezing also is of diagnostic significance. Intermittent wheezing suggests a bronchospastic, allergic, or asthmatic cause, while persistent wheezing raises the suspicion of a fixed bronchial obstruction.

Symptomatic triggers of wheezing, such as exposures to allergens, chemicals, cigarette smoke, and strong odors, and seasonal occurrence of distress are highly suggestive of asthma. Wheezing that follows several minutes of exercise indicates a diagnosis of exercise-induced asthma, while wheezing that usually accompanies respiratory tract infections is classified as asthmatic bronchitis.

Figure. Lung Capacities and Volumes in the Normal State and in Three Abnormal Conditions*

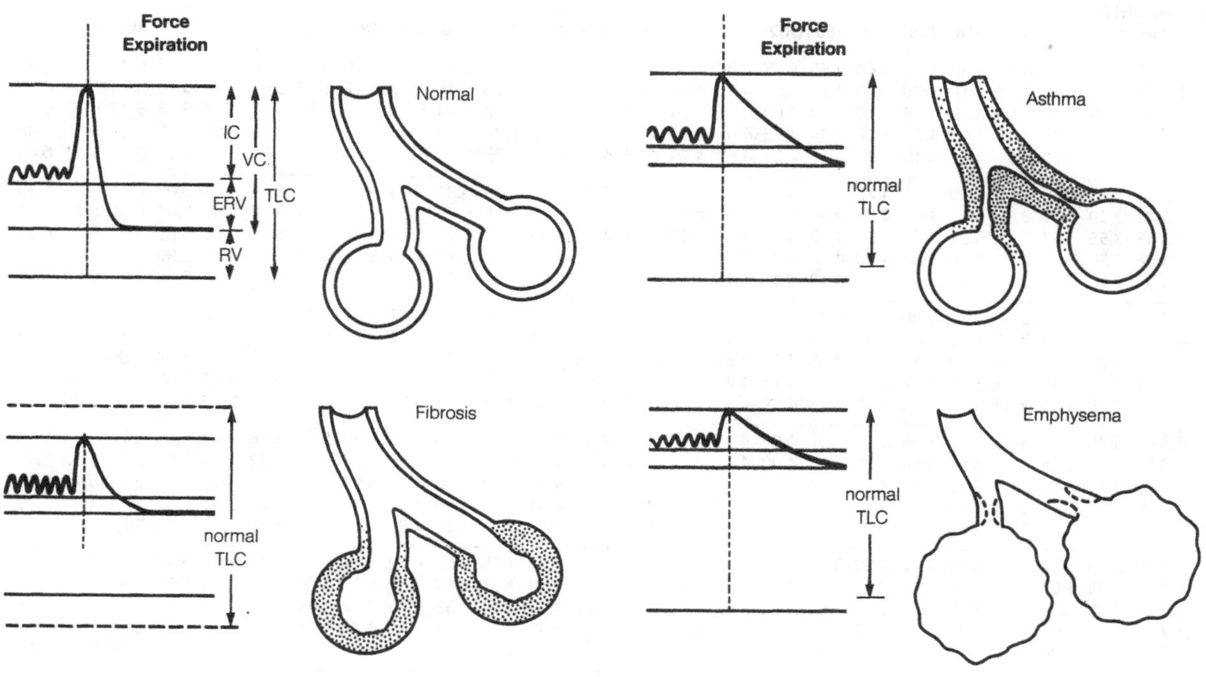

IC-inspiratory capacity, **VC**-vital capacity, **TLC**-total lung capacity, **RV**-residual volume, **ERV**-expiratory reserve volume.
* Residual volume, and therefore total lung capacity, cannot be measured by spirometry alone.

Tobacco Use

The most common cause of self-inflicted respiratory impairment is cigarette smoking. While there is variable individual susceptibility to the adverse effects of cigarette smoke, a discernible dose-response relationship is known. The examining physician should standardize data collection regarding dose by inquiring about the age when the patient started smoking, age at quitting or current age if the smoking continues, and the average number of packs smoked per day.

Multiplying the number of years of smoking by the number of packs smoked per day produces the standard measure, pack-years of cigarette smoking. This information can be used in assessing the impact of personal habits on respiratory impairment and may aid in the apportionment of respiratory abnormality among various deleterious factors. Cigarette smoking is the most significant causative factor in the development of chronic bronchitis, emphysema, and lung cancer. Chronic exposure to environmental tobacco smoke may also be a factor in the genesis of these conditions.

Occupational History

Environmental exposures in the workplace often are cited as causative or contributory factors in the development of respiratory impairment. To evaluate the possible effect of these exposures, it is important to obtain a complete occupational history from the patient. A major part of the history consists of a chronologic description of work activities beginning with the year of first employment and includes names of employers, the specific types of work performed, the materials used by the patient, and the potentially toxic materials present at the workplaces. An estimate of frequency and intensity of exposure to each substance is needed to assess its significance. Information about the use of respiratory protective devices is important and should be elicited. The number of years the devices were used with each employer should be recorded.

In addition to information on workplace exposures, the physician should obtain information about hobbies or leisure-time activities that might involve exposure to organic or inorganic chemicals or substances with potentially adverse effects on the respiratory tract; these might include paints, solvents, glues, and pesticides.

Physical Examination

Although a thorough physical examination is mandatory to reach valid conclusions about an individual's impairment, certain portions of the examination are particularly pertinent in evaluating the respiratory system. Vital signs should be measured after the

Table 2. Predicted Normal FVC Values (Liters) for *Men* (BTPS)*

Age	Height (cm) 146	148	150	152	154	156	158	160	162	164	166	168	170	172	174	176	178	180	182	184	186	188	190	192	194
18	3.72	3.84	3.96	4.08	4.20	4.32	4.44	4.56	4.68	4.80	4.92	5.04	5.16	5.28	5.40	5.52	5.64	5.76	5.88	6.00	6.12	6.24	6.36	6.48	6.60
20	3.68	3.80	3.92	4.04	4.16	4.28	4.40	4.52	4.64	4.76	4.88	5.00	5.12	5.24	5.36	5.48	5.60	5.72	5.84	5.96	6.08	6.20	6.32	6.44	6.56
22	3.64	3.76	3.88	4.00	4.12	4.24	4.36	4.48	4.60	4.72	4.84	4.96	5.08	5.20	5.32	5.44	5.56	5.68	5.80	5.92	6.04	6.16	6.28	6.40	6.52
24	3.60	3.72	3.84	3.95	4.08	4.20	4.32	4.44	4.56	4.68	4.80	4.92	5.04	5.16	5.28	5.40	5.52	5.64	5.76	5.88	6.00	6.12	6.24	6.36	6.48
26	3.55	3.67	3.79	3.91	4.03	4.15	4.27	4.39	4.51	4.63	4.75	4.87	4.99	5.11	5.23	5.35	5.47	5.59	5.71	5.83	5.95	6.07	6.19	6.31	6.43
28	3.51	3.63	3.75	3.87	3.99	4.11	4.23	4.35	4.47	4.59	4.71	4.83	4.95	5.07	5.19	5.31	5.43	5.55	5.67	5.79	5.91	6.03	6.15	6.27	6.39
30	3.47	3.59	3.71	3.83	3.95	4.07	4.19	4.31	4.43	4.55	4.67	4.79	4.91	5.03	5.15	5.27	5.39	5.51	5.63	5.75	5.87	5.99	6.11	6.23	6.35
32	3.43	3.55	3.67	3.79	3.91	4.03	4.15	4.27	4.39	4.51	4.63	4.75	4.87	4.99	5.11	5.23	5.35	5.47	5.59	5.71	5.83	5.95	6.07	6.19	6.31
34	3.38	3.50	3.62	3.74	3.86	3.98	4.10	4.22	4.34	4.46	4.58	4.70	4.82	4.94	5.06	5.18	5.30	5.42	5.54	5.66	5.78	5.90	6.02	6.14	6.26
36	3.34	3.46	3.58	3.70	3.82	3.94	4.06	4.18	4.30	4.42	4.54	4.66	4.78	4.90	5.02	5.14	5.26	5.38	5.50	5.62	5.74	5.86	5.98	6.10	6.22
38	3.30	3.42	3.54	3.66	3.78	3.90	4.02	4.14	4.26	4.38	4.50	4.62	4.74	4.86	4.98	5.10	5.22	5.34	5.46	5.58	5.70	5.82	5.94	6.06	6.18
40	3.25	3.37	3.49	3.61	3.73	3.85	3.97	4.09	4.21	4.33	4.45	4.57	4.69	4.81	4.93	5.05	5.17	5.29	5.41	5.53	5.65	5.77	5.89	6.01	6.13
42	3.21	3.33	3.45	3.57	3.69	3.81	3.93	4.05	4.17	4.29	4.41	4.53	4.65	4.77	4.89	5.01	5.13	5.25	5.37	5.49	5.61	5.73	5.85	5.97	6.09
44	3.17	3.29	3.41	3.53	3.65	3.77	3.89	4.01	4.13	4.25	4.37	4.49	4.61	4.73	4.85	4.97	5.09	5.21	5.33	5.45	5.57	5.69	5.81	5.93	6.05
46	3.13	3.25	3.37	3.49	3.61	3.73	3.85	3.97	4.09	4.21	4.33	4.45	4.57	4.69	4.81	4.93	5.05	5.17	5.29	5.41	5.53	5.65	5.77	5.89	6.01
48	3.08	3.20	3.32	3.44	3.56	3.68	3.80	3.92	4.04	4.16	4.28	4.40	4.52	4.64	4.76	4.88	5.00	5.12	5.24	5.36	5.48	5.60	5.72	5.84	5.96
50	3.04	3.16	3.28	3.40	3.52	3.64	3.76	3.88	4.00	4.12	4.24	4.36	4.48	4.60	4.72	4.84	4.96	5.08	5.20	5.32	5.44	5.56	5.68	5.80	5.92
52	3.00	3.12	3.24	3.36	3.48	3.60	3.72	3.84	3.96	4.08	4.20	4.32	4.44	4.56	4.68	4.80	4.92	5.04	5.16	5.28	5.40	5.52	5.64	5.76	5.88
54	2.95	3.07	3.19	3.31	3.43	3.55	3.67	3.79	3.91	4.03	4.15	4.27	4.39	4.51	4.63	4.75	4.87	4.99	5.11	5.23	5.35	5.47	5.59	5.71	5.83
56	2.91	3.03	3.15	3.27	3.39	3.51	3.63	3.75	3.87	3.99	4.11	4.23	4.35	4.47	4.59	4.71	4.83	4.95	5.07	5.19	5.31	5.43	5.55	5.67	5.79
58	2.87	2.99	3.11	3.23	3.35	3.47	3.59	3.71	3.83	3.95	4.07	4.19	4.31	4.43	4.55	4.67	4.79	4.91	5.03	5.15	5.27	5.39	5.51	5.63	5.75
60	2.83	2.95	3.07	3.19	3.31	3.43	3.55	3.67	3.79	3.91	4.03	4.15	4.27	4.39	4.51	4.63	4.75	4.87	4.99	5.11	5.23	5.35	5.47	5.59	5.71
62	2.78	2.90	3.02	3.14	3.26	3.38	3.50	3.62	3.74	3.86	3.98	4.10	4.22	4.34	4.46	4.58	4.70	4.82	4.94	5.06	5.18	5.30	5.42	5.54	5.66
64	2.74	2.86	2.98	3.10	3.22	3.34	3.46	3.58	3.70	3.82	3.94	4.06	4.18	4.30	4.42	4.54	4.66	4.78	4.90	5.02	5.14	5.26	5.38	5.50	5.62
66	2.70	2.82	2.94	3.06	3.18	3.30	3.42	3.54	3.66	3.78	3.90	4.02	4.14	4.26	4.38	4.50	4.62	4.74	4.86	4.98	5.10	5.22	5.34	5.46	5.58
68	2.65	2.77	2.89	3.01	3.13	3.25	3.37	3.49	3.61	3.73	3.85	3.97	4.09	4.21	4.33	4.45	4.57	4.69	4.81	4.93	5.05	5.17	5.29	5.41	5.53
70	2.61	2.73	2.85	2.97	3.09	3.21	3.33	3.45	3.57	3.69	3.81	3.93	4.05	4.17	4.29	4.41	4.53	4.65	4.77	4.89	5.01	5.13	5.25	5.37	5.49
72	2.57	2.69	2.81	2.93	3.05	3.17	3.29	3.41	3.53	3.65	3.77	3.89	4.01	4.13	4.25	4.37	4.49	4.61	4.73	4.85	4.97	5.09	5.21	5.33	5.45
74	2.53	2.65	2.77	2.89	3.01	3.13	3.25	3.37	3.49	3.61	3.73	3.85	3.97	4.09	4.21	4.33	4.45	4.57	4.69	4.81	4.93	5.05	5.17	5.29	5.41

*FVC in liters = 0.0600 H – 0.0214 A – 4.650. R^2 = 0.54, SEE = 0.644, 95% confidence interval = 1.115. Note: Do not subtract the confidence interval from the value indicated by the table.

Definitions of abbreviations: R^2 = coefficient of determination, SEE = standard error of estimate, H = height in cm, and A = age in years. BTPS = body temperature, ambient pressure and saturated with water vapor at these conditions.

Adapted from Crapo et al.[2]

patient has had an opportunity to relax and become accustomed to the surroundings. The physician should note the use of accessory muscles of respiration and the patient's body habitus. A breathing pattern characterized by pursing the lips during expiration suggests the presence of chronic obstructive pulmonary disease (COPD).

The thoracic cage should be inspected for vertebral or rib cage deformity, wasting of the intercostal muscles, a barrel shape that may indicate hyperinflation of the chest, and movement of the ribs with inspiration and expiration. Percussion of the chest is carried out to ascertain hyperresonance or consolidation and assess diaphragmatic motion.

Auscultation may reveal decreased breath sounds, crackles, wheezes, or rhonchi. The intensity, quality, and location of wheezing, rhonchi, and rales should be described, as well as whether they are heard during inspiration, expiration, or both. Crackles may be present in two thirds of persons with chronic interstitial disease; these usually occur during late inspiration.

Early inspiratory crackles may be heard in diseases of airflow obstruction and particularly in bronchiolitis obliterans. The presence of wheezing cannot be excluded until the physician performs auscultation during both quiet breathing and forced expiration. Diffuse, bilateral, expiratory wheezing indicates generalized bronchospasm, while unilateral or localized wheezing may be caused by partial bronchial obstruction due to an endobronchial tumor or pressure on the wall of the bronchus.

Cyanosis, indicated by a bluish discoloration of the lips, is a striking but unreliable indicator of severe pulmonary impairment. Poor lighting in the examination room, anemia, and skin pigmentation can interfere with assessing its magnitude. Suspicion of cyanosis calls for a pulse oximetry test or arterial blood gas analysis.

Digital clubbing is characterized by loss of the angle at the junction of the cuticle and the nail, softening of the nail bed, increased curvature of the nail, and widening of the distal portion of the fingers

Table 3. Predicted Normal FVC Values for *Women* (BTPS).*

Age	Height (cm)																							
	146	148	150	152	154	156	158	160	162	164	166	168	170	172	174	176	178	180	182	184	186	188	190	192	194
18	3.19	3.29	3.39	3.48	3.58	3.68	3.78	3.88	3.98	4.07	4.17	4.27	4.37	4.47	4.56	4.66	4.76	4.86	4.96	5.06	5.15	5.25	5.35	5.45	5.55
20	3.15	3.24	3.34	3.44	3.54	3.64	3.74	3.83	3.93	4.03	4.13	4.23	4.32	4.42	4.52	4.62	4.72	4.82	4.91	5.01	5.11	5.21	5.31	5.41	5.50
22	3.10	3.20	3.30	3.40	3.50	3.59	3.69	3.79	3.89	3.99	4.09	4.18	4.28	4.38	4.48	4.58	4.67	4.77	4.87	4.97	5.07	5.17	5.26	5.36	5.46
24	3.06	3.16	3.26	3.35	3.45	3.55	3.65	3.75	3.85	3.94	4.04	4.14	4.24	4.34	4.43	4.53	4.63	4.73	4.83	4.93	5.02	5.12	5.22	5.32	5.42
26	3.02	3.12	3.21	3.31	3.41	3.51	3.61	3.70	3.80	3.90	4.00	4.10	4.20	4.29	4.39	4.49	4.59	4.69	4.78	4.88	4.98	5.08	5.18	5.28	5.37
28	2.97	3.07	3.17	3.27	3.37	3.46	3.56	3.66	3.76	3.86	3.96	4.05	4.15	4.25	4.35	4.45	4.54	4.64	4.74	4.84	4.94	5.04	5.13	5.23	5.33
30	2.93	3.03	3.13	3.23	3.32	3.42	3.52	3.62	3.72	3.81	3.91	4.01	4.11	4.21	4.31	4.40	4.50	4.60	4.70	4.80	4.89	4.99	5.09	5.19	5.29
32	2.89	2.99	3.08	3.18	3.28	3.38	3.48	3.57	3.67	3.77	3.87	3.97	4.07	4.16	4.26	4.36	4.46	4.56	4.65	4.75	4.85	4.95	5.05	5.15	5.24
34	2.84	2.94	3.04	3.14	3.24	3.34	3.43	3.53	3.63	3.73	3.83	3.92	4.02	4.12	4.22	4.32	4.42	4.51	4.61	4.71	4.81	4.91	5.00	5.10	5.20
36	2.80	2.90	3.00	3.10	3.19	3.29	3.39	3.49	3.59	3.68	3.78	3.88	3.98	4.08	4.18	4.27	4.37	4.47	4.57	4.67	4.76	4.86	4.96	5.06	5.16
38	2.76	2.86	2.95	3.05	3.15	3.25	3.35	3.45	3.54	3.64	3.74	3.84	3.94	4.03	4.13	4.23	4.33	4.43	4.53	4.62	4.72	4.82	4.92	5.02	5.11
40	2.71	2.81	2.91	3.01	3.11	3.21	3.30	3.40	3.50	3.60	3.70	3.79	3.89	3.99	4.09	4.19	4.29	4.38	4.48	4.58	4.68	4.78	4.87	4.97	5.07
42	2.67	2.77	2.87	2.97	3.06	3.16	3.26	3.36	3.46	3.56	3.65	3.75	3.85	3.95	4.05	4.14	4.24	4.34	4.44	4.54	4.64	4.73	4.83	4.93	5.03
44	2.63	2.73	2.82	2.92	3.02	3.12	3.22	3.32	3.41	3.51	3.61	3.71	3.81	3.90	4.00	4.10	4.20	4.30	4.40	4.49	4.59	4.69	4.79	4.89	4.98
46	2.58	2.68	2.78	2.88	2.98	3.08	3.17	3.27	3.37	3.47	3.57	3.67	3.76	3.86	3.96	4.06	4.16	4.25	4.35	4.45	4.55	4.65	4.75	4.84	4.94
48	2.54	2.64	2.74	2.84	2.93	3.03	3.13	3.23	3.33	3.43	3.52	3.62	3.72	3.82	3.92	4.01	4.11	4.21	4.31	4.41	4.51	4.60	4.70	4.80	4.90
50	2.50	2.60	2.69	2.79	2.89	2.99	3.09	3.19	3.28	3.38	3.48	3.58	3.68	3.78	3.87	3.97	4.07	4.17	4.27	4.36	4.46	4.56	4.66	4.76	4.86
52	2.46	2.55	2.65	2.75	2.85	2.95	3.04	3.14	3.24	3.34	3.44	3.54	3.63	3.73	3.83	3.93	4.03	4.12	4.22	4.32	4.42	4.52	4.62	4.71	4.81
54	2.41	2.51	2.61	2.71	2.80	2.90	3.00	3.10	3.20	3.30	3.39	3.49	3.59	3.69	3.79	3.89	3.98	4.08	4.18	4.28	4.38	4.47	4.57	4.67	4.77
56	2.37	2.47	2.57	2.66	2.76	2.86	2.96	3.06	3.15	3.25	3.35	3.45	3.55	3.65	3.74	3.84	3.94	4.04	4.14	4.23	4.33	4.43	4.53	4.63	4.73
58	2.33	2.42	2.52	2.62	2.72	2.82	2.91	3.01	3.11	3.21	3.31	3.41	3.50	3.60	3.70	3.80	3.90	4.00	4.09	4.19	4.29	4.39	4.49	4.58	4.68
60	2.28	2.38	2.48	2.58	2.68	2.77	2.87	2.97	3.07	3.17	3.26	3.36	3.46	3.56	3.66	2.76	3.85	3.95	4.05	4.15	4.25	4.34	4.44	4.54	4.64
62	2.24	2.34	2.44	2.53	2.63	2.73	2.83	2.93	3.02	3.12	3.22	3.32	3.42	3.52	3.61	3.71	3.81	3.91	4.01	4.11	4.20	4.30	4.40	4.50	4.60
64	2.20	2.29	2.39	2.49	2.59	2.69	2.79	2.88	2.98	3.08	3.18	3.28	3.37	3.47	3.57	3.67	3.77	3.87	3.96	4.06	4.16	4.26	4.36	4.45	4.55
66	2.15	2.25	2.35	2.45	2.55	2.64	2.74	2.84	2.94	3.04	3.14	3.23	3.33	3.43	3.53	3.63	3.72	3.82	3.92	4.02	4.12	4.22	4.31	4.41	4.51
68	2.11	2.21	2.31	2.40	2.50	2.60	2.70	2.80	2.90	2.99	3.09	3.19	3.29	3.39	3.48	3.58	3.68	3.78	3.88	3.98	4.07	4.17	4.27	4.37	4.47
70	2.07	2.16	2.26	2.36	2.46	2.56	2.66	2.75	2.85	2.95	3.05	3.15	3.24	3.34	3.44	3.54	3.64	3.74	3.83	3.93	4.03	4.13	4.23	4.33	4.42
72	2.02	2.12	2.22	2.32	2.42	2.51	2.61	2.71	2.81	2.91	3.01	3.10	3.20	3.30	3.40	3.50	3.59	3.69	3.79	3.89	3.99	4.09	4.18	4.28	4.38
74	1.98	2.08	2.18	2.27	2.37	2.47	2.57	2.67	2.77	2.86	2.96	3.06	3.16	3.26	3.36	3.45	3.55	3.65	3.75	3.85	3.94	4.04	4.14	4.24	4.34

*FVC in liters = 0.0491H – 0.0216 A – 3.590. R^2 = 0.74, SEE = 0.393, 95% confidence interval = 0.676. Note: Do not subtract the confidence interval from the value indicated by the table.

Definitions of abbreviations: R^2 = coefficient of determination, SEE = standard error of estimate, H = height in cm, and A = age in years. BTPS = body temperature, ambient pressure and saturated with water vapor at these conditions.

Adapted from Crapo et al.[2]

or toes. Diseases of the chest associated with clubbing include pulmonary fibrosis, bronchiectasis, bronchogenic carcinoma, pleural tumors, lung abscess, empyema, and cyanotic congenital heart disease.

Chest Roentgenograms

The initial roentgenographic examination should include posteroanterior and lateral views of the chest taken in full inspiration. Chest roentgenographic findings often correlate poorly with physiologic findings in diseases with airflow limitation, such as asthma and emphysema. Chronic roentgenographic abnormalities of the chest may be classified as parenchymal, cardiovascular, pleural, or osseous. Parenchymal changes can be subdivided further into those causing hyperinflation and those characterized by fibrosis.

The physiologic abnormalities associated with hyperinflation are obstructive airway diseases, and those diseases associated with fibrosis restrict lung volume. In roentenographic terms, chronic obstructive pulmonary disease shows hyperinflation and pulmonary parenchymal destruction and is characterized by flattening of the diaphragm, vascular attenuation, increased anteroposterior diameter of the chest, and increased retrosternal airspace. Hyperinflation caused by asthma is usually transient. No correlation between the ability to work and lung hyperinflation has been demonstrated.

Fibrotic changes in the lungs may be localized or diffuse. Because of the redundancy of pulmonary tissue in the normal individual, diffuse fibrotic disease is much more likely to cause impairment than is localized disease. Diffuse, fibrotic abnormalities assume the characteristic roentgenographic appearance of being either rounded (nodular) or linear (reticular). Specific diagnostic information is obtained by describing both the type and the predominant location of fibrotic changes. For example, silicosis produces rounded opacities that predominate in the upper lung, while asbestosis produces linear opacities that predominate in the lower lung.

Table 4. Predicted Normal FEV_1 Values for *Men**

Age	Height (cm) 146	148	150	152	154	156	158	160	162	164	166	168	170	172	174	176	178	180	182	184	186	188	190	192	194
18	3.42	3.50	3.58	3.66	3.75	3.83	3.91	3.99	4.08	4.16	4.24	4.33	4.41	4.49	4.57	4.66	4.74	4.82	4.91	4.99	5.07	5.15	5.24	5.32	5.40
20	3.37	3.45	3.53	3.61	3.70	3.78	3.86	3.95	4.03	4.11	4.19	4.28	4.36	4.44	4.53	4.61	4.69	4.77	4.86	4.94	5.02	5.11	5.19	5.27	5.35
22	3.32	3.40	3.48	3.57	3.65	3.73	3.81	3.90	3.98	4.06	4.15	4.23	4.31	4.39	4.48	4.56	4.64	4.73	4.81	4.89	4.97	5.05	5.14	5.22	5.30
24	3.27	3.35	3.43	3.52	3.60	3.68	3.77	3.85	3.93	4.01	4.10	4.18	4.26	4.35	4.43	4.51	4.59	4.68	4.76	4.84	4.92	5.01	5.09	5.17	5.26
26	3.22	3.30	3.39	3.47	3.55	3.63	3.72	3.80	3.88	3.97	4.05	4.13	4.21	4.30	4.38	4.46	4.54	4.63	4.71	4.79	4.88	4.90	5.04	5.12	5.21
28	3.17	3.25	3.34	3.42	3.50	3.59	3.67	3.75	3.83	3.92	4.00	4.08	4.16	4.25	4.33	4.41	4.50	4.58	4.66	4.74	4.83	4.91	4.99	5.08	5.16
30	3.12	3.21	3.29	3.37	3.45	3.54	3.62	3.70	3.78	3.87	3.95	4.03	4.12	4.20	4.28	4.36	4.45	4.53	4.61	4.70	4.78	4.86	4.94	5.03	5.11
32	3.07	3.16	3.24	3.32	3.40	3.49	3.57	3.65	3.74	3.82	3.90	3.98	4.07	4.15	4.23	4.32	4.40	4.48	4.56	4.65	4.73	4.81	4.90	4.98	5.06
34	3.02	3.11	3.19	3.27	3.36	3.44	3.52	3.60	3.69	3.77	3.85	3.94	4.02	4.10	4.18	4.27	4.35	4.43	4.52	4.60	4.68	4.76	4.85	4.93	5.01
36	2.98	3.06	3.14	3.22	3.31	3.39	3.47	3.56	3.64	3.72	3.80	3.89	3.97	4.05	4.14	4.22	4.30	4.38	4.47	4.55	4.63	4.71	4.80	4.88	4.96
38	2.93	3.01	3.09	3.18	3.26	3.34	3.42	3.51	3.59	3.67	3.76	3.84	3.92	4.00	4.09	4.17	4.25	4.33	4.42	4.50	4.58	4.67	4.75	4.83	4.91
40	2.88	2.96	3.04	3.13	3.21	3.29	3.38	3.46	3.54	3.62	3.71	3.79	3.87	3.95	4.04	4.12	4.20	4.29	4.37	4.45	4.53	4.62	4.70	4.78	4.87
42	2.83	2.91	3.00	3.08	3.16	3.24	3.33	3.41	3.49	3.57	3.66	3.74	3.82	3.91	3.99	4.07	4.15	4.24	4.32	4.40	4.49	4.57	4.65	4.73	4.82
44	2.78	2.86	2.95	3.03	3.11	3.19	3.28	3.36	3.44	3.53	3.61	3.69	3.77	3.86	3.94	4.02	4.11	4.19	4.27	4.35	4.44	4.52	4.60	4.69	4.77
46	2.73	2.81	2.90	2.98	3.06	3.15	3.23	3.31	3.39	3.48	3.56	3.64	3.73	3.81	3.89	3.97	4.06	4.14	4.22	4.31	4.39	4.47	4.55	4.64	4.72
48	2.68	2.77	2.85	2.93	3.01	3.10	3.18	3.26	3.35	3.43	3.51	3.59	3.68	3.76	3.84	3.93	4.01	4.09	4.17	4.25	4.34	4.42	4.50	4.59	4.67
50	2.63	2.72	2.80	2.88	2.97	3.05	3.13	3.21	3.30	3.38	3.46	3.55	3.63	3.71	3.79	3.88	3.96	4.04	4.12	4.21	4.29	4.37	4.46	4.54	4.62
52	2.59	2.67	2.75	2.83	2.92	3.00	3.08	3.17	3.25	3.33	3.41	3.50	3.58	3.66	3.74	3.83	3.91	3.99	4.08	4.16	4.24	4.32	4.41	4.49	4.57
54	2.54	2.62	2.70	2.79	2.87	2.95	3.03	3.12	3.20	3.28	3.36	3.45	3.53	3.61	3.70	3.78	3.86	3.94	4.03	4.11	4.19	4.28	4.36	4.44	4.52
56	2.49	2.57	2.65	2.74	2.82	2.90	2.98	3.07	3.15	3.23	3.32	3.40	3.48	3.56	3.65	3.73	3.81	3.90	3.98	4.06	4.14	4.23	4.31	4.39	4.48
58	2.44	2.52	2.60	2.69	2.77	2.85	2.94	3.02	3.10	3.18	3.27	3.35	3.43	3.52	3.60	3.68	3.76	3.85	3.93	4.01	4.10	4.18	4.26	4.34	4.43
60	2.39	2.47	2.55	2.64	2.72	2.80	2.89	2.97	3.05	3.14	3.22	3.30	3.38	3.47	3.55	3.63	3.72	3.80	3.88	3.96	4.05	4.13	4.21	4.29	4.38
62	2.34	2.42	2.51	2.59	2.67	2.76	2.84	2.92	3.00	3.09	3.17	3.25	3.34	3.42	3.50	3.58	3.67	3.75	3.83	3.91	4.00	4.08	4.16	4.25	4.33
64	2.29	2.38	2.46	2.54	2.62	2.71	2.79	2.87	2.96	3.04	3.12	3.20	3.29	3.37	3.45	3.53	3.62	3.70	3.78	3.87	3.95	4.03	4.11	4.20	4.28
66	2.24	2.33	2.41	2.49	2.58	2.66	2.74	2.82	2.91	2.99	3.07	3.15	3.24	3.32	3.40	3.49	3.57	3.65	3.73	3.82	3.90	3.98	4.07	4.15	4.23
68	2.20	2.28	2.36	2.44	2.53	2.61	2.69	2.77	2.86	2.94	3.02	3.11	3.19	3.27	3.35	3.44	3.52	3.60	3.69	3.77	3.85	3.93	4.02	4.10	4.18
70	2.15	2.23	2.31	2.39	2.48	2.56	2.64	2.73	2.81	2.89	2.97	3.06	3.14	3.22	3.31	3.39	3.47	3.55	3.64	3.72	3.80	3.89	3.97	4.05	4.13
72	2.10	2.18	2.26	2.35	2.43	2.51	2.59	2.68	2.76	2.84	2.93	3.01	3.09	3.17	3.26	3.34	3.42	3.51	3.59	3.67	3.75	3.84	3.92	4.00	4.08
74	2.05	2.13	2.21	2.30	2.38	2.46	2.55	2.63	2.71	2.79	2.88	2.96	3.04	3.13	3.21	3.29	3.37	3.46	3.54	3.62	3.70	3.79	3.87	3.95	4.04

*FEV_1 in liters = 0.0414 H – 0.0244 A – 2.190. R^2 = 0.64, SEE = 0.486, 95% confidence interval = 0.842.

Definitions of abbreviations: R^2 = coefficient of determination, SEE = standard error of estimate, H = height in cm, and A = age in years. BTPS = body temperature, ambient pressure and saturated with water vapor at these conditions.

Adapted from Crapo et al.[2]

A standardized method of classifying roentgenographic abnormalities associated with fibrotic diseases caused by the pneumoconioses has been adopted by the International Labor Organization (ILO). Knowledge and proficiency in use of the method is certified by the B-reader Examination administered by the National Institute of Occupational Safety and Health. Despite the objective nature of the ILO classification system, the correlation of interpretations and readings with physiologic measures of impairment is poor.

Evidence of cardiovascular abnormalities associated with chronic pulmonary disease is provided by roentgenograms suggesting pulmonary hypertension and cor pulmonale. Pulmonary hypertension is indicated by bilateral enlargement of the main pulmonary arteries and rapid tapering of the peripheral vessels. Cor pulmonale is suggested by enlargement of the right ventricle and the changes of pulmonary hypertension. The presence of pulmonary hypertension and cor pulmonale should be confirmed by additional clinical and laboratory tests.

Pleural thickening usually is not associated with respiratory impairment. However, in an unusual case of diffuse massive thickening, respiratory movement may be impeded and a restrictive abnormality may result.

Spine Abnormalities

Osseous abnormalities of the spine may produce respiratory impairment due to mechanical factors involving the size of the chest cavity and restriction of rib motion. Kyphoscoliosis is the most common of these abnormalities. It is characterized by curvature of the vertebral column from side to side in the frontal plane (scoliosis), and curving from the dorsal to the ventral aspect in the sagittal plane (kyphosis). The severity of curvature is most commonly measured by the Cobb method. With this method, posteroanterior and lateral roentgenograms of the spine are used to measure the angles of curvature. Only severe angles of curvature, that is, Cobb angles greater than 100°, are likely to lead to respiratory

Table 5. Predicted Normal FEV_1 Values for *Women**

Age	Height (cm)																								
	146	148	150	152	154	156	158	160	162	164	166	168	170	172	174	176	178	180	182	184	186	188	190	192	194
18	2.96	3.02	3.09	3.16	3.23	3.30	3.37	3.43	3.50	3.57	3.64	3.71	3.78	3.85	3.91	3.98	4.05	4.12	4.19	4.26	4.32	4.39	4.46	4.53	4.60
20	2.91	2.97	3.04	3.11	3.18	3.25	3.32	3.38	3.45	3.52	3.59	3.66	3.73	3.79	3.86	3.93	4.00	4.07	4.14	4.20	4.27	4.34	4.41	4.48	4.55
22	2.85	2.92	2.99	3.06	3.13	3.20	3.26	3.33	3.40	3.47	3.54	3.61	3.67	3.74	3.81	3.88	3.95	4.02	4.09	4.15	4.22	4.29	4.36	4.43	4.50
24	2.80	2.87	2.94	3.01	3.08	3.15	3.21	3.28	3.35	3.42	3.49	3.56	3.62	3.69	3.76	3.83	3.90	3.97	4.03	4.10	4.17	4.24	4.31	4.38	4.44
26	2.75	2.82	2.89	2.96	3.03	3.09	3.16	3.23	3.30	3.37	3.44	3.50	3.57	3.64	3.71	3.78	3.85	3.91	3.98	4.05	4.12	4.19	4.26	4.33	4.39
28	2.70	2.77	2.84	2.91	2.97	3.04	3.11	3.18	3.25	3.32	3.39	3.45	3.52	3.59	3.66	3.73	3.80	3.86	3.93	4.00	4.07	4.14	4.21	4.27	4.34
30	2.65	2.72	2.79	2.86	2.92	2.99	3.06	3.13	3.20	3.27	3.33	3.40	3.47	3.54	3.61	3.68	3.74	3.81	3.88	3.95	4.02	4.09	4.15	4.22	4.29
32	2.60	2.67	2.74	2.80	2.87	2.94	3.01	3.08	3.15	3.21	3.28	3.35	3.42	3.49	3.56	3.63	3.69	3.76	3.83	3.90	3.97	4.04	4.10	4.17	4.24
34	2.55	2.62	2.68	2.75	2.82	2.89	2.96	3.03	3.10	3.16	3.23	3.30	3.37	3.44	3.51	3.57	3.64	3.71	3.78	3.85	3.92	3.98	4.05	4.12	4.19
36	2.50	2.57	2.63	2.70	2.77	2.84	2.91	2.98	3.04	3.11	3.18	3.25	3.32	3.39	3.45	3.52	3.59	3.66	3.73	3.80	3.87	3.93	4.00	4.07	4.14
38	2.45	2.51	2.58	2.65	2.72	2.79	2.86	2.92	2.99	3.06	3.13	3.20	3.27	3.34	3.40	3.47	3.54	3.61	3.68	3.75	3.81	3.88	3.95	4.02	4.09
40	2.40	2.46	2.53	2.60	2.67	2.74	2.81	2.87	2.94	3.01	3.08	3.15	3.22	3.28	3.35	3.42	3.49	3.56	3.63	3.69	3.76	3.83	3.90	3.97	4.04
42	2.34	2.41	2.48	2.55	2.62	2.69	2.75	2.82	2.89	2.96	3.03	3.10	3.17	3.23	3.30	3.37	3.44	3.51	3.58	3.64	3.71	3.78	3.85	3.92	3.99
44	2.29	2.36	2.43	2.50	2.57	2.64	2.70	2.77	2.84	2.91	2.98	3.05	3.11	3.18	3.25	3.32	3.39	3.46	3.52	3.59	3.66	3.73	3.80	3.87	3.93
46	2.24	2.31	2.38	2.45	2.52	2.58	2.65	2.72	2.79	2.86	2.93	2.99	3.06	3.13	3.20	3.27	3.34	3.41	3.47	3.54	3.61	3.68	3.75	3.82	3.88
48	2.19	2.26	2.33	2.40	2.46	2.53	2.60	2.67	2.74	2.81	2.88	2.94	3.01	3.08	3.15	3.22	3.29	3.35	3.42	3.49	3.56	3.63	3.70	3.76	3.83
50	2.14	2.21	2.28	2.35	2.41	2.48	2.55	2.62	2.69	2.76	2.82	2.89	2.96	3.03	3.10	3.17	3.23	3.30	3.37	3.44	3.51	3.58	3.65	3.71	3.78
52	2.09	2.16	2.23	2.29	2.36	2.43	2.50	2.57	2.64	2.70	2.77	2.84	2.91	2.98	3.05	3.12	3.18	3.25	3.32	3.39	3.46	3.53	3.59	3.66	3.73
54	2.04	2.11	2.18	2.24	2.31	2.38	2.45	2.52	2.59	2.65	2.72	2.79	3.86	2.93	3.00	3.06	3.13	3.20	3.27	3.34	3.41	3.47	3.54	3.61	3.68
56	1.99	2.06	2.12	2.19	2.26	2.33	2.40	2.47	2.53	2.60	2.67	2.74	2.81	2.88	2.94	3.01	3.08	3.15	3.22	3.29	3.36	3.42	3.49	3.56	3.63
58	1.94	2.00	2.07	2.14	2.21	2.28	2.35	2.42	2.48	2.55	2.62	2.69	2.76	2.83	2.89	2.96	3.03	3.10	3.17	3.24	3.30	3.37	3.44	3.51	3.58
60	1.89	1.95	2.02	2.09	2.16	2.23	2.30	2.36	2.43	2.50	2.57	2.64	2.71	2.77	2.84	2.91	2.98	3.05	3.12	3.18	3.25	3.32	3.39	3.46	3.53
62	1.83	1.90	1.97	2.04	2.11	2.18	2.24	2.31	2.38	2.45	2.52	2.59	2.66	2.72	2.79	2.86	2.93	3.00	3.07	3.13	3.20	3.27	3.34	3.41	3.48
64	1.78	1.85	1.92	1.99	2.06	2.13	2.19	2.26	2.33	2.40	2.47	2.54	2.60	2.67	2.74	2.81	2.88	2.95	3.01	3.08	3.15	3.22	3.29	3.36	3.42
66	1.73	1.80	1.87	1.94	2.01	2.07	2.14	2.21	2.28	2.35	2.42	2.48	2.55	2.62	2.69	2.76	2.83	2.90	2.96	3.03	3.10	3.17	3.24	3.31	3.37
68	1.68	1.75	1.82	1.89	1.95	2.02	2.09	2.16	2.23	2.30	2.37	2.43	2.50	2.57	2.64	2.71	2.78	2.84	2.91	2.98	3.05	3.12	3.19	3.25	3.32
70	1.63	1.70	1.77	1.84	1.90	1.97	2.04	2.11	2.18	2.25	2.31	2.38	2.45	2.52	2.59	2.66	2.72	2.79	2.86	2.93	3.00	3.07	3.14	3.20	3.27
72	1.58	1.65	1.72	1.78	1.85	1.92	1.99	2.06	2.13	2.19	2.26	2.33	2.40	2.47	2.54	2.61	2.67	2.74	2.81	2.88	2.95	3.02	3.08	3.15	3.22
74	1.53	1.60	1.67	1.73	1.80	1.87	1.94	2.01	2.08	2.14	2.21	2.28	2.35	2.42	2.49	2.55	2.62	2.69	2.76	2.83	2.90	2.96	3.03	3.10	3.17

*FEV_1 in liters = 0.0342 H – 0.0255 A – 1.578. $R^2 = 0.80$, SEE = 0.326, 95% confidence interval = 0.561.

Definitions of abbreviations: R^2 = coefficient of determination, SEE = standard error of estimate, H = height in cm, and A = age in years. BTPS = body temperature, ambient pressure and saturated with water vapor at these conditions.

Adapted from Crapo et al.[2]

failure. Even when severe spinal deformities are present, respiratory decompensation usually does not occur until middle age or later.

Respiratory compromise is produced by the combined effects of restrictive lung volume, decreased cross-sectional area of the vascular bed, and age-related decrease in chest wall compliance. Progressive stiffness of the chest wall with advancing age increases the work of breathing and leads to hypoventilation. This in turn produces hypoxia and hypercapnia. Hypoxia or oxygen lack is a powerful vasoconstrictor of pulmonary hypertension, and it further decreases the vascular cross-section, leading eventually to cor pulmonale. The presence of impairment should be judged on the bases described in Sections 5.2 (at right) and 5.3 (p. 163) of this chapter.

5.2 Physiologic Tests of Pulmonary Function: Techniques, Use, and Interpretation

Forced Respiratory Maneuvers (Simple Spirometry)
Physiologic testing of pulmonary function is the quantitative basis on which the evaluation of respiratory system impairment rests. A forced expiratory maneuver must be performed during the examination and evaluation of each patient for permanent pulmonary impairment. The testing and spirometry must be performed on standardized equipment calibrated according to, and using techniques described in, the 1987 ATS Statement on Standardization of Spirometry.[1]

Measurements are made from at least three acceptable spirometric tracings of forced expiration: forced vital capacity (FVC), forced expiratory volume in the first second (FEV_1), and the ratio of these measurements (FEV_1/FVC). The maneuvers should be performed at least three times, and the results of the two

Table 6. Predicted Normal Single-Breath D_{CO} Values for *Men* (STPD)*

Age	Height (cm) 146	148	150	152	154	156	158	160	162	164	166	168	170	172	174	176	178	180	182	184	186	188	190	192	194
18	29.8	30.6	31.4	32.2	33.1	33.9	34.7	35.5	36.3	37.1	38.0	38.8	39.6	40.4	41.2	42.1	42.9	43.7	44.5	45.4	46.2	47.0	47.8	48.6	49.4
20	29.3	30.2	31.0	31.8	32.6	33.4	34.3	35.1	35.9	36.7	37.5	38.4	39.2	40.0	40.8	41.6	42.5	43.3	44.1	44.9	45.7	46.6	47.4	48.2	49.0
22	28.9	29.7	30.6	31.4	32.2	33.0	33.8	34.7	35.5	36.3	37.1	37.9	38.8	39.6	40.4	41.2	42.0	42.9	43.7	44.5	45.3	46.1	47.0	47.8	48.6
24	28.5	29.3	30.1	31.0	31.8	32.6	33.4	34.2	35.1	35.9	36.7	37.5	38.3	39.2	40.0	40.8	41.6	42.4	43.3	44.1	44.9	45.7	46.5	47.4	48.2
26	28.1	28.9	29.7	30.5	31.4	32.2	33.0	33.8	34.6	35.5	36.3	37.1	37.9	38.7	39.6	40.4	41.2	42.0	42.8	43.7	44.5	45.3	46.1	46.9	47.8
28	27.7	28.5	29.3	30.1	30.9	31.8	32.6	33.4	34.2	35.0	35.9	36.7	37.5	38.3	39.1	40.0	40.8	41.6	42.4	43.2	44.1	44.9	45.7	46.5	47.3
30	27.2	28.1	28.9	29.7	30.5	31.3	32.2	33.0	33.8	34.6	35.4	36.3	37.1	37.9	38.7	39.6	40.4	41.2	42.0	42.8	43.6	44.5	45.3	46.1	46.9
32	26.8	27.6	28.5	29.3	30.1	30.9	31.7	32.6	33.4	34.2	35.0	35.8	36.7	37.5	38.3	39.1	39.9	40.8	41.6	42.4	43.2	44.1	44.9	45.7	46.5
34	26.4	27.2	28.1	28.9	29.7	30.5	31.3	32.1	33.0	33.8	34.6	35.4	36.2	37.1	37.9	38.7	39.5	40.4	41.2	42.0	42.8	43.6	44.4	45.3	46.1
36	26.0	26.8	27.6	28.4	29.3	30.1	30.9	31.7	32.5	33.4	34.2	35.0	35.8	36.6	37.5	38.3	39.1	39.9	40.7	41.6	42.4	43.2	44.0	44.8	45.7
38	25.6	26.4	27.2	28.0	28.8	29.7	30.5	31.3	32.1	32.9	33.8	34.6	35.4	36.2	37.0	37.9	38.7	39.5	40.3	41.1	42.0	42.8	43.6	44.4	45.2
40	25.1	26.0	26.8	27.6	28.4	29.2	30.1	30.9	31.7	32.5	33.3	34.2	35.0	35.8	36.6	37.4	38.3	39.1	39.9	40.7	41.5	42.4	43.2	44.0	44.8
42	24.7	25.5	26.4	27.2	28.0	28.8	29.6	30.5	31.3	32.1	32.9	33.7	34.6	35.4	36.2	37.0	37.8	38.7	39.5	40.3	41.1	41.9	42.8	43.6	44.4
44	24.3	25.1	25.9	26.8	27.6	28.4	29.2	30.0	30.9	31.7	32.5	33.3	34.1	35.0	35.8	36.6	37.4	38.2	39.1	39.9	40.7	41.5	42.3	43.2	44.0
46	23.9	24.7	25.5	26.3	27.2	28.0	28.8	29.6	30.4	31.3	32.1	32.9	33.7	34.6	35.4	36.2	37.0	37.8	38.6	39.5	40.3	41.1	41.9	42.7	43.6
48	23.5	24.3	25.1	25.9	26.7	27.6	28.4	29.2	30.0	30.8	31.7	32.5	33.3	34.1	34.9	35.8	36.6	37.4	38.2	39.1	39.9	40.7	41.5	42.3	43.1
50	23.1	23.9	24.7	25.5	26.3	27.1	28.0	28.8	29.6	30.4	31.2	32.1	32.9	33.7	34.5	35.4	36.2	37.0	37.8	38.6	39.4	40.3	41.1	41.9	42.7
52	22.6	23.4	24.3	25.1	25.9	26.7	27.6	28.4	29.2	30.0	30.8	31.6	32.5	33.3	34.1	34.9	35.7	36.6	37.4	38.2	39.0	39.9	40.7	41.6	42.3
54	22.2	23.0	23.8	24.7	25.5	26.3	27.1	27.9	28.8	29.6	30.4	31.2	32.0	32.9	33.7	34.5	35.3	36.1	37.0	37.8	38.6	39.4	40.2	41.1	41.9
56	21.8	22.6	23.4	24.2	25.1	25.9	26.7	27.5	28.3	29.2	30.0	30.8	31.6	32.4	33.3	34.1	34.9	35.7	36.5	37.4	38.2	39.0	39.8	40.6	41.5
58	21.4	22.2	23.0	23.8	24.6	25.5	26.3	27.1	27.9	28.7	29.6	30.4	31.2	32.0	32.8	33.7	34.5	35.3	36.1	36.9	37.8	38.6	39.4	40.2	41.0
60	20.9	21.8	22.6	23.4	24.2	25.0	25.9	26.7	27.5	28.3	29.1	30.0	30.8	31.6	32.4	33.2	34.1	34.9	35.7	36.5	37.3	38.2	39.0	39.8	40.6
62	20.5	21.3	22.2	23.0	23.8	24.6	25.4	26.3	27.1	27.9	28.7	29.5	30.4	31.2	32.0	32.8	33.6	34.5	35.3	36.1	36.9	37.7	38.6	39.4	40.2
64	20.1	20.9	21.7	22.6	23.4	24.2	25.0	25.8	26.7	27.5	28.3	29.1	29.9	30.8	31.6	32.4	33.2	34.1	34.9	35.7	36.5	37.3	38.1	39.0	39.8
66	19.7	20.5	21.3	22.1	23.0	23.8	24.6	25.4	26.2	27.1	27.9	28.7	29.5	30.4	31.2	32.0	32.8	33.6	34.4	35.3	36.1	36.9	37.7	38.6	39.4
68	19.3	20.1	20.9	21.7	22.6	23.4	24.2	25.0	25.8	26.6	27.5	28.3	29.1	29.9	30.7	31.6	32.4	38.2	34.0	34.9	35.7	36.5	37.3	38.1	38.9
70	18.8	19.7	20.5	21.3	22.1	22.9	23.8	24.6	25.4	26.2	27.0	27.9	28.7	29.5	30.3	31.1	32.0	32.8	33.6	34.4	35.2	36.1	36.9	37.7	38.5
72	18.4	19.2	20.1	20.9	21.7	22.5	23.3	24.2	25.0	25.8	26.6	27.4	28.3	29.1	29.9	30.7	31.5	32.4	33.2	34.0	34.8	35.6	36.5	37.3	38.1
74	18.0	18.8	19.6	20.5	21.3	22.1	22.9	23.7	24.6	25.4	26.2	27.0	27.8	28.7	29.5	30.3	31.1	31.9	32.8	33.6	34.4	35.2	36.0	36.9	37.7

*D_{CO} in mL/min/mm Hg = 0.410 H – 0.210 A – 26.31. R^2 = 0.60, SEE = 4.82, 95% confidence interval = 8.2.

Definitions of abbreviations: R^2 = coefficient of determination, SEE = standard error of estimate, H = height in cm, and A = age in years. STPD = temperature 0°C, pressure 760 mm Hg and dry (0 water vapor).

The regression analysis has been normalized to a standard hemoglobin of 146 g/L by means of Cotes' modification of the relationship described by Roughton and Forster.

Adapted from Crapo and Morris.[4]

best FVC efforts should be within 5% of each other. The tracing with the highest FVC and the tracing with the highest FEV_1 should be used to calculate the FEV_1/FVC ratio, even if these measurements occur on different expiratory efforts.

If wheezing is heard on chest examination, or the initial spirogram shows that obstruction is present, or the FEV_1/FVC ratio is below 0.70, spirometry should be repeated after the administration of an inhaled bronchodilator. The spirogram indicating the best effort, either before or after administration of the bronchodilator, should be used to determine FVC and FEV_1 and the presence of permanent impairment.

Measurements of FVC and FEV_1 should be compared to the values obtained from healthy subjects or reference values. Such values for both men and women are presented in Tables 2 through 5 (pp. 156 through 159).[2] To find the average or "predicted" value, find the patient's age in the left-hand column and the height along the top row; the predicted value lies at the intersection of the appropriate row and column.

North American whites have larger spirometric values for a given age and height than North American blacks. According to the ATS Task Force for Interpretation of Pulmonary Function,[3] the following adjustments for predicted lung function in black persons should be followed: values given for predicted normal FVC in Tables 2 and 3 should be multiplied by 0.88; values for predicted normal FEV_1 in Tables 4 and 5 should be multiplied by 0.88; values for normal single-breath carbon monoxide diffusing capacity (D_{co}) in Table 6 (above) should be multiplied by 0.93.[4]

Current information indicates there is a tendency for Hispanics, Native Americans, and Asians to have lower lung function values than North American whites. The cause and the magnitude of this difference are not yet well established, however, and no recommendation for the proportional adjustment

Table 7. Predicted Normal Single-Breath D_{CO} Values for *Women* (STPD):*

Age	Height (cm)																								
	146	148	150	152	154	156	158	160	162	164	166	168	170	172	174	176	178	180	182	184	186	188	190	192	194
18	26.0	26.5	27.0	27.6	28.1	28.6	29.2	29.7	30.2	30.8	31.3	31.9	32.4	32.9	33.5	34.0	34.5	35.1	35.6	36.1	36.7	37.2	37.7	38.3	38.8
20	25.7	26.2	26.7	27.3	27.8	28.4	28.9	29.4	30.0	30.5	31.0	31.6	32.1	32.6	33.2	33.7	34.2	34.8	35.3	35.8	36.4	36.9	37.4	38.0	38.5
22	25.4	25.9	26.5	27.0	27.5	28.1	28.6	29.1	29.7	30.2	30.7	31.3	31.8	32.3	32.9	33.4	33.9	34.5	35.0	35.5	36.1	36.6	37.1	37.7	38.2
24	25.1	25.6	26.2	26.7	27.2	27.8	28.3	28.8	29.4	29.9	30.4	31.0	31.5	32.0	32.6	33.1	33.6	34.2	34.7	35.2	35.8	36.3	36.8	37.4	37.9
26	24.8	25.3	25.9	26.4	26.9	27.5	28.0	28.5	29.1	29.6	30.1	30.7	31.2	31.7	32.3	32.8	33.3	33.9	34.4	34.9	35.5	36.0	36.5	37.1	37.6
28	24.5	25.0	25.6	26.1	26.6	27.2	27.7	28.2	28.8	29.3	29.8	30.4	30.9	31.4	32.0	32.5	33.0	33.6	34.1	34.6	35.2	35.7	36.2	36.8	37.3
30	24.2	24.7	25.3	25.8	26.3	26.9	27.4	27.9	28.5	29.0	29.5	30.1	30.6	31.1	31.7	32.2	32.7	33.3	33.8	34.3	34.9	35.4	35.9	36.5	37.0
32	23.9	24.4	25.0	25.5	26.0	26.6	27.1	27.6	28.2	28.7	29.2	29.8	30.3	30.8	31.4	31.9	32.4	33.0	33.5	34.1	34.6	35.1	35.7	36.2	36.7
34	23.6	24.1	24.7	25.2	25.7	26.3	26.8	27.3	27.9	28.4	28.9	29.5	30.0	30.6	31.1	31.6	32.2	32.7	33.2	33.8	34.3	34.8	35.4	35.9	36.4
36	23.3	23.8	24.4	24.9	25.4	26.0	26.5	27.1	27.6	28.1	28.7	29.2	29.7	30.3	30.8	31.3	31.9	32.4	32.9	33.5	34.0	34.5	35.1	35.6	36.1
38	23.0	23.6	24.1	24.6	25.2	25.7	26.2	26.8	27.3	27.8	28.4	28.9	29.4	30.0	30.5	31.0	31.6	32.1	32.6	33.2	33.7	34.2	34.8	35.3	35.8
40	22.7	23.3	23.8	24.3	24.9	25.4	25.9	26.5	27.0	27.5	28.1	28.6	29.1	29.7	30.2	30.7	31.3	31.8	32.3	32.9	33.4	33.9	34.5	35.0	35.5
42	22.4	23.0	23.5	24.0	24.6	25.1	25.6	26.2	26.7	27.2	27.8	28.3	28.8	29.4	29.9	30.4	31.0	31.5	32.0	32.6	33.1	33.6	34.2	34.7	35.2
44	22.1	22.7	23.2	23.7	24.3	24.3	25.3	25.9	26.4	26.9	27.5	28.0	28.5	29.1	29.6	30.1	30.7	31.2	31.7	32.3	32.8	33.3	33.9	34.4	34.9
46	21.8	22.4	22.9	23.4	24.0	24.5	25.0	25.6	26.1	26.6	27.2	27.7	28.2	28.8	29.3	29.8	30.4	30.9	31.4	32.0	32.5	33.0	33.6	34.1	34.6
48	21.5	22.1	22.6	23.1	23.7	24.2	24.7	25.3	25.8	26.3	26.9	27.4	27.9	28.5	29.0	29.5	30.1	30.6	31.1	31.7	32.2	32.8	33.3	33.8	34.4
50	21.2	21.8	22.3	22.8	23.4	23.9	24.4	25.0	25.5	26.0	26.6	27.1	27.6	28.2	28.7	29.3	29.8	30.3	30.9	31.4	31.9	32.5	33.0	33.5	34.1
52	20.9	21.5	22.0	22.5	23.1	23.5	24.1	24.7	25.2	25.8	26.3	26.8	27.4	27.9	28.4	29.0	29.5	30.0	30.6	31.1	31.6	32.2	32.7	33.2	33.8
54	20.6	21.2	21.7	22.3	22.8	23.3	23.9	24.4	24.9	25.5	26.0	26.5	27.1	27.6	28.1	28.7	29.2	29.7	30.3	30.8	31.3	31.9	32.4	32.9	33.5
56	20.4	20.9	21.4	22.0	22.5	23.0	23.6	24.1	24.6	25.2	25.7	26.2	26.8	27.3	27.8	28.4	28.9	29.4	30.0	30.5	31.0	31.6	32.1	32.6	33.2
58	20.1	20.6	21.1	21.7	22.2	22.7	23.3	23.8	24.3	24.9	25.4	25.9	26.5	27.0	27.5	28.1	28.6	29.1	29.7	30.2	30.7	31.3	31.8	32.3	32.9
60	19.8	20.3	20.8	21.4	21.9	22.4	23.0	23.5	24.0	24.6	25.1	25.6	26.2	26.7	27.2	27.8	28.3	28.8	29.4	29.9	30.4	31.0	31.5	32.0	32.6
62	19.5	20.0	20.5	21.1	21.6	22.1	22.7	23.2	23.7	24.3	24.8	25.3	25.9	26.4	26.9	27.5	28.0	28.5	29.1	29.6	30.1	30.7	31.2	31.7	32.3
64	19.2	19.7	20.2	20.8	21.3	21.8	22.4	22.9	23.4	24.0	24.5	25.0	25.6	26.1	26.6	27.2	27.7	28.2	28.8	29.3	29.8	30.4	30.9	31.5	32.0
66	18.9	19.4	19.9	20.5	21.0	21.5	22.1	22.6	23.1	23.7	24.2	24.1	25.3	25.8	26.3	26.9	27.4	28.0	28.5	29.0	29.6	30.1	30.6	31.2	31.7
68	18.6	19.1	19.6	20.2	20.7	21.2	21.8	22.3	22.8	23.4	23.9	24.5	25.0	25.5	26.1	26.6	27.1	27.7	28.2	28.7	29.3	29.8	30.3	30.9	31.4
70	18.3	18.8	19.3	19.9	20.4	21.0	21.5	22.0	22.6	23.1	23.5	24.2	24.7	25.2	25.8	26.3	26.8	27.4	27.9	28.4	29.0	29.5	30.0	30.6	31.1
72	18.0	18.5	19.1	19.6	20.1	20.7	21.2	21.1	22.3	22.8	23.3	23.9	24.4	24.9	25.5	26.0	26.5	27.1	27.6	28.1	28.7	29.2	29.7	30.3	30.8
74	17.7	18.2	18.8	19.3	19.8	20.4	20.9	21.4	22.0	22.5	23.0	23.6	24.1	24.6	25.2	25.7	26.2	26.8	27.3	27.8	28.4	28.9	29.4	30.0	30.5

*D_{CO} in mL/min/mm Hg = 0.267 H – 0.148 A – 10.34. R^2 = 0.60, SEE = 3.40, 95% confidence interval = 5.74.

Definitions of abbreviations: R^2 = coefficient of determination, SEE = standard error of estimate, H = height in cm, and A = age in years. STPD = temperature 0°C, pressure 760 mm Hg and dry (0 water vapor).

The regression analysis has been normalized to a standard hemoglobin of 125 g/L (the original equation was normalized to a standard hemoglobin of 146 g/d) by means of Cotes' modification of the relationship described by Roughton and Forster.

Adapted from Crapo and Morris.[4]

of predicted lung function can be made at the present time.

The FEV_1/FVC ratio is helpful in the *diagnosis* of obstructive airway disease. However, according to the most recent ATS statement on the interpretation of pulmonary function testing, that ratio is not useful in assessing the severity of that type of disease.[5] Rather, the severity should be judged on the basis of the absolute value of FEV_1 or the percentage of predicted value of FEV_1.

Diffusing Capacity of Carbon Monoxide (D_{CO})

The single-breath D_{CO} should be used for the evaluation of all levels of impairment. The method for performing single-breath D_{CO} described by the ATS[6] should be followed.

The D_{CO} measurement provides information on the efficiency of gas transfer across the lung. Several physiologic factors affect the gas transfer process, including the thickness of the alveolar-capillary membrane, surface area available for gas exchange, solubility of the gas, pulmonary capillary blood volume, hematocrit, concentration gradient of the test gas across the alveolar-capillary membrane, and availability of binding sites on the hemoglobin.

Mechanical factors involved in the test procedure affect the results, including speed of inhalation of the test gas, depth of inspiration, period of breath-holding, and speed of expiration. Cigarette smoking can elevate the amount of carbon monoxide in the blood, causing as much as 10% to 12% saturation of the hemoglobin and a decrease in the D_{CO}. Therefore, the patient should be instructed not to smoke for at least 8 hours before the test.

While mechanical factors generally are controlled by automation of the D_{CO} test, it is clear that many extrapulmonary factors are important in interpreting the results. Minor decreases in D_{CO} measurements occur in asymptomatic persons and do not decrease

Table 8. Classes of Respiratory Impairment.*

	Class 1: **0%, no impairment of the whole person**	**Class 2:** **10-25%, mild impairment of the whole person**	**Class 3:** **26-50%, moderate impairment of the whole person**	**Class 4:** **51-100%, severe impairment of the whole person**
FVC FEV_1 FEV_1/FVC (%) D_{CO}	FVC ≥ 80% of predicted; *and* FEV_1 ≥ 80% of predicted; *and* FEV_1/FVC ≥ 70%; *and* D_{CO} ≥ 70% of predicted.	FVC between 60% and 79% of predicted; *or* FEV_1 between 60% and 79% of predicted; *or* D_{CO} between 60% and 69% of predicted.	FVC between 51% and 59% of predicted; *or* FEV_1 between 41% and 59% of predicted; *or* D_{CO} between 41% and 59% of predicted.	FVC ≤ 50% of predicted; *or* FEV_1 ≤ 40% of predicted; *or* D_{CO} ≤ 40% of predicted.
	or	**or**	**or**	**or**
$\dot{V}O_2$ Max	> 25 mL/(kg • min); *or* > 7.1 METS	Between 20 and 25 mL/(kg • min); *or* 5.7-7.1 METS	Between 15 and 20 mL/(kg • min); *or* 4.3-5.7 METS	< 15 mL/(kg • min); *or* < 1.05 L/min; *or* < 4.3 METS

*FVC = forced vital capacity, FEV_1 = forced expiratory volume in the first second, D_{CO} = diffusing capacity of carbon monoxide. The D_{CO} is primarily of value for persons with restrictive lung disease. In classes 2 and 3, if the FVC, FEV_1 and FEV_1/FVC ratio are normal and the D_{CO} is between 41% and 79%, then an exercise test is required.

$\dot{V}O_2$ Max, or measured exercise capacity, is useful in assessing whether a person's complaint of dyspnea (see Table 1) is a result of respiratory or other conditions. A person's cardiac and conditioning status must be considered in performing the test and in interpreting the results.

their ability to work. Exercise-induced hypoxia rarely occurs when the D_{co} is greater than 60% of the predicted value.

Reference values for population-based average results for D_{co} are presented in Tables 6 and 7 (pp. 160 and 161).[4] These tables are to be used in a manner similar to the tables on spirometry. A laboratory that performs the D_{co} under conditions or with procedures that are different from the ATS recommendations should either develop and verify its own prediction equations or use an accepted and verified equation.

The classification of testing results for FVC, FEV_1, FEV_1/FVC, and D_{co} is given in Table 8 (above). In evaluating the cause of abnormality in any of the listed measures, the physician should consider the possible contribution of extrapulmonary factors to respiratory system impairment. For example, obesity may decrease the forced vital capacity, and anemia may decrease the D_{co}. However, only pulmonary dysfunction should be considered in evaluating impairment according to Table 8. Impairments of other organ systems may be evaluated according to the criteria given in other *Guides* chapters and then *combined* with the respiratory system impairment using the Combined Values Chart (p. 322).

Measured Exercise Capacity

Exercise capacity measurements may be used as an adjunctive or accessory means of assessing the severity and cause of exercise intolerance. When properly performed and interpreted, these tests can help differentiate pulmonary impairment from cardiac impairment or the effects of physical deconditioning. Since these studies are more difficult to perform, frequently more expensive, and sometimes more invasive than conventional tests, they should be used sparingly and only when they are likely to clarify the nature of an impairment.[7] Ordinarily, exercise capacity measurements should not be used to study individuals with normal results on routine pulmonary function tests. Similarly, they should not be used when an individual's spirometry and D_{co} measurements indicate severe impairment, because the additional information will not be helpful in assessing ability to work or carry out daily activities. Finally, exercise testing is not recommended for an individual who, in the opinion of the examining physician, has a medical contraindication such as unstable cardiac disease.

Measured exercise testing may be done when an individual whose daily activities require sustained moderate exertion or frequent heavy exertion complains of shortness of breath, and the physician has reason to believe that the usual tests may have underestimated the impairment. Exercise capacity is measured by the uptake of oxygen (VO_2) in mL(kg·min), or in METS, a unit of expended energy equal to 3.5 mL(kg·min) oxygen consumption. The MET is discussed in the chapter on the cardiovascular system (p. 169). Generally, an individual can sustain a work level equal to 40% of his or her measured maximum VO_2 for an 8-hour period. Table 9 (p. 163) shows the relationship between work intensity and oxygen consumption.

Assessment of Arterial Oxygenation

Arterial blood gas analysis should be used sparingly in the evaluation of pulmonary impairment because of its invasive nature. In addition, the results of arterial blood gas analysis may be outside the normal range for reasons other than pulmonary disease. For example, the arterial PO_2 may be decreased because of the altitude at which the sample was taken or the patient's obesity or breathholding. In general, for most persons with obstructive lung disease, the FEV_1 correlates better with exercise capacity than does the arterial PO_2. For purposes of evaluating permanent impairment, hypoxia must be documented on two occasions at least 4 weeks apart.

An arterial blood gas determination may indicate the presence of severe impairment even when an individual is stable and receiving optimal therapy. When a patient is examined at rest while breathing room air at sea level, an arterial PO_2 of less than 60 mm Hg is evidence of severe impairment, if the patient also has one or more of the secondary conditions related to arterial hypoxemia, such as pulmonary hypertension, cor pulmonale, increasingly severe hypoxemia during exercise testing, or erythrocytosis. An arterial PO_2 of less than 55 mm Hg in a resting patient breathing room air at sea level is by itself strong evidence of severe impairment.

Table 9. Classification of Prolonged Physical Work Intensity by Oxygen Consumption.*

Work intensity for 70-kg person*	Oxygen consumption		Excess energy expenditure
Light work	7 mL/kg	≤ 0.5 Liter/min	≤ 2 METS
Moderate work	8-15 mL/kg	0.6-1.0 Liter/min	2-4 METS
Heavy work	16-20 mL/kg	1.1-1.5 Liter/min	5-6 METS
Very heavy work	21-30 mL/kg	1.6-2.0 Liter/min	7-8 METS
Arduous work	> 30 mL/kg	> 2.0 Liter/min	> 8 METS

*Adapted from Astrand P, Rodahl K.[8]

5.3 Criteria for Evaluating Permanent Impairment

Table 8 (p. 162) presents criteria for estimating the extent of permanent impairment. Spirometry and D_{CO} must be performed on each individual being studied. The VO_2 max will be performed rarely and is not often necessary for identifying classes of impairment. If the patient is to be considered to have no impairment, all of the listed criteria except for VO_2 max must be met. For all other classes, at least one of the listed criteria must be fulfilled.

Sleep Disorders, Asthma, Lung Cancer, and Other Impairments

Certain respiratory conditions may cause impairment that is not readily quantifiable by testing pulmonary functioning, spirometry, diffusing capacity, or measured exercise testing. Sleep disorders are examples of conditions of this type.

Although the lungs and respiratory system may be structurally and functionally normal while the individual is awake, the breathing pattern during sleep is altered and periods of apnea (cessation of air flow at the nose and mouth) may occur throughout the night. In the normal individual, alterations in respiratory drive and ventilatory mechanics occur during the various stages of sleep. In normal non-rapid eye movement sleep, there is an overall reduction in respiratory drive, while in normal rapid eye movement sleep, respiratory drive is irregular and tone in the muscles of the rib cage and muscles of the upper airways is inhibited. In patients with disordered breathing during sleep, periods of apnea occur and lead to episodes of hypoxia and hypercapnia. Arousal from sleep under these circumstances is effected by reticular and cortical activation in the brain. While the arousal is a protective response, the resulting fragmentation of the normal sleep pattern produces restless and unrefreshing sleep, morning headache, daytime sleepiness, intellectual impairment, and personality changes.

Two major subgroups of sleep apnea are recognized. Obstructive sleep apnea is characterized by occlusion of the upper respiratory tract by sleep-induced relaxation of the oropharyngeal muscles, which allows the tongue and palate to rest against the posterior pharyngeal wall. Air ceases to flow through the nose and mouth despite continued respiratory efforts by muscles of the chest wall and diaphragm. Arousal leads to improvement in muscle tone of the upper airway, which dilates the pharynx and allows passage of air into the lungs. The apneic period is usually terminated by loud snoring. Approximately 75% of patients with obstructive sleep apnea are obese. The concept that obesity narrows the upper airway is reinforced by the observation that weight loss decreases the severity of obstructive sleep apnea.

A distinct but related abnormality is the obesity-hypoventilation syndrome (also known as pickwickian syndrome). In this condition, a heavy chest wall increases the work of breathing and worsens the effect of a decreased central respiratory drive. These combined abnormalities cause hypoventilation during wakefulness as well as during sleep. Hypoxia and hypercapnia constantly are present and commonly lead to pulmonary hypertension and cor pulmonale. Patients with the obesity-hypoventilation syndrome may have obstructive sleep apnea as well.

The second major subgroup of these disorders is central sleep apnea. Episodic apneas during sleep are characterized by a total cessation of respiratory effort rather than an obstruction to air flow. Although the genesis of the disorder is in the central nervous system, the clinical and physiologic effects of disruption of sleep patterns and the hypoxia and hypercapnia are similar to the effects seen in obstructive sleep apnea. The manifestations of the abnormality

Table 10. Impairments Not Directly Related to Lung Functions.

Asthma	Asthma presents a difficult problem in impairment evaluation because results of pulmonary function studies may be normal or near normal between attacks. Despite the intermittent nature of the disease, severe impairment may be diagnosed when the individual is receiving optimum medical therapy and has physiologic test results in the severely impaired range on three successive tests performed at least 1 week apart. The frequency of attacks also should be taken into consideration when deciding on the level of impairment. Persons whose asthma causes less than severe impairment, or whose asthma appears to be related to a class of chemicals or to a specific substance, such as toluene diisocyanate, may need to be evaluated for employability or the presence of an employment-related disability. In such a case the person should have spirometric testing before and immediately after work to determine whether an impairment related to workplace exposure occurs. The testing should be performed on at least three occasions. The physician's thorough documentation of the nature of the asthmatic condition and the compilation of the nonmedical evidence, such as that relating to occupation activities, specific chemicals that may be involved, and other circumstances of work, are crucial to the determination of work-related disability (see Glossary).
Hypersensitivity pneumonitis	A person with this condition may need to be removed from exposure to the causative agent or to other agents with similar sensitizing properties. This would help the person avoid future attacks and chronic sequelae.
Pneumoconiosis	Although a pneumoconiosis may cause no physiologic impairment, its presence usually requires the patient's removal from exposure to the dust causing the condition.
Lung cancers	All persons with lung cancers are considered to be severely impaired at the time of diagnosis. At a reevaluation 1 year after the diagnosis is established, if the person is found to be free of all evidence of tumor recurrence, then he or she should be rated according to the physiologic measures in Table 8 (p. 162). If there is evidence of tumor, the person remains "severely impaired." If the tumor recurs at a later date, the person immediately is considered to be severely impaired. Table 11 (p. 165) may be used to describe further the capabilities of a patient with lung cancer.

are chronic alveolar hypoventilation with persistent arterial blood gas abnormalities, pulmonary hypertension, and cor pulmonale. It is not uncommon to see the obstructive and central types of sleep apnea in the same individual.

Screening for the presence or absence of sleep apnea can be performed by overnight pulse oximetry, which monitors episodes of oxyhemoglobin desaturation during sleep. Differentiation between obstructive and central sleep apnea and finer definition of the severity of the disorder require formal polysomnography, which involves evaluating or monitoring the electroencephalogram, electro-oculogram, submental electromyogram, impedance plethysmography of the chest, and abdominal movements, as well as oximetry and transcutaneous carbon dioxide level. Objective measurement of daytime sleepiness requires a sleep latency test that measures time to onset of sleep in a dark, quiet room.

Even when arterial blood gases are normal during the daytime and pulmonary hemodynamics are unaltered, untreated sleep apnea is a cause of severe impairment. Daytime sleepiness, intellectual impairment, and personality changes make these individuals unlikely candidates for gainful employment.

Effective treatment for obstructive sleep apnea often can be accomplished by weight loss and nocturnal use of a device that delivers continuous positive airway pressure through the nose to splint open the oropharynx during sleep. The treatment of central sleep apnea is less well defined. Nocturnal use of a mechanical ventilator, either through a tracheostomy or by negative pressure applied to the external chest wall (cuirass ventilator), has been effective in some cases. Patients with documented sleep apnea who have received effective therapy should be reevaluated by polysomnography before they are judged to be severely impaired.

Table 10 (above) highlights some other conditions in which impairment is not readily quantifiable and provides some general comments. Impairments in persons with these conditions should be evaluated by physicians with expertise in lung disease, and the impairment estimate should be left to the physician's judgment.

It is important to recognize that such conditions as asthma, hypersensitivity pneumonitis, and pneumoconiosis may require that the individual refrain from working in a specific occupational setting where he or she is exposed to the offending agent. This does not necessarily indicate that the individual has permanent pulmonary impairment in occupational settings other than those causing the abnormality.

Table 11 (p. 165), based on the Karnofsky Scale, provides a scale by which the overall capabilities of a patient with cancer may be judged.[9]

5.4 Examples of Permanent Respiratory Impairment

Class 1: Impairment of the Whole Person, 0%

Example: A 50-year-old delivery truck driver, who had been in that occupation for the past 25 years, was referred because he had become too short of breath to carry three boxes up a flight of stairs. Three months before referral he had been hospitalized for treatment of an anteroseptal myocardial infarction. He had been allowed to return to work after beginning a progressive exercise program. He had been smoking cigarettes at age 15 years, smoked one pack per day, and stopped 3 months before evaluation (exposure was 35 pack-years).

At physical examination, the patient was 188 cm (6 ft 2 in) tall and weighed 86.4 kg (190 lb). Breath sounds and results of cardiac examination were normal. The chest roentgenogram showed left ventricular enlargement and normal lungs. Pulmonary function studies showed the following:

Study	Observed	Predicted	Observed/ Predicted (%)
FVC (L)	5.28	5.56	95
FEV_1 (L)	3.85	4.37	88
FEV_1/FVC (%)	73	—	—
D_{CO}	—	—	91

Maximum exercise VO_2 was 18 mL/kg.

Diagnosis: Inadequate cardiac output resulting from myocardial infarction.

Respiratory system impairment: Class 1, no impairment.

Comment: Although the patient was a smoker, pulmonary function studies indicated he was in class 1 and had no respiratory impairment (Table 8, p. 162). Evaluation of cardiovascular system impairment was arranged.

Table 11. Scale for Judging Cancer Patients' Capabilities*

Grade	Description
0	Fully active, able to carry on all predisease activities without restrictions
1	Restricted in physically strenuous activity but ambulatory and able to carry out light tasks, such as light work in home or office
2	Requires occasional to considerable care for most needs and frequent medical care
3	Capable only of limited self-care and confined to bed or chair at least half of waking hours
4	Almost totally impaired, cannot care for self, and totally confined to bed or chair

*Adapted from Moossa et al.[9]

Class 2: Impairment of the Whole Person, 10% through 25%

Example: A 58-year-old advertising executive had experienced a daily cough productive of morning sputum for several years. She had no dyspnea, chest pain, or hemoptysis but noted some wheezing, especially with colds. She had smoked continuously from age 16 to age 58 years, using 1½ packs per day from age 16 years to age 58. There was no history of asthma or pneumonia. She knew of no exposures to hazardous dusts, chemicals, or fumes.

On physical examination, the patient's height was 168 cm (5 ft 6 in) and her weight was 61 kg (135 lb). There was an expiratory wheeze with forced exhalation. Otherwise the results of physical examination were normal. The chest roentgenogram was normal. Pulmonary function studies showed the following:

Study	Observed	Predicted	Observed/ Predicted (%)
FVC (L)	2.73	3.41	80
FEV_1 (L)	1.83	2.69	68
FEV_1/FVC (%)	67	—	—
D_{CO}	—	—	73

Exercise VO_2 max was 26 mL/kg.

Diagnosis: Chronic bronchitis with mild airflow obstruction.

Respiratory system impairment: Class 2, mild (Table 8, p. 162).

Class 3: Impairment of the Whole Person, 26% through 50%

Example: A 60-year-old man, who had worked as an insulator for 40 years, complained of increasing dyspnea of 5 years' duration. He had difficulty keeping up with other workers his age, and he usually had to stop on the second flight when walking up stairs. He denied cough, wheezing, or chest pain. He had never smoked cigarettes. There was no history of asthma, pneumonia, or other medical disorders, and he took no medications. As an insulator, he had mixed powdered asbestos with water and applied it to pipes and steel beams for the first 20 years of his working life.

Examination disclosed that the patient was 170 cm (5 ft 7 in) tall and weighed 70.5 kg (155 lb). There was questionable finger clubbing. He had bilateral, end-inspiratory, fine crackles. The results of cardiac examination were normal. The chest roentegenogram showed moderately pronounced, small, linear, irregular opacities at the lung bases. Small, bilateral, pleural plaques were present. Pulmonary function studies showed the following:

Study	Observed	Predicted	Observed/ Predicted (%)
FVC (L)	2.35	4.27	55
FEV_1 (L)	2.10	3.38	62
FEV_1/FVC (%)	89	—	—
D_{CO}	16.0	30.8	52

Exercise VO_2 max was 16 mL/kg.

Diagnosis: Asbestosis.

Respiratory system impairment: Class 3, moderate (Table 8, p. 162).

Comment: This man had interstitial lung disease with crackles on examination, decreased vital capacity, and decreased gas exchange by diffusion capacity measurement. The oxygen uptake was decreased, probably because of pulmonary dysfunction.

Class 4: Impairment of the Whole Person, 51% through 100%

Example: A 62-year-old bookkeeper had worked in a vegetable-processing plant for 38 years and gradually developed shortness of breath during a 10-year period. The dyspnea became so severe that he was not able to perform routine daily activities, such as driving to and from work, walking on level ground, or dressing himself. He had an occasional, nonproductive cough but no wheezing, chest pain, or hemoptysis. He had begun smoking at age 12 years, smoked 2½ packs per day, and had been able to stop 6 months previously. He had no history of other disorders or other exposures to hazardous dusts, chemicals, or fumes.

On physical examination, the man was 180 cm (5 ft 11 in) tall and weighed 69.5 kg (153 lb). Breath sounds were absent, and no crackles or wheezes were heard. No other signs were present. A chest roentgenogram showed hyperinflated lungs and lack of airway-vascular markings. Pulmonary function studies showed the following:

Study	Observed	Predicted	Observed/ Predicted (%)
FVC (L)	2.94	4.82	61
FEV_1 (L)	1.16	3.75	31
FEV_1/FVC (%)	39	—	—
D_{CO} or Dsb, mL/min	12.8	34.5	37

Exercise VO_2 max was 10 mL/kg.

Diagnosis: Emphysema.

Respiratory system impairment: Class 4, severe (Table 8, p. 162).

Special Condition: Asthma

Example: A 58-year-old woman had developed asthma as a child. She was able to work as an inspector for a computer company for 15 years, but 3 years ago she had begun to have exacerbations of asthma about once monthly. Also, she noted dyspnea while walking on level ground after a few steps, and she complained of a morning cough. She had never smoked cigarettes. She had been taking bronchodilators for many years and inhaled corticosteroid therapy for 3 years. The work environment was not dusty, and there were no fumes associated with her work.

On physical examination, the woman was 160 cm (5 ft 3 in) tall and weighed 56.8 kg (125 lb). There was no finger clubbing. Expiratory wheezes were heard throughout the lungs. Results of cardiac examination and a chest roentengenogram were normal. Pulmonary function studies showed the following:

Study	Observed	Observed after broncho-dilator	Predicted	After broncho-dilator/ predicted (%)
FVC_1 (L)	2.08	2.12	3.01	70
FEV_1 (L)	1.14	1.18	2.42	47
FEV_1/FVC (%)	55	—	—	—
D_{CO}	18.0	—	—	76

Diagnosis: Asthma with fixed airflow obstruction.

Respiratory system impairment: Class 3, moderate (Table 8, p. 162).

Comment: The pulmonary function studies showed a moderate degree of fixed airflow obstruction, but when combined with the frequency of exacerbations, the impairment might be judged to be severe.

References

1. American Thoracic Society Committee on Proficiency Standards for Pulmonary Function Laboratories. Standardization of spirometry-1987 update. *Am Rev Respir Dis.* 1987;136:1285-1298.

2. Crapo RO, Morris AH, Gardner PM. Reference spirometric values using techniques and equipment that meet ATS recommendations. *Am Rev Respir Dis.* 1981;123:659-664.

3. American Thoracic Society Ad Hoc Committee on Impairment/Disability Criteria. Evaluation of impairment/disability secondary to respiratory disorders. *Am Rev Respir Dis.* 1986;134:1205-1209.

4. Crapo RO, Morris AH. Standardized single breath normal values for carbon monoxide diffusing capacity. *Am Rev Respir Dis.* 1981;123:185-190.

5. American Thoracic Society. Lung function testing: selection of reference values and interpretative strategies. *Am Rev Respir Dis.* 1991;144:1202-1218.

6. American Thoracic Society D_{lco} Standardization Conference. Single breath carbon monoxide diffusing capacity (transfer factor) recommendations for a standard technique. *Am Rev Respir Dis.* 1987;136: 1299-1307.

7. Carlson DJ, Ries AL, Kaplan PM. Prediction of maximum exercise tolerance in patients with COPD. *Chest.* 1991;100:307-311.

8. Astrand, P, Rodahl K. *Textbook of Work Physiology.* New York, NY. McGraw Hill; 1977:462.

9. Moossa AR, Robson MC, Schimpff SC, eds. *Comprehensive Textbook of Oncology.* Baltimore, Md: Williams & Wilkins; 1986:67.

Chapter 6

The Cardiovascular System

The purpose of this chapter is to provide the physician with criteria for evaluating permanent impairments of the cardiovascular system as they affect the individual's ability to perform the activities of daily living. The cardiovascular system consists of the heart, the aorta, the systemic arteries, and the pulmonary arteries. Impairment of this system includes abnormal elevation of pressure either in the aorta, which is called systemic hypertension, or in the pulmonary artery, which is called pulmonary hypertension. The coronary and peripheral circulations are considered to be part of the cardiovascular system. Impairment from disorders of the cerebral circulation is considered in the chapter on the nervous system.

Before using the information in this chapter, the *Guides* user should become familiar with Chapters 1 and 2 and the Glossary, which discuss the purposes of the *Guides* and the situations in which they are useful and provide basic definitions. Chapter 2 describes methods for examining patients and preparing reports. A medical evaluation report should include information such as that shown below.

A. Medical Evaluation
- History of medical condition(s)
- Results of most recent clinical evaluation
- Assessment of current clinical status and statement of further medical plans
- Diagnosis

B. Analysis of Findings
- Impact of medical condition on daily activities
- Explanation for concluding that the condition is stable, has been present for a period of months, and is not amenable to further therapy
- Explanation for concluding that the individual is or is not likely to suffer further impairment by engaging in usual activities
- Explanation for concluding that accommodations or restrictions are or are not warranted

C. Comparison of Analysis with Impairment Criteria
- Description of major findings and how they relate to specific impairment criteria
- Explanation of each impairment estimate
- Summary of estimates
- Overall whole-person impairment estimate

Symptomatic Limitation

In this chapter reference is made to the limiting of daily activities because of symptoms. Information about such limitation is subjective, and it is open to interpretation on the part of both the patient and the examiner. Therefore, the examiner should attempt to obtain objective data about the extent of the limitation before attempting to estimate the degree of permanent impairment. When estimating the extent of an impairment, the physician should use the functional classifications in Table 1 (p. 170).

Table 1. Functional Classification of Cardiac Disease*

Class	Description
1	Patient has cardiac disease but no resulting limitation of physical activity; ordinary physical activity does not cause undue fatigue, palpitation, dyspnea, or anginal pain.
2	Patient has cardiac disease resulting in slight limitation of physical activity; patient is comfortable at rest and in the performance of ordinary, light, daily activities; greater than ordinary physical activity, such as heavy physical exertion, results in fatigue, palpitation, dyspnea, or anginal pain.
3	Patient has cardiac disease resulting in marked limitation of physical activity; patient is comfortable at rest. Ordinary physical activity results in fatigue, palpitation, dyspnea, or anginal pain.
4	Patient has cardiac disease resulting in inability to carry on any physical activity without discomfort. Symptoms of inadequate cardiac output, pulmonary congestion, systemic congestion, or anginal syndrome may be present, even at rest; if any physical activity is undertaken, discomfort is increased.

*Adapted from: Criteria Committee of the New York Heart Association: *Diseases of the Heart and Blood Vessels: Nomenclature and Criteria for Diagnosis*, ed 6. Boston, Mass: Little Brown & Co; 1964. This well-established classification is preferred over the newer classification introduced in the seventh edition.

Exercise Testing

In most circumstances, the physician should attempt to quantitate limitations due to symptoms by observing the patient during exercise. The most widely used and standardized exercise protocols involve the use of a motor-driven treadmill with varying grades and speeds. The protocols vary slightly, but they all attempt to relate the exercise to excess energy expended and to functional class. The excess energy expended is usually expressed in terms of the "MET," which represents the multiples of resting metabolic energy used for any given activity. One MET is considered to be 3.5 mL/(kg/min). The 70-kg man who burns 1.2 kcal/min while sitting at rest uses approximately 3 METS when walking 4 km/h.

Table 2 (p. 171) displays the relationship of excess energy expenditures in METS to functional class according to the protocols of several investigators. With all protocols, the exercise periods last for 2 or 3 minutes; the time periods are represented in the table by boxes with numbers giving the estimated METS involved.

Estimations of excess energy expenditure also can be made with a bicycle ergometer (Table 3, p. 171). Some laboratories are equipped to measure oxygen consumption and carbon dioxide production during exercise. Data acquired with these techniques may provide the most accurate view of a patient's exercise capacity.

The functional capacity of an individual patient depends on age, sex, and level of training. The functional class determined by means of Tables 2 and 3 (p. 171) may not be applicable to patients at the ends of the age spectrum, such as a 20-year-old athlete or an inactive 70-year-old woman. Therefore, it may be useful to calculate a "percentage functional aerobic capacity" that is achieved on an exercise test. Standard charts are available for the various exercise protocols for determining the percentage functional aerobic capacity based on total exercise duration, age, sex, and level of training.

A major problem with the use of any exercise-testing technique to attempt to quantitate an individual's functional capacity is the marked variability in patients' abilities and willingness to cooperate. Therefore, the physician must estimate the individual's cooperation and effort during the test; some patients will continue longer than they should, while others will stop after minimal effort because they feel fatigued.

Knowledge of the status of the left ventricle is important in the examination and evaluation of a patient with cardiac disease. Two phases of left ventricular function contribute to the patient's symptoms and condition: systolic function, which is the ability of the heart to pump out blood during contraction, and diastolic function, the process by which the heart fills with blood during relaxation of the myocardium and a passive filling phase.

A clinically used measure of systolic function is the "ejection fraction," which is the percentage of blood the heart is able to eject during one beat. The ejection fraction may be measured by echocardiography, radionuclide angiography, or left ventriculography and is normally greater than 55%. Mild systolic dysfunction may be defined as ejection fractions of 40% to 50%, moderate systolic dysfunction as 30% to 40%, and severe systolic dysfunction as less than 30%.

Although diastolic dysfunction may contribute to the signs and symptoms of heart failure, there are no well-accepted techniques for its measurement. Diastolic dysfunction is usually diagnosed clinically, if there are elevated filling pressures that result in heart failure in the absence of systolic dysfunction, or valvular abnormalities that could account for the heart failure.

In the illustrative cases of impairment in this chapter, any historical, physical examination, or laboratory information or data not described should be considered to be within normal limits.

Table 2. Relationship of METS and Functional Class According to Five Treadmill Protocols*

METS	1.6	2	3	4	5	6	7	8	9	10	11	12	13	14	15	16
Treadmill tests																
Ellestad																
Miles per hour					1.7	3.0			4.0						5.0	
% grade					10	10			10						10	
Bruce																
Miles per hour					1.7		2.5		3.4				4.2			
% grade					10		12		14				16			
Balke																
Miles per hour				3.4	3.4	3.4	3.4	3.4	3.4	3.4	3.4	3.4	3.4	3.4	3.4	3.4
% grade				2	4	6	8	10	12	14	16	18	20	22	24	26
Balke																
Miles per hour			3.0	3.0	3.0	3.0	3.0	3.0	3.0	3.0	3.0	3.0				
% grade			0	2.5	5	7.5	10	12.5	15	17.5	20	22.5				
Naughton																
Miles per hour	1.0	2.0	2.0	2.0	2.0	2.0	2.0									
% grade	0	0	3.5	7	10.5	14	17.5									
METS	**1.6**	**2**	**3**	**4**	**5**	**6**	**7**	**8**	**9**	**10**	**11**	**12**	**13**	**14**	**15**	**16**
Clinical status																
Symptomatic patients	←						→									
Diseased, recovered		←					→									
Sedentary healthy				←						→						
Physically active					←											→
Functional class	IV	←	III	→	← II	→	←				I and Normal					→

*Adapted from: Fox SM III, Naughton JP, Haskell WL. Physical activity and the prevention of coronary heart disease. *Ann Clin Res.* 1971; 3:404-432.

Table 3. Energy Expenditure in METS During Bicycle Ergometry*

Body weight		Work rate on bicycle ergometer, kg m^{-1} min^{-1}, (Watts)												
kg	(lb)	75 (12)	150 (25)	300 (50)	450 (75)	600 (100)	750 (125)	900 (150)	1050 (175)	1200 (200)	1350 (225)	1500 (250)	1650 (275)	1800 (300)
20	(44)	4.0	6.0	10.0	14.0	18.0	22.0							
30	(66)	3.4	4.7	7.3	10.0	12.7	15.3	17.9	20.7	23.3				
40	(88)	3.0	4.0	6.0	8.0	10.0	12.0	14.0	16.0	18.0	20.0	22.0		
50	(110)	2.8	3.6	5.2	6.8	8.4	10.0	11.5	13.2	14.8	16.3	18.0	19.6	21.1
60	(132)	2.7	3.3	4.7	6.0	7.3	8.7	10.0	11.3	12.7	14.0	15.3	16.7	18.0
70	(154)	2.6	3.1	4.3	5.4	6.6	7.7	8.8	10.0	11.1	12.2	13.4	14.0	15.7
80	(176)	2.5	3.0	4.0	5.0	6.0	7.0	8.0	9.0	10.0	11.0	12.0	13.0	14.0
90	(198)	2.4	2.9	3.8	4.7	5.6	6.4	7.3	8.2	9.1	10.0	10.9	11.8	12.6
100	(220)	2.4	2.8	3.6	4.4	5.2	6.0	6.8	7.6	8.4	9.2	10.0	10.8	11.6
110	(242)	2.4	2.7	3.4	4.2	4.9	5.6	6.3	7.1	7.8	8.5	9.3	10.0	10.7
120	(264)	2.3	2.7	3.3	4.0	4.7	5.3	6.0	6.7	7.3	8.0	8.7	9.3	10.0

*Source: American College of Sports Medicine. *Guidelines for Graded Exercise Testing and Exercise Prescription.* Philadelphia, Pa: Lea and Febiger; 1975:17.

6.1 Valvular Heart Disease

Valvular heart disease may be caused by congenital, rheumatic, infectious, or traumatic factors, or a combination of factors. Valvular disease may result in (1) pressure hypertrophy of the left or right ventricle, resulting in elevated filling pressures, myocardial ischemia, and eventual left ventricular dysfunction with signs and symptoms of congestive heart failure; (2) volume hypertrophy of the left or right ventricle, resulting in ventricular dilatation and eventual irreversible myocardial dysfunction with signs and symptoms of congestive heart failure; (3) obstruction to inflow of the ventricles causing congestion of organs, even in the absence of ventricular dysfunction; or (4) decreased cardiac output.

Valvular heart disease can be detected and its severity assessed by a thorough history and physical examination. The severity of a stenotic valve lesion can be assessed by physical examination and should be confirmed by either Doppler echocardiography or cardiac catheterization. A valve gradient measures the pressure drop across a stenotic valve and is proportional to the severity of obstruction. Since the valve gradient is influenced by the cardiac output, a valve area is calculated that takes into consideration both the pressure gradient and the cardiac output. There may be technical limitations to these derived variables. Their correlation with the severity of the stenosis is shown in Table 4 (below).

Table 4. Severity of Valve Stenosis.*

Severity of stenosis†	Mean valve gradient (mm Hg)	Valve area† (cm^2)
Aortic valve		
Mild	<25	>1.2
Moderate	25-50	0.7-1.2
Severe	>50	<0.7
Mitral valve		
Mild	<5	>1.5
Moderate	5-10	1.0-1.5
Severe	>10	<1.0

*Cardiac catheterization may be required for a semiquantitative estimate of the valve lesion's severity; the catheterization can provide a view of the contrast medium's intensity as it flows in regrograde fashion across the regurgitating valve into the receiving heart chamber. The estimate is obtained with aortic root angiography to assess the severity of aortic valve regurgitation and with left ventriculography to assess the severity of mitral valve regurgitation.

†Severity of stenosis may be indexed also to body surface area.

The severity of a regurgitant valve lesion is more difficult to assess than that of a stenotic lesion. A qualitative assessment may be made by physical examination and Doppler echocardiography. Although Doppler echocardiography may help the physician determine whether a regurgitant lesion is mild or severe, this technique's inherent limitations preclude an accurate assessment of intermediate grades of severity.

The severity of valvular heart disease can be reduced, but not fully reversed, by catheter-based interventional procedures, operative repair, or replacement of the valve with a prosthetic device. After any of these procedures, sufficient time from the date of operation must elapse to allow maximum recovery of the heart, lungs, and other organs before permanent impairment due to the valvular disease is estimated. The Glossary (p. 315) defines a "permanent" impairment.

In addition, medications may affect the severity of valvular heart disease, especially limitations due to symptoms. Therefore, sufficient time must be allowed for medications to be introduced and adjusted and to exert their effects before an estimate of permanent impairment is made.

The impairment criteria for valvular heart disease are given in Table 5 (p. 173).

Criteria for Evaluating Impairment Resulting from Valvular Disease

Class 1: Impairment of the Whole Person, 0% to 10%
For a patient to be in class 1, *all* of the following criteria must be met: (1) evidence exists by physical examination or laboratory test of valvular heart disease; (2) the patient has no symptoms in performance of ordinary daily activities (5 METS; Table 2, p. 171); (3) the patient has no symptoms with moderately heavy exertion (7 to 10 METS); (4) the patient does not require continuous treatment, except for intermittent antibiotic prophylaxis for surgical or dental treatments; (5) the patient does not have evidence of congestive heart failure; (6) the patient does not have evidence of ventricular dysfunction; and (7) in the patient who has recovered from valvular heart surgery or a catheter-based interventional procedure, criteria 1 through 6 are met.

Example 1: A 22-year-old woman had a midsystolic click and a late systolic murmur. She had no symptoms, and there were no signs of cardiac enlargement, congestive heart failure, or cardiac rhythm disturbance. Physical examination showed slight pectus excavatum. A chest roentgenogram and electrocardiogram (ECG) were normal. An echocardiogram indicated prolapse of the mitral valve and normal left atrial and left ventricular size and function.

Diagnosis: Mitral valve prolapse syndrome.

Impairment: 0% impairment of the whole person.

Comment: If the ECG showed definite T-wave abnormalities, or the echocardiogram showed slight enlargement of the left atrium or left ventricle, then the valve disorder would be estimated to be a 1% to 9% impairment, depending on the severity of the abnormality as shown by the laboratory studies.

A patient with a murmur of aortic regurgitation but with no symptoms or signs of cardiac enlargement on examination, chest roentgenogram, or ECG, and no signs of congestive heart failure, may be estimated to have an impairment of 1% to 9%. However, a measurement of left ventricular size and function should be performed by either two-dimensional echocardiography or radionuclide angiography to rule out significant left ventricular dilation or dysfunction, which may be present even with the above findings.

Table 5. Impairment Classification for Valvular Heart Disease.

Class 1: **0%-9% impairment of the whole person**	**Class 2:** **10%-29% impairment of the whole person**	**Class 3:** **30%-49% impairment of the whole person**	**Class 4:** **50%-100% impairment of the whole person**
Patient has evidence by physical examination or laboratory studies of valvular heart disease, but no symptoms in the performance of ordinary daily activities or even on moderately heavy exertion (functional class 1); **and** Patient does not require continuous treatment, although prophylactic antibiotics may be recommended at time of surgical procedure to reduce risk of bacterial endocarditis; **and** Patient remains free of signs of congestive heart failure; **and** There are no signs of ventricular dysfunction or dilation, and severity of stenosis or regurgitation is estimated to be mild; METS >7; TMET (Bruce protocol) >6 min; **and** In patient who has recovered from valvular heart surgery, all of above criteria are met.	Patient has evidence by physical examination or laboratory studies of valvular heart disease, and there are no symptoms in performance of daily activities, but symptoms develop on moderately heavy physical exertion (functional class 2); **or** Patient requires moderate dietary adjustment or drugs to prevent symptoms or to remain free of signs of congestive heart failure or other consequences of valvular heart disease, such as syncope, chest pain, and emboli; **or** Patient has signs or laboratory evidence of cardiac chamber dysfunction and/or dilation, severity of stenosis or regurgitation is estimated to be moderate, and surgical correction is not feasible or advisable; METS >5 but <7; TMET (Bruce protocol) >3 min; **or** Patient has recovered from valvular heart surgery and meets above criteria.	Patient has signs of valvular heart disease and has slight to moderate symptomatic discomfort during performance of ordinary daily activities (functional class 3); **and** Dietary therapy or drugs do not completely control symptoms or prevent congestive heart failure; **and** Patient has signs or laboratory evidence of cardiac chamber dysfunction or dilation, severity of stenosis or regurgitation is estimated to be moderate or severe, and surgical correction is not feasible; METS >2 but <5; TMET (Bruce protocol) >1 min; **or** Patient has recovered from heart valve surgery but continues to have symptoms and signs of congestive heart failure including cardiomegaly.	Patient has signs by physical examination of valvular heart disease, and symptoms at rest or in performance of less than ordinary daily activities (functional class 4); **and** Dietary therapy and drugs cannot control symptoms or prevent signs of congestive heart failure; **and** Patient has signs or laboratory evidence of cardiac chamber dysfunction or dilation, severity of stenosis or regurgitation is estimated to be moderate or severe, and surgical correction is not feasible; METS <1; TMET <1 min; **or** Patient has recovered from valvular heart surgery but continues to have symptoms or signs of congestive heart failure.

A patient with the signs of mild aortic stenosis due to a bicuspid valve might be estimated to have an impairment of 1% to 9%, if there were no symptoms, no evidence of left ventricular hypertrophy on examination or ECG, and no signs of congestive heart failure. A Doppler echocardiogram may be helpful in confirming that the degree of stenosis is only mild.

Example 2: A 30-year-old woman had recovered from mitral commissurotomy, was asymptomatic, and had returned to an active life. She had had rheumatic fever at age 8 years and had had no recurrences.

Physical examination revealed a well-healed surgical wound without tenderness. The heart rate was 80 beats per minute and regular. There were no abnormal precordial pulsations or signs of congestive heart failure. The first heart sound was loud; an opening snap was heard approximately 100 milliseconds after the second heart sound, and there was a short rumble in mid-diastole. A grade 1/6 to 2/6 holosystolic murmur was heard at the apex.

A chest roentgenogram showed a heart of normal size and no signs of pulmonary congestion. An ECG showed minimal P-wave abnormalities. An echocardiogram showed slight enlargement of the left atrium and no enlargement or dysfunction of the ventricles.

Diagnosis: Mitral stenosis and postmitral commissurotomy.

Impairment: 5% to 9% impairment of the whole person.

Comment: The estimated degree of impairment will depend on the estimated severity or abnormality of mitral regurgitation, residual stenosis, heart rhythm, and other signs. Echocardiography, cardiac catheterization, and angiography are not necessary and should not be obtained solely to help estimate the impairment.

Class 2: Impairment of the Whole Person, 10% to 30%

A patient belongs in class II when the following criteria are met: (1) the patient has evidence of valvular heart disease by physical examination or laboratory evaluation; (2) the patient has no symptoms in performance of ordinary daily activities (5 METS; see Table 2, p. 171); and (3) the patient has symptoms with moderately heavy exertion (7 METS), that is, the patient is in functional class 2 (Table 1, p. 170); *or* the patient requires continuous drug therapy for prevention of one or more of the following: (a) symptoms (functional class 2, see Table 1, p. 170);

(b) congestive heart failure; (c) syncope; (d) chest pain; (e) emboli; *or* the patient has hypertrophy and/or dilatation of one or more cardiac chambers according to objective evidence, but left ventricular systolic function is maintained *and* the severity of stenosis or regurgitation is estimated to be moderate (see Table 4, p. 172, for severity definitions).

Surgical correction may not be necessary or feasible, or the patient may have recovered from valvular surgery and now meets the above criteria. Standard evaluation includes exercise testing, echocardiogram, ECG, and chest roentgenogram; cardiac catheterization and angiography data may be available.

Example 1: A 63-year-old man had been noted during a routine examination 5 years earlier to have the murmur of aortic regurgitation and mild heart failure. He was an office worker who played 18 holes of golf regularly, using a powered cart. His physician had advised him to restrict salt intake.

At examination the patient's blood pressure was 160/50 mm Hg, the pulse was 70 beats per minute and regular, and the peripheral pulses were bounding. There were no signs of congestive heart failure. The apical impulse was just outside the midclavicular line, was slightly larger than normal, and was slightly prolonged. There was a grade 3/6 harsh, short, systolic ejection murmur in the aortic area and a grade 3/6 long, decrescendo, diastolic murmur along the left lower sternal border. A faint, mid-diastolic rumble was heard at the apex. The first and second heart sounds were normal.

An ECG showed tall R waves in V5 and V6 with low but upright T waves. A chest roentgenogram showed prominence of the apical portion of the cardiac silhouette and no cardiomegaly or pulmonary congestion. An echocardiogram showed an aortic root of normal size, delicate aortic valve leaflets, fluttering of the anterior leaflet of the mitral valve, normal left ventricular function, and ventricular volumes and volume indices at the upper limits of normal. Doppler echocardiography showed moderate aortic regurgitation with no stenosis.

Diagnosis: Moderately severe aortic regurgitation of uncertain cause.

Impairment: 20% to 24% impairment of the whole person.

Comment: The patient was asymptomatic but impaired. His impairment would be estimated to be greater if there were cardiomegaly or deeply inverted T waves in leads I, L, V5, and V6 on the ECG, or if the echocardiogram showed a dilated left ventricle or left ventricular systolic dysfunction. Cardiac catheterization and angiography were not necessary to estimate the degree of his impairment.

Example 2: A 66-year-old woman had had several syncopal episodes 3 years earlier, had been found to have severe calcific stenosis of the aortic valve, and had undergone aortic valve replacement with a large Bjork-Shiley prosthesis. She returned to an active life, which included walking 2 miles each morning. She took oral anticoagulants to maintain the prothrombin time in the therapeutic range, the level being tested every 3 weeks. She took antibiotics before dental or operative procedures but no other medication.

Physical examination disclosed normal blood pressure and pulse and no signs of heart failure. The apical impulse had a slightly sustained quality. On auscultation, a grade 1/6 early systolic murmur was heard in the first right intercostal space. The first heart sound was normal, and there was a crisp, closing click of the prosthetic valve at the second heart sound.

An ECG showed a normal rhythm and QRS pattern and low T waves in leads I, L, V5, and V6. A chest roentgenogram showed slight prominence of the apex of the heart, a properly positioned prosthesis, and no evidence of pulmonary congestion. An echocardiogram disclosed ventricles of normal size with thickening of the left ventricular wall, a properly positioned prosthesis with a mean gradient of 10 mm Hg across the prosthesis, and slight regurgitation. The left ventricle had a normal cavity, mild hypertrophy of the wall, and normal systolic function.

Diagnosis: Calcific aortic stenosis, probably related to congenital bicuspid aortic valve, and valve replacement.

Impairment: 20% impairment of the whole person.

Comment: The degree of impairment in this patient would be greater if (1) a diastolic decrescendo murmur were audible; (2) the systolic gradient across the prosthesis were greater than Doppler-derived normal values for the type of prosthesis; or (3) left ventricular systolic dysfunction were present. Cardiac catheterization was not necessary in this patient to estimate the degree of impairment.

Class 3: Impairment of the Whole Person, 30% to 50%

A patient belongs in Class 3 when (1) the patient has signs of valvular heart disease and has slight to moderate symptomatic discomfort during the performance of ordinary daily activities (functional class 3); *and* (2) dietary therapy or drugs do not completely control symptoms or prevent congestive heart failure; *and* (3) the patient has signs or laboratory evidence of cardiac chamber dysfunction or dilation, the severity of the stenosis or regurgitation is estimated to be moderate or severe, and surgical correction is not feasible; *or* (4) the patient has recovered from heart valve surgery but continues to have symptoms and signs of congestive heart failure including cardiomegaly.

Example 1: A 71-year-old man with idiopathic thrombocytopenia that did not respond to medications had had moderate exertional dyspnea for the past 2 years despite the continued use of diuretics and digoxin. He was comfortable at rest, but he became short of breath when climbing to the second floor. He slept on two pillows and had not awakened short of breath since the dose of diuretics had been increased 1 year earlier.

Physical examination showed a patient able to lie flat comfortably. Blood pressure was 110/80 mm Hg, and pulse rate was 84 beats per minute and irregular. The venous pressure was normal, and there was no edema. Breath sounds were harsh at each base, but there were no rales. The apical impulse was large, hyperdynamic, and displaced to the anterior axillary line. There was a slight parasternal heave. The first and second heart sounds were loud, and a grade 4/6 holosystolic murmur was heard at the lower sternal border, apex, and axilla. A third heart sound was audible.

The ECG showed atrial fibrillation with an irregular ventricular response of about 80 per minute. There were low T waves, but the QRS pattern was normal. The chest roentgenogram showed cardiomegaly with a large left atrium. There was prominence of the vasculature of the upper lobes. An echocardiogram showed mild enlargement of the left ventricle with hyperdynamic systolic function and moderate enlargement of the left atrium. A flail mitral leaflet was visualized by two-dimensional echocardiography, and severe mitral regurgitation was shown by Doppler echocardiography. Estimated peak systolic pulmonary artery pressure by Doppler echocardiography was 50 mm Hg.

Diagnosis: Severe mitral regurgitation due to mitral valve prolapse.

Impairment: 50% impairment of the whole person.

Comment: Greater exercise tolerance and less cardiomegaly would suggest a lower degree of impairment. Reduced systolic function suggests a higher degree of impairment. Cardiac catheterization was not necessary to estimate this patient's degree of impairment.

Example 2: A 60-year-old woman had had surgery to replace the aortic and mitral valves 1 year earlier. Despite taking oral anticoagulants, digoxin, and diuretics and restricting salt in her diet, the woman did not have much stamina. She tired easily and had to rest each afternoon. Ankle edema sometimes developed, but it cleared promptly after she took an extra diuretic tablet. She slept on one pillow and had no nocturnal dyspnea. While able to do light housework, the patient did not feel well enough to return to work as a seamstress. Her weight remained about 6.8 kg below her preoperative weight.

Physical examination showed the patient to be comfortable when lying flat. Blood pressure was 110/70 mm Hg; pulse was 80 beats per minute and irregular. Venous pressure was normal, and there was no edema. The lungs were clear. The apical impulse was enlarged, located at the anterior axillary line, and was sustained through all of systole; there was no parasternal heave. The prosthetic valve sounds were normal. A grade 1/6 early systolic murmur was heard in the first right interspace and along the left sternal border.

The ECG showed atrial fibrillation with an irregular ventricular response of about 80 per minute. A chest roentgenogram showed cardiomegaly with left ventricular and left atrial enlargement. There was prominence of the vasculature in the upper lobes. An echocardiogram showed no evidence of prosthetic valve malfunction or displacement. There was slight enlargement of the ventricles and left atrium. Left ventricular systolic function was normal. A treadmill exertion test using the Bruce protocol showed that the patient could complete stage I of the protocol but could not proceed to stage II because of fatigue and shortness of breath (5 METS).

Diagnosis: Aortic and mitral valve disease, probably rheumatic in origin; surgical replacement of valves.

Impairment: 40% impairment of the whole person.

Comment: The treadmill exertion test was useful in providing objective data about the degree of impairment. With the Bruce protocol, the functional class may be denoted objectively as class I if greater than 6 minutes of exertion can be achieved; class II if 3 to 6 minutes can be achieved; class III if 1 to 3 minutes can be achieved; and class IV if less than 1 minute can be achieved.

Class 4: Impairment of the Whole Person, 50% to 100%

A patient belongs in Class 4 when (1) the patient has signs by physical examination of valvular heart disease and symptoms at rest or in the performance of less than ordinary daily activities (functional class 4); *and* (2) dietary therapy and drugs cannot control symptoms or prevent signs of congestive heart failure; *and* (3) the patient has signs or laboratory evidence of cardiac chamber dysfunction and/or dilation, the severity of the stenosis or regurgitation is estimated to be moderate or severe, and surgical correction is not feasible; *or* (4) the patient has recovered from valvular heart surgery but continues to have symptoms or signs of congestive heart failure.

Example 1: A 45-year-old woman had been treated for congestive heart failure for 10 years. In spite of properly using diuretics and digoxin and, for the past year, a peripheral vasodilator, the patient continued to become breathless with minimal exertion. Even going to the bathroom caused breathlessness and fatigue. The patient slept on three pillows. For years, her ankles had been swollen, and during the past year her abdomen had become protuberant.

Physical examination showed a woman who was pale and weak. Her face was thin and showed temporal depression, and jaundice was present. She was breathing 22 times per minute, and blood pressure was 110/70 mm Hg; the pulse rate was about 80 beats per minute and irregular. The patient preferred the sitting position, and in that position the neck veins were distended to the mid-neck and showed prominent V waves.

There were rales at both lung bases. There was a parasternal heave. On auscultation there was a grade 3/6 harsh, systolic murmur in the second right interspace; this murmur was long but stopped in late systole. After a time gap, a long, loud, decrescendo, diastolic murmur was heard. At the lower sternal border and at the apex were a blowing holosystolic murmur and a mid-diastolic rumble, respectively. The first heart sound was diminished, and the second heart sound was loud in the second left interspace. The liver was large and pulsatile, and it had a span of approximately 12 cm. Ascites and pitting edema of the thighs, sacral area, and legs were present.

The ECG showed atrial fibrillation and an irregular ventricular response of about 80 per minute. There was low voltage of the QRS and T waves. The chest roentgenogram showed massive cardiomegaly suggesting enlargement of all chambers. There was prominence of the vasculature in the upper lobes, and Kerley B lines were seen on both sides. The echocardiogram showed enlargement of all chambers. The left ventricular ejection fraction was 20%. Heavy calcification of both the aortic and mitral valves was shown by two-dimensional echocardiography. Doppler echocardiography revealed severe aortic stenosis; also present were mitral regurgitation, tricuspid regurgitation, moderate aortic regurgitation, and mitral stenosis. The pulmonary artery systolic pressure was 70 mm Hg.

Diagnosis: Aortic and mitral stenosis and regurgitation, and tricuspid regurgitation.

Impairment: 95% or 100% impairment of the whole person.

Example 2: A 50-year-old man with mitral valve disease had had advanced symptoms and signs of heart failure resulting in congestion of the pulmonary and systemic circulations and had undergone mitral valve replacement 2 years earlier. Since then, despite restriction of activities and salt and the use of digoxin and diuretics, his activities remained limited by dyspnea on minimal exertion. Vigorous use of diuretics eliminated peripheral edema but resulted in chemical evidence of pre-renal azotemia. The patient was able to walk a city block at a normal pace, drive an automobile, and sleep comfortably, but he became breathless after climbing one flight of stairs.

Physical examination showed a comfortable man with a blood pressure of 110/70 mm Hg; pulse was 80 beats per minute and irregular. The venous pressure was normal, and there was no peripheral edema. There were rales at the left base. The apical impulse was normal, but there was a parasternal heave. The prosthetic valve sounds were normal, but there was a grade 1/6 holosystolic murmur at the apex.

An ECG showed atrial fibrillation with irregular ventricular response at about 80 per minute and low T waves. A chest roentgenorgram showed cardiomegaly with enlargement of the left and right ventricles and left atrium. There was prominence of the pulmonary vasculature in all lung fields. No Kerley B lines were seen. The prosthetic valve was properly positioned. An echocardiogram showed enlargement of the ventricles and the left atrium. Moderate global reduction of left ventricular systolic function with an ejection fraction of 30% was present. The prosthetic valve was well seated; a normal mean gradient of 5 mm Hg across the valve and a normal mild degree of periprosthetic regurgitation were present.

Cardiac catheterization and angiography disclosed a left ventricular pressure of 110/18 mm Hg and a mean left atrial pressure of 20 mm Hg. The pulmonary artery pressure was 45/18 mm Hg. A left ventricular angiogram showed mild mitral regurgitation and reduction of ventricular contraction.

Diagnosis: Mitral valve replacement with a prosthesis; left ventricular dysfunction. The cause is probably rheumatic.

Impairment: 80% impairment of the whole person.

Comment: Cardiac catheterization was not necessary to establish the degree of impairment.

6.2 Coronary Heart Disease

Coronary heart disease is most commonly due to arteriosclerosis of the coronary arteries, a complex process that results in reduced coronary blood flow. Other causes of limited or reduced coronary blood flow include coronary artery spasm, emboli, congenital abnormalities, and trauma. Also, inflammatory processes and arthritis can obstruct the coronary arteries, especially the coronary ostia.

Reduced coronary flow may result in injury to the myocardium and lead to infarction or diffuse fibrosis. The degree of the patient's impairment is determined by the consequences of both the reduced coronary blood flow and the reduced ventricular function. Reduced coronary blood flow also can cause angina pectoris, which itself may impair a person's ability to perform usual activities. In addition, reduced coronary blood flow and myocardial damage may cause cardiac arrhythmias, which are discussed in Section 6.7 (p. 194).

The physician must obtain a detailed history to estimate the degree of impairment due to coronary heart disease. The physical examination may contribute to estimating the severity of the disorder, especially to estimating the degree of impairment of ventricular function. In most patients, laboratory studies will also be necessary. Studies obtained at rest, during exercise, and after exercise are especially useful in examining patients suspected of having coronary heart disease. Coronary angiography may be necessary in some patients.

Impairment due to coronary heart disease can be reduced but not eliminated by diet, exercise training programs, cessation of cigarette smoking, use of medications, and surgical procedures. Sufficient time must be allowed for these measures to have an effect before an estimate of permanent impairment is made. Impairment criteria are given in Table 6 (p. 178).

Criteria for Evaluating Permanent Impairment Resulting from Coronary Heart Disease

Class 1: Impairment of the Whole Person, 0% to 10%
Because of the serious implications of reduced coronary blood flow, it is not reasonable to classify the degree of impairment as 0% to 10% in any patient who has symptoms of coronary heart disease corroborated by physical examination or laboratory tests. This class of impairment should be reserved for the patient with an equivocal history of angina pectoris on whom coronary angiography is performed, or for a patient on whom coronary angiography is performed for other reasons, and in whom a less than 50% reduction in the cross-sectional area of a coronary artery is found.

Class 2: Impairment of the Whole Person, 10% to 30%
A patient belongs in class 2 when (1) the patient has a history of myocardial infarction or angina pectoris that is documented by appropriate laboratory studies, but at the time of evaluation the patient has no symptoms while performing ordinary daily activities or even moderately heavy physical exertion (functional class 1); *and* (2) the patient may require moderate dietary adjustment or medication to prevent angina or to remain free of signs and symptoms of congestive heart failure; *and* (3) the patient is able to walk on the treadmill or bicycle ergometer and obtain a heart rate of 90% of the predicted maximum rate without developing significant ST-segment shift, ventricular tachycardia, or hypotension; if the patient is uncooperative or unable to exercise because of disease affecting another organ system, this requirement may be omitted; *or* (4) the patient has recovered from coronary artery surgery or angioplasty, remains asymptomatic during ordinary daily activities, and is able to exercise as outlined above. If the patient is taking a beta-adrenergic blocking agent, he or she should be able to exercise on the treadmill or bicycle ergometer to a level estimated to cause an energy expenditure of at least 7 METS as a substitute for the heart rate target.

Any of the exercise protocols in Table 2 (p. 171) may be used. The maximum and 90% of maximum predicted heart rates by age and sex group are presented in Table 7 (p. 178).

Example 1: A 50-year-old man had had an acute myocardial infarction 8 months earlier. He had been hospitalized for 10 days, at which time serial ECGs showed classic changes of an inferior wall infarction. After recovering, the patient returned to his work as an attendant in a service station. The man was following a diet to maintain a weight of 72 kg, which was 11 kg less than his weight 1 year previously. He had no symptoms and was receiving no medication.

Physical examination and chest roentgenograms were normal. The ECG showed Q waves in leads 2, 3, and F and flat T waves in the same leads. When the man exercised, his heart rate was 152 beats per minute, he had an adequate rise in blood pressure, and there were no ECG pattern changes indicating ischemia or arrhythmias.

Diagnosis: Recent inferior wall myocardial infarction.

Impairment: 20% impairment of the whole person.

Comment: An uncomplicated recovery from an *anterior* wall infarction would be estimated as a 29% impairment.

Table 6. Impairment Classification for Coronary Heart Disease.

Class 1: **0%-9% impairment of the whole person**	**Class 2:** **10%-29% impairment of the whole person**	**Class 3:** **30%-49% impairment of the whole person**	**Class 4:** **50%-100% impairment of the whole person**
Because of serious implications of reduced coronary blood flow, it is not reasonable to classify degree of impairment as 0 through 9 in any patient who has symptoms of coronary heart disease corroborated by physical examination or laboratory tests; this class of impairment should be reserved for patients with equivocal histories of angina pectoris on whom coronary angiography is performed, or for patients on whom coronary angiography is performed for other reasons and in whom less than 50% reduction in cross sectional area of coronary artery is found; METS determination is not applicable.	Patient has a history of myocardial infarction or angina pectoris documented by appropriate laboratory studies, but at time of evaluation, patient has no symptoms while performing ordinary daily activities or even moderately heavy physical exertion (functional class 1); **and** Patient may require moderate dietary adjustment or medication to prevent angina or to remain free of signs and symptoms of congestive heart failure; **and** Patient is able to walk on the treadmill or bicycle ergometer and obtain heart rate of 90% of predicted maximum heart rate without developing significant ST-segment shift, ventricular tachycardia, or hypotension; if patient is uncooperative or unable to exercise because of disease affecting another organ system, this requirement may be omitted; METS >7; **or** Patient has recovered from coronary artery surgery or angioplasty, remains asymptomatic during ordinary daily activities, and is able to exercise as outlined above; if patient is taking a beta-adrenergic blocking agent, he or she should be able to walk on treadmill to level estimated to cause energy expenditure of at least 7 METS as substitute for heart rate target.	Patient has history of myocardial infarction documented by appropriate laboratory studies, or angina pectoris documented by changes on resting or exercise ECG or radioisotope study suggestive of ischemia; **or** Patient has either fixed or dynamic focal obstruction of at least 50% of coronary artery, angiography, and function testing; **and** Patient requires moderate dietary adjustment or drugs to prevent frequent angina or to remain free of symptoms and signs of congestive heart failure but may develop angina pectoris after moderately heavy physical exertion (functional class 2); METS >5 but <7; **or** Patient has recovered from coronary artery surgery or angioplasty, continues to require treatment, and has symptoms described above.	Patient has history of myocardial infarction that is documented by appropriate laboratory studies, or angina pectoris documented by changes on resting ECG or radioisotope study highly suggestive of myocardial ischemia; **or** Patient has either fixed or dynamic focal obstruction of at least 50% of one or more coronary arteries, demonstrated by angiography and function testing; **and** Patient requires moderate dietary adjustments or drugs to prevent angina or to remain free of symptoms and signs of congestive heart failure, but continues to develop symptoms of angina pectoris or congestive heart failure during ordinary daily activities (functional class 3 or 4), or there are signs or laboratory evidence of cardiac enlargement and abnormal ventricular function; METS <5; **or** Patient has recovered from coronary artery bypass surgery or angioplasty and continues to require treatment and have symptoms as described above.

Table 7. Maximal and 90% of Maximal Achievable Heart Rate, by Age and Sex*

		Heart rate (beats/min) by Age (y)							
		30	35	40	45	50	55	60	65
Men	Maximal	193	191	189	187	184	182	180	178
	90% Maximal	173	172	170	168	166	164	162	160
Women	Maximal	190	185	181	177	172	168	163	159
	90% Maximal	171	167	163	159	155	151	147	143

*Source: Sheffield LH. Exercise stress testing. In Braunwald E, ed. *Heart Disease: A Textbook of Cardiovascular Medicine.* 3rd ed. Philadelphia, Pa: WB Saunders Co; 1988:227.

Example 2: A 52-year-old woman had undergone coronary artery bypass surgery 6 months earlier for relief of angina. A vein graft had been placed into the left anterior descending coronary artery and another into the right coronary artery. Preoperative coronary angiography had shown no significant obstruction in the circumflex coronary artery. After surgery, the patient did well and had worked for 14 months as a service specialist for an insurance firm. She had had no symptoms but had avoided heavy physical exertion. She was taking 0.3 g of aspirin daily but no other medications. An exercise test 10 days earlier showed a heart rate of 144 beats per minute after 10 minutes of exercise under the Bruce protocol and no ST-segment shifts or arrhythmias.

Physical examination showed a well-healed scar and a normal heart. The resting ECG showed low T waves in leads I, L, V4, V5, and V6 and no Q waves. The chest roentgenogram was normal.

Diagnosis: Coronary heart disease with coronary artery bypass surgery.

Impairment: 15% impairment of the whole person.

Class 3: Impairment of the Whole Person, 30% to 50%

A patient belongs in class 3 when (1) the patient has a history of myocardial infarction that is documented by appropriate laboratory studies, or of angina pectoris that is documented by changes on a resting or exercise ECG or radioisotope study that are suggestive of ischemia; *or* (2) the patient has either a fixed or dynamic focal obstruction of at least 50% of a coronary artery, demonstrated by angiography; *and* (3) the patient requires moderate dietary adjustment or drugs to prevent frequent episodes of angina or to remain free of symptoms and signs of congestive heart failure, but may develop angina pectoris or symptoms of congestive heart failure after moderately heavy physical exertion (5 to 7 METS, functional class 2); *or* (4) the patient has recovered from coronary artery surgery or angioplasty, continues to require treatment, and has the symptoms described above.

Example 1: A 60-year-old family physician had suffered an acute anterior wall myocardial infarction 12 months earlier. He had the classic history of chest pain, diaphoresis, and weakness, and typical ECG and enzyme changes. After discharge from the hospital, the patient entered a rehabilitation program, but even after 3 months he continued to experience fatigue and breathlessness after a brisk walk of 20 to 30 minutes. The patient returned to work but limited his practice and accepted no new patients.

An ECG 3 months previously recorded a heart rate of 140 beats per minute after 10 minutes of exercise and ST-segment elevation in leads I, L, and V3 through V6. After exercising, the patient was tired but experienced no chest pain. A radiosotope angiogram revealed a large anterior aneurysm of the left ventricle and good function of the inferior wall of the left ventricle. The patient was placed on a regimen of a low-salt diet; digoxin, 0.25 mg daily; and hydrochlorothiazide, 25 mg three times per week.

On physical examination, the patient was comfortable, and there were no signs of heart failure. Blood pressure was 135/85 mm Hg, and the pulse was regular. There was a large, sustained impulse above and lateral to the left nipple, centered in the third intercostal space at the anterior axillary line. A fourth heart sound was present.

The ECG showed a Q wave in leads I, L, and V1 through V4. A chest roentgenogram showed cardiac enlargement and clear lung fields.

Diagnosis: Anterior left ventricular aneurysm secondary to coronary heart disease.

Impairment: 45% impairment of the whole person.

Example 2: A 62-year-old woman had undergone quadruple coronary artery bypass surgery 13 months earlier, but she continued to experience retrosternal chest discomfort if she hurried while doing usual activities. She was likely to experience discomfort in the morning and when outdoors in the cold. She enjoyed walking but usually experienced discomfort if she hurried up a steep hill going to church. She was able to care for her house and perform other activities without symptoms, if she did not rush. She was on a diet, and she took a beta-adrenergic blocking agent and oral nitrates.

At the latest physical examination, she was comfortable and had no signs of congestive heart failure. Blood pressure was 110/70 mm Hg, and pulse was regular at 62 beats per minute. The apical impulse was normal, and there were no gallops or murmurs.

An ECG showed low T waves in all leads, and the chest roentgenogram was normal. An exercise ECG recorded a heart rate of 118 beats per minute after 6 minutes of exercise. The patient experienced retrosternal discomfort during the last minute of exercise, and there was 1.5 mm of ST-segment depression in leads V4 through V6 at 1 and 2 minutes after exercise.

A coronary angiogram showed 90% or greater obstruction of all three coronary arteries. The grafts to the right, circumflex, and left anterior descending coronary arteries were patent, but the graft to the diagonal branch of the left anterior descending coronary artery could not be visualized.

Diagnosis: Coronary heart disease and continued chest discomfort after coronary artery bypass surgery.

Impairment: 45% impairment of the whole person.

Class 4: Impairment of the Whole Person, 50% to 100%

A patient belongs in class 4 when (1) the patient has history of a myocardial infarction that is documented by appropriate laboratory studies, or angina pectoris that has been documented by changes on a resting ECG or radioisotope study that are highly suggestive of myocardial ischemia; *or* (2) the patient has either fixed or dynamic focal obstruction of at least 50% of one or more coronary arteries demonstrated by angiography; *and* (3) moderate dietary adjustments or drugs are required to prevent angina or to remain free of symptoms and signs of congestive heart failure, but the patient continues to develop symptoms of angina pectoris or congestive heart failure during ordinary daily activities (functional class 3 or 4), and there are signs or laboratory evidence of cardiac enlargement and abnormal ventricular function; *or* (4) the patient has recovered from coronary artery bypass surgery or angioplasty and continues to require treatment and have symptoms as described above.

Example 1: A 42-year-old man had suffered an anteroseptal myocardial infarction 15 months earlier. Two years ago he had had an inferior wall myocardial infarction. During the past 6 months he had continued to have episodes of retrosternal discomfort on minimal exertion and sometimes at rest, despite the use of adequate doses of beta-adrenergic blocking agents, oral and sublingual nitrates, and, more recently, a calcium-channel blocking agent. He rarely went a full day without an episode of chest discomfort, which usually lasted 1 to 10 minutes.

On examination, the patient was comfortable at rest. His blood pressure was 120/80 mm Hg, and his resting pulse rate was 54 beats per minute. There were no signs of congestive heart failure. The apical impulse was enlarged, sustained, and displaced laterally to the anterior axillary line at the fifth intercostal space. The first heart sound was soft and there was a prominent fourth heart sound. A grade 2/6 holosystolic murmur was present at the apex.

The resting ECG showed Q waves in leads 2, 3 and F, a QS pattern in VI through V3, and a QR in V4; the T waves were low in all leads. The chest roentgenogram showed marked cardiomegaly and prominence of the vasculature in the upper lung fields. During exercise, the patient developed pain and ST depression in I, L, V5, and V6 after 2 minutes. The ejection fraction fell from 30% to 25% as measured by the multigated blood pool scan.

Diagnosis: Angina pectoris and left ventricular failure due to coronary heart disease.

Impairment: 90% impairment of the whole person.

Example 2: A 46-year-old woman had had quadruple coronary artery bypass surgery 11 months earlier but continued to have pain each day and to be weak and breathless after minimal exertion. She slept on three pillows; she often awakened short of breath and had to sit in a chair for the remainder of the night. These symptoms continued despite treatment with digitalis, diuretics, nitrates, calcium-channel blocking agents, and hydralazine.

On examination, there was evidence of weight loss. The patient preferred the sitting position. Blood pressure was 110/70 mm Hg, and the heart rate was 92 beats per minute. The neck veins distended when hand pressure was applied to the abdomen, even when the upper part of the examining table was at a 45° angle. The apical impulse was enlarged, sustained, and displaced to the anterior axillary line, and a parasternal heave was present. There were rales at both lung bases and dullness at the right lung base. The first heart sound was soft, and there was a prominent third heart sound. A grade 2/6 holosystolic murmur was present at the apex.

The ECG showed a QS pattern in Vl through V4, prominent Q waves in V5 and V6, and low R waves throughout. The T waves were inverted in I, L, and Vl through V5 and low elsewhere. The chest roentgenogram showed marked cardiomegaly, increased vascular markings in the upper lung fields, and a small, right-sided pleural effusion.

Coronary angiography showed total occlusion of the left anterior descending coronary artery and 90% blockage in both the right and circumflex coronary arteries. The graft to the right coronary artery and the graft to one of the branches of the circumflex artery were patent, but the graft to the other branch of the circumflex artery and the graft to the anterior descending artery were not visualized. The ventriculogram showed an ejection fraction of 20%; there was akinesis of the entire anterior wall and poor contraction elsewhere.

Diagnosis: Angina pectoris and left ventricular failure after coronary artery bypass surgery.

Impairment: 95% to 100% impairment of the whole person.

6.3 Congenital Heart Disease

In recent years, surgical procedures designed to correct or improve the circulation of infants and children with congenital cardiac disorders have allowed many of the children to live to adulthood. Many of these surgically treated patients continue to have less than perfect functioning of the heart and circulation and are therefore impaired.

Congenital heart disease may be recognized by history and physical examination, but often the exact diagnosis and the patient's functional impairment require special studies, including ECG, chest roentgenogram, radioisotope studies, echocardiography, hemodynamic measurements, and angiography. A classification of limitations due to symptoms is found in Table 1 (p. 170).

The criteria for evaluating impairment due to congenital heart disease are given in Table 8 (p. 181).

Criteria for Evaluating Impairment Resulting from Congenital Heart Disease

Class 1: Impairment of the Whole Person, 0% to 10%
A patient belongs in class 1 when (1) the patient has evidence by physical examination or laboratory studies of congenital heart disease and has no symptoms in the performance of ordinary daily activities or even on moderately heavy physical exertion; *and* (2) continuous treatment is not required, although

Table 8. Impairment Classification for Congenital Heart Disease.

Class 1: **0%-9% impairment of the whole person**	**Class 2:** **10%-29% impairment of the whole person**	**Class 3:** **30%-49% impairment of the whole person**	**Class 4:** **50%-100% impairment of the whole person**
Patient has evidence by physical examination or laboratory studies of congenital heart disease and has no symptoms in performance of ordinary daily activities or even on moderately heavy physical exertion; **and** Continuous treatment is not required, although prophylactic antibiotics may be recommended after surgical procedures to reduce risk of bacterial endocarditis; and patient remains free of signs of congestive heart failure and pain; **and** There are no signs of cardiac chamber dysfunction or dilation; evidence of residual valvular stenosis or regurgitation is estimated to be mild; there is no evidence of right-to-left shunt; a small left-to-right shunt may be present, but Qp/Qs is less than 1.5:1.0; **or** In patient who has recovered from corrective heart surgery, all of above criteria are met.	Patient has evidence by physical examination or laboratory studies of congenital heart disease, has no symptoms in performance of ordinary daily activities, but has symptoms with moderately heavy physical exertion (functional class 2); **or** Patient requires moderate dietary adjustments or drugs to prevent symptoms or to remain free of signs of congestive heart failure or other consequences of congenital heart disease, such as syncope, chest pain, emboli, or cyanosis; **or** There are signs or laboratory findings of cardiac chamber dysfunction or dilation, or severity of valvular stenosis or regurgitation is estimated to be moderate; there is no evidence of right-to-left shunt; moderate-sized left-to-right shunt may be present with Qp/Qs of less than 2.0:1.0; or there is evidence of moderate elevation of pulmonary vascular resistance, which should be less than one-half systemic vascular resistance; **or** Patient has recovered from surgery for treatment of congenital heart disease and meets above criteria for impairment.	Patient has evidence by physical examination or laboratory studies of congenital heart disease and experiences symptoms during performance of ordinary daily activities (functional class 3); **and** Diet modification and drugs do not completely control symptoms or prevent signs of congestive heart failure; **and** There are signs or laboratory evidence of cardiac chamber dysfunction or dilation; or the severity of valvular stenosis or regurgitation is estimated to be moderate or severe; or there is evidence of a right-to-left shunt or evidence of left-to-right shunt with pulmonary flow being greater than 2 times the systemic flow; or pulmonary vascular resistance is elevated to greater than one-half systemic vascular resistance; **or** Patient has recovered from surgery for treatment of congenital heart disease but continues to have functional class 3 symptoms; or continues to have signs of congestive failure or cyanosis, and there is evidence of cardiomegaly and significant residual valvular stenosis or regurgitation, left-to-right shunt, right-to-left shunt, or elevated pulmonary vascular resistance.	Patient has signs of congenital heart disease and experiences symptoms of congestive heart failure at less than ordinary daily activities (functional class 4); **and** Dietary therapy and drugs do not prevent symptoms or signs of congestive heart failure; **and** There is evidence from physical examination or laboratory studies of cardiac dilation, or chamber dysfunction or dilation, or pulmonary vascular resistance remains elevated at greater than one-half systemic vascular resistance; or severity of valvular stenosis or regurgitation is estimated to be moderate to severe; or there is left-to-right shunt with pulmonary flow being greater than 2 times systemic flow; or there is left-to-right shunt with pulmonary vascular resistance being elevated to greater than one-half systemic vascular resistance; or there is right-to-left shunt; **or** Patient has recovered from heart surgery for treatment of congenital heart disease and continues to have symptoms or signs of congestive heart failure causing impairment as outlined above.

prophylactic antibiotics may be recommended after surgical procedures to reduce the risk of bacterial endocarditis, and the patient remains free of signs of congestive heart failure and cyanosis; *and* (3) there are no signs of cardiac chamber dysfunction or dilation; the evidence of residual valvular stenosis or regurgitation is estimated to be mild; there is no evidence of a right-to-left shunt, and if a left-to-right shunt is present, it is mild (Qp/Qs ratio <1.5:1.0); the pulmonary vascular resistance is estimated to be normal; *or* (4) in the patient who has recovered from corrective heart surgery, all of the above criteria are met.

Example 1: A 22-year-old woman was known to have had a loud systolic murmur along the left sternal border since childhood. She had undergone cardiac catheterization at the ages of 2 and 18 years, and on both occasions a 20-mm Hg gradient was noted between the right ventricle and the pulmonary artery. She also had normal pulmonary artery pressures, no evidence of shunts, and normal cardiac output. She never had symptoms referable to the cardiovascular system.

Physical examination showed the patient to be comfortable without signs of heart failure or cyanosis. The precordium was without heaves, thrills, or taps. The first heart sound was normal; the second heart sound was widely split and varied with respiration. There was a grade 3/6 systolic murmur that ended well short of the second heart sound; the murmur was loudest in the second left intercostal space, and an early systolic click was present that varied with respiration. There were no diastolic murmurs or gallops. The chest roentgenogram and ECG were normal.

Diagnosis: Mild pulmonary valve stenosis.

Impairment: 9% impairment of the whole person.

Comment: If the gradient were greater than 40 mm Hg according to Doppler echocardiography, or if the ECG showed right ventricular hypertrophy, then the patient would be in a higher category of impairment and would be a suitable candidate for percutaneous balloon valvuloplasty or surgical treatment of the stenosis.

An asymptomatic patient with a small ventricular septal defect might be estimated to be at the upper end of class 1 impairment, but if bacterial endocarditis had ever been present, the impairment rating would be higher. Also at the upper end of class 1 might be a patient with a small atrial septal defect and normal pressures in all cardiac chambers and great vessels, or a patient with anomalous venous return from a small segment of the lung.

Example 2: A 25-year-old woman had undergone repair of an atrial septal defect 10 years earlier. There were no complications, and the patient remained asymptomatic and returned to an active life.

Physical examination showed a well-healed wound over the sternum without tenderness. There were no abnormal precordial pulsations or signs of congestive heart failure. The first heart sound was normal. The second heart sound was widely split, and there was variation with respiration in the degree of splitting. A grade 2/6 early systolic ejection murmur was heard along the left sternal border.

The ECG showed an incomplete right bundle-branch block pattern. The chest roentgenogram was normal. The echocardiogram showed mild enlargement of the right ventricle and reduced motion of the ventricular septum. No shunt at the atrial level was seen on two-dimensional or Doppler echocardiography. The pulmonary artery systolic pressure by Doppler echocardiography was normal. Findings on cardiac catheterization and angiography were normal.

Diagnosis: Atrial septal defect with surgical closure.

Impairment: 5% impairment of the whole person.

Comment: If a very small left-to-right shunt were demonstrated postoperatively, or the residual pulmonary artery pressures were mildly elevated, then the degree of impairment might be raised to 6% to 9%. Cardiac catheterization and angiography were not necessary for evaluating this patient's impairment.

Class 2: Impairment of the Whole Person, 10% to 30%

A patient belongs in class 2 when (1) the patient has evidence by physical examination or laboratory studies of congenital heart disease, has no symptoms in the performance of ordinary activities, and has symptoms with moderately heavy physical exertion (functional class 2); *or* (2) the patient requires moderate dietary adjustments or drugs to prevent symptoms or to remain free of signs of congestive heart failure or other consequences of congenital heart disease, such as syncope, chest pain, emboli, or cyanosis; *or* (3) there are signs or laboratory evidence of cardiac chamber dysfunction or dilation, or the severity of valvular stenosis or regurgitation is estimated to be moderate; or there is evidence of a small to moderate left-to-right shunt with Qp/Qs less than 2.0:1.0 and no evidence of right-to-left shunt; or there is evidence of moderate elevation of the pulmonary vascular resistance, which should be less than one-half the systemic vascular resistance; *or* (4) the patient has recovered from surgery for the treatment of congenital heart disease and meets the above criteria for impairment.

Example 1: A 35-year-old woman had had a systolic murmur and abnormal cardiac sounds for many years. She had led a relatively normal life but avoided participation in sports at the advice of physicians. During the past year she noted becoming weak and tired with heavy exercising, but she was still able to perform daily activities without limitations. The palpitations were not associated with symptoms of inadequate cerebral perfusion and were never sustained. There was no history of cyanosis, breathlessness, or peripheral edema.

On examination, the patient was comfortable and had no cyanosis. There was elevation of venous pressure to 15 cm without large V waves, and the liver was enlarged to a width of 12 cm. The lungs were clear. There were no thrills, taps, or heaves in the precordium. The first heart sound was loud and was followed by a very loud, sharp sound in early systole that was heard best along the left sternal border. The second heart sound was loud, and there was an early diastolic sound heard best at the mid-precordium. A holosystolic murmur was heard along the left sternal border that increased in intensity with inspiration.

The ECG demonstrated a right bundle-branch block pattern, and the R wave in V1 was very low. A broad, notched P wave in leads III and F and inverted T waves in V1 and V2 were present. There were occasional premature atrial beats. The chest roentgenogram showed marked enlargement of the cardiac silhouette, particularly to the right of the sternum. The pulmonary vasculature was normal. An echocardiogram showed features consistent with Ebstein's anomaly of the tricuspid valve. The tricuspid valve was markedly displaced into a small right ventricle, and severe tricuspid regurgitation was present. No right-to-left shunt was present by Doppler echocardiography.

Cardiac catheterization and angiography demonstrated a mean right atrial pressure of 7 mm Hg with V waves of 15 mm Hg. Right ventricular and pulmonary artery pressures were normal. There was no evidence of a shunt.

Diagnosis: Ebstein's anomaly of the tricuspid valve.

Impairment: 25% impairment of the whole person.

Comment: If the patient had had a right-to-left shunt, then the estimated impairment would be considerably higher. If the patient had had a cardiac arrhythmia that caused symptoms, the impairment would have been estimated according to the criteria for arrhythmias, and impairment percents due to congenital heart disease and the arrhythmia would have been *combined* (Combined Values Chart, p. 322).

Cardiac catheterization was not necessary to determine the degree of this patient's impairment. Exercise testing might have been useful.

Example 2: A 42-year-old man had undergone open heart surgery 15 years earlier for the treatment of tetralogy of Fallot. The procedure resulted in relief of pulmonary stenosis, placement of a pericardial bridge in the outflow tract of the right ventricle, and closure of the ventricular septal defect. After the operation, the patient did well without medication and achieved his present position as dispatcher for a trucking firm.

At examination, the man appeared healthy. Blood pressure was 110/70 mm Hg, and the pulse was regular at 70 beats per minute. There were no signs of congestive heart failure, and the precordium was normal. The first heart sound was normal. The second heart sound was louder than normal, and it was followed by a mid-diastolic, scratchy murmur heard in the second and third left intercostal spaces. There was a short, grade 2/6 ejection systolic murmur heard in the same places.

The ECG showed right bundle-branch block. A chest roentgenogram showed an apical prominence at the left side of the cardiac silhouette. Echocardiography showed thickening of the right ventricular wall and dilation of the right ventricular cavity with diminished ventricular septal motion. The right ventricular outflow tract was patent and had an 8-mm Hg gradient. The right ventricular systolic pressure was 30 mm Hg. No shunt was shown by Doppler echocardiography.

Diagnosis: Tetralogy of Fallot with surgical relief of pulmonary valve stenosis and closure of the ventricular septal defect.

Impairment: 15% to 20% impairment of the whole person.

Comment: Had there been evidence of a shunt, the estimated impairment would have been greater. Also, if a conduit or prosthesis had been placed in the pulmonary outflow tract, or if significant symptoms had been present, the rating would have been greater. Cardiac catheterization was not necessary in this instance to determine the degree of impairment.

Class 3: Impairment of the Whole Person, 30% to 50%

A patient belongs in class 3 when (1) the patient has evidence by physical examination or laboratory studies of congenital heart disease and experiences symptoms during the performance of ordinary daily activities (functional class 3); *and* (2) diet modifications and drugs do not completely control symptoms or prevent signs of congestive heart failure; *and* (3) there are signs or laboratory evidence of cardiac chamber dysfunction or dilation; or valvular stenosis or regurgitation is estimated to be moderate or severe; or there is evidence of a right-to-left shunt; or there is evidence of a left-to-right shunt with the pulmonary flow being greater than two times the systemic flow; or the pulmonary vascular resistance is elevated to greater than one-half the systemic vascular resistance; *or* (4) the patient has recovered from surgery for the treatment of congenital heart disease but continues to have functional class 3 symptoms; or the patient continues to have signs of congestive failure or cyanosis, and there is evidence of cardiomegaly and significant residual valvular stenosis or regurgitation, left-to-right shunt, right-to-left shunt, or elevated pulmonary vascular resistance.

Example 1: A 52-year-old woman had Ebstein's anomaly of the tricuspid valve; the diagnosis had been made years ago with the aid of echocardiography, cardiac catheterization, and angiography. During the past several years, she had had increasing breathlessness during daily activities, such as climbing stairs, mopping, or cleaning. Also, she had noticed ankle edema and increased abdominal girth. The use of diuretics had diminished the edema and ascites. The patient restricted the salt in her diet and took digitalis.

On examination, the patient appeared well, but there was duskiness of the lips and the fingernails. The neck veins were markedly distended, and the liver was 14 cm wide and slightly pulsatile. The lungs were clear. The precordium showed an active parasternal area without a heave. The first heart sound was loud and was followed by a loud, early systolic sound along the left sternal border. The second heart sound was widely split and was followed by an early diastolic sound. There was a holosystolic murmur that increased with inspiration and was heard best at the left of the sternum. A diastolic murmur was heard best during inspiration and along the left sternal border.

The ECG showed right bundle-branch block with low R waves in V1 and prominent P waves. The chest roentgenogram showed a greatly enlarged cardiac silhouette, especially to the right of the sternum. The pulmonary vasculature was normal. An echocardiogram showed typical changes of Ebstein's anomaly of the tricuspid valve. Doppler echocardiography revealed a small right-to-left shunt across the atrial septum.

Diagnosis: Ebstein's anomaly of the tricuspid valve.

Impairment: 49% impairment of the whole person.

Example 2: A 20-year-old man had undergone a Mustard procedure 10 years earlier for treatment of transposition of the great vessels. In infancy he had had a Blalock-Hanlon procedure. After the Mustard procedure, he did moderately well, but he never developed satisfactory stamina, tiring easily and being unable to participate in such activities as tennis and hiking.

On examination, the patient appeared healthy but underweight and had no cyanosis. The neck veins were distended and showed a prominent A wave. The liver was not enlarged and there was no peripheral edema. The lungs were clear. There were parasternal and apical heaves at the precordium. There was a holosystolic murmur at the left sternal border, and a fourth heart sound was present.

The ECG showed tall R-wave voltage in all of the precordial leads. The chest roentgenogram showed moderate cardiomegaly. The echocardiogram showed signs of a properly functioning intra-atrial baffle. Both ventricular cavities were enlarged, but there was good ventricular function. Cardiac catheterization and angiography demonstrated an elevated right mean atrial pressure of 12 mm Hg with A waves of 20 mm Hg. Right ventricular and pulmonary artery systolic pressures were 30 to 35 mm Hg.

Diagnosis: Transposition of the great vessels and Mustard procedure.

Impairment: 40% to 49% impairment of the whole person.

Comment: If significant arrhythmias were to complicate the postoperative period, they would be evaluated according to the criteria in the section on arrhythmias, and the impairments for congenital heart disease and arrhythmia would be combined (Combined Values Chart, p. 322) to determine whole-person impairment from cardiac disease.

Class 4: Impairment of the Whole Person, 50% to 100%

A patient belongs in class 4 when (1) the patient has signs of congenital heart disease and experiences symptoms of congestive heart failure at less than ordinary daily activities (functional class 4); *and* (2) dietary therapy and drugs do not prevent symptoms or signs of congestive heart failure; *and* (3) there is evidence from physical examination or laboratory studies of cardiac chamber hypertrophy or dilation; or the pulmonary vascular resistance remains elevated at greater than one-half the systemic vascular resistance; or the severity of the valvular stenosis or regurgitation is estimated to be moderate to severe; or there is left-to-right shunt with the pulmonary flow being greater than two times the systemic flow; or there is a left-to-right shunt with the pulmonary vascular resistance being elevated to greater than one-half the systemic vascular resistance; or there is a right-to-left shunt; *or* (4) the patient has recovered from heart surgery for the treatment of congenital heart disease and continues to have symptoms or signs of congestive heart failure causing impairment as outlined above.

Example 1: A 23-year-old woman in whom Eisenmenger's complex had been diagnosed 10 years earlier had been followed up regularly. Cardiac catheterization and angiography had demonstrated a ventricular septal defect and pulmonary vascular resistance equal to systemic vascular resistance. Recently the woman's activities became markedly limited because of fatigue on minimal exertion. Peripheral edema of recent onset responded to diuretic therapy.

On examination, the woman had mild cyanosis that intensified with exertion. There were prominent A waves in the neck veins, but there was no jugular venous distention when the patient was placed at a 45° angle. The liver was not enlarged and there was no peripheral edema. The lungs were clear. There was a forceful, sustained, parasternal heave. The first heart sound was normal, and the second was narrowly split. There was a marked increase in the second component of the second sound. There was a short, early systolic ejection murmur along the left sternal border.

The ECG showed right ventricular hypertrophy and peaked P waves in leads II, III, and F. A chest roentgenogram showed evidence of right ventricular hypertrophy, marked prominence of the proximal portion of the pulmonary arteries, and greatly diminished pulmonary vascular markings in the periphery of the lung fields.

Diagnosis: Eisenmenger's complex with ventricular septal defect and elevated pulmonary vascular resistance.

Impairment: 95% to 100% impairment of the whole person.

Example 2: A 35-year-old man with tetralogy of Fallot had had a Blalock-Taussig systemic to pulmonary artery anastomosis as a child, which had been ligated during a second operative procedure years later. At that time, pulmonary stenosis was relieved by removing muscle in the outflow area of the right ventricle, and the ventricular septal defect was closed. After the second operation the patient did not do well but continued to tire easily. Significant peripheral edema and ascites responded to the use of diuretics. The man was comfortable during light work activities about the home but became weak and breathless on more vigorous exertion.

At examination, a prominent V wave in the neck veins was seen. The liver was 14 cm across. There was palpable cardiac activity parasternally but no sustained heave. There was a grade 3/6 holosystolic murmur along the left sternal border and a mid-diastolic murmur in the second left interspace. The first heart sound was normal, and the second heart sound was single and loud. The ECG showed right bundle-branch block. The chest roentgenogram showed cardiomegaly and a right pleural effusion. The echocardiogram showed a dilated, poorly functioning right ventricle with severe tricuspid regurgitation. No residual right ventricular outflow obstruction was visualized. No residual ventricular septal defect was seen by two-dimensional or Doppler echocardiography.

Diagnosis: Tetralogy of Fallot with surgical relief of the pulmonary stenosis and closure of the ventricular septal defect, followed by development of tricuspid regurgitation and heart failure.

Impairment: 80% to 90% impairment of the whole person.

6.4 Hypertensive Cardiovascular Disease

Elevated pressure within the systemic arterial system is known as hypertension. A transient elevation of arterial pressure is the normal physiologic response to exercise and excitement, but a sustained elevation of pressure is not normal and can lead to damage of arterial walls and damage of the organs supplied by these vessels, especially the brain and the kidneys. Also, sustained increased pressure may lead to aortic dissection and rupture. Elevated pressure in the arterial system, if sustained, greatly increases the work of the left ventricle. Initially this leads to compensatory hypertrophy, but eventually it may cause left ventricle failure, with all of the attendant complications, and then death.

The cause of hypertension in most patients is not understood, and in those instances the disorder is called "essential" or "primary" hypertension. In some patients other disorders can be established as the cause of the hypertension, in which case the disorder is termed "secondary" hypertension. An organized approach to detect secondary disorders is warranted, because their correction may lead to elimination or amelioration of the hypertension. Secondary hypertension may be due to coarctation of the aorta, renal artery obstruction, renal parenchymal disease, hyperaldosteronism, Cushing's disease, rare endocrine disorders such as pheochromocytoma, and chronic nocturnal hypoxia resulting from sleep apnea syndromes.

In the patient in whom an identifiable disorder causes the hypertension, an evaluation of a permanent impairment should not be undertaken until a period of months has elapsed and the disorder is stable and unlikely to change. If other organs are affected, as with the kidneys in chronic renal disease, then the percent of impairment due to the hypertension should be *combined* with that due to the other organ system (Combined Values Chart, p. 322) to estimate the total whole-person impairment.

Drugs with acceptable side effects are available that can maintain blood pressure within the normal range in most patients without correctable causes of hypertension. Estimates of impairment due to hypertension should be delayed until after drug therapy has been adjusted to achieve optimum blood pressure control with minimal side effects.

Before classifying a patient as having hypertensive cardiovascular disease, the physician should make several determinations of the arterial pressure. Hypertensive cardiovascular disease is not necessarily present when a patient exhibits transient or irregular episodes of elevated arterial pressure; these episodes can be associated with an emotional or environmental stimulus or with signs or symptoms of cardiovascular system hyperactivity. Most authorities agree that hypertensive cardiovascular disease is present when the diastolic pressure is repeatedly in excess of 90 mm Hg before antihypertensive therapy has been started.

Impairment criteria for hypertensive cardiovascular disease are given in Table 9 (p. 187).

Criteria for Evaluating Impairment Resulting from Hypertensive Cardiovascular Disease

Class 1: Impairment of the Whole Person, 0% to 10%
A patient belongs in class 1 when (1) the patient has no symptoms and the diastolic pressures are repeatedly in excess of 90 mm Hg; *and* (2) the patient is taking antihypertensive medications but has *none* of the following abnormalities: (*a*) abnormal results of urinalysis or renal function tests; (*b*) history of hypertensive cerebrovascular disease; (*c*) evidence of left ventricular hypertrophy; or (*d*) hypertensive vascular abnormalities of the optic fundus, except minimal narrowing of arterioles.

Example: A 26-year-old ophthalmology resident had been told when he was 18 years old that his blood pressure was "high." Numerous determinations of blood pressure made during medical school confirmed the presence of hypertension. An employment examination at the beginning of his residency confirmed the elevated blood pressure, and he was sent for a diagnostic workup and treatment. No cause for the elevated blood pressure was found. The patient was asymptomatic, and he was started on a regimen of restricted salt intake, weight control, and regular exercise. His blood pressure remained elevated, and an antihypertensive medication was prescribed.

At a recent examination, the patient's blood pressure in the sitting position was 160/105 mm Hg in each arm and 170/105 mm Hg in the right leg. The arterial pulses were of good quality. A week later the pressures were the same. All other physical findings were normal; the patient's weight was normal for his height. The ECG and chest roentgenogram were normal. Serum electrolyte levels, including the serum urea nitrogen (SUN) and serum creatinine levels, and results of urinalysis were normal.

Diagnosis: Essential hypertension.

Impairment: 5% impairment of the whole person.

Comment: It may be necessary to alter the antihypertensive medication to effect a reduction in the patient's blood pressure.

Class 2: Impairment of the Whole Person, 10% to 30%
A patient belongs in class 2 when (1) the patient has no symptoms and the diastolic pressures are repeatedly in excess of 90 mm Hg; *and* (2) the patient is taking antihypertensive medication and has *any* of the following abnormalities: (*a*) proteinuria and abnormalities of the urinary sediment, but no impairment of renal function as measured by SUN and serum creatinine determinations; (*b*) history of hypertensive cerebrovascular damage; (*c*) definite hypertensive changes in the retinal arterioles, including crossing defects or old exudates.

Example: A 40-year-old woman had had elevated blood pressure during a pregnancy at age 32 years, but the pressure had been normal 3 weeks and 12 months post partum. Recently she had had bleeding between menstrual periods. Her gynecologist found her blood pressure to be in the range of 150/100 mm to 160/105 Hg on several occasions. Leg blood pressures were elevated. The woman was placed on a low-salt diet and an exercise program.

Findings of a thorough physical examination were normal, as were the ECG and chest roentgenogram. Serum electrolyte levels were normal, including the SUN and creatinine levels. Urinalysis showed 2+ proteinuria, and the sediment showed one to three red blood cells per high power field. Proteinuria was confirmed on two occasions. A 24-hour urine collection yielded 1400 mg of protein.

Diagnosis: Essential hypertension with proteinuria.

Impairment: 15% impairment of the whole person.

Comment: If the blood pressure remains elevated, an antihypertensive medication should be prescribed.

Class 3: Impairment of the Whole Person, 30% to 50%
A patient belongs in class 3 when (1) the patient has no symptoms and the diastolic pressure readings are consistently in excess of 90 mm Hg; *and* (2) the patient is taking antihypertensive medication and has *any* of the following abnormalities: (*a*) diastolic pressure readings usually in excess of 120 mm Hg; (*b*) proteinuria or abnormalities in the urinary sediment, with evidence of impaired renal function as measured by elevated SUN or serum creatinine level or by creatinine clearance below 50%; (c) hypertensive cerebrovascular damage with permanent neurologic

Table 9. Impairment Classification for Hypertensive Cardiovascular Disease.

Class 1: **0%-9% impairment of the whole person**	**Class 2:** **10%-29% impairment of the whole person**	**Class 3:** **30%-49% impairment of the whole person**	**Class 4:** **50%-100% impairment of the whole person**
Patient has no symptoms but diastolic pressures are repeatedly > 90 mm Hg; **and** Patient is normotensive with antihypertensive medications and has *none* of the following abnormalities: (1) abnormal urinalysis or renal function tests; (2) history of hypertensive cerebrovascular disease; (3) evidence of left ventricular hypertrophy; (4) hypertensive vascular abnormalities of optic fundus, except minimal narrowing of arterioles.	Patient has no symptoms but diastolic pressures are repeatedly > 90 mm Hg; **and** Patient is taking antihypertensive medication and has *any* of the following abnormalities: (1) proteinuria and abnormalities of the urinary sediment, but no impairment of renal function as measured by serum urea nitrogen (SUN) and serum creatinine determinations; (2) history of hypertensive cerebrovascular damage; (3) definite hypertensive changes in retinal arterioles, including crossing defects or old exudates.	Patient has no symptoms but diastolic pressure readings are consistently > 90 mm Hg; **and** Patient is taking antihypertensive medication and has *any* of the following abnormalities: (1) diastolic pressure readings usually > 120 mm Hg; (2) proteinuria or abnormalities in urinary sediment, with evidence of impaired renal function as measured by elevated SUN and serum creatinine, or by creatinine clearance below 50%; (3) hypertensive cerebrovascular damage with permanent neurologic residual; (4) left ventricular hypertrophy according to findings of physical examination, echocardiography, ECG, or chest roentgenogram, but no symptoms, signs, or evidence by chest roentgenogram of congestive heart failure; (5) retinopathy, with definite hypertensive changes in arterioles, such as "copper" or "silver wiring," or arteriovenous crossing changes, with or without hemorrhages and exudates.	Patient has a diastolic pressure consistently > 90 mm Hg; **and** Patient is taking antihypertensive medication and has *any 2* of the following abnormalities: (1) diastolic pressure readings usually > 120 mm Hg; (2) proteinuria and abnormalities in urinary sediment, with impaired renal function and evidence of nitrogen retention as measured by elevated SUN and serum creatinine or by creatinine clearance below 50%; (3) hypertensive cerebrovascular damage with permanent neurologic deficits; (4) left ventricular hypertrophy; (5) retinopathy as manifested by hypertensive changes in arterioles, retina, or optic nerve; (6) history of congestive heart failure; **or** Patient has left ventricular hypertrophy with persistence of congestive heart failure despite digitalis and diuretics.

residual; (d) left ventricular hypertrophy according to findings of physical examination, ECG, echocardiogram, or chest roentgenogram, but no symptoms, signs, or other evidence of congestive heart failure; or (*e*) retinopathy with definite hypertensive changes in the arterioles, such as "copper" or "silver wiring" or arteriovenous nicks with or without hemorrhages and exudates.

Example: A 48-year-old man had a long history of severe hypertension and took therapeutic drugs intermittently. He had had no symptoms until 1 year earlier, when he developed breathlessness on exertion, orthopnea, and occasional nocturnal dyspnea. These symptoms improved after the administration of digitalis and diuretics. However, the man still became breathless on heavy exertion and occasionally awakened with breathlessness.

Examination disclosed a comfortable patient with blood pressure of 170/95 mm Hg and pulse rate of 84 beats per minute. There were no signs of congestive heart failure. In the fundus there were increased light reflexes from the arterioles and arteriovenous crossing depressions but no hemorrhages or exudates; the disk was flat. The left ventricular impulse was enlarged and sustained but in the normal position. The first heart sound was normal, and the second was increased in intensity. There was a fourth heart sound.

The ECG showed left ventricular hypertrophy with tall R waves in the lateral chest leads and inverted T waves in the same leads. A chest roentgenogram showed mild cardiomegaly and normal pulmonary vasculature. The serum electrolyte levels and results of urinalysis were normal.

Diagnosis: Essential hypertension and hypertensive heart disease with history of congestive heart failure.

Impairment: 40% to 50% impairment of the whole person.

Class 4: Impairment of the Whole Person, 50% to 100%

A patient belongs in class 4 when (1) the patient has a diastolic pressure consistently in excess of 90 mm Hg; *and* (2) the patient is taking antihypertensive medication and has *any two* of the following abnormalities: (*a*) diastolic pressure readings usually in excess of 120 mm Hg; (*b*) proteinuria and abnormalities in the urinary sediment, with impaired renal function and evidence of nitrogen retention as measured by elevated SUN and serum creatinine levels or by creatinine clearance below 50%; (*c*) hypertensive cerebrovascular damage with permanent neurologic deficits; (*d*) left ventricular hypertrophy; (*e*) retinopathy as manifested by hypertensive changes in the arterioles, retina, or optic nerve; (*f*) history of congestive heart failure; *or* (3) the patient has left ventricular hypertrophy and persisting congestive heart failure despite taking digitalis and diuretics.

Example 1: A 48-year-old man had been admitted to the hospital 8 months earlier with headaches, blurred vision, and breathlessness of 2 weeks' duration. His blood pressure was 260/160 mm Hg in the arms and legs. He was drowsy, but he had no localizing neurologic signs.

The patient's fundi showed arterial spasm, hemorrhages, and bilateral papilledema. Results of examination of the heart, lungs, and abdomen and the chest roentgenogram were normal. The ECG showed low T waves in the lateral chest leads; the SUN level was 14.3 mmol/L (40 mg/dL) and the serum creatinine level, 203 μmol/L (2.3 mg/dL). Results of urinalysis were abnormal, showing 3+ proteinuria, numerous red blood cells, and occasional white blood cells.

The patient's symptoms and papilledema cleared with treatment, and he remained asymptomatic. He took three antihypertensive drugs faithfully, but his diastolic blood pressure remained above 120 mm Hg.

Diagnosis: Essential hypertension with a history of hypertensive encephalopathy.

Impairment: 55% impairment of the whole person.

Comment: If the diastolic pressure and renal function had returned to normal but any one of the other findings had persisted, the estimated impairment would have been less.

Example 2: A 62-year-old woman had received treatment for high blood pressure for 10 years. Despite taking drugs and following a restricted salt and weight control diet, she had continued to have elevation of blood pressure. Two years earlier she had developed congestive heart failure, which improved with the use of digitalis and diuretics. Six months ago she had begun to have marked tiredness and breathlessness with ordinary activity, and her ankles remained swollen.

Examination disclosed a comfortable woman with blood pressure of 180/100 mm Hg in the arms and legs. There was edema of the ankles and lower legs. Fundus examination showed increased light reflexes of arterioles with arteriovenous crossing compressions and no hemorrhages or exudates; the disks were flat. The apical impulse was enlarged, sustained, and displaced to the anterior axillary line. The first heart sound was normal, the second heart sound was increased, and there was a fourth heart sound. Rales were heard at both lung bases. There was edema of the ankles and pretibial area.

The ECG showed a deep S wave in V2, but the height of the R waves in V5 and V6 was normal. There were low T waves in I, L, and V4 through V6. The chest roentgenogram showed cardiomegaly and prominence of the pulmonary vasculature in the upper lung fields. The serum electrolyte, SUN, creatinine levels, and results of urinalysis were normal.

Diagnosis: Essential hypertension with congestive heart failure.

Impairment: 80% impairment of the whole person.

6.5 Cardiomyopathies

Cardiomyopathies lead to impairment by causing abnormal ventricular function. Abnormal ventricular function may be the result of (1) systolic dysfunction; (2) diastolic dysfunction; or (3) a combination of both phenomena. A patient with these abnormalities may be asymptomatic, or the abnormalities may lead to pulmonary or systemic organ congestion and decreased cardiac output. Abnormal ventricular function related to coronary heart disease, valvular heart disease, and hypertensive heart disease are considered in other parts of this chapter. Cardiomyopathies may cause arrhythmias, which also are considered elsewhere in this chapter. Some cardiomyopathies are reversible. Every effort should be made to identify the reversible forms and to treat them appropriately over an adequate period of time. When the conditions are stable, they may be evaluated in terms of permanent impairment.

There are many mechanisms by which the cardiomyopathies arise, but the conditions may be divided conveniently into three major types: (1) dilated or congestive; (2) hypertrophic; and (3) restrictive. The disorders can be recognized in most patients by taking careful histories and performing careful physical examinations. In most patients, it is appropriate to supplement these procedures with selected laboratory studies.

Impairment criteria for cardiomyopathies are given in Table 10 (p. 189).

Table 10. Impairment Classification for Cardiomyopathies.

Class 1: **0%-9% impairment of the whole person**	**Class 2:** **10%-29% impairment of the whole person**	**Class 3:** **30%-49% impairment of the whole person**	**Class 4:** **50%-100% impairment of the whole person**
Patient is asymptomatic and there is evidence of impaired left ventricular function from clinical examination or laboratory studies; **and** There is no evidence of congestive heart failure from physical examination or laboratory studies.	Patient is asymptomatic and there is evidence of impaired left ventricular function from physical examination or laboratory studies; **and** Moderate dietary adjustment or drug therapy is necessary for patient to be free of symptoms and signs of congestive heart failure; **or** Patient has recovered from surgery for treatment of hypertrophic cardiomyopathy or has recovered from successful heart transplantation and meets above criteria.	Patient develops symptoms of congestive heart failure on greater than ordinary daily activities (functional class 2) and there is evidence of abnormal ventricular function from physical examination or laboratory studies; **and** Moderate dietary restriction or use of drugs is necessary to minimize patient's symptoms, or to prevent appearance of signs of congestive heart failure or evidence of it by laboratory study; **or** Patient has recovered from surgery for treatment of hypertrophic cardiomyopathy or has recovered from successful heart transplantation and meets above criteria.	Patient is symptomatic during ordinary daily activities despite appropriate use of dietary adjustment and drugs (functional class 3 or 4) and there is evidence of abnormal ventricular function from physical examination or laboratory studies; **or** There are persistent signs of congestive heart failure despite use of dietary adjustment and drugs; **or** Patient has recovered from surgery for treatment of hypertrophic cardiomyopathy or has recovered from successful heart transplantation and meets above criteria.

Criteria for Evaluating Impairment Resulting from Cardiomyopathy

Class 1: Impairment of the Whole Person, 0% to 10%

A patient belongs in class 1 when (1) the patient is asymptomatic, and there is evidence from examination or laboratory tests of impaired left ventricular function; *and* (2) *no* evidence exists of congestive heart failure, including evidence from physical examination and laboratory studies.

Example: One year earlier a 26-year-old woman, a lawyer, had been delivered of a normal infant, but 3 days post partum she developed signs of pulmonary congestion. She was normotensive. There was no evidence of valvular heart disease, and the ECG was within normal limits except for sinus tachycardia. She was treated successfully with digitalis and diuretics. During the next several months, the woman returned to full activities and had no symptoms. Six months ago the treatment with digitalis and diuretics was discontinued. The woman was advised to avoid subsequent pregnancies. She led a normal life, working in her profession and taking care of her family and home.

At examination, the woman had no signs of congestive failure. Blood pressure was 110/70 mm Hg, and pulse was regular at 70 beats per minute. The precordium was quiet, without ventricular heaves. The heart sounds were normal. The ECG was normal. The chest roentgenogram demonstrated slight cardiomegaly without chamber enlargement. Echocardiography showed a slightly enlarged left ventricle with mild global hypokinesis and an ejection fraction of 55%. On exercise testing, the woman was able to achieve 95% of her functional aerobic capacity with ECG changes, but the ejection fraction fell to 50%.

Diagnosis: Postpartum cardiomyopathy.

Impairment: 9% impairment of the whole person.

Comment: If the woman had had symptoms, she would be estimated to have greater impairment. If the heart size were normal, and the ejection fraction were normal at rest and increased on exercise, then the estimate of impairment would be less than 9%.

Class 2: Impairment of the Whole Person, 10% to 30%

A patient belongs in class 2 when (1) the patient is asymptomatic and there is evidence of impaired left ventricular function from physical examination or laboratory studies; *and* (2) moderate dietary adjustment or drug therapy is necessary for the patient to be free of symptoms and signs of congestive heart failure; *or* (3) the patient has recovered from surgery for the treatment of hypertrophic cardiomyopathy or has undergone a successful heart transplantation and meets criteria in (1) and (2) above.

Example 1: A 59-year-old man had consumed excessive amounts of alcohol for many years and also had nutritional deficiencies. He had been admitted to the hospital 1 year earlier with severe pulmonary congestion. A thorough evaluation indicated that the congestion probably was due to left ventricular failure attributable to a combination of excessive alcohol intake and poor nutrition. The man's condition responded promptly to nutritional treatment, digitalis, diuretics, and angiotensin-converting enzyme inhibitors. He learned to avoid alcohol and returned to a fully active life, working as a greenskeeper on a golf course. He was seen regularly by his physician, who elected to continue prescribing angiotensin-converting enzyme inhibitors and moderate salt restriction because of a persistent gallop rhythm.

On examination, the patient appeared comfortable and had no signs of congestive heart failure. Blood pressure was 120/80 mm Hg, and pulse was regular at 70 beats per minute. At the precordium, the apical impulse was larger than normal, slightly sustained, and displaced to the anterior axillary line. There was no parasternal heave. The first and second heart sounds were normal. A third heart sound was present at the apex. The ECG showed small R waves and low T waves in the lateral chest leads. The chest roentgenogram showed moderate cardiomegaly with no specific chamber enlargement. The echocardiogram at rest had an ejection fraction of 40%, and this remained at 40% after exercise. The patient was able to achieve 75% of his functional aerobic capacity on exercise testing. There were no ECG changes during exercise.

Diagnosis: Cardiomyopathy, probably alcoholic and nutritional.

Impairment: 25% impairment of the whole person.

Example: An 18-year-old man, whose father had hypertrophic cardiomyopathy, was examined by his physician and found to have evidence of hypertrophic cardiomyopathy. The patient had no heart-related symptoms and was an active participant in sports.

On examination, the young man appeared healthy and had no evidence of congestive heart failure. Blood pressure was 130/70 mm Hg, and the pulse was regular at 70 beats per minute. Carotid pulses were brisk, and the apical impulse was normal. There was a grade 2/6 midsystolic murmur heard best along the left sternal border and also an S_4 gallop.

The ECG showed prominent Q waves and high voltage. A chest roentgenogram showed a heart of normal size. An echocardiogram showed marked thickening of the ventricular septum and some thickening of the posterior ventricular wall. The mitral valve motion was normal, and the ejection fraction was 80%. There was systolic anterior motion of the mitral valve, and Doppler echocardiography showed a 40-mm Hg gradient across the left ventricular outflow tract. A 48-hour Holter monitor showed no evidence of ventricular tachycardia.

Diagnosis: Hypertrophic cardiomyopathy.

Impairment: 20% impairment of the whole person.

Comment: The patient was advised to avoid strenuous physical exertion, and the importance of follow-up evaluation was stressed. If significant ventricular tachycardia were present on Holter monitoring, antiarrhythmic therapy might be indicated. In this situation, the degree of impairment would be estimated according to the specific criteria for arrhythmias and impairment due to cardiomyopathy, and the impairment percents would be *combined* (Combined Values Chart, p. 322).

Class 3: Impairment of the Whole Person, 30% to 50%

A patient belongs in class 3 when (1) the patient develops symptoms of congestive heart failure with greater than ordinary daily activities (functional class 2) and there is evidence of abnormal ventricular function from physical examination or laboratory studies; *and* (2) moderate dietary restriction or the use of drugs is necessary to minimize the patient's symptoms, or to prevent the appearance of signs of congestive heart failure or evidence of it by laboratory study; *or* (3) the patient has recovered from surgery for the treatment of hypertrophic cardiomyopathy, or has recovered from heart transplantation and meets the criteria described above.

Example: A 54-year-old woman had been treated by her physician for the past 3 years for symptoms of congestive heart failure and inadequate cardiac output. Two years ago she had undergone cardiac catheterization and cineangiography, which demonstrated no evidence of coronary artery or valvular disease. Ventricular function then was poor; the end-diastolic pressure was elevated to 18 mm Hg, and the ejection fraction was 30%. The patient subsequently was treated with angiotensin-converting enzyme inhibitors. During the past year, the patient's condition was stable, and she was able to do kitchen work, go shopping, and drive an automobile. She became breathless on climbing a flight of stairs and preferred to sleep on two pillows.

At examination, the patient's blood pressure was 110/70 mm Hg, and the pulse was regular at 70 beats per minute. There was a markedly enlarged apical impulse, which was sustained and displaced laterally to the anterior axillary line. An early diastolic impulse was palpable after the systolic impulse. The first heart sound was diminished, the second heart sound was normal, and there was a prominent third heart sound.

The ECG showed low T waves in all leads. There was a QS pattern in V1 and V2. The chest roentgenogram showed marked cardiomegaly with some distention of the pulmonary vessels in the upper lobes. Echocardiography showed a moderately dilated left ventricle with an ejection fraction of 30% and an enlarged left atrium.

Diagnosis: Idiopathic cardiomyopathy.

Impairment: 49% impairment of the whole person.

Class 4: Impairment of the Whole Person, 50% to 100%

A patient belongs in class 4 when (1) the patient is symptomatic during ordinary daily activities despite the appropriate use of dietary adjustment and drugs (functional class 3 or 4), and there is evidence of abnormal ventricular function from physical examination or laboratory studies; *or* (2) there are persistent signs of congestive heart failure despite the use of dietary adjustment and drugs; *or* (3) the patient has recovered from surgery for the treatment of hypertrophic cardiomyopathy or has recovered from heart transplantation and meets the above criteria.

Example: A 38-year-old woman had received a diagnosis of hypertrophic cardiomyopathy at age 30 years. For several years she had frequently experienced chest pain, despite the use of beta-adrenergic blocking agents. Nitrates were not effective and seemed to worsen her pain. Because of the angina, the woman had undergone cardiac surgery to remove a large portion of the ventricular septum. After the operation, she had continued to experience angina almost on a daily basis. Many of the episodes occurred at rest, but they also could be provoked by sexual intercourse or running up stairs, despite large doses of beta-blockers. Two months ago she had experienced several syncopal spells after exercising.

Examination showed a patient who was comfortable at rest. Her blood pressure was 140/80 mm Hg, and the pulse was regular at 52 beats per minute. The carotid pulse was quick and "jerky" bilaterally. The lungs were clear. There was no peripheral edema. There was a sustained apical impulse that was moderately enlarged and displaced laterally to the anterior axillary line. A grade 3/6 long, almost holosystolic murmur was heard best at the left mid-precordium and poorly transmitted to the left axilla. The first and second heart sounds were normal, and a fourth heart sound was present.

The ECG showed a sinus rhythm with Q waves in leads I, L, and V3 and low T waves in the lateral chest leads, I, and L. A chest roentgenogram showed moderate cardiomegaly. An exercise ECG showed ST-segment depression on I, L, and V4 through V6 at a heart rate of 75 beats per minute, a low rate because the patient was receiving beta-adrenergic blocking agents. She was limited to achieving 40% of her functional aerobic capacity on the treadmill exertion test. A resting thallium 201 perfusion scan showed the ventricular septum to be thick.

Echocardiography showed a thick ventricular septum and hyperdynamic systolic function. There was a residual 50-mm Hg left ventricular outflow gradient by Doppler echocardiography with severe mitral regurgitation. The left atrium was enlarged.

Diagnosis: Hypertrophic cardiomyopathy, with resection of a portion of the left ventricular septum.

Impairment: 85% to 95% impairment of the whole person.

6.6 Pericardial Heart Disease

Diseases of the pericardium include inflammation (1) associated with systemic illnesses, such as lupus erythematosus; (2) in reaction to mechanical forces, such as trauma or irradiation; (3) with no obvious cause (idiopathic pericarditis); (4) associated with infections caused by viruses or bacteria; (5) after open-heart surgery (postcardiotomy syndrome). The pericardium may also be affected by tumors.

Recurrent pericarditis is a known entity that can lead to disabling episodes of fevers and pleuritic chest pain. Since chest pain itself is nonspecific, evidence of pericarditis must be documented by the presence of a pericardial effusion on echocardiography or laboratory evidence of active inflammation, such as an increase in the erythrocyte sedimentation rate.

The most common pericardial disorder leading to permanent impairment is constrictive pericarditis. Surgical removal of the thickened pericardium may significantly reduce symptoms and improve the overall condition of the patient who has constrictive pericarditis. It is mandatory to allow sufficient time for the patient to recover from a surgical procedure and to have a stable condition before assessing permanent impairment.

While pain and compromise of cardiac function because of tamponade can cause some impairment, they are rare as causes of permanent impairment; however, recurrent episodes of pericarditis with tamponade, or pericardial disease related to tumors, may lead to permanent impairment. It is important to allow adequate time for resolution of an acute illness, generally a period of months, before assessing permanent impairment.

Table 11. Impairment Classification for Pericardial Disease.

Class 1: 0%-9% impairment of the whole person	Class 2: 10%-29% impairment of the whole person	Class 3: 30%-49% impairment of the whole person	Class 4: 50%-100% impairment of the whole person
Patient has no symptoms in performance of ordinary daily activities or moderately heavy physical exertion, but does have evidence from either physical examination or laboratory studies of pericardial heart disease; **and** Continuous treatment is not required, and there are no signs of cardiac enlargement, or of congestion of lungs or other organs; **or** In patient who has had surgical removal of pericardium, there are no adverse consequences of surgical removal and patient meets criteria above.	Patient has no symptoms in performance of ordinary daily activities, but does have evidence from either physical examination or laboratory studies of pericardial heart disease; **and** Moderate dietary adjustment or drugs are required to keep the patient free of symptoms and signs of congestive heart failure; **or** Patient has signs or laboratory evidence of cardiac chamber hypertrophy or dilation; **or** Patient has recovered from surgery to remove pericardium and meets criteria above.	Patient has slight to moderate discomfort in performance of greater than ordinary daily activities (functional class 2) despite dietary or drug therapy, and patient has evidence from physical examination or laboratory studies of pericardial heart disease; **and** Physical signs are present, or there is laboratory evidence of cardiac chamber enlargement, or there is evidence of significant pericardial thickening and calcification; **or** Patient has recovered from surgery to remove pericardium but continues to have the symptoms, signs, and laboratory evidence described above.	Patient has symptoms on performance of ordinary daily activities (functional class 3 or 4) despite using appropriate dietary restrictions or drugs, and evidence from physical examination or laboratory studies of pericardial heart disease; **and** Patient has signs or laboratory evidence of congestion of lungs or other organs; **or** Patient has recovered from surgery to remove the pericardium and continues to have symptoms, signs, and laboratory evidence described above.

Diagnosis of pericardial disease is made by history; identifying a pericardial friction rub or early diastolic pericardial knock; demonstrating pericardial effusion, thickening, or calcification on an echocardiogram, or showing a thickened pericardium with such imaging modalities as computed tomography or magnetic resonance imaging; or findings at cardiac catheterization.

Criteria for evaluating permanent impairments related to pericardial diseases are given in Table 11 (above).

Criteria for Evaluating Impairment Resulting from Pericardial Heart Disease

Class 1: Impairment of the Whole Person, 0% to 10%

A patient belongs in class 1 when (1) the patient has no symptoms in the performance of ordinary daily activities or moderately heavy physical exertion, but does have past or present evidence from physical examination or laboratory studies of pericardial heart disease; *and* (2) continuous treatment is not required, and there are no signs of left ventricular enlargement or dysfunction, or of congestion of the lungs or other organs; *or* (3) in the patient who has had surgical removal of the pericardium, there are no adverse consequences of the removal and the patient meets the criteria above.

Example: A 28-year-old male postal clerk had experienced an acute, self-limited, febrile illness 15 months earlier, associated with anterior chest pain and a pericardial friction rub; the diagnosis was acute pericarditis. The echocardiogram at that time showed a small pericardial effusion. The man's illness resolved with curtailed physical activities and the taking of aspirin for 3 weeks. He then returned to work and led a normal life without symptoms.

Diagnosis: Acute benign idiopathic pericarditis.

Impairment: 0% impairment of the whole person.

Comment: Though it is possible that constrictive pericarditis might develop later, most patients like the one described would experience no long-term disorder contributing to permanent impairment.

Class 2: Impairment of the Whole Person, 10% to 30%

A patient belongs in class 2 when (1) the patient has no symptoms in the performance of ordinary activities but has evidence from either physical examination or laboratory studies of pericardial heart disease; *and* (2) moderate dietary adjustment or drugs are required to keep the patient free of symptoms and signs of congestive heart failure; *or* (3) the patient has signs or laboratory evidence of left ventricular enlargement or dysfunction; *or* (4) the patient has recovered from surgery to remove the pericardium and meets the criteria above.

Example: A 32-year-old woman had experienced an episode of viral pericarditis 1 year earlier with fever and pleuritic pain. An echocardiogram performed at that time demonstrated a moderate-sized, circumferential, pericardial effusion. The erythrocyte sedimentation rate and white blood cell count were elevated, but there was no evidence of bacterial or fungal infection. A pericardial tap was performed, which showed no evidence of bacteria. The autoimmune workup was negative. The woman was treated with nonsteroidal anti-inflammatory agents for 4 weeks and had resolution of symptoms.

During the past year, the woman had several recurrences of chest pain, each time with an effusion on echocardiography and an elevated erythrocyte sedimentation rate. The chest pain was so severe that she could not carry out daily activities. Each time she was treated with nonsteroidal anti-inflammatory drugs for 4-6 weeks. The condition was stable for about 10 months.

An examination showed that the patient was comfortable and had no signs or symptoms of congestive heart failure. The heart sounds were normal without murmurs or extra heart sounds. No pericardial rub was audible.

An ECG showed flat T-wave abnormalities. A chest roentgenogram showed the heart to be of normal size and the lung fields clear. Echocardiography revealed a small residual pericardial effusion.

Diagnosis: Recurrent idiopathic pericarditis.

Impairment: 15% impairment of the whole person. Recurrent episodes may occur. If the episodes become more frequent, long-term administration of medications may be indicated, such as salicylates, nonsteroidal anti-inflammatory drugs, steroids, or colchicine.

Class 3: Impairment of the Whole Person, 30% to 50%

A patient belongs in class 3 when (1) the patient has slight to moderate discomfort in the performance of greater than ordinary daily activities (functional class 2) despite dietary or drug therapy, and the patient has evidence from physical examination or laboratory studies of pericardial heart disease; *and* (2) physical signs are present, or there is laboratory evidence of cardiac chamber enlargement or evidence of significant pericardial thickening and calcification; *or* (3) the patient has recovered from surgery to remove the pericardium but continues to have the symptoms, signs, and laboratory findings described above.

Example: A 45-year-old real estate broker and school teacher had had a pericardiectomy for constrictive pericarditis 10 years earlier and had a good recovery. He continued to have some limitation of activity characterized by weakness and breathlessness on heavy physical exertion, but he worked regularly.

On physical examination, the man's venous pressure was normal, and there was no edema. The blood pressure was normal and the pulse was regular. There were no ventricular heaves, thrills, or taps. The first heart sound was normal, and the second heart sound was diminished. There were no extra sounds or rubs.

The ECG demonstrated low-voltage QRS and T waves in all leads. The chest roentgenogram showed considerable cardiomegaly and some calcification at the posterior aspect of the heart. The lung fields were clear. Echocardiography showed thickening of the pericardium and moderate diminution of right and left ventricular contraction; the left ventricular ejection fraction was 45%.

Diagnosis: Constrictive pericarditis with pericardiectomy.

Impairment: 30% impairment of the whole person.

Comment: If the patient had had more limitation of activities, a level of impairment greater than 30% might have been assigned.

Class 4: Impairment of the Whole Person, 50% to 100%

A patient belongs in class 4 when (1) the patient has symptoms on performance of ordinary daily activities (functional class 3 or 4), despite using appropriate dietary restriction or drugs, and evidence from physical examination or laboratory studies of pericardial heart disease; *and* (2) the patient has signs or laboratory evidence of congestion of the lungs or other organs; *or* (3) the patient has recovered from surgery to remove the pericardium and continues to have the symptoms, signs, and laboratory evidence described above.

Example: One year earlier a 62-year-old man had had profound ascites, peripheral edema, weight loss, and signs of pulmonary congestion that were attributed to constrictive pericarditis. Pericardiectomy relieved the severe ascites and peripheral edema. However, the man continued to have fatigue and breathlessness with ordinary activity and was unable to climb a flight of stairs without resting. He was relatively comfortable when walking on a level surface and doing light household activities.

On examination, the man was comfortable. The neck veins were normal, and there was no peripheral edema or ascites. Evidence of marked weight loss remained. There were no ventricular heaves, thrills, or taps in the precordium. The heart sounds were diminished, and there were no murmurs or extra sounds.

An ECG showed low voltage of the QRS and T waves. The chest roentgenogram showed marked cardiomegaly and some distention of pulmonary vasculature in the upper lobes. The echocardiogram demonstrated reduction of ventricular function and a left ventricular ejection fraction of 40%.

Diagnosis: Constrictive pericarditis with pericardiectomy.

Impairment: 75% impairment of the whole person.

Comment: If the patient had had symptoms with minimal daily activities, or if he had had signs of overt congestion at the time of evaluation, then the degree of impairment might have been as high as 95% to 100%, which is considered to represent total impairment and a near-mortal condition.

6.7 Arrhythmias

Arrhythmias may occur in patients with structurally and functionally normal hearts or in patients with any type of organic heart disease. An arrhythmia is defined as one or more heart beats generated at a site other than the sinus node. An impulse that is generated in the sinus node but is not transmitted normally through the conducting system is considered an arrhythmia of the conduction defect type.

Arrhythmias tend to fluctuate remarkably in the frequency with which they occur. Thus, the arrhythmia must be adequately documented and the frequency with which it occurs must be estimated. The associated symptoms may be different from the symptoms of other forms of heart disease. Arrhythmias may cause syncope, weakness and fatigue, palpitation, dizziness, light-headedness, chest heaviness, or shortness of breath, or combinations of those symptoms.

The degree of impairment from cardiac arrhythmias often will have to be *combined* with the degree of impairment due to an underlying heart disease; this should be done according to the Combined Values Chart (p. 322). After instituting therapy for the arrhythmias, one should allow a prolonged period of time to pass, usually months, for the patient's condition to stabilize before estimating the degree of permanent impairment.

Criteria for evaluating impairments related to arrhythmias are given in Table 12 (p. 195).

Criteria for Evaluating Impairment Resulting from Arrhythmias

Class 1: Impairment of the Whole Person, 0% to 10%
A patient belongs in class 1 when (1) the patient is asymptomatic during ordinary activities and a cardiac arrhythmia is documented by ECG; *and* (2) there is no documentation of three or more consecutive ectopic beats or periods of asystole greater than 2.0 seconds, and both the atrial and ventricular rates are maintained between 50 and 100 beats per minute; *and* (3) there is no evidence of organic heart disease.

Example: A 56-year-old man without symptoms had frequent premature beats during an annual physical examination. The results of the remainder of the examination were normal. An ECG showed frequent premature complexes. The chest roentgenogram was normal.

Diagnosis: Atrial premature complexes.

Impairment: 0% impairment of the whole person.

Class 2: Impairment of the Whole Person, 10% to 30%
A patient belongs in class 2 when (1) the patient is asymptomatic during ordinary daily activities and a cardiac arrhythmia is documented by ECG; *and* (2) moderate dietary adjustment, or the use of drugs or an artificial pacemaker, is required to prevent symptoms related to the cardiac arrhythmia; *or* (3) the arrhythmia persists and there is organic heart disease.

Example 1: An asymptomatic 62-year-old man had atrial fibrillation with an irregular ventricular response of about 85 beats per minute during an examination 1 year earlier. The remainder of the examination results were normal, including ECG, chest roentgenogram, and echocardiogram.

Diagnosis: Atrial fibrillation.

Impairment: 15% impairment of the whole person.

Comment: If it were necessary for the patient to take digitalis to maintain the ventricular response between 50 and 100 beats per minute, the estimated impairment would be slightly greater.

Example 2: A 52-year-old plumber had had recurring syncope 8 months earlier and was treated with insertion of a permanent artificial pacemaker. After treatment, the patient felt well and continued to work.

On examination, the man appeared well and showed no signs of congestive heart failure. His pulse was regular at 72 beats per minute, and blood pressure was 120/80 mm Hg. There were no ventricular heaves, thrills, or taps in the precordium. The heart sounds were of good quality, and there were no murmurs.

The ECG showed complete capture of the heart by the artificial pacemaker, running at 72 beats per minute. A rare premature ventricular beat was sensed by the pacemaker, and the pacemaker was properly inhibited.

Diagnosis: Adams-Stokes attacks in a patient with complete heart block, which was managed with a properly functioning artificial pacemaker.

Impairment: 20% impairment of the whole person.

Class 3: Impairment of the Whole Person, 30% to 50%

A patient belongs in class 3 when (1) the patient has symptoms despite the use of dietary therapy or drugs or of an artificial pacemaker, and a cardiac arrhythmia is documented with ECG; *and* (2) the patient is able to lead an active life, and the symptoms caused by the arrhythmia are limited to infrequent palpitations and episodes of lightheadedness or other symptoms of temporarily inadequate cardiac output.

Example: A 44-year-old airline ground crew member experienced recurrent episodes of a sensation of rapid heart action accompanied by lightheadedness. The episodes lasted 5 to 15 minutes. While vagal-type maneuvers occasionally terminated such episodes, usually the episodes stopped for no obvious reason. During the episodes, the patient felt weak and could not perform any type of physical activity. Usually he would lie down and try breathholding and other maneuvers. He never experienced frank syncope.

The patient underwent Holter monitoring and was found to have atrial tachycardia of 155 beats per minute during one of the symptomatic episodes. The ECG showed typical patterns of the Wolff-Parkinson-White syndrome. The patient was started on a regimen of quinidine sulfate, 300 mg every 6 hours, but he continued to have an occasional episode. After the dose was increased to 400 mg, the patient became free of symptoms. He continued on that regimen for 13 months, at which time his impairment status was evaluated. His stools were loose, but he experienced no abdominal pain.

Table 12. Impairment Classification for Cardiac Arrhythmias.*

Class 1: **0%-9% impairment of the whole person**	**Class 2:** **10%-29% impairment of the whole person**	**Class 3:** **30%-49% impairment of the whole person**	**Class 4:** **50%-100% impairment of the whole person**
Patient is asymptomatic during ordinary activities and a cardiac arrhythmia is documented by ECG; **and** There is no documentation of three or more consecutive ectopic beats or periods of asystole greater than 1.5 seconds, and both atrial and ventricular rates are maintained between 50 and 100 beats per minute; **and** There is no evidence of organic heart disease; **or** Patient has recovered from surgery or a catheter procedure to correct arrhythmia and above critera are met.	Patient is asymptomatic during ordinary daily activities and a cardiac arrhythmia is documented by ECG; **and** Moderate dietary adjustment, or use of drugs, or an artificial pacemaker, is required to prevent symptoms related to the cardiac arrhythmia; **or** Arrhythmia persists and there is organic heart disease; **or** Patient has recovered from surgery or a catheter procedure to correct arrhythmia and meets above criteria for impairment.	Patient has symptoms despite use of dietary therapy or drugs or of an artificial pacemaker, and a cardiac arrhythmia is documented with ECG; **and** Patient is able to lead an active life and symptoms due to arrhythmia are limited to infrequent palpitations and episodes of lightheadedness, or other symptoms of temporarily inadequate cardiac output; **or** Patient has recovered from surgery, a catheter procedure, or implantable cardioverter difibrillator placement to treat arrhythmia and meets above criteria for impairment.	Patient has symptoms due to documented cardiac arrhythmia that are constant and interfere with ordinary daily activities (functional class 3 or 4); **or** Patient has frequent symptoms of inadequate cardiac output documented by ECG to be due to frequent episodes of cardiac arrhythmia; **or** Patient continues to have episodes of syncope that are either due to, or have a high probability of being related to arrhythmia. To fit into this category of impairment, symptoms must be present despite use of dietary therapy, drugs, or artificial pacemakers; **or** Patient has recovered from surgery, a catheter procedure, or implantable cardioverter defibrillator placement to treat arrhythmia and continues to have symptoms causing impairment as outlined above.

*If an arrhythmia is the result of organic heart disease, the arrhythmia should be evaluated separately and its impairment rating should be *combined* with the impairment rating for the organic heart disease using the Combined Values Chart (p. 322).

Diagnosis: Wolff-Parkinson-White syndrome with atrial tachycardia, adequately controlled by quinidine.

Impairment: 30% impairment of the whole person.

Comment: If the patient were to continue to have palpitations, or even a rare episode associated with symptoms of inadequate cerebral perfusion, then the degree of estimated impairment might be as high as 49%.

Class 4: Impairment of the Whole Person, 50% to 100%

A patient belongs in class 4 when (1) the patient has symptoms caused by documented cardiac arrhythmia that are constant and interfere with ordinary daily activities (functional class 3 or 4); *or* (2) the patient has frequent symptoms of inadequate cardiac output documented by ECG and caused by frequent episodes of cardiac arrhythmia; *or* (3) the patient has episodes of syncope that are either due to, or have a high probability of being related to, the arrhythmia. To fit into class 4, the patient's symptoms must be present despite the use of dietary therapy, drugs, or artificial pacemakers.

Example: A 28-year-old mother of three had experienced episodes of rapid heart action for more than 10 years. These were associated with an uncomfortable retrosternal pressure, a fainting sensation, and general weakness. She had had several spells of unconsciousness, during which her husband had had to use cardiopulmonary resuscitation. During all episodes, the tachyarrhythmia ended spontaneously within 30 minutes, and external electrical conversion was not been necessary.

The patient had taken a number of antiarrhythmic medications, and for the past 5 months she had been taking quinidine sulfate, 300 mg every 6 hours; procainamide, 750 mg every 4 hours; and propranolol, 160 mg twice daily. This regimen had controlled the arrhythmia fairly well. Previous use of verapamil had failed to prevent the arrhythmia. The patient continued to have episodes about once a month, none associated with loss of consciousness. She had developed serologic abnormalities characteristic of lupus erythematosus and had occasional swelling of the small joints in the hands, that had responded to low doses of corticosteroids.

A thorough evaluation of the patient's cardiovascular system revealed no evidence of valvular or myocardial disease. An interval ECG showed a normal pattern and rhythym; ECGs taken during the episodes of palpitations showed a rapid regular rhythm at about 200 to 250 beats per minute. Electrophysiologic studies demonstrated no abnormal conduction problems. Ventricular tachycardia was easily induced, its pattern being similar to that recorded during one of the spontaneous episodes.

Diagnosis: Recurrent ventricular tachycardia.

Impairment: 90% impairment of the whole person.

Comment: The degree of impairment would depend on how often the patient had episodes and the nature of the symptoms the episodes produced.

6.8 Vascular Diseases Affecting the Extremities

Permanent impairment resulting from peripheral vascular disorders most commonly results from (1) diseases of the arteries that reduce blood flow and lead to one or more of the following: intermittent claudication, pain at rest, minor trophic changes, ulceration, gangrene, loss of the extremity, and Raynaud's phenomenon; (2) diseases of the veins resulting in one or more of the following: pain, edema, induration, stasis dermatitis, and ulceration; or (3) disorders of the lymphatics, leading to chronic lymphedema that may be complicated by recurrent acute infection.

The causative factors most commonly encountered in patients with arterial disorders are arteriosclerosis, trauma, and inflammatory processes, such as thromboangiitis obliterans. The venous system is most frequently affected by varicose veins, thrombosis, and chronic deep venous insufficiency. Diseases of the lymphatic system that most frequently cause impairment are obstructive lesions of an inflammatory or neoplastic origin.

Noninvasive laboratory studies are valuable in confirming occlusive arterial disease or venous abnormalities of the extremities. An estimate of the functional impairment imposed by occlusive peripheral arterial disease can be made by determining ankle or arm systolic pressure indices before, and 1 minute after, standard exercises, for instance, walking on a treadmill at 2 miles per hour up a 10% grade for 5 minutes, or less strenuous exercising if the patient's symptoms warrant it.

Before the evaluation of impairment, a specific diagnosis of vascular disease should be established. The estimated amount of the impairment depends on the the extent and severity of the lesions rather than on the specific diagnosis.

The criteria for evaluating impairment due to vascular diseases of the upper extremity are found in Table 13 (p. 197), and the criteria for vascular impairments of the lower extremity are found in Table 14 (p. 198).

To change an upper-extremity impairment percent to a whole-person impairment percent, use Table 3, p. 20. To change a lower-extremity impairment percent to a whole-person impairment percent, multiply it by 0.4, as explained in Sec. 3.2 (p. 75).

Table 13. Impairment of the Upper Extremity Due to Peripheral Vascular Disease.

Class 1: **0%-9% impairment of the upper extremity**	**Class 2:** **10%-39% impairment of the upper extremity**	**Class 3:** **40%-69% impairment of the upper extremity**	**Class 4:** **70%-89% impairment of the upper extremity**	**Class 5:** **90%-100% impairment of the upper extremity**
Patient experiences neither intermittent claudication nor pain at rest; **or** Patient experiences only transient edema; **and** On physical examination not more than the following findings are present: loss of pulses; minimal loss of subcutaneous tissue of fingertips; calcification of arteries as detected by radiographic examination; asymptomatic dilation of arteries or of veins, not requiring surgery and not resulting in curtailment of activity; **or** Raynaud's phenomenon that occurs with exposure to temperatures lower than 0°C (32°F) but is readily controlled by medication.	Patient experiences intermittent claudication on severe usage of the upper extremity; **or** There is persistent edema of a moderate degree, controlled by elastic supports; **or** There is vascular damage evidenced by a sign such as a healed, painless stump of an amputated digit showing evidence of persistent vascular disease, or a healed ulcer; **or** Raynaud's phenomenon occurs on exposure to temperatures lower than 4°C (39°F) but is controlled by medication.	Patient experiences intermittent claudication on mild upper extremity usage; **or** There is marked edema that is only partially controlled by elastic supports; **and** There is vascular damage evidenced by a healed amputation of 2 or more digits of 1 extremity, with evidence of persisting vascular disease or superficial ulceration; **or** Raynaud's phenomenon occurs on exposure to temperatures lower than 10°C (50°F), and it is only partially controlled by medication.	Patient experiences intermittent claudication on mild upper extremity usage; **or** There is marked edema that cannot be controlled by elastic supports; **or** There is vascular damage as evidenced by signs such as an amputation at or above a wrist, or amputation of 2 or more digits of both extremities with evidence of persistent vascular disease; or persistent widespread or deep ulceration involving 1 extremity; **or** Raynaud's phenomenon occurs on exposure to temperatures lower than 15°C (59°F), and it is only partially controlled by medication.	Patient experiences severe and constant pain at rest; **or** There is vascular damage evidenced by signs such as amputation at or above the wrists of both extremities, or amputation of all digits of both extremities with evidence of persistent, widespread, or deep ulceration involving both upper extremities; **or** Raynaud's phenomenon occurs on exposure to temperatures lower than 20°C (68°F) and is poorly controlled by medication.

Class 1: Impairment of the Upper Extremity, 0% to 10%

Example: A 25-year-old man who worked as a meat cutter had noted Raynaud's phenomenon of his fingers for the past year. Results of physical examination and laboratory studies were normal. The blanching of his digits occurred only on exposure to cold when the temperature was less than 0°C (32°F) or with extreme emotional stress. The regular use of prazosin, 1 mg twice daily, relieved the problem.

Diagnosis: Raynaud's phenomenon.

Impairment: 0% impairment of the upper extremity.

Class 2: Impairment of the Lower Extremity, 10% to 40%

Example: A 36-year-old man had developed progressive swelling of both lower extremities during the past 8 years; the edema did not recede overnight. During this period he experienced multiple episodes of acute malaise with chills and fever requiring antibiotic therapy for relief. The febrile episodes occurred four to eight times a year.

The man had leg edema that receded incompletely with elevation for 3 days and was incompletely controlled with the regular use of a heavy-duty, fitted leotard. The recurrent febrile episodes were prevented by treatment of the dermatophytosis and monthly injections of a long-acting penicillin.

On examination, the man had firm edema of both legs and feet and of the toes. There was interdigital fissuring, typical of dermatophytosis, bilaterally.

Diagnosis: Lymphedema of both legs secondary to recurring lymphangitis.

Impairment: 20% impairment of the lower extremity.

Comment: The moderate degree of edema is incompletely controlled by the elastic support.

Class 3: Impairment of the Upper Extremity, 40% to 70%

Example: A 45-year-old female homemaker and part-time secretary had had Raynaud's phenomenon as a result of scleroderma for the past 9 years. She had had ulcerations of the tips of her index and ring fingers of both hands, but these healed with conservative measures and the regular use of prazosin, 1 mg three times daily. However, the Raynaud's phenomenon occurred at progressively warmer temperatures and finally occurred on exposure to temperatures lower than 10°C (50°F).

Table 14. Impairment of the Lower Extremity Due to Peripheral Vascular Disease.

Class 1: **0%-9% impairment of the lower extremity**	**Class 2:** **10%-39% impairment of the lower extremity**	**Class 3:** **40%-69% impairment of the lower extremity**	**Class 4:** **70%-89% impairment of the lower extremity**	**Class 5:** **90%-100% impairment of the lower extremity**
Patient experiences neither intermittent claudication nor pain at rest; **or** Patient experiences only transient edema; **and** On physical examination not more than the following findings are present: loss of pulses; minimal loss of subcutaneous tissue; calcification of arteries as detected by radiographic examination; asymptomatic dilation of arteries or of veins, not requiring surgery and not resulting in curtailment of activity.	Patient experiences intermittent claudication on walking at least 100 yards at an average pace; **or** There is persistent edema of a moderate degree, controlled by elastic supports; **or** There is vascular damage evidenced by a sign, such as a that of a healed, painless stump of an amputated digit showing evidence of persistent vascular disease or a healed ulcer.	Patient experiences intermittent claudication on walking as few as 25 yards and no more than 100 yards at average pace; **or** There is marked edema that is only partially controlled by elastic supports; **and** There is vascular damage evidenced by a sign such as healed amputation of two or more digits of one extremity, with evidence of persisting vascular disease or superficial ulceration.	Patient experiences intermittent claudication on walking less than 25 yards, or the patient experiences intermittent pain at rest: **or** Patient has marked edema that cannot be controlled by elastic supports; **or** There is vascular damage as evidenced by signs such as an amputation at or above an ankle, or amputation of two or more digits of two extremities with evidence of persistent vascular disease, or persistent widespread or deep ulceration involving one extremity.	Patient experiences severe and constant pain at rest; **or** There is vascular damage evidenced by signs such as amputation at or above the ankles of two extremities, or amputation of all digits of two or more extremities with evidence of persistent, widespread, or deep ulceration involving two or more extremities.

Diagnosis: Scleroderma with Raynaud's phenomenon and multiple digital ulcerations.

Impairment: 50% impairment of the upper extremity.

Comment: The vasospasm occurs on exposure to temperatures lower than 10°C (50°F), and there is evidence of persistent vascular damage manifested by the multiple digital ulcerations.

Class 4: Impairment of the Lower Extremity, 70% to 90%

Example: A 24-year-old man had experienced recurrent thrombophlebitis in both lower extremities during the past 3 years. One year ago he developed venous stasis ulceration of the right ankle, which required bed rest and later skin grafting to effect healing. When on his feet, he developed marked bilateral leg and ankle edema, despite the use of full-length, fitted elastic stockings. He was treated with long-term oral anticoagulant therapy to prevent further venous thrombosis.

Diagnosis: Recurrent thrombophlebitis with bilateral chronic postphlebitic deep venous insufficiency.

Impairment: 80% impairment of the lower extremity.

Comment: Because of the marked, postphlebitic deep venous insufficiency, venous stasis ulceration occurred, and dependent leg edema is poorly controlled by elastic support.

Class 5: Impairment of the Lower Extremity, 90% to 100%

Example: A 56-year-old insulin-dependent diabetic man had had symptomatic arteriosclerosis obliterans in both lower extremities for the past 9 years. His walking capacity had gradually shortened to less than 25 feet because of calf pain. In addition, during the past few months he had developed painful, nonhealing ulcers of the right great toe and right heel; the pain was particularly severe at night. He had a history of myocardial infarction, and at present he had class III angina pectoris. He also had progressing renal insufficiency with a creatinine level of 407 μmol/L (4.6 mg/dL).

Diagnosis: Arteriosclerosis obliterans with ischemic ulceration and ischemic rest pain in a diabetic man, who also has severe coronary artery disease and moderate renal insufficiency.

Impairment: 95% impairment of the lower extremity.

Comment: The severe occlusive peripheral arterial disease would warrant a procedure to restore pulsatile flow to the right leg. The renal insufficiency makes arteriography hazardous, and the coronary disease markedly increases the surgical risk. A renal transplant may be considered.

References

1. Rahimtoola SH. Perspective on valvular heart disease: an update. *J Am Coll Cardiol.* 1989;14:1-23.

2. Nobuyoshi M, Hamasaki N, Kimura T, et al. Indications, complications, and short-term clinical outcome of percutaneous transvenous mitral commissurotomy. *Circulation.* 1989;80:782-792.

3. Jaffe WM, Roche AHG, Coverdale HA, et al. Clinical evaluation vs. Doppler echocardiography in quantitative assessment of valvular heart disease. *Circulation.* 1988;78:267-275.

4. Centman EM, Braunwald E. Acute MI management in the 1990s. *Hosp Pract.* 1990;25:15-94.

5. Thoreson RW, Ackerman M. Cardiac rehabilitation: basic principles and psychosocial factors. *Rehab Counsel Bull.* 1981;24:223-257.

6. Perloff JK (chairman), et al. Congenital heart disease after childhood: an expanding patient population. Bethesda Conference Report. *J Am Coll Cardiol.* 1991;18:312-342.

7. 1988 Joint National Committee. The 1988 report of the Joint National Committee on Detection, Evaluation and Treatment of High Blood Pressure. *Arch Intern Med.* 1988;148:1023-1038.

8. Engler R, Ray R, Higgins CB, et al. Clinical assessment and follow-up functional capacity in patients with chronic congestive cardiomyopathy. *Am J Cardiol.* 1982;49:1832-1837.

9. Szlachcic J, Massie BM, Kramer BL, et al. Correlates and prognostic implication of exercise capacity in chronic congestive heart failure. *Am J Cardiol.* 1985;55:1037-1042.

10. Goldman L, Hashimoto B, Cook EF et al. Comparative reproducibility and validity of systems for assessing cardiovascular functional class: advantages of a new specific activity scale. *Circulation.* 1981;64:1227-1233.

11. Hatle LK, Appleton CP, Popp RL. Differentiation of constrictive pericarditis and restrictive cardiomyopathy by Doppler echocardiography. *Circulation.* 1989;79:357-370.

12. Cardiac Arrhythmia Suppression Trial (CAST) Investigators. Preliminary report: effect of encainide and flecainide on mortality in a randomized trial of arrhythmia suppression after myocardial infarction. *N Engl J Med.* 1989;321:406-412.

13. Stroke Prevention in Atrial Fibrillation Study. Preliminary report of the Stroke Prevention in Atrial Fibrillation Study. *N Engl J Med.* 1990;322:863-868.

14. Wildus DM, Osterman FA. Evaluation and percutaneous management of atherosclerotic peripheral vascular disease. *JAMA.* 1989;261:3148-3154.

15. Coffman JD. Intermittent claudication: be conservative. *N Engl J Med.* 1991;325:577-578.

16. Aguire FV, Pearson AC, Lewen MK, et al. Usefulness of Doppler echocardiography in the diagnosis of congestive heart failure. *Am J Cardiol.* 1989;63:1098-1102.

17. Nishimura RA, Miller FA, Callahan MJ, et al. Doppler echocardiography: therapy instrumentation, technique, and application. *Mayo Clin Proc.* 1985;60:321-343.

18. Edwards BS. Recent advances in cardiac transplantation. *Curr Opin Cardiol.* 1990;5:295-299.

19. Reed CJ, Yacoub MH. Determinants of left ventricular function one year after cardiac transplantation. *Br Heart J.* 1988;59:397-402.

Chapter 7

The Hematopoietic System

The hematopoietic system deals with red blood cells, white blood cells, platelets, and coagulation proteins, and it includes the immune defense system. Abnormalities may be quantitative, with too few elements being produced, as in aplastic anemia, or too many elements, as in polycythemia; or they may be qualitative, with faulty production, as in congenital hemolytic anemia and hemophilia.

Disorders may be hereditary or acquired. Hereditary defects frequently involve only a single cell line, as with the red blood cells in hereditary spherocytosis, or a single protein, as with factor VIII deficiency in hemophilia. Acquired disorders are more likely to involve several cell lines, as with leukemia, or several proteins, as with disseminated intravascular coagulation. Disorders do not necessarily imply impairment. Rather, impairment depends on the severity of the defect and the mode of clinical expression.

In this chapter, general reference is made to symptoms and to limitations of the patient's daily activities caused by the hematologic abnormality. The limitations fit into one of the following categories:

(1) *none*—there are no symptoms despite laboratory abnormalities, and the usual activities of daily living can be performed;

(2) *minimal*—some signs or symptoms of disease are present, and there is some difficulty in performing the usual activities of daily living;

(3) *moderate*—signs and symptoms of disease are present, and difficulty is experienced in performing the usual activities of daily living, which now require varying amounts of assistance from others; and

(4) *marked*—signs and symptoms of disease are present, and assistance is needed in performing most to all daily activities.

Before using the information in this chapter, the evaluator should read Chapters 1 and 2 and the Glossary, which provide a general discussion of the purpose of the *Guides* and of the situations in which they are useful. Chapters 1 and 2 consider techniques for examining the patient and preparing an evaluation report. The report should include information such as that in the following outline.

A. Medical Evaluation
- History of medical condition(s)
- Results of most recent clinical evaluation
- Assessment of clinical status and statement of further medical plans
- Diagnoses

B. Analysis of Findings
- Impact of medical condition on life activities
- Explanation for concluding that the condition is stable, not amenable to further therapy, and unlikely to change in the next year
- Explanation for concluding that the individual is or is not likely to suffer further impairment by engaging in usual activities
- Explanation for concluding that accommodations or restrictions are or are not warranted

C. Comparison of Analysis with Impairment Criteria
- Description of clinical findings and how these findings relate to specific criteria
- Explanation of each impairment estimate
- Summary of all impairment estimates
- Overall whole-person permanent impairment estimate

7.1 Permanent Impairment Related to Anemia

The effects of chronic anemia on function depend on the degree of compensatory response by the cardiovascular system. The symptoms of anemia include shortness of breath on exertion, lightheadedness, and fatigability. Regardless of the pathogenesis of the anemia, impairment is related to the inability to deliver adequate oxygen to tissues. The heart compensates for the anemia by increasing cardiac output through an increase in heart rate, and there is further compensation through increased extraction of oxygen by the tissues; that is, an increased arteriovenous difference. Therefore, mild anemia with a hemoglobin level of about 100 g/L may be associated with little impairment in a patient who has a normal cardiovascular system.

Greater degrees of anemia may be associated with increasing impairment that leads, in succession, to lack of stamina, fatigue on exertion, fatigue at rest, and even dyspnea at rest. Thus, there are no specific concentrations of hemoglobin that determine impairment in a given patient. Impairment is measured instead in terms of the limitations of cardiovascular response. Because anemia can be treated successfully by transfusion, impairment may be lessened by that measure.

Iron-deficiency anemia and the megaloblastic anemias usually are reversible with proper management and would not be associated with impairment on recovery. An important exception is the patient with combined-system disease, who has neurologic symptoms that become irreversible because proper therapy was given too late. Gait disturbance may render such an individual severely impaired. Such disturbances are considered in the *Guides* chapters on the musculoskeletal and nervous systems. Some hemolytic anemias are reversible by appropriate therapy, such as steroids or splenectomy, which may totally or almost totally eliminate the impairments.

Patients with *sickle cell anemia* often have disabling symptoms, which are related to the sickling of the red blood cells rather than to the anemia per se. Painful crises, which usually last several days and involve the limbs, trunk, or abdomen, may represent an impairment of 10% to 30% if they occur relatively infrequently, for instance, once per month or less often, or an impairment of 30% to 70% if they occur more frequently. Vascular occlusive disease and increased susceptibility to infection may be other sources of moderate to severe impairments.

Persistent hemolytic anemia may cause impairment, the degree of which is related to the severity of the anemia. The same considerations of impairment apply to anemias caused by defective functioning of the bone marrow, that is, aplastic anemia or refractory anemia. Persistent refractory anemia may cause impairment regardless of cause; the degree of impairment is related to the severity of the anemia and the need for transfusions.

Under the best circumstances, that is, with normal survival of transfused red blood cells, the beneficial effects of transfusions last 6 to 8 weeks. In patients with hemolytic anemias caused by serum factors, and in some patients who have received transfusions many times, the survival of transfused cells becomes shortened, and transfusions must be repeated at shorter intervals of 1 to 5 weeks. As hemolysis becomes more severe, impairment increases.

Table 1 provides criteria for estimating permanent impairments resulting from anemia.

Table 1. Criteria for Evaluating Permanent Impairment Related to Anemia.

Symptoms	Hemoglobin level (g/L)	Transfusion requirement	Impairment (%)
None	100 - 120	None	0
Minimal	80 - 100	None	10 - 29
Moderate to marked	50 - 80*	2-3 U every 4-6 wks †	30 - 69
Moderate to marked	50 - 80*	2-3 U every 2 wks †	70 -100

*Level before transfusion.
†Implies hemolysis of transfused blood.

7.2 Permanent Impairment Related to Polycythemia

Polycythemia vera is manifested by elevated hematocrit values, that is, values above 0.52 in men and above 0.49 in women, and by red blood cell volumes above 36 mL/kg in men and 32 mL/kg in women. Normal arterial oxygen tension, an enlarged spleen, slight elevation of the white blood cell and platelet counts, and increased leukocyte alkaline phosphatase are frequently seen.

Myelofibrosis often develops in patients who have had polycythemia for many years; it may also arise spontaneously in patients who have not had a previous hematologic disorder. While some patients remain relatively asymptomatic for several years, others develop disabling symptoms, such as easy fatigability, weakness, weight loss, perspiration, low-grade fever, and a large spleen.

Currently, no therapy exists to relieve the symptoms of myelofibrosis. Transfusions may be needed for severe anemia. Erythrocytosis and increased red blood cell volume may be seen in subjects who do not have true polycythemia but who smoke more than two packs of cigarettes a day; increased carbon monoxide levels are characteristic of this so-called smoker's polycythemia.

7.3 Permanent Impairment Related to White Blood Cell Diseases or Abnormalities

The primary function of the white blood cells (leukocytes) is to provide protection against invading microorganisms, foreign proteins, and other materials. Three separate white blood cell "families" interact to provide this protection. In addition to the cells in the circulation, each white blood cell family has a fixed tissue component that not only provides the renewal or precursor pool, but also functions at fixed sites, such as the bone marrow, spleen, and lymph nodes. The white blood cell families are the granulocytes, lymphocytes, and monocytes-macrophages. Abnormalities in the white blood cells are expressed in terms of both numbers and alterations in function.

Granulocytes

The major function of the granulocytes is to protect against infection through the phagocytosis of invading organisms. Thus, granulocytes function primarily at the site of tissue invasion, and the observation or enumeration of granulocytes in the circulation is in reality a view of traffic to tissues. Survival of granulocytes in the circulation is brief, the half-life being approximately 6 hours. When granulocytes leave the circulation, they generally do not return. The granulocyte precursor pool is in the bone marrow, where a very large production capacity exists.

Granulocyte abnormalities of function are most commonly congenital, although acquired functional abnormalities may result from the use of or exposure to drugs or toxins. Defective granulocyte function is recognized by the occurrence of frequent infections. The evaluation of impairment under such circumstances is based on the type, frequency, and severity of the recurring infections. These may vary from furunculosis, which has no impact on functional capacity, to recurring septicemias. In general, an affected individual will have a reasonably consistent pattern of infection that makes characterization on clinical grounds reliable.

Quantitative granulocyte abnormalities are of two different forms. The first is granulocytopenia. Since granulocytes in the circulation are really in transit to the tissues, large reserves of granulocytes are usually available; significant infections due to low numbers are uncommon, unless the circulating granulocyte count is less than 0.50×10^9/L. In the absence of reversibility, chronic neutropenia with counts below 0.50×10^9/L is associated with substantially increased risk of infection, and impairment is defined in terms of the infection.

The other form of quantitative granulocyte impairment is leukemia. Both acute granulocytic leukemia and chronic granulocytic leukemia result in impaired function of the patient and limited life expectancy, even with currently available therapy. The evaluation of the degree of impairment is based on the presence of symptoms and physical findings, the requirement for and frequency of therapy, and the ability to carry out activities of daily living.

Lymphocytes

The major function of the lymphocytes is to provide humoral and cellular defense mechanisms. The circulating lymphocytes have their origin in lymphoid tissues, that is, the bone marrow, spleen, lymph nodes, and thymus. Two-way traffic between the circulation and these tissues is known. Lymphocytes are cell types with heterogeneous functions.

Of the two major subgroups, the "T," or thymus-derived, lymphocytes are primarily responsible for cellular immunity and are involved in delayed hypersensitivity reactions and with tissue grafts. The

"B," or bursa-derived, lymphocytes are primarily responsible for humoral immunity related to their production of immunoglobulins and biologically active kinins. Each of these subgroups is heterogeneous.

Lymphocyte abnormalities of function and number occur. Acquired defects in function have been identified in Hodgkin's disease, in connective-tissue diseases, and in patients who have been exposed to ionizing radiation. In general, the clinical clue to altered function is the presence of recurrent infections.

Determining failure of end functions, such as generalized deficiencies of immunoglobulins or failure of delayed hypersensitivity reactions, has provided the best documentation of defective lymphocyte function or numbers. The evaluation of impaired function due to lymphopenia must be based on the severity of the impairment as it is signaled by recurrent infection. Finally, it should be emphasized that some diseases that are called "autoimmune" may be due to functionally altered or numerically predominant subsets of lymphocytes.

Abnormalities of lymphocytes are associated with three forms of neoplastic transformation. (1) *Leukemias* include chronic lymphatic leukemia, acute lymphatic leukemia, and hairy cell leukemia. (2) *Lymphomas* include Hodgkin's disease, non-Hodgkin's lymphoma, and mycosis fungoides. (3) *Multiple myeloma and macroglobulinemia* are the third form of neoplastic transformation.

Chronic lymphatic leukemia, hairy cell leukemia, and some so-called low-grade lymphomas may be relatively indolent, require no initial therapy unless severe and irreversible, and constitute no impairment for several years. Similarly, multiple myeloma and macroglobulinemia may be asymptomatic initially and manifested only by certain laboratory abnormalities and constitute no impairment. However, some patients have great impairment because of recurrent gastrointestinal tract bleeding. Impairment in these disorders may be related to developing anemia, the need for chemotherapy or radiation to enlarging lymph nodes or, in the case of multiple myeloma, bone pain. Intestinal bleeding and bone pain are considered in the *Guides* chapters on the digestive system, the musculoskeletal system, and pain.

Infection by the human immunodeficiency virus (HIV) creates a progressive and ultimately fatal disease process with a complex course and widely variable degrees of functional impairment. As the primary cells infected by HIV include circulating and tissue-bound T lymphocytes ($CD4^+$ or T4 cells) and monocytes-macrophages, it is appropriate to consider HIV disease as a primary hematologic disorder. Infection with HIV itself can create symptomatic organ dysfunction resulting in impairment and can also cause impairment as a result of immune deficiency complicated by secondary infectious and malignant disease. Essentially every organ system can be affected by HIV disease, and not uncommonly several systems are affected simultaneously. The degree of impairment is, then, a complex product of the symptoms caused by primary HIV infection, the severity of disease in any single system, and the number of organ systems contributing to the overall disease.

Symptoms of HIV infection include, among others, chronic fever, fatigue, wasting, diarrhea, and dementia. Principal organ systems affected by complications of infection include the pulmonary, hematopoietic, neurologic, renal, and gastrointestinal systems. In addition, many of the drugs used to treat HIV disease and its complications are toxic and commonly contribute to functional impairment.

The overall stage of HIV disease is determined by the peripheral $CD4^+$ cell count. Important milestones are a $CD4^+$ cell count less than $0.50 \times 10^9/L$ (500 cells/mm^3), which indicates the need to initiate antiretroviral therapy; a cell count below $0.20 \times 10^9/L$, indicating an increased risk of opportunistic infection and meeting the definition by the federal Centers for Disease Control (CDC) for acquired immunodeficiency syndrome; and a count below $0.05 \times 10^9/L$, which indicates a risk near death. These milestones are only somewhat useful in assessing impairment. Impairment must be determined after careful consideration of the patient's symptomatic status, which can vary considerably even within one of the $CD4^+$ cell-defined stages.

If several organ systems are involved in the patient's HIV infection process, the whole-person impairment percentages related to the several systems are *combined* by means of the Combined Values Chart (p. 322).

Monocytes-Macrophages

The major function of the monocyte-macrophage family is to ingest foreign proteins, remove cellular debris and particulate material, and modulate immune responses. This functional unit of circulating monocytes and fixed macrophages, called "histiocytes," is structurally associated with endothelial cells and fibroblasts in the reticuloendothelial system. Recognition of this system is based primarily on the phagocytic capacity of monocytes and macrophages.

At present, knowledge about functional defects in the monocyte-macrophage system is limited. The degree of impairment of the system can be correlated with the nature, type, and extent of infection.

A second abnormality of the system is seen in the lipid storage diseases, in which the macrophages become repositories for lipids, and cellular and organ hyperplasia occurs in the spleen, lymph nodes, and bone marrow. Impairment from these disorders depends on the nature of the lipid and the rate of deposition.

Neoplastic transformation of this family occurs primarily as acute monocytic leukemia, a relatively rare form of leukemia. A more chronic variant, leukemic reticuloendotheliosis, is a recently recognized variant. The exact cell of origin is not clear, but the condition behaves as a form of chronic neoplastic transformation.

7.4 The Spleen and Splenectomy

A normal spleen cleanses the blood of bacteria and other foreign matter. Splenectomy removes a quarter of the total lymphoid tissue and the major mass of macrophages. As a consequence of splenectomy, some functional abnormalities may develop. These include impaired clearance of certain encapsulated bacteria, such as the pneumococcus. Occasionally, patients develop overwhelming infections after splenectomy. This occurs in fewer than 2% of patients in whom the organ has been removed and is confined mostly to the first 2 years after the operation. The incidence is greatly reduced by the prophylactic administration of the polyvalent pneumococcal vaccine.

Splenectomy leads to some subtle, albeit clinically silent, morphologic abnormalities of red blood cells and a slight elevation of the platelet count. Splenectomized patients do not have ordinary infections more frequently than normal subjects do.

7.5 Criteria for Evaluating Permanent Impairment of the White Blood Cell Systems

Class 1: Impairment of the Whole Person, 0% to 15%

A patient belongs in class 1 when (1) there are symptoms or signs of leukocyte abnormality; *and* (2) no, or infrequent, treatment is needed; *and* (3) all or most of the activities of daily living can be performed.

Example 1: A 50-year-old man with no previous symptoms was admitted to the hospital after an injury. Routine examination of the blood disclosed a leukocyte count of $18.0 \times 10^9/L$, of which 82% were lymphocytes. Erythrocyte and platelet counts were within normal limits. The physician's diagnosis was leukemia, but no treatment was given. The patient recovered from the injury and resumed normal activities.

Diagnosis: Chronic lymphocytic leukemia.

Impairment: 0% impairment.

Example 2: A healthy 21-year-old man suffered a ruptured spleen in an automobile crash. A splenectomy was performed. The postoperative course was uneventful. Within 2 months the patient returned to his usual daily activities. He was examined for permanent impairment 8 months after hospital discharge.

Diagnosis: Status post splenectomy for splenic rupture.

Impairment: 0% impairment.

Class 2: Impairment of the Whole Person, 15% to 30%

A person belongs in class 2 when (1) there are symptoms and signs of leukocyte abnormality; *and* (2) although continuous treatment is required, most of the activities of daily living can be performed.

Example: A 40-year-old man complained of pain and tightness in the left upper abdominal quadrant and of a 3.6-kg weight loss. He was found to have splenomegaly, the spleen extending 12 cm below the left costal margin, and a leukocyte count of $150.0 \times 10^9/L$, with many myelocytes and progranulocytes. After treatment, the spleen extended below the costal margin only 4 cm, and the leukocyte count fell to the normal range. With daily medication, the patient's condition remained in remission. Periodic adjustment of the dosage according to laboratory data was required. While in remission 6 months after onset of the illness, the patient underwent an impairment evaluation.

Diagnosis: Chronic granulocytic leukemia.

Impairment: 15% impairment of the whole person.

Class 3: Impairment of the Whole Person, 30% to 55%

A patient belongs in class 3 when (1) continuous treatment is required; *and* (2) there is interference with the performance of daily activities, which requires occasional assistance from others.

Example 1: A 55-year-old woman complained of weakness and dyspnea. The patient was found to have a hemoglobin level of 70 g/L, hematocrit of 0.21, leukocyte count of $82.0 \times 10^9/L$, reticulocytes of 13%, and positive Coombs' antiglobulin test. Although the anemia responded well to treatment, during the subsequent year the patient developed progressive cachexia, extreme weight loss, profound weakness, and fever.

Diagnosis: Chronic lymphocytic leukemia with autoimmune hemolytic anemia.

Impairment: 40% impairment due to the leukemia and 0% impairment due to the anemia controlled by therapy, which combine to give a 40% whole-person impairment.

Example 2: A 28-year-old man was found by lymph node biopsy to have Hodgkin's disease. Although he responded at first to treatment with ionizing radiation, recurrence of generalized lymphadenopathy below and above the diaphragm, pruritus, chills, and fever necessitated continuous chemotherapy. He became profoundly weak because of anemia that responded temporarily to drug treatment and transfusions.

Diagnosis: Hodgkin's disease, recurrent, active.

Impairment: 50% impairment from the advanced Hodgkin's disease, which is to be *combined* by means of the Combined Values Chart (p. 322) with an appropriate impairment percentage for anemia to determine the whole-person impairment.

Class 4: Impairment of the Whole Person, 55% to 95%

A patient belongs in class 4 when (1) there are symptoms and signs of leukocyte abnormality; *and* (2) continuous treatment is required; *and* (3) difficulty is experienced in the performance of the activities of daily living, which requires continuous care from others.

Example: A 55-year-old man during a period of 10 months developed profound weakness, chills, night sweats, and fever. He had gingival hypertrophy, nosebleeds, splenomegaly such that the spleen extended 4 cm below the costal margin, and ecchymoses. Hematologic values included a hemoglobin level of 40 g/L, a white blood cell count of 12.0×10^9/L with 80% blast forms, and a platelet count of 18.0×10^9/L. He responded partially to treatment, and when evaluated 6 months later, his condition was relatively stable. However, he required continuous observation, frequent blood transfusions, and continuing assistance with daily activities.

Diagnosis: Acute leukemia.

Impairment: 90% impairment of the whole person.

7.6 Hemorrhagic Disorders and Platelets

Hemorrhagic disorders include coagulation disorders and diseases affecting platelets. Thrombocytopenia does not constitute an impairment, unless it is severe and not reversible by steroids, splenectomy, or other therapeutic regimens. Qualitative platelet defects rarely cause impairment, unless there is serious bleeding. The latter may occur in some of the rare congenital disorders. Von Willebrand's disease is frequently mild, with bleeding occurring only after trauma or surgery; in general, that condition does not constitute an impairment. However, some patients have great impairment because of recurrent gastrointestinal tract bleeding.

Hemorrhagic disorders are either congenital or acquired. In the great majority of hereditary disorders, the basic hemostatic defect remains unchanged throughout the patient's life. Patients with severe hereditary blood coagulation disorders may require prophylactic therapy; this may help them participate in activities, such as bicycling, which they might otherwise have to avoid because of the threat of trauma. Moreover, many patients require frequent home treatment to control bleeding that interferes with their daily activities. Patients with such severe disorders would have 15% to 50% whole-person impairments, depending on the frequency of treatment and the extent of interference with their normal activities.

A patient with an inherited bleeding disorder may develop complications from recurrent hemorrhage, such as joint dysfunction. An impairment from such a complication should be evaluated in accordance with criteria in the *Guides* chapter on the musculoskeletal system (p. 13). If impairments of several organ systems exist, the whole-person impairment percents should be *combined* by means of the Combined Values Chart (p. 322).

Example: A 21-year-old man had severe factor VIII deficiency, or hemophilia A. He frequently had spontaneous bleeding into large joints and muscles, which required home therapy with intravenous factor VIII concentrate two times per week. In addition, because of past joint hemorrhages, he had significant chronic dysfunction of his left knee, right ankle, and both elbows. The frequent joint and muscle hemorrhages and the need for continuous medical treatment interfered with his usual activities.

Diagnosis: Severe hemophilia A with permanent joint dysfunction secondary to recurrent bleeding.

Impairment: 40% impairment for the underlying bleeding disorder, which is to be *combined* by means of the Combined Values Chart (p. 322) with whatever percentages of joint impairment exist.

Persons with autoimmune thrombocytopenia may require long-term immunosuppressive therapy, which in itself can lead to the dysfunction of several organ systems and hamper daily living activities. Complications resulting from the therapy should be evaluated according to the criteria for evaluating impairment of the particular body system or organ affected and *combined* with the impairment percentage for the appropriate blood platelet disorder, by means of the Combined Values Chart (p. 322).

Acquired blood clotting defects are usually secondary to severe underlying conditions, such as chronic liver disease. Patients with venous or arterial thromboembolic disease who receive anticoagulant therapy with a vitamin K antagonist, such as warfarin sodium, need to avoid activities that might lead to trauma. In these patients there might be an estimated 0% to 10% impairment of the whole person.

Example: A 49-year-old woman had chronic idiopathic autoimmune thrombocytopenia of 5 years' duration. She had a splenectomy, and during 4 of the past 5 years she received corticosteroids and other immunosuppressive drugs. At the time of examination, she was not taking any medication, and her platelet count was $30.0 \times 10^9/L$. Except for bruising easily, she had no significant bleeding problem. She had severe osteoporosis and compression fractures of the T12 and L1 vertebrae. These caused her to have chronic low-back pain that interfered significantly with her daily activities.

Diagnosis: Chronic idiopathic autoimmune thrombocytopenic purpura.

Impairment: 0% impairment for the underlying bleeding disorder, which is to be *combined* with whatever percentage of impairment is estimated to arise from the vertebral fractures and osteoporosis.

7.7 Inherited Thrombotic Disorders

Individuals with specific protein deficiencies, for instance, antithrombin III, protein C, or protein S deficiencies, may be at increased risk of developing thrombotic complications. It is estimated that 10% to 20% of young patients who present with venous thrombosis have one of these deficiencies. Lifelong warfarin sodium prophylaxis may be needed and would constitute a slight impairment of 5% to 10%.

References

1. Wyngaarden JB, Smith LH Jr, eds. *Cecil's Textbook of Medicine.* 18th ed. Philadelphia, Pa: WB Saunders Co; 1988.

2. Wilson JD, Braunwald E, Isselbacher KJ, eds. *Harrison's Principles of Internal Medicine.* 12th ed. New York, NY: McGraw-Hill; 1991.

3. Kelley WN. *Textbook of Internal Medicine.* Philadelphia, Pa: JB Lippincott Co; 1989.

4. Rapaport SI. *Introduction to Hematology.* 2nd ed. Philadelphia, Pa: JB Lippincott Co; 1987.

5. Council on Scientific Affairs, American Medical Association. *Information on AIDS for the Practicing Physician.* Chicago, Ill: American Medical Association; 1992.

Chapter 8

The Visual System

The purpose of this chapter is to provide criteria and a method for evaluating permanent impairments of the visual system and relating them to permanent impairment of the whole person. The visual system consists of the eyes, ocular adnexa, and visual pathways.

Visual impairment occurs in the presence of a deviation from normal in one or more of the functions of the eye, which include (1) corrected visual acuity for near and far objects; (2) visual field perception; and (3) ocular motility with diplopia. Evaluation of visual impairment is based on evaluation of the three functions. Although not all of the functions are equally important, vision is imperfect without coordination of all three. Other ocular functions and disturbances are considered to the extent that they affect one or more of the three functions. Impairment percents representing the functions are *combined* (Combined Values Chart, p.322).

If an ocular or adnexal disturbance or deformity interferes with visual function and is not reflected in diminished visual acuity, decreased visual fields, or ocular motility with diplopia, the significance of the disturbance or deformity should be evaluated by the examining physician. In that situation, the physician may *combine* an additional 5% to 10% impairment with the impaired visual function of the involved eye. Abnormalities that might result in such impairments include media opacities, corneal or lens opacities, and abnormalities resulting in such symptoms as epiphora, photophobia, or metamorphopsia.

Permanent deformities of the orbit, such as scars or cosmetic defects that do not alter ocular function, also may be considered to be factors causing whole-person impairments as high as 10%. If facial disfigurement due to scarring above the upper lip is evaluated by means of the chapter in the *Guides* on the ear, nose, throat, and related structures, then any overlapping impairment percentage due to ocular scarring should be subtracted from the greater value.

Equipment

The following equipment is necessary to test the functions of the visual system.

1. *Visual Acuity Test Charts:* For distance vision tests, the Snellen test chart with nonserif block letters or numbers, the illiterate E chart, or Landolt's broken-ring chart are acceptable. For near vision, charts with print similar to that of the Snellen chart, with Revised Jaeger Standard print, or with American point-type notation for use at 35 cm (14 in) are acceptable.

The 10 equally difficult block letters (D, K, R, H, V, C, N, Z, S, and O) of Louise L. Sloan are recommended for testing distance vision. Each letter subtends a visual angle of 5 minutes and a stroke width of 1 minute.

2. *Visual Field Testing:* The standard for testing visual fields is the traditional stimulus III-4e of the Goldmann perimeter. Other acceptable perimeters and stimuli are listed in Table 1 (p. 210). The tangent screen may be used for diplopia testing.

3. *Refraction Equipment:* The necessary equipment consists of a phoropter or a combination of hand-held lenses and a retinoscope.

Table 1. Stimuli Equivalent to the Goldmann Kinetic Stimulus.

	Phakic	Aphakic
Goldmann (kinetic)	III-4e	IV-4e
ARC perimeter (kinetic)	3 mm white at radius 330 mm	6 mm white at radius 330 mm
Allergan-Humphrey (static, size 3)	10 dB	6 dB
Octopus (static, size 3)	7 dB	3 dB

Preparation for Medical Evaluation

Before using the information in this chapter, the reader should become familiar with Chapters 1 and 2 and the Glossary, which discuss the purpose of the *Guides* and the situations in which they are useful and also provide basic definitions. Chapters 1 and 2 discuss the methods for examining patients and preparing reports. A medical evaluation report should include information such as the following.

A. Medical Evaluation

- History of medical condition
- Results of most recent clinical evaluation
- Assessment of current clinical status and statement of further medical plans
- Diagnosis

B. Analysis of Findings

- Impact of medical condition on life activities
- Explanation for concluding that the condition is stable and unlikely to change during the next year
- Explanation for concluding that the individual is or is not likely to suffer further impairment by engaging in ordinary activities
- Explanation for concluding that accommodations or restrictions are or are not warranted

C. Comparison of Analysis with Impairment Criteria

- Description of clinical findings and how these findings relate to specific criteria
- Explanation of each impairment estimate
- Summary of all impairment estimates
- Overall estimate of whole-person impairment

8.1 Central Visual Acuity

Test chart illumination of at least 5 foot-candles is recommended to attain a distinct contrast of 0.85 or greater and a comfortable luminance of approximately 85 ± 5 candelas per square meter. The chart or reflecting surface should not be dirty or discolored. The far test distance simulates infinity at 6 m (20 ft) or at no less than 4 m (13 ft 1 in). The near test distance should be fixed at 35 cm (14 in) in keeping with the Revised Jaeger Standard. Adequate and comfortable illumination must be diffused onto the test card at a level about three times greater than that of usual room illumination. Table 2 (p. 211) shows standards for distance and near visual acuity.

There are no universally accepted standards for contrast and glare sensitivity testing and glare disability testing. Thus, the results of such testing are not incorporated in visual tests of central visual acuity. However, such testing, if it is done with generally accepted methods, may be the basis for an additional impairment of visual function of the involved eye as high as 10%.

Central vision should be measured and recorded for distance and for near objects, without correction and with best corrected conventional spectacle refraction. If a patient is well adapted to contact lenses and wishes to wear them, best corrected vision with contact lenses is acceptable as the basis for estimating impairment. In certain ocular conditions, particularly in the presence of corneal abnormalities, contact lens-corrected vision may be better than that which can be obtained with spectacle correction. If the patient does not already wear contact lenses, it is not necessary to fit a contact lens to determine best corrected visual acuity.

Visual acuity for distance should be recorded in the Snellen notation, using a fraction in which the numerator is the test distance in feet or meters and the denominator is the distance at which the smallest letter discriminated by the patient would subtend 5 minutes of arc and at which an eye with 20/20 vision would see that letter. The fraction notation is one of convenience that does not indicate percentage of visual acuity. A similar Snellen notation using centimeters or inches, or a comparable Revised Jaeger Standard or American point type notation, may be used in designating near visual acuity.

The values shown in Table 2 (p. 211) for distance and near visual acuity and loss were used to develop Table 3. Table 3 (p. 212) combines both types of loss to derive an overall estimate of loss of central vision in an eye. Using Table 3, the examiner identifies the Snellen rating for near vision along the top row and the Snellen rating for distance along the first column. Reading down from the former

Table 2. Visual Acuity Notations with Corresponding Percentages of Loss of Central Vision.

For Distance			
English	**Snellen notations**		**% Loss**
	Metric 6	**Metric 4**	
20/15	6/5	4/3	0
20/20	6/6	4/4	0
20/25	6/7.5	4/5	5
20/30	6/10	4/6	10
20/40	6/12	4/8	15
20/50	6/15	4/10	25
20/60	6/20	4/12	35
20/70	6/22	4/14	40
20/80	6/24	4/16	45
20/100	6/30	4/20	50
20/125	6/38	4/25	60
20/150	6/50	4/30	70
20/200	6/60	4/40	80
20/300	6/90	4/60	85
20/400	6/120	4/80	90
20/800	6/240	4/160	95

For Near				
Near Snellen		**Revised Jaeger Standard**	**American point-type**	**% Loss**
Inches	**Centimeters**			
14/14	35/35	1	3	0
14/18	35/45	2	4	0
14/21	35/53	3	5	5
14/24	35/60	4	6	7
14/28	35/70	5	7	10
14/35	35/88	6	8	50
14/40	35/100	7	9	55
14/45	35/113	8	10	60
14/60	35/150	9	11	80
14/70	35/175	10	12	85
14/80	35/200	11	13	87
14/88	35/220	12	14	90
14/112	35/280	13	21	95
14/140	35/350	14	23	98

and across from the latter, the examiner locates two impairment values for loss of central vision where the column and row cross. It can be seen that each impairment percentage for loss of central vision is the mean of the impairment percentages for the losses of distance acuity and near visual acuity. Tables 2 and 3 were developed in 1955 by the Council on Industrial Health of the American Medical Association.

Monocular aphakia or monocular pseudophakia is considered to be an additional central vision impairment. If either is present, the remaining central vision is decreased by 50%, as shown by Table 3 (p. 212). With monocular pseudophakia, despite a normal Snellen acuity, there is more light scattering and a greater likelihood of glare, diminished contrast sensitivity, and spherical aberration than with a normal phakic eye. Also, capsular opacification, lens decentralization with visualization of the lens edge or positioning hole, or pupillary abnormalities may occur, and there is total loss of accomodation. For these reasons an initial 50% impairment in the central visual acuity of the pseudophakic eye is allowed, with which the observed impairment for loss of central vision is *combined* (Combined Values Chart, p. 322, and Table 3, p. 212).

Determining the Loss of Central Vision in One Eye
First, measure and record the best central visual acuity for distance and the best acuity for near vision, with and without conventional corrective spectacles or contact lenses.

Then consult Table 3 (p. 212) to derive the overall loss, combining the values for best corrected near and distance acuities. Allow, if indicated, for the additional loss of central vision that results from monocular aphakia or pseudophakia.

Example: A 55-year-old man's Snellen rating for distance vision of the left eye was 20/30, and the rating for near vision of the same eye was 14/24. The man's native lens was present. Table 3 (p. 212) indicates that the loss of central vision of the eye was 9%.

8.2 Visual Fields

While central visual acuity represents the ability to discern fine details, visual field acuity represents visual ability over a wider breadth of view while the subject is looking straight ahead. There are two elements to the visual field evaluation. One is the peripheral-most location at which a standard object can be detected. The other is the quality of visual functioning at every point within the field of view.

For the purpose of evaluating impairment in a standard fashion, a patient's visual field is evaluated as the ability to see a standard stimulus, either in terms of the peripheral-most extent along eight meridians at which the stimulus is seen (method 1) or in terms of the proportion of a predefined region in which the standard stimulus is or is not visible (method 2).

With either method, tests that have been performed for medical diagnosis may be used for calculation of impairment or to determine that a certain level of impairment has been exceeded. Sometimes, however, the available test results are not adequate for this purpose, so a specific examination must be done to allow determination of impairment. Figure 1 (p. 213) shows a type of chart that is used to measure visual fields.

The traditional standard stimulus is the III-4e kinetic stimulus of the Goldmann perimeter. The IV-4e stimulus should be used in aphakic patients without a lens implant or contact lens. The equivalent stimuli with other instruments are given in Table 1 (p. 210).

Table 3. Loss (in %) of Central Vision* in a Single Eye.

Snellen rating for distance in feet	Approximate Snellen rating for near in inches													
	14/14	14/18	14/21	14/24	14/28	14/35	14/40	14/45	14/60	14/70	14/80	14/88	14/112	14/140
20/15	0	0	3	4	5	25	27	30	40	43	44	45	48	49
	50	50	52	52	53	63	64	65	70	72	72	73	74	75
20/20	0	0	3	4	5	25	27	30	40	43	44	46	48	49
	50	50	52	52	53	63	64	65	70	72	72	73	74	75
20/25	3	3	5	6	8	28	30	33	43	45	46	48	50	52
	52	52	53	53	54	64	65	67	72	73	73	74	75	76
20/30	5	5	8	9	10	30	32	35	45	48	49	50	53	54
	53	53	54	54	55	65	66	68	73	74	74	75	76	77
20/40	8	8	10	11	13	33	35	38	48	50	51	53	55	57
	54	54	55	56	57	67	68	69	74	75	76	77	78	79
20/50	13	13	15	16	18	38	40	43	53	55	56	58	60	62
	57	57	58	58	59	69	70	72	77	78	78	79	80	81
20/60	16	16	18	20	22	41	44	46	56	59	60	61	64	65
	58	58	59	60	61	70	72	73	78	79	80	81	82	83
20/70	18	18	21	22	23	43	46	48	58	61	62	63	66	67
	59	59	61	61	62	72	73	74	79	81	81	82	83	84
20/80	20	20	23	24	25	45	47	50	60	63	64	65	68	69
	60	60	62	62	63	73	74	75	80	82	82	83	84	85
20/100	25	25	28	29	30	50	52	55	65	68	69	70	73	74
	63	63	64	64	65	75	76	78	83	84	84	85	87	87
20/125	30	30	33	34	35	55	57	60	70	73	74	75	78	79
	65	65	67	67	68	78	79	80	85	87	87	88	89	90
20/150	34	34	37	38	39	59	61	64	74	77	78	79	82	83
	67	67	68	69	70	80	81	82	87	88	89	90	91	92
20/200	40	40	43	44	45	65	67	70	80	83	84	85	88	89
	70	70	72	72	73	83	84	85	90	91	92	93	94	95
20/300	43	43	45	46	48	68	70	73	83	85	86	88	90	92
	72	72	73	73	74	84	85	87	91	93	93	94	95	96
20/400	45	45	48	49	50	70	72	75	85	88	89	90	93	94
	73	73	74	74	75	85	86	88	93	94	94	95	97	97
20/800	48	48	50	51	53	73	75	78	88	90	91	93	95	97
	74	74	75	76	77	87	88	89	94	95	96	97	98	99

*Upper number shows % loss of central vision without allowance for monocular aphakia or monocular pseudophakia; lower number shows % loss of central vision with allowance for monocular aphakia or monocular pseudophakia.

Determining Loss of Monocular Visual Fields

In method 1 of measuring the visual field, the peripheral-most extent over which the static stimulus is seen is noted in each of eight principal meridians. The normal extent of these meridians is given in Table 4 (at right); the total extent summed over eight meridians is 500. To calculate the percentage of retained vision, one adds the extent of the visual field along each of the eight meridians, considering the maximum normal values for the meridians given in Table 4, then divides by 5 to determine the percentage of visual field perception that remains. One must subtract the percentage of visual field remaining from 100% to obtain the percentage of visual field lost.

Table 4. Normal Visual Fields for Eight Principal Meridians.

Direction of vision	Degrees of field
Temporally	85
Down temporally	85
Direct down	65
Down nasally	50
Nasally	60
Up nasally	55
Direct up	45
Up temporally	55
Total	500

Figure 1. Example of Perimetric Charts Used to Plot Extent or Outline of Visual Field Along Eight Principal Meridians Separated by 45° Intervals.

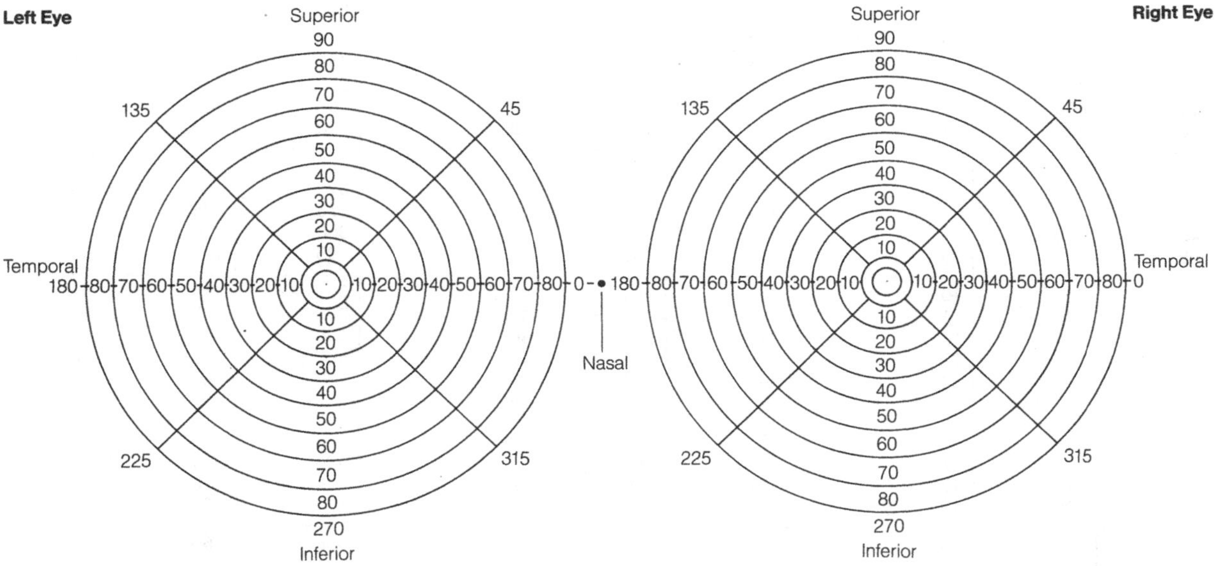

Table 5 (p. 214) tabulates the losses of monocular visual fields calculated by this method.

If the boundary of the visual field coincides with a principal meridian, as in hemianopia or nasal step, the value used for that meridian is the midpoint. Thus, in a hemianopic patient in whom the vertical meridian is split by the III-4e isopter from the point of fixation (0°) up to 40°, that meridian is given a value of 20°. In the case of a nasal step extending from 30° to 60° with the standard stimulus, a value of 45° is used for the nasal meridian.

If a meridian passes through a scotoma, the width of the scotoma is subtracted from the maximum number of degrees for that meridian. The visual field loss in each eye is increased by 5% for an inferior quadrant loss and by 10% for an inferior hemianopic loss, because major loss of a visual field below has more of a functional consequence than an equivalent field loss above. The increase of 5% or 10% is *added* to the percentage representing the visual field loss.

In method 2, an Esterman grid is used (Figs. 2A and 2B, p. 215). The extent over which the standard stimulus is seen or not seen in an ordinary monocular field test is transferred onto the Esterman 100 unit monocular grid. A simple count of the number of dots seen within the field among the 100 dots that are in the grid gives the percentage of retained vision. A count of the number of dots *not* seen gives the percentage lost. The Esterman grid is available from the American Academy of Ophthalmology, 655 Beech St., P.O. Box 7424, San Francisco, CA 94120-7424.

When it is available, a binocular field test performed with both eyes open and the chin in the middle of the instrument is preferred if method 2 is to be used, except for patients with one eye or those with a strabismic deviation of one eye (heterotropia). The binocular field result is determined by using the Esterman 120-unit binocular grid, and the dot count is multiplied by 5/6 to obtain the percentage of retained or lost field.

Some automated machines can perform a test of one or two eyes with a method corresponding to method 2, presenting the standard stimulus at the 100 or 120 prescribed locations and recording the result.

If a medical test of visual fields is already available, it may or may not be valid for determining visual impairment. Kinetic visual field tests should not be used if the standard stimulus was not among those plotted. An exception may occur if a stimulus stronger than the standard was plotted and the field is quite restricted. The loss is gauged by calculating the percentage of loss with the stronger stimulus; then it is certain that the percentage loss with the standard stimulus would be greater.

Another way of using a previously determined diagnostic field occurs if it covers only part of the maximum visual field, for example, only the central 30°. Methods 1 and 2 will yield the desired percentage calculation only if the patient can visualize the standard stimulus within the tested region. Thus, if the

Table 5. Loss of Monocular Visual Field.

Total degrees Lost	Total degrees Retained	% of Loss
0	500*	0
5	495	1
10	490	2
15	485	3
20	480	4
25	475	5
30	470	6
35	465	7
40	460	8
45	455	9
50	450	10
55	445	11
60	440	12
65	435	13
70	430	14
75	425	15
80	420	16
85	415	17
90	410	18
95	405	19
100	400	20
105	395	21
110	390	22
115	385	23
120	380	24
125	375	25
130	370	26
135	365	27
140	360	28
145	355	29
150	350	30
155	345	31
160	340	32
165	335	33
170	330	34
175	325	35
180	320	36
185	315	37
190	310	38
195	305	39
200	300	40
205	295	41
210	290	42
215	285	43
220	280	44
225	275	45
230	270	46
235	265	47
240	260	48
245	255	49
250	250	50
255	245	51
260	240	52
265	235	53
270	230	54
275	225	55
280	220	56
285	215	57
290	210	58
295	205	59
300	200	60
305	195	61
310	190	62
315	185	63
320	180	64
325	175	65
330	170	66
335	165	67
340	160	68
345	155	69
350	150	70
355	145	71
360	140	72
365	135	73
370	130	74
375	125	75
380	120	76
385	115	77
390	110	78
395	105	79
400	100	80
405	95	81
410	90	82
415	85	83
420	80	84
425	75	85
430	70	86
435	65	87
440	60	88
445	55	89
450	50	90
455	45	91
460	40	92
465	35	93
470	30	94
475	25	95
480	20	96
485	15	97
490	10	98
495	5	99
500	0	100

*Or more.

10-decibel (dB) stimulus of the Allergan-Humphrey instrument is seen only inside 15° along all eight meridians but is not seen outside 15°, in considering the 20° or 30° field one may calculate that the retained vision is 24% (15° x 8/5). However, if the 10-dB stimulus is seen out to the edge of the 30° field along each meridian and for an unknown extent beyond, one cannot calculate the percentage of retained vision or visual loss. In such an instance, one can document the loss only if the visual field examination covers a larger field.

If an automated central field examination is normal, it is acceptable as documentation that the entire field is normal, if the ocular history and examination do not suggest lesions that would affect the outer extent of the field.

Figure 2A. Esterman 120-unit *Binocular* Scoring Grid* for Use with Both Eyes Open.

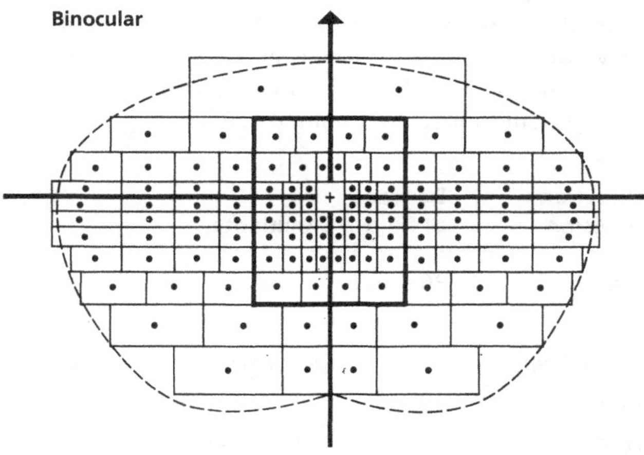

Figure 2B. Esterman 100-unit *Monocular* Scoring Grid* for Arc and Bowl Perimeter or Similar Automated Instrument Providing Full Monocular Field Analysis.

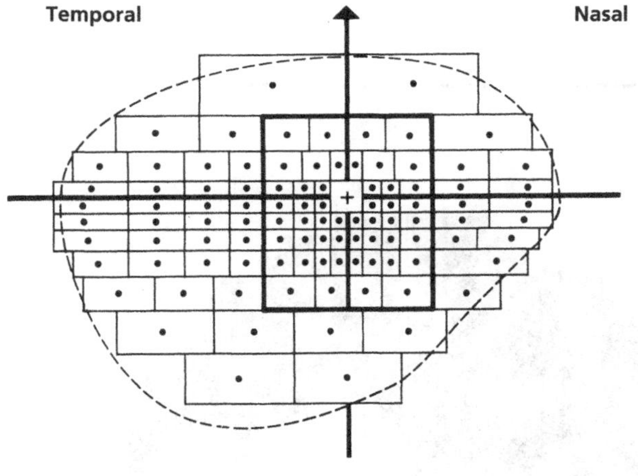

*Grids may be obtained from the American Academy of Ophthalmology, 655 Beech St., San Francisco, CA 94120-7424.

Examples of determining visual field impairments follow.

Example 1: Determine the visual field impairment and percentage of retained visual field in Field 1, right eye (below) using method 1.

Direction of vision	Degrees of field	Comments
Temporally	77	
Down temporally	84	
Direct down	55	65° maximum from table, minus 10° of scotoma between 15° and 25°
Down nasally	50	Not 55°, because maximum from table is 50°
Nasally	37	Midway between 22° and 52°
Up nasally	15	
Direct up	10	
Up temporally	33	40° peripheral extent, minus 7° excluded by isopter between 10° and 17°
Total	361	361 divided by 5 = 72

Thus, the retained visual field is 72%, and the impairment is 28%.

Field 1.

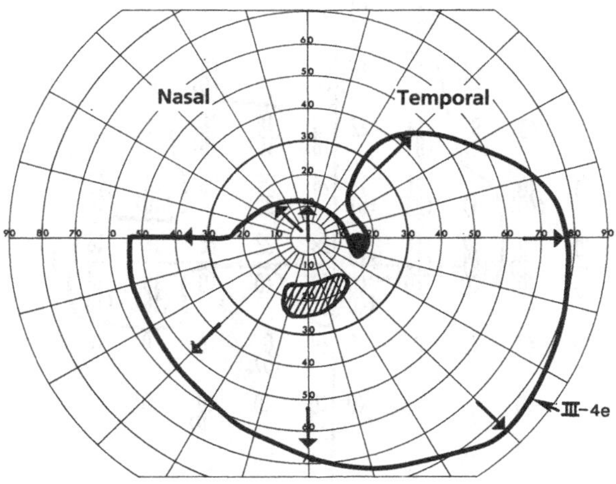

Example 2: Determine the percentage of field loss in Field 2, left eye (below) using method 2.

Solution: Twenty-seven of the dots are excluded by the standard isopter. This is considered to be a 27% visual field loss, with 73% of the visual field retained.

Field 2

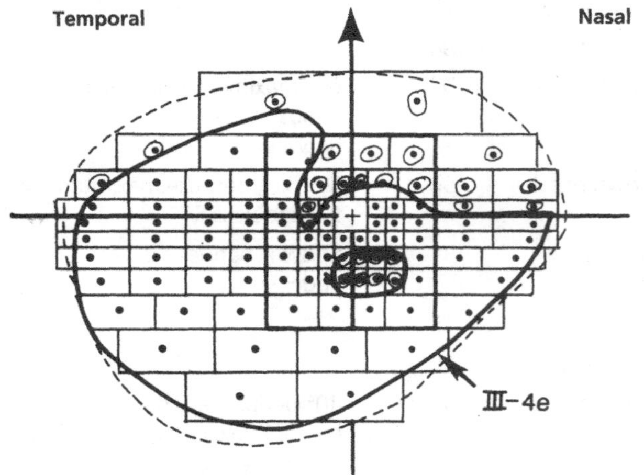

Example 3: Calculate the visual field using Method 1 and the diagnostic results shown in Field 3, right eye (below).

A line is drawn around the location where visibility is better than 10 dB, the standard stimulus for the Humphrey Visual Field Analyzer. Although the field may extend slightly beyond the 30° edge of the tested region, it is obvious that the field is quite restricted. The eight meridians are summed as follows.

Direction of vision	Degrees of field	Comments
Temporally	30	
Down temporally	5	
Direct down	3	Midpoint between 6 and 0°
Down nasally	0	
Nasally	8	Midpoint between 15 and 0°
Up nasally	15	
Direct up	17.5	
Up temporally	20	
Total	98.5	98.5 divided by 5 = 19.7, or about 20%

Thus, the patient retains 20% of the visual field and has an 80% loss.

Field 3

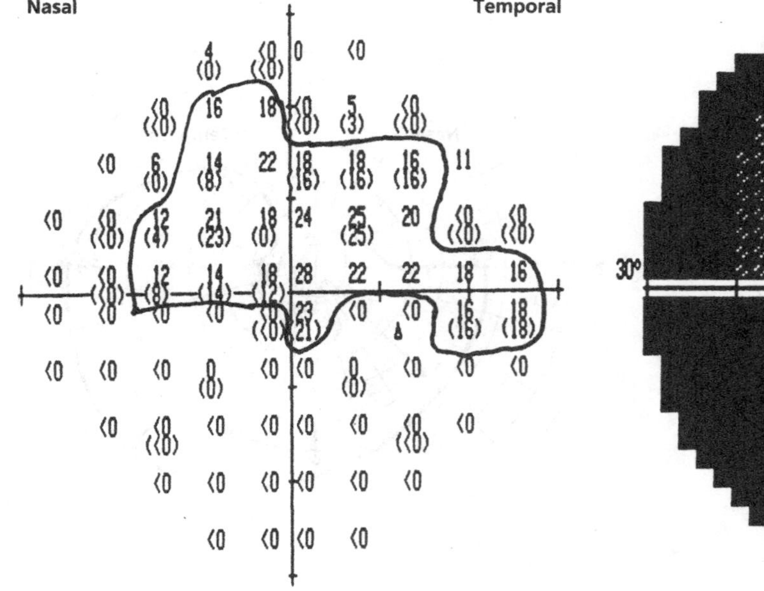

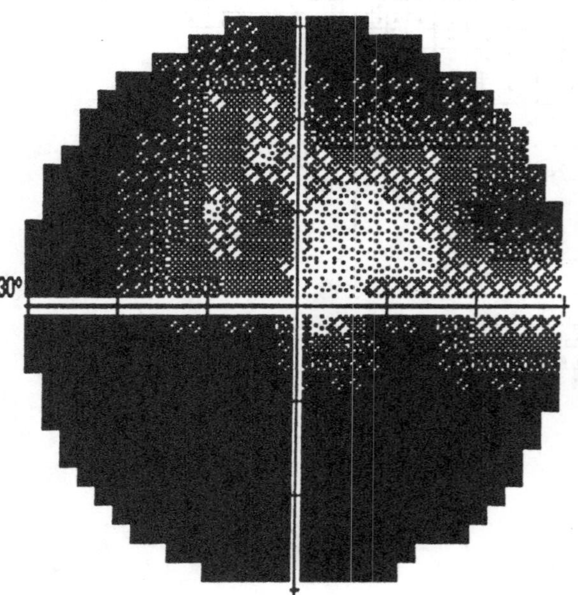

8.3 Abnormal Ocular Motility and Binocular Diplopia

Unless a patient has diplopia within 30° of the center of fixation, the diplopia rarely causes significant visual impairment. An exception is diplopia on looking downward. The extent of diplopia in the various directions of gaze is determined on an arc perimeter at 33 cm or with a bowl perimeter. A tangent screen also is acceptable for evaluating the central 30°. Examination is made in each of the eight major meridians by using a small test light or the projected light of approximately Goldmann III-4e without adding colored lenses or correcting prisms.

To determine the impairment of ocular motility, the patient is seated with both eyes open and the chin resting in the chin rest and centered so that the eyes are equidistant from the sides of the central fixation target.

The presence of diplopia is then plotted along the eight meridians of a suitable visual field chart (Fig. 1, p. 213). The impairment percentage for loss of ocular motility due to diplopia in the meridian of maximum impairment, according to Fig. 3 (below), is *combined* with any other visual impairment (Combined Values Chart, p. 322).

Example 1: Diplopia within the central 20° is estimated to be a 100% impairment of ocular motility (Fig. 3, below). This is equivalent to the total loss of vision of one eye, which is estimated to be a 25% impairment of the visual system and a 24% whole-person impairment (Table 6, p. 218).

Figure 3. Percentage Loss of Ocular Motility of One Eye in Diplopia Fields.

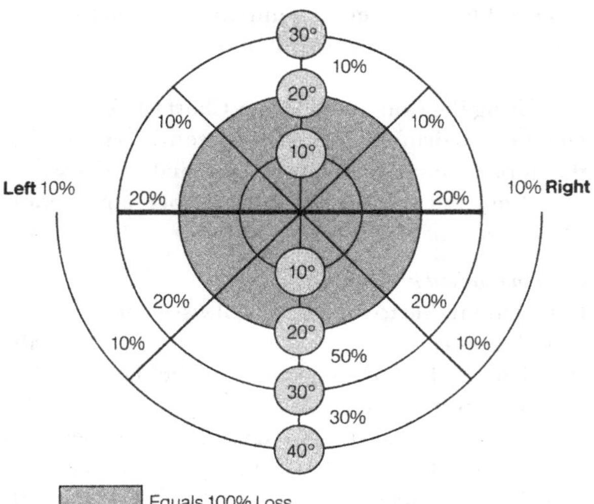

Example 2: Diplopia on looking horizontally off center from 20° to 30° is equivalent to 20% loss of ocular motility. Diplopia of the same eye when looking diagonally from 30° to 40° is equivalent to 10% loss of ocular motility. The impairments from diplopia are added, and the total loss of ocular motility is 30%.

8.4 Steps in Determining Impairment of the Visual System and of the Whole Person

Step 1: Determine and record the percentage loss of central vision for each eye separately, combining the losses of near and distance vision.

Step 2: Determine and record the percentage loss of visual field for each eye separately (monocular) or for both eyes together (binocular).

Step 3: Determine and record the percentage loss of ocular motility.

Procedure with Monocular Visual Fields Test

If the percentage loss of visual field is calculated for each eye separately (monocular), *combine* (Combined Values Chart, p. 322) the percentage loss of central vision with the percentage loss of visual field in each eye and record the values.

Example 1:

Right Eye

Loss of central vision
(both near and distance) 56%
Loss of visual field 32%
56% *combined* with 32%
(Combined Values Chart, p. 322) 70%
Thus, the estimated impairment of the right eye is 70%.

Left Eye

Loss of central vision
(both near and distance) 46%
Loss of visual field 32%
46% *combined* with 32%
(Combined Values Chart, p. 322) 63%
Estimated impairment of the left eye is 63%.

Again using the Combined Values Chart (p. 322), *combine* the percentage for impairment of ocular motility with the combined value for central vision and visual field in the eye manifesting the greater impairment, the right eye in example 1. Disregard the loss of ocular motility in the other eye.

Table 6. Impairment of the Visual System as It Relates to Impairment of the Whole Person.

% Impairment of the											
Visual system	**Whole person**	**Visual system**	**Whole person**	**Visual system**	**Whole person**	**Visual system**	**Whole person**	**Visual system**	**Whole person**	**Visual system**	**Whole person**
0	0	15	14	30	28	45	42	60	57	75	71
1	1	16	15	31	29	46	43	61	58	76	72
2	2	17	16	32	30	47	44	62	59	77	73
3	3	18	17	33	31	48	45	63	59	78	74
4	4	19	18	34	32	49	46	64	60	79	75
5	5	20	19	35	33	50	47	65	61	80	76
6	6	21	20	36	34	51	48	66	62	81	76
7	7	22	21	37	35	52	49	67	63	82	77
8	8	23	22	38	36	53	50	68	64	83	78
9	8	24	23	39	37	54	51	69	65	84	79
10	9	25	24	40	38	55	52	70	66	85	80
11	10	26	25	41	39	56	53	71	67	86	81
12	11	27	25	42	40	57	54	72	68	87	82
13	12	28	26	43	41	58	55	73	69	88	83
14	13	29	27	44	42	59	56	74	70	89	84
										90-100	85

	% Impairment of the	
	Visual system	**Whole person**
Total loss of vision of one eye	25	24
Total loss of vision of both eyes	100	85

Example 2:
In the patient described above, the eye with the greater motility loss has a 25% motility impairment.

Right Eye
Impairment of central vision and visual field 70%
Loss of ocular motility 25%
70% *combined* with 25%
(Combined Values Chart, p. 322) 78%

The examiner may *combine* as much as a 10% impairment for an ocular abnormality or dysfunction that he or she believes is not adequately reflected in the visual acuity, visual fields, or diplopia testing (Combined Values Chart, p. 322). In the above example, an impairment of 78% combined with a 10% impairment would result in a visual impairment of the right eye of 80%.

Step 4: After determining the level of impairment of each eye, use Table 7 (p. 219) to determine visual system impairment. In the above example, considering impairments of 80% and 63%, impairment of the visual system is seen from Table 7 to be 67%.

Step 5: Consult Table 6 (above) to ascertain the impairment of the whole person that is contributed by impairment of the visual system. A 67% impairment of the patient's visual system, as shown in the example above, is equivalent to a 63% impairment of the whole person (Table 6).

Procedure with Binocular Esterman Field Test
If the percentage loss of visual fields is determined for both eyes together by means of the Esterman binocular grid, consult Table 7 (p. 219) to ascertain the impairment of the visual system due to loss of central vision.

Example 3:
Right Eye
Loss of central vision for both near and distance is 56%
Left Eye
Loss of central vision for both near and distance is 46%
From Table 7 it is seen that impairment due to the loss of central vision of both eyes is 49%

Using the Combined Values Chart (p. 322), *combine* the impairment due to loss of central vision with the impairment due to binocular visual field loss.

Binocular visual field testing is not recommended when loss of ocular motility is present.

With the patient in example 3:
Impairment due to loss of central vision of both eyes is 49%
Impairment due to binocular visual field loss is determined to be 20%
Combine the central vision and visual field losses (Combined Values Chart); the impairment of the visual system is 59%

Table 7. Visual System Impairment for Both Eyes.

The values in this table are based on the following formula:

$$\frac{3 \times \text{impairment value of better eye} + \text{impairment value of worse eye}}{4} = \text{impairment of visual system}$$

The guides to the table are percentage impairment values for each eye. The percentage for the worse eye is read at the side of the table. The percentage for the better eye is read at the bottom of the table. At the intersection of the column for the worse eye and the column for the better eye is the impairment of visual system value.

For example, when there is 60% impairment of one eye and 30% impairment of the other eye, read down the side of the table until you come to the larger value (60%). Then follow across the row until it is intersected by the column designated by 30% at the bottom of the page. At the intersection of these two columns is printed the number 38. This number (38) represents the percentage impairment of the visual system when there is 60% impairment of one eye and 30% impairment of the other eye.

If bilateral aphakia is present and corrected central vision has been used in evaluation, impairment of the visual system is weighted by an additional 25% decrease in the value of the remaining corrected vision. For example, a 38% impairment (62% remaining) would be increased to 38% + (25%) (62%) = 54%.

% Impairment worse eye	0	1	2	3	4	5	6	7	8	9	10	11	12	13	14	15	16	17	18	19	20	21	22	23	24	25	26	27	28	29	30	31	32	33	34	35	36	37	38	39	40	41	42	43	44	45	46	47	48	49
0	0																																																	
1	0	1																																																
2	1	1	2																																															
3	1	2	2	3																																														
4	1	2	3	3	4																																													
5	1	2	3	4	4	5																																												
6	2	2	3	4	5	5	6																																											
7	2	3	3	4	5	6	6	7																																										
8	2	3	4	4	5	6	7	7	8																																									
9	2	3	4	5	5	6	7	8	8	9																																								
10	3	3	4	5	6	6	7	8	9	9	10																																							
11	3	4	4	5	6	7	7	8	9	10	10	11																																						
12	3	4	5	5	6	7	8	8	9	10	11	11	12																																					
13	3	4	5	6	6	7	8	9	9	10	11	12	12	13																																				
14	4	4	5	6	7	7	8	9	10	10	11	12	13	13	14																																			
15	4	5	5	6	7	8	8	9	10	11	11	12	13	14	14	15																																		
16	4	5	6	6	7	8	9	9	10	11	12	12	13	14	15	15	16																																	
17	4	5	6	7	7	8	9	10	10	11	12	13	13	14	15	16	16	17																																
18	5	5	6	7	8	8	9	10	11	11	12	13	14	14	15	16	17	17	18																															
19	5	6	6	7	8	9	9	10	11	12	12	13	14	15	15	16	17	18	18	19																														
20	5	6	7	7	8	9	10	10	11	12	13	13	14	15	16	16	17	18	19	19	20																													
21	5	6	7	8	8	9	10	11	11	12	13	14	14	15	16	17	17	18	19	20	20	21																												
22	6	6	7	8	9	9	10	11	12	12	13	14	15	15	16	17	18	18	19	20	21	21	22																											
23	6	7	7	8	9	10	10	11	12	13	13	14	15	16	16	17	18	19	19	20	21	22	22	23																										
24	6	7	8	8	9	10	11	11	12	13	14	14	15	16	17	17	18	19	20	20	21	22	23	23	24																									
25	6	7	8	9	9	10	11	12	12	13	14	15	15	16	17	18	18	19	20	21	21	22	23	24	24	25																								
26	7	7	8	9	10	10	11	12	13	13	14	15	16	16	17	18	19	19	20	21	22	22	23	24	25	25	26																							
27	7	8	8	9	10	11	11	12	13	14	14	15	16	17	17	18	19	20	20	21	22	23	23	24	25	26	26	27																						
28	7	8	9	9	10	11	12	12	13	14	15	15	16	17	18	18	19	20	21	21	22	23	24	24	25	26	27	27	28																					
29	7	8	9	10	10	11	12	13	13	14	15	16	16	17	18	19	19	20	21	22	22	23	24	25	25	26	27	28	28	29																				
30	8	8	9	10	11	11	12	13	14	14	15	16	17	17	18	19	20	20	21	22	23	23	24	25	26	26	27	28	29	29	30																			
31	8	9	9	10	11	12	12	13	14	15	15	16	17	18	18	19	20	21	21	22	23	24	24	25	26	27	27	28	29	30	30	31																		
32	8	9	10	10	11	12	13	13	14	15	16	16	17	18	19	19	20	21	22	22	23	24	25	25	26	27	28	28	29	30	31	31	32																	
33	8	9	10	11	11	12	13	14	14	15	16	17	17	18	19	20	20	21	22	23	23	24	25	26	26	27	28	29	29	30	31	32	32	33																
34	9	9	10	11	12	12	13	14	15	15	16	17	18	18	19	20	21	21	22	23	24	24	25	26	27	27	28	29	30	30	31	32	33	33	34															
35	9	10	10	11	12	13	13	14	15	16	16	17	18	19	19	20	21	22	22	23	24	25	25	26	27	28	28	29	30	31	31	32	33	34	34	35														
36	9	10	11	11	12	13	14	14	15	16	17	17	18	19	20	20	21	22	23	23	24	25	26	26	27	28	29	29	30	31	32	32	33	34	35	35	36													
37	9	10	11	12	12	13	14	15	15	16	17	18	18	19	20	21	21	22	23	24	24	25	26	27	27	28	29	30	30	31	32	33	33	34	35	36	36	37												
38	10	10	11	12	13	13	14	15	16	16	17	18	19	19	20	21	22	22	23	24	25	25	26	27	28	28	29	30	31	31	32	33	34	34	35	36	37	37	38											
39	10	11	11	12	13	14	14	15	16	17	17	18	19	20	20	21	22	23	23	24	25	26	26	27	28	29	29	30	31	32	32	33	34	35	35	36	37	38	38	39										
40	10	11	12	12	13	14	15	15	16	17	18	18	19	20	21	21	22	23	24	24	25	26	27	27	28	29	30	30	31	32	33	33	34	35	36	36	37	38	39	39	40									
41	10	11	12	13	13	14	15	16	16	17	18	19	19	20	21	22	22	23	24	25	25	26	27	28	28	29	30	31	31	32	33	34	34	35	36	37	37	38	39	40	40	41								
42	11	11	12	13	14	14	15	16	17	17	18	19	20	20	21	22	23	23	24	25	26	26	27	28	29	29	30	31	32	32	33	34	35	35	36	37	38	38	39	40	41	41	42							
43	11	12	12	13	14	15	15	16	17	18	18	19	20	21	21	22	23	24	24	25	26	27	27	28	29	30	30	31	32	33	33	34	35	36	36	37	38	39	39	40	41	42	42	43						
44	11	12	13	13	14	15	16	16	17	18	19	19	20	21	22	22	23	24	25	25	26	27	28	28	29	30	31	31	32	33	34	34	35	36	37	37	38	39	40	40	41	42	43	43	44					
45	11	12	13	14	14	15	16	17	17	18	19	20	20	21	22	23	23	24	25	26	26	27	28	29	29	30	31	32	32	33	34	35	35	36	37	38	38	39	40	41	41	42	43	44	44	45				
46	12	12	13	14	15	15	16	17	18	18	19	20	21	21	22	23	24	24	25	26	27	27	28	29	30	30	31	32	33	33	34	35	36	36	37	38	39	39	40	41	42	42	43	44	45	45	46			
47	12	13	13	14	15	16	16	17	18	19	19	20	21	22	22	23	24	25	25	26	27	28	28	29	30	31	31	32	33	34	34	35	36	37	37	38	39	40	40	41	42	43	43	44	45	46	46	47		
48	12	13	14	14	15	16	17	17	18	19	20	20	21	22	23	23	24	25	26	26	27	28	29	29	30	31	32	32	33	34	35	35	36	37	38	38	39	40	41	41	42	43	44	44	45	46	47	47	48	
49	12	13	14	15	15	16	17	18	18	19	20	21	21	22	23	24	24	25	26	27	27	28	29	30	30	31	32	33	33	34	35	36	36	37	38	39	39	40	41	42	42	43	44	45	45	46	47	48	48	49

% Impairment better eye

% Impairment worse eye

	0	1	2	3	4	5	6	7	8	9	10	11	12	13	14	15	16	17	18	19	20	21	22	23	24	25	26	27	28	29	30	31	32	33	34	35	36	37	38	39	40	41	42	43	44	45	46	47	48	49	
50	13	13	14	15	16	16	17	18	19	19	20	21	22	22	23	24	25	25	26	27	28	28	29	30	31	31	32	33	34	34	35	36	37	37	38	39	40	40	41	42	43	43	44	45	46	46	47	48	49	49	**50**
51	13	14	14	15	16	17	17	18	19	20	20	21	22	23	23	24	25	26	26	27	28	29	29	30	31	32	32	33	34	35	35	36	37	38	38	39	40	41	41	42	43	44	44	45	46	47	47	48	49	50	**51**
52	13	14	15	15	16	17	18	18	19	20	21	21	22	23	24	24	25	26	27	27	28	29	30	30	31	32	33	33	34	35	36	36	37	38	39	39	40	41	42	42	43	44	45	45	46	47	48	48	49	50	**52**
53	13	14	15	16	16	17	18	19	19	20	21	22	22	23	24	25	25	26	27	28	28	29	30	31	31	32	33	34	34	35	36	37	37	38	39	40	40	41	42	43	43	44	45	46	46	47	48	49	49	50	**53**
54	14	14	15	16	17	17	18	19	20	20	21	22	23	23	24	25	26	26	27	28	29	29	30	31	32	32	33	34	35	35	36	37	38	38	39	40	41	41	42	43	44	44	45	46	47	47	48	49	50	50	**54**
55	14	15	15	16	17	18	18	19	20	21	21	22	23	24	24	25	26	27	27	28	29	30	30	31	32	33	33	34	35	36	36	37	38	39	39	40	41	42	42	43	44	45	45	46	47	48	48	49	50	51	**55**
56	14	15	16	16	17	18	19	19	20	21	22	22	23	24	25	25	26	27	28	28	29	30	31	31	32	33	34	34	35	36	37	37	38	39	40	40	41	42	43	43	44	45	46	46	47	48	49	49	50	51	**56**
57	14	15	16	17	17	18	19	20	20	21	22	23	23	24	25	26	26	27	28	29	29	30	31	32	32	33	34	35	35	36	37	38	38	39	40	41	41	42	43	44	44	45	46	47	47	48	49	50	50	51	**57**
58	15	15	16	17	18	18	19	20	21	21	22	23	24	24	25	26	27	27	28	29	30	30	31	32	33	33	34	35	36	36	37	38	39	39	40	41	42	42	43	44	45	45	46	47	48	48	49	50	51	51	**58**
59	15	16	16	17	18	19	19	20	21	22	22	23	24	25	25	26	27	28	28	29	30	31	31	32	33	34	34	35	36	37	37	38	39	40	40	41	42	43	43	44	45	46	46	47	48	49	49	50	51	52	**59**
60	15	16	17	17	18	19	20	20	21	22	23	23	24	25	26	26	27	28	29	29	30	31	32	32	33	34	35	35	36	37	38	38	39	40	41	41	42	43	44	44	45	46	47	47	48	49	50	50	51	52	**60**
61	15	16	17	18	18	19	20	21	21	22	23	24	24	25	26	27	27	28	29	30	30	31	32	33	33	34	35	36	36	37	38	39	39	40	41	42	42	43	44	45	45	46	47	48	48	49	50	51	51	52	**61**
62	16	16	17	18	19	19	20	21	22	22	23	24	25	25	26	27	28	28	29	30	31	31	32	33	34	34	35	36	37	37	38	39	40	40	41	42	43	43	44	45	46	46	47	48	49	49	50	51	52	52	**62**
63	16	17	17	18	19	20	20	21	22	23	23	24	25	26	26	27	28	29	29	30	31	32	32	33	34	35	35	36	37	38	38	39	40	41	41	42	43	44	44	45	46	47	47	48	49	50	50	51	52	53	**63**
64	16	17	18	18	19	20	21	21	22	23	24	24	25	26	27	27	28	29	30	30	31	32	33	33	34	35	36	36	37	38	39	39	40	41	42	42	43	44	45	45	46	47	48	48	49	50	51	51	52	53	**64**
65	16	17	18	19	19	20	21	22	22	23	24	25	25	26	27	28	28	29	30	31	31	32	33	34	34	35	36	37	37	38	39	40	40	41	42	43	43	44	45	46	46	47	48	49	49	50	51	52	52	53	**65**
66	17	17	18	19	20	20	21	22	23	23	24	25	26	26	27	28	29	29	30	31	32	32	33	34	35	35	36	37	38	38	39	40	41	41	42	43	44	44	45	46	47	47	48	49	50	50	51	52	53	53	**66**
67	17	18	18	19	20	21	21	22	23	24	24	25	26	27	27	28	29	30	30	31	32	33	33	34	35	36	36	37	38	39	39	40	41	42	42	43	44	45	45	46	47	48	48	49	50	51	51	52	53	54	**67**
68	17	18	19	19	20	21	22	22	23	24	25	25	26	27	28	28	29	30	31	31	32	33	34	34	35	36	37	37	38	39	40	40	41	42	43	43	44	45	46	46	47	48	49	49	50	51	52	52	53	54	**68**
69	17	18	19	20	20	21	22	23	23	24	25	26	26	27	28	29	29	30	31	32	32	33	34	35	35	36	37	38	38	39	40	41	41	42	43	44	44	45	46	47	47	48	49	50	50	51	52	53	53	54	**69**
70	18	18	19	20	21	21	22	23	24	24	25	26	27	27	28	29	30	30	31	32	33	33	34	35	36	36	37	38	39	39	40	41	42	42	43	44	45	45	46	47	48	48	49	50	51	51	52	53	54	54	**70**
71	18	19	19	20	21	22	22	23	24	25	25	26	27	28	28	29	30	31	31	32	33	34	34	35	36	37	37	38	39	40	40	41	42	43	43	44	45	46	46	47	48	49	49	50	51	52	52	53	54	55	**71**
72	18	19	20	20	21	22	23	23	24	25	26	26	27	28	29	29	30	31	32	32	33	34	35	35	36	37	38	38	39	40	41	41	42	43	44	44	45	46	47	47	48	49	50	50	51	52	53	53	54	55	**72**
73	18	19	20	21	21	22	23	24	24	25	26	27	27	28	29	30	30	31	32	33	33	34	35	36	36	37	38	39	39	40	41	42	42	43	44	45	45	46	47	48	48	49	50	51	51	52	53	54	54	55	**73**
74	19	19	20	21	22	22	23	24	25	25	26	27	28	28	29	30	31	31	32	33	34	34	35	36	37	37	38	39	40	40	41	42	43	43	44	45	46	46	47	48	49	49	50	51	52	52	53	54	55	55	**74**
75	19	20	20	21	22	23	23	24	25	26	26	27	28	29	29	30	31	32	32	33	34	35	35	36	37	38	38	39	40	41	41	42	43	44	44	45	46	47	47	48	49	50	50	51	52	53	53	54	55	56	**75**
76	19	20	21	21	22	23	24	24	25	26	27	27	28	29	30	30	31	32	33	33	34	35	36	36	37	38	39	39	40	41	42	42	43	44	45	45	46	47	48	48	49	50	51	51	52	53	54	54	55	56	**76**
77	19	20	21	22	22	23	24	25	25	26	27	28	28	29	30	31	31	32	33	34	34	35	36	37	37	38	39	40	40	41	42	43	43	44	45	46	46	47	48	49	49	50	51	52	52	53	54	55	55	56	**77**
78	20	20	21	22	23	23	24	25	26	26	27	28	29	29	30	31	32	32	33	34	35	35	36	37	38	38	39	40	41	41	42	43	44	44	45	46	47	47	48	49	50	50	51	52	53	53	54	55	56	56	**78**
79	20	21	21	22	23	24	24	25	26	27	27	28	29	30	30	31	32	33	33	34	35	36	36	37	38	39	39	40	41	42	42	43	44	45	45	46	47	48	48	49	50	51	51	52	53	54	54	55	56	57	**79**
80	20	21	22	22	23	24	25	25	26	27	28	28	29	30	31	31	32	33	34	34	35	36	37	37	38	39	40	40	41	42	43	43	44	45	46	46	47	48	49	49	50	51	52	52	53	54	55	55	56	57	**80**
81	20	21	22	23	23	24	25	26	26	27	28	29	29	30	31	32	32	33	34	35	35	36	37	38	38	39	40	41	41	42	43	44	44	45	46	47	47	48	49	50	50	51	52	53	53	54	55	56	56	57	**81**
82	21	21	22	23	24	24	25	26	27	27	28	29	30	30	31	32	33	33	34	35	36	36	37	38	39	39	40	41	42	42	43	44	45	45	46	47	48	48	49	50	51	51	52	53	54	54	55	56	57	57	**82**
83	21	22	22	23	24	25	25	26	27	28	28	29	30	31	31	32	33	34	34	35	36	37	37	38	39	40	40	41	42	43	43	44	45	46	46	47	48	49	49	50	51	52	52	53	54	55	55	56	57	58	**83**
84	21	22	23	23	24	25	26	26	27	28	29	29	30	31	32	32	33	34	35	35	36	37	38	38	39	40	41	41	42	43	44	44	45	46	47	47	48	49	50	50	51	52	53	53	54	55	56	56	57	58	**84**
85	21	22	23	24	24	25	26	27	27	28	29	30	30	31	32	33	33	34	35	36	36	37	38	39	39	40	41	42	42	43	44	45	45	46	47	48	48	49	50	51	51	52	53	54	54	55	56	57	57	58	**85**
86	22	22	23	24	25	25	26	27	28	28	29	30	31	31	32	33	34	34	35	36	37	37	38	39	40	40	41	42	43	43	44	45	46	46	47	48	49	49	50	51	52	52	53	54	55	55	56	57	58	58	**86**
87	22	23	23	24	25	26	26	27	28	29	29	30	31	32	32	33	34	35	35	36	37	38	38	39	40	41	41	42	43	44	44	45	46	47	47	48	49	50	50	51	52	53	53	54	55	56	56	57	58	59	**87**
88	22	23	24	24	25	26	27	27	28	29	30	30	31	32	33	33	34	35	36	36	37	38	39	39	40	41	42	42	43	44	45	45	46	47	48	48	49	50	51	51	52	53	54	54	55	56	57	57	58	59	**88**
89	22	23	24	25	25	26	27	28	28	29	30	31	31	32	33	34	34	35	36	37	37	38	39	40	40	41	42	43	43	44	45	46	46	47	48	49	49	50	51	52	52	53	54	55	55	56	57	58	58	59	**89**
90	23	23	24	25	26	26	27	28	29	29	30	31	32	32	33	34	35	35	36	37	38	38	39	40	41	41	42	43	44	44	45	46	47	47	48	49	50	50	51	52	53	53	54	55	56	56	57	58	59	59	**90**
91	23	24	24	25	26	27	27	28	29	30	30	31	32	33	33	34	35	36	36	37	38	39	39	40	41	42	42	43	44	45	45	46	47	48	48	49	50	51	51	52	53	54	54	55	56	57	57	58	59	60	**91**
92	23	24	25	25	26	27	28	28	29	30	31	31	32	33	34	34	35	36	37	37	38	39	40	40	41	42	43	43	44	45	46	46	47	48	49	49	50	51	52	52	53	54	55	55	56	57	58	58	59	60	**92**
93	23	24	25	26	26	27	28	29	29	30	31	32	32	33	34	35	35	36	37	38	38	39	40	41	41	42	43	44	44	45	46	47	47	48	49	50	50	51	52	53	53	54	55	56	56	57	58	59	59	60	**93**
94	24	24	25	26	27	27	28	29	30	30	31	32	33	33	34	35	36	36	37	38	39	39	40	41	42	42	43	44	45	45	46	47	48	48	49	50	51	51	52	53	54	54	55	56	57	57	58	59	60	60	**94**
95	24	25	25	26	27	28	28	29	30	31	31	32	33	34	34	35	36	37	37	38	39	40	40	41	42	43	43	44	45	46	46	47	48	49	49	50	51	52	52	53	54	55	55	56	57	58	58	59	60	61	**95**
96	24	25	26	26	27	28	29	29	30	31	32	32	33	34	35	35	36	37	38	38	39	40	41	41	42	43	44	44	45	46	47	47	48	49	50	50	51	52	53	53	54	55	56	56	57	58	59	59	60	61	**96**
97	24	25	26	27	27	28	29	30	30	31	32	33	33	34	35	36	36	37	38	39	39	40	41	42	42	43	44	45	45	46	47	48	48	49	50	51	51	52	53	54	54	55	56	57	57	58	59	60	60	61	**97**
98	25	25	26	27	28	28	29	30	31	31	32	33	34	34	35	36	37	37	38	39	40	40	41	42	43	43	44	45	46	46	47	48	49	49	50	51	52	52	53	54	55	55	56	57	58	58	59	60	61	61	**98**
99	25	26	26	27	28	29	29	30	31	32	32	33	34	35	35	36	37	38	38	39	40	41	41	42	43	44	44	45	46	47	47	48	49	50	50	51	52	53	53	54	55	56	56	57	58	59	59	60	61	62	**99**
100	25	26	27	27	28	29	30	30	31	32	33	33	34	35	36	36	37	38	39	39	40	41	42	42	43	44	45	45	46	47	48	48	49	50	51	51	52	53	54	54	55	56	57	57	58	59	60	60	61	62	**100**
	0	**1**	**2**	**3**	**4**	**5**	**6**	**7**	**8**	**9**	**10**	**11**	**12**	**13**	**14**	**15**	**16**	**17**	**18**	**19**	**20**	**21**	**22**	**23**	**24**	**25**	**26**	**27**	**28**	**29**	**30**	**31**	**32**	**33**	**34**	**35**	**36**	**37**	**38**	**39**	**40**	**41**	**42**	**43**	**44**	**45**	**46**	**47**	**48**	**49**	

% Impairment better eye

% Impairment better eye

% Impairment worse eye	50	51	52	53	54	55	56	57	58	59	60	61	62	63	64	65	66	67	68	69	70	71	72	73	74	75	76	77	78	79	80	81	82	83	84	85	86	87	88	89	90	91	92	93	94	95	96	97	98	99	100
50	50																																																		
51	50	51																																																	
52	51	51	52																																																
53	51	52	52	53																																															
54	51	52	53	53	54																																														
55	51	52	53	54	54	55																																													
56	52	52	53	54	55	55	56																																												
57	52	53	53	54	55	56	56	57																																											
58	52	53	54	54	55	56	57	57	58																																										
59	52	53	54	55	55	56	57	58	58	59																																									
60	53	53	54	55	56	56	57	58	59	59	60																																								
61	53	54	54	55	56	57	57	58	59	60	60	61																																							
62	53	54	55	55	56	57	58	58	59	60	61	61	62																																						
63	53	54	55	56	56	57	58	59	59	60	61	62	62	63																																					
64	54	54	55	56	57	57	58	59	60	60	61	62	63	63	64																																				
65	54	55	55	56	57	58	58	59	60	61	61	62	63	64	64	65																																			
66	54	55	56	56	57	58	59	59	60	61	62	62	63	64	65	65	66																																		
67	54	55	56	57	57	58	59	60	60	61	62	63	63	64	65	66	66	67																																	
68	55	55	56	57	58	58	59	60	61	61	62	63	64	64	65	66	67	67	68																																
69	55	56	56	57	58	59	59	60	61	62	62	63	64	65	65	66	67	68	68	69																															
70	55	56	57	57	58	59	60	60	61	62	63	63	64	65	66	66	67	68	69	69	70																														
71	55	56	57	58	58	59	60	61	61	62	63	64	64	65	66	67	67	68	69	70	70	71																													
72	56	56	57	58	59	59	60	61	62	62	63	64	65	65	66	67	68	68	69	70	71	71	72																												
73	56	57	57	58	59	60	60	61	62	63	63	64	65	66	66	67	68	69	69	70	71	72	72	73																											
74	56	57	58	58	59	60	61	61	62	63	64	64	65	66	67	67	68	69	70	70	71	72	73	73	74																										
75	56	57	58	59	59	60	61	62	62	63	64	65	65	66	67	68	68	69	70	71	71	72	73	74	74	75																									
76	57	57	58	59	60	60	61	62	63	63	64	65	66	66	67	68	69	69	70	71	72	72	73	74	75	75	76																								
77	57	58	58	59	60	61	61	62	63	64	64	65	66	67	67	68	69	70	70	71	72	73	73	74	75	76	76	77																							
78	57	58	59	59	60	61	62	62	63	64	65	65	66	67	68	68	69	70	71	71	72	73	74	74	75	76	77	77	78																						
79	57	58	59	60	60	61	62	63	63	64	65	66	66	67	68	69	69	70	71	72	72	73	74	75	75	76	77	78	78	79																					
80	58	58	59	60	61	61	62	63	64	64	65	66	67	67	68	69	70	70	71	72	73	73	74	75	76	76	77	78	79	79	80																				
81	58	59	59	60	61	62	62	63	64	65	65	66	67	68	68	69	70	71	71	72	73	74	74	75	76	77	77	78	79	80	80	81																			
82	58	59	60	60	61	62	63	63	64	65	66	66	67	68	69	69	70	71	72	72	73	74	75	75	76	77	78	78	79	80	81	81	82																		
83	58	59	60	61	61	62	63	64	64	65	66	67	67	68	69	70	70	71	72	73	73	74	75	76	76	77	78	79	79	80	81	82	82	83																	
84	59	59	60	61	62	62	63	64	65	65	66	67	68	68	69	70	71	71	72	73	74	74	75	76	77	77	78	79	80	80	81	82	83	83	84																
85	59	60	60	61	62	63	63	64	65	66	66	67	68	69	69	70	71	72	72	73	74	75	75	76	77	78	78	79	80	81	81	82	83	84	84	85															
86	59	60	61	61	62	63	64	64	65	66	67	67	68	69	70	70	71	72	73	73	74	75	76	76	77	78	79	79	80	81	82	82	83	84	85	85	86														
87	59	60	61	62	62	63	64	65	65	66	67	68	68	69	70	71	71	72	73	74	74	75	76	77	77	78	79	80	80	81	82	83	83	84	85	86	86	87													
88	60	60	61	62	63	63	64	65	66	66	67	68	69	69	70	71	72	72	73	74	75	75	76	77	78	78	79	80	81	81	82	83	84	84	85	86	87	87	88												
89	60	61	61	62	63	64	64	65	66	67	67	68	69	70	70	71	72	73	73	74	75	76	76	77	78	79	79	80	81	82	82	83	84	85	85	86	87	88	88	89											
90	60	61	62	62	63	64	65	65	66	67	68	68	69	70	71	71	72	73	74	74	75	76	77	77	78	79	80	80	81	82	83	83	84	85	86	86	87	88	89	89	90										
91	60	61	62	63	63	64	65	66	66	67	68	69	69	70	71	72	72	73	74	75	75	76	77	78	78	79	80	81	81	82	83	84	84	85	86	87	87	88	89	90	90	91									
92	61	61	62	63	64	64	65	66	67	67	68	69	70	70	71	72	73	73	74	75	76	76	77	78	79	79	80	81	82	82	83	84	85	85	86	87	88	88	89	90	91	91	92								
93	61	62	62	63	64	65	65	66	67	68	68	69	70	71	71	72	73	74	74	75	76	77	77	78	79	80	80	81	82	83	83	84	85	86	86	87	88	89	89	90	91	92	92	93							
94	61	62	63	63	64	65	66	66	67	68	69	69	70	71	72	72	73	74	75	75	76	77	78	78	79	80	81	81	82	83	84	84	85	86	87	87	88	89	90	90	91	92	93	93	94						
95	61	62	63	64	64	65	66	67	67	68	69	70	70	71	72	73	73	74	75	76	76	77	78	79	79	80	81	82	82	83	84	85	85	86	87	88	88	89	90	91	91	92	93	94	94	95					
96	62	62	63	64	65	65	66	67	68	68	69	70	71	71	72	73	74	74	75	76	77	77	78	79	80	80	81	82	83	83	84	85	86	86	87	88	89	89	90	91	92	92	93	94	95	95	96				
97	62	63	63	64	65	66	66	67	68	69	69	70	71	72	72	73	74	75	75	76	77	78	78	79	80	81	81	82	83	84	84	85	86	87	87	88	89	90	90	91	92	93	93	94	95	96	96	97			
98	62	63	64	64	65	66	67	67	68	69	70	70	71	72	73	73	74	75	76	76	77	78	79	79	80	81	82	82	83	84	85	85	86	87	88	88	89	90	91	91	92	93	94	94	95	96	97	97	98		
99	62	63	64	65	65	66	67	68	68	69	70	71	71	72	73	74	74	75	76	77	77	78	79	80	80	81	82	83	83	84	85	86	86	87	88	89	89	90	91	92	92	93	94	95	95	96	97	98	98	99	
100	63	63	64	65	66	66	67	68	69	69	70	71	72	72	73	74	75	75	76	77	78	78	79	80	81	81	82	83	84	84	85	86	87	87	88	89	90	90	91	92	93	93	94	95	96	96	97	98	99	99	100

Consult Table 6 (p. 218) to ascertain the impairment of the whole person that is contributed by the visual system.

In example 3, the 59% visual system impairment is equivalent to a 56% whole-person impairment (Table 6).

8.5 Other Conditions

Up to an additional 10% impairment may be *combined* with the whole-person impairment related to the visual system for such conditions as permanent deformities of the orbit, scars, and other cosmetic deformities that do not otherwise alter ocular function. *Combine* the estimates by means of the Combined Values Chart (p. 322).

Example:

Impairment due to loss of central vision of both eyes	49%
Impairment due to binocular visual field loss	20%
Impairment of visual system (Combined Values Chart, p. 322)	59%
Impairment of whole person related to visual system (Table 6, p. 218)	56%
10% impairment for orbital scar and deformity	10%
Whole-person impairment (Combined Values Chart)	60%

References

1. Sloan LL. New test charts for the measurement of visual acuity. *Am J Ophthalmol.* 1959;48:808-813.

2. Report of Working Group 39, Committee on Vision, National Academy of Sciences. Recommended standard procedures for the clinical measurement and specification of visual acuity. *Adv Ophthalmol.* 1980;41:103-143.

3. Esterman B. Grid for scoring visual field, II perimeter. *Arch Ophthalmol.* 1968;79:400-406.

4. Keeney AH, Duerson HL Jr. Collated near-vision test card. *Am J Ophthalmol.* 1958;46:592-594.

5. Keeney AH. *Ocular Examination: Basis and Technique.* 2nd ed. St Louis, Mo: CV Mosby Co; 1976.

6. Newell FW. *Ophthalmology: Principles and Concepts.* 7th ed. St Louis, Mo: CV Mosby Co; 1992.

7. Esterman B. Functional scoring of the binocular visual field. *Ophthalmology.* 1982;89:1226-1234.

8. Esterman B, Blance E, Wallach M, Bonelli A. Computerized scoring of the functional field: preliminary report. *Doc Ophthalmol Proc Ser.* 1985;42:333-339.

9. Anderson DR. *Perimetry: With and Without Automation.* 2nd ed. St Louis, Mo: CV Mosby Co; 1987.

10. American Academy of Ophthalmology. Contrast sensitivity and glare testing in the evaluation of anterior segment disease. *Ophthalmology.* 1990;97:1233-1237.

11. Frisen L. *Clinical Tests of Vision.* New York, NY: Raven Press; 1990.

Chapter 9

Ear, Nose, Throat, and Related Structures

The purpose of this chapter is to provide criteria for use in evaluating permanent impairments resulting from the principal dysfunctions of the ear, nose, throat, and related structures. Although these structures have multiple functions, some of which are closely allied, permanent impairments of the structures usually result from clinically established deviations from normal in one or more of the following functions: (1) hearing; (2) equilibrium; (3) respiration; (4) mastication, including temporomandibular joint function; (5) olfaction and taste; (6) speech; and (7) facial features and their movements.

Before using this chapter, the reader should peruse Chapters 1 and 2 and the Glossary, which discuss the purpose of the *Guides* and the situations in which they are useful. Chapters 1 and 2 also discuss the methods and techniques for evaluating a patient and present a format for the evaluation report. The medical report on a permanent impairment should include the information outlined below.

A. Medical Evaluation
- History of medical condition(s)
- Results of most recent clinical evaluation
- Assessment of current clinical status and statement of further medical plans
- Diagnosis

B. Analysis of Findings
- Impact of medical condition(s) on life activities
- Explanation for concluding that the condition is stable and is unlikely to change in future months
- Explanation for concluding that the individual is or is not likely to suffer further impairment by engaging in usual activities
- Explanation for concluding that accommodations or restrictions are or are not warranted

C. Comparison of Analysis with Impairment Criteria
- Description of clinical findings and how these findings relate to specific criteria
- Explanation of each impairment percentage
- List of organ system impairments and percentages
- Overall whole-person impairment percentage

9.1 The Ear

The ear consists of the auricle, the external canal, the tympanic membrane, the eustachian tube, the mastoid, the internal ear, central nervous system pathways, and the auditory cortex.

The functions of the ear are hearing and equilibrium, which are considered in the following paragraphs. The criteria for evaluating hearing impairment are relatively specific. In contrast, the criteria for evaluating disturbances of equilibrium are more general.

Disturbances of the ear, such as chronic otorrhea, otalgia, and tinnitus, are not measurable. Therefore, the physician should estimate an impairment percentage based on the severity of those conditions and the degree to which they interfere with functions of the ear, and a percentage that is consistent with established values.[1]

Tinnitus in the presence of unilateral or bilateral hearing loss may impair speech discrimination; therefore, an impairment percentage up to 5% may be added to the impairment for hearing loss.

9.1a Hearing

The following criteria have been adapted from information provided by the American Academy of Otolaryngology-Head and Neck Surgery.[2] Impairment of an individual's hearing is determined according to evaluation of the individual's binaural hearing impairment. In using these criteria, the abbreviations and definitions given below should be kept in mind.

1. Permanent hearing impairment: This is reduced hearing sensitivity that is outside the range of normal. Hearing should be evaluated after maximum rehabilitation has been achieved and when the impairment is nonprogressive.

Prosthetic devices *must not* be used during the evaluation of hearing sensitivity. The reason for this dictum is that the use of such devices might give a false impression of patients' sensitivities and distort the need to take hearing conservation or other measures that might be indicated.

2. Permanent binaural hearing impairment: This is a binaural hearing loss that interferes with the individual's ability to carry out the activities of daily living.

3. Intensity: This is measured in decibels (dB).

4. Frequency: This is measured in cycles per second, or hertz (Hz).

5. Hearing threshold level for pure tones: This is defined as the number of decibels above a standard audiometric zero level for a given frequency at which the listener's threshold of hearing lies. It is the reading on the hearing level (HL) dial of an audiometer that is calibrated according to American National Standards Institute (ANSI) audiometer specifications S3.6-1989.[3]

6. Estimated hearing level for speech: This is the arithmetic mean of the hearing threshold levels at the four test frequencies, 500, 1000, 2000, and 3000 Hz, which may be considered to represent everyday auditory stimuli. Because of the present limitations of speech audiometry, the hearing loss for speech is estimated from measurements made with a pure-tone audiometer.

7. Evaluation of monaural hearing impairment: If the average of the hearing levels at 500, 1000, 2000, and 3000 Hz is 25 dB or less, according to 1989 ANSI standards, no impairment is considered to exist in the ability to hear everyday sounds under everyday listening conditions (Table 1, p. 225). At the other extreme, if the average of the hearing levels at 500, 1000, 2000, and 3000 Hz is over 91.7 dB, the impairment for hearing everyday speech is considered to be total, that is, 100%.

According to the above standards for monaural hearing impairment, for every decibel that the average hearing level or loss for speech exceeds 25 dB, 1.5% of monaural impairment is assigned. Thus, with an average hearing level loss of 67 dB above 25 dB, monaural impairment is 100% (Table 1, p. 225).

This method of evaluating hearing impairment should be applied only to adults who have acquired language skills. Evidence suggests that language acquisition by children who do not have language skills may be delayed when the average hearing level is in the range of 15 to 25 dB.

8. Evaluation of binaural hearing impairment: The evaluation of binaural hearing impairment in adults is derived from the pure-tone audiogram and is always based on the functioning of both ears.

Binaural impairment is determined by means of the following formula: binaural hearing impairment (%) = [5 x (% hearing impairment in better ear) + (% hearing impairment in poorer ear)] ÷ 6.

If it is necessary to convert a monaural impairment to a binaural impairment, it should be done with the use of the formula above, allowing 0% impairment for the better ear.

Table 2 (p. 226) is derived from the formula given above. Table 3 (p. 228) converts binaural hearing impairment to impairment of the whole person.

9.1b Objective Techniques for Determining Hearing Impairments

In determining impairments, the following steps should be taken.

1. Test each ear separately with a pure-tone audiometer and record the hearing levels at 500, 1000, 2000, and 3000 Hz. It is necessary that the hearing level for each frequency be determined in every patient. The following rules apply for extreme values:

a. If the hearing level at a given frequency is greater than 100 dB or is beyond the range of the audiometer, the level should be taken as 100 dB.

b. If the hearing level for a given frequency is better than normal, the level should be taken as 0 dB.

2. Total the four decibel hearing levels for each ear separately. In the examples of patients A and B below, hearing levels are determined according to ANSI S3.6-1989 standards.

3. Consult Table 1 (at right) to determine the percentages of monaural hearing impairment(s).

In patient A, the right-ear hearing level is 140 dB, which equates to a 15% hearing impairment (Table 1, at right). The left-ear hearing level is 220 dB, which equates to a 45% hearing impairment.

In patient B, the right-ear hearing level is 370 dB, which is equivalent to a 100% hearing impairment. The left-ear hearing level is 340 dB, which equates to a 90% hearing impairment.

Patient A

Frequency, Hz	Hearing level, dB Left ear	Right ear
500	30	15
1000	45	25
2000	60	45
3000	85	55
DSHL*	220	140

Patient B

Frequency, Hz	Hearing level, dB Left ear	Right ear
500	75	80
1000	80	90
2000	90	100
3000	95	100
DHSL*	340	370

*Decibel sum of the hearing threshold levels.

Table 1. Monaural Hearing Loss and Impairment (%)*

DSHL†	%	DSHL	%	DSHL	%
100	0.0	190	33.8	285	69.3
		195	35.6	290	71.2
105	1.9	200	37.5	295	73.1
110	3.8			300	75.0
115	5.6	205	39.4		
120	7.5	210	41.2	305	76.9
		215	43.1	310	78.8
125	9.4	220	45.0	315	80.6
130	11.2			320	82.5
135	13.1	225	46.9		
140	15.0	230	48.9	325	84.4
		235	50.5	330	86.2
145	16.9	240	52.5	335	88.1
150	18.8			340	90.0
155	20.6	245	54.4		
160	22.5	250	56.2	345	90.9
		255	58.1	350	93.8
165	24.4	260	60.0	355	95.6
170	26.2			360	97.5
175	28.1	265	61.9		
180	30.0	270	63.8	365	99.4
		275	65.6	368	100.0
185	31.9	280	67.5	or greater	

*Audiometers are calibrated to ANSI 3.6-1989 standard reference levels.
†Decibel sum of the hearing threshold levels at 500, 1000, 2000, and 3000 Hz.

4. Consult Table 2 (p. 226) to determine the percentage of binaural hearing impairment.

In patient A, a DSHL of 140 (better ear) and a DSHL of 220 (poorer ear) *combine* to give a 20% binaural hearing impairment.

In patient B, a DSHL of 340 (better ear) and a DSHL of 30 (poorer ear) combine to give a 92% binaural hearing impairment. *Note:* the maximum value of 368 DSHL is used.

5. Consult Table 3 (p. 228) to determine the impairment of the whole person.

In patient A, a 20% binaural hearing impairment is equivalent to a 7% impairment of the whole person.

In patient B, a 92% binaural hearing impairment is equivalent to a 32% impairment of the whole person.

Table 2. Computation of Binaural Hearing Impairment*

Worse ear

ANSI 1969	100	105	110	115	120	125	130	135	140	145	150	155	160	165	170	175	180	185	190	195	200	205	210	215	220	225	230
100	0																										
105	0.3	1.9																									
110	0.6	2.2	3.8																								
115	0.9	2.5	4.1	5.6																							
120	1.3	2.8	4.4	5.9	7.5																						
125	1.6	3.1	4.7	6.3	7.8	9.4																					
130	1.9	3.4	5	6.6	8.1	9.7	11.3																				
135	2.2	3.8	5.3	6.9	8.4	10	11.6	13.1																			
140	2.5	4.1	5.6	7.2	8.8	10.3	11.9	13.4	15																		
145	2.8	4.4	5.9	7.5	9.1	10.6	12.2	13.8	15.3	16.9																	
150	3.1	4.7	6.3	7.8	9.4	10.9	12.5	14.1	15.6	17.2	18.8																
155	3.4	5	6.6	8.1	9.7	11.3	12.8	14.4	15.9	17.5	19.1	20.6															
160	3.8	5.3	6.9	8.4	10	11.6	13.1	14.7	16.3	17.8	19.4	20.9	22.5														
165	4.1	5.6	7.2	8.8	10.3	11.9	13.4	15	16.6	18.1	19.7	21.3	22.8	24.4													
170	4.4	5.9	7.5	9.1	10.6	12.2	13.8	15.3	16.9	18.4	20	21.6	23.1	24.7	26.3												
175	4.7	6.3	7.8	9.4	10.9	12.5	14.1	15.6	17.2	18.8	20.3	21.9	23.4	25	26.6	28.1											
180	5	6.6	8.1	9.7	11.3	12.8	14.4	15.9	17.5	19.1	20.6	22.2	23.8	25.3	26.9	28.4	30										
185	5.3	6.9	8.4	10	11.6	13.1	14.7	16.3	17.8	19.4	20.9	22.5	24.1	25.6	27.2	28.8	30.3	31.9									
190	5.6	7.2	8.8	10.3	11.9	13.4	15	16.6	18.1	19.7	21.3	22.8	24.4	25.9	27.5	29.1	30.6	32.2	33.8								
195	5.9	7.5	9.1	10.6	12.2	13.8	15.3	16.9	18.4	20	21.6	23.1	24.7	26.3	27.8	29.4	30.9	32.5	34.1	35.6							
200	6.3	7.8	9.4	10.9	12.5	14.1	15.6	17.2	18.8	20.3	21.9	23.4	25	26.6	28.1	29.7	31.3	32.8	34.4	35.9	37.5						
205	6.6	8.1	9.7	11.3	12.8	14.4	15.9	17.5	19.1	20.6	22.2	23.8	25.3	26.9	28.4	30	31.6	33.1	34.7	36.3	37.8	39.4					
210	6.9	8.4	10	11.6	13.1	14.7	16.3	17.8	19.4	20.9	22.5	24.1	25.6	27.2	28.8	30.3	31.9	33.4	35	36.6	38.1	39.7	41.3				
215	7.2	8.8	10.3	11.9	13.4	15	16.6	18.1	19.7	21.3	22.8	24.4	25.9	27.5	29.1	30.6	32.2	33.8	35.3	36.9	38.4	40	41.6	43.1			
220	7.5	9.1	10.6	12.2	13.8	15.3	16.9	18.4	20	21.6	23.1	24.7	26.3	27.8	29.4	30.9	32.5	34.1	35.6	37.2	38.8	40.3	41.9	43.4	45		
225	7.8	9.4	10.9	12.5	14.1	15.6	17.2	18.8	20.3	21.9	23.4	25	26.6	28.1	29.7	31.3	32.8	34.4	35.9	37.5	39.1	40.6	42.2	43.8	45.3	46.9	
230	8.1	9.7	11.3	12.8	14.4	15.9	17.5	19.1	20.6	22.2	23.8	25.3	26.9	28.4	30	31.6	33.1	34.7	36.3	37.8	39.4	40.9	42.5	44.1	45.6	47.2	48.8
235	8.4	10	11.6	13.1	14.7	16.3	17.8	19.4	20.9	22.5	24.1	25.6	27.2	28.8	30.3	31.9	33.4	35	36.6	38.1	39.7	41.3	42.8	44.4	45.9	47.5	49.1
240	8.8	10.3	11.9	13.4	15	16.6	18.1	19.7	21.3	22.8	24.4	25.9	27.5	29.1	3.06	32.2	33.8	35.3	36.9	38.4	40	41.6	43.1	44.7	46.3	47.8	49.4
245	9.1	10.6	12.2	13.8	15.3	16.9	18.4	20	21.6	23.1	24.7	26.3	27.8	29.4	30.9	32.5	34.1	35.6	37.2	38.8	40.3	41.9	43.4	45	46.6	48.1	49.7
250	9.4	10.9	12.5	14.1	15.6	17.2	18.8	20.3	21.9	23.4	25	26.6	28.1	29.7	31.3	32.8	34.4	35.9	37.5	39.1	40.6	42.2	43.8	45.3	46.9	48.4	50
255	9.7	11.3	12.8	14.4	15.9	17.5	19.1	20.6	22.2	23.8	25.3	26.9	28.4	30	31.6	33.1	34.7	36.3	37.8	39.4	40.9	42.5	44.1	45.6	47.2	48.8	50.3
260	10	11.6	13.1	14.7	16.3	17.8	19.4	20.9	22.5	24.1	25.6	27.2	28.8	30.3	31.9	33.4	35	36.6	38.1	39.7	41.3	42.8	44.4	45.9	47.5	49.1	50.6
265	10.3	11.9	13.4	15	16.6	18.1	19.7	21.3	22.8	24.4	25.9	27.5	29.1	30.6	32.2	33.8	35.3	36.9	38.4	40	41.6	43.1	44.7	46.3	47.8	49.4	50.9
270	10.6	12.2	13.8	15.3	16.9	18.4	20	21.6	23.1	24.7	26.3	27.8	29.4	30.9	32.5	34.1	35.6	37.2	38.8	40.3	41.9	43.4	45	46.6	48.1	49.7	51.3
275	10.9	12.5	14.1	15.6	17.2	18.8	20.3	21.9	23.4	25	26.6	28.1	29.7	31.3	32.8	34.4	35.9	37.5	39.1	40.6	42.2	43.8	45.3	46.9	48.4	50	51.6
280	11.3	12.8	14.4	15.9	17.5	19.1	20.6	22.2	23.8	25.3	26.9	28.4	30	31.6	33.1	34.7	36.3	37.8	39.4	40.9	42.5	44.1	45.6	47.2	48.8	50.3	51.9
285	11.6	13.1	14.7	16.3	17.8	19.4	20.9	22.5	24.1	25.6	27.2	28.8	30.3	31.9	33.4	35	36.6	38.1	39.7	41.3	42.8	44.4	45.9	47.5	49.1	50.6	52.2
290	11.9	13.4	15	16.6	18.1	19.7	21.3	22.8	24.4	25.9	27.5	29.1	30.6	32.2	33.8	35.3	36.9	38.4	40	41.6	43.1	44.7	46.3	47.8	49.4	50.9	52.5
295	12.2	13.8	15.3	16.9	18.4	20	21.6	23.1	24.7	26.3	27.8	29,4	30.9	32.5	34.1	35.6	37.2	38.8	40.3	41.9	43.4	45	46.6	48.1	49.7	51.3	52.8
300	12.5	14.1	15.6	17.2	18.8	20.3	21.9	23.4	25	26.6	28.1	29.7	31.3	32.8	34.4	35.9	37.5	39.1	40.6	42.2	43.8	45.3	46.9	48.4	50	51.6	53.1
305	12.8	14.4	15.9	17.5	19.1	20.6	22.2	23.8	25.3	26.9	28.4	30	31.6	33.1	34.7	36.3	37.8	39.4	40.9	42.5	44.1	45.6	47.2	48.8	50.3	51.9	53.4
310	13.1	14.7	16.3	17.8	19.4	20.9	22.5	24.1	25.6	27.2	28.8	30.3	31.9	33.4	35	36.6	38.1	39.7	41.3	42.8	44.4	45.9	47.5	49.1	50.6	52.2	53.8
315	13.4	15	16.6	18.1	19.7	21.3	22.8	24.4	25.9	27.5	29.1	30.6	32.2	33.8	35.3	36.9	38.4	40	41.6	43.1	44.7	46.3	47.8	49.4	50.9	52.5	54.1
320	13.8	15.3	16.9	18.4	20	21.6	23.1	24.7	26.3	27.8	29.4	30.9	32.5	34.1	35.6	37.2	38.8	40.3	41.9	43.4	45	46.6	48.1	49.7	51.3	52.8	54.4
325	14.1	15.6	17.2	18.8	20.3	21.9	23.4	25	26.6	28.1	29.7	31.3	32.8	34.4	35.9	37.5	39.1	40.6	42.2	43.8	45.3	46.9	48.4	50	51.6	53.1	54.7
330	14.4	15.9	17.5	19.1	20.6	22.2	23.8	25.3	26.9	28.4	30	31.6	33.1	34.7	36.3	37.8	39.4	40.9	42.5	44.1	45.6	47.2	48.8	50.3	51.9	53.4	55
335	14.7	16.3	17.8	19.4	20.9	22.5	24.1	25.6	27.2	28.8	30.3	31.9	33.4	35	36.6	38.1	39.7	41.3	42.8	44.4	45.9	47.5	49.1	50.6	52.2	53.8	55.3
340	15	16.6	18.1	19.7	21.3	22.8	24.4	25.9	27.5	29.1	30.6	32.2	33.8	35.3	36.9	38.4	40	41.6	43.1	44.7	46.3	47.8	49.4	50.9	52.5	54.1	55.6
345	15.3	16.9	18.4	20	21.6	23.1	24.7	26.3	27.8	29.4	30.9	32.5	34.1	35.6	37.2	38.8	40.3	41.9	43.4	45	46.6	48.1	49.7	51.3	52.8	54.4	55.9
350	15.6	17.2	18.8	20.3	21.9	23.4	25	26.6	28.1	29.7	31.3	32.8	34.4	35.9	37.5	39.1	40.6	42.2	43.8	45.3	46.9	48.4	50	51.6	53.1	54.7	56.3
355	15.9	17.5	19.1	20.6	22.2	23.8	25.3	26.9	28.4	30	31.6	33.1	34.7	36.3	37.8	39.4	40.9	42.5	44.1	45.6	47.2	48.8	50.3	51.9	53.4	55	56.6
360	16.3	17.8	19.4	20.9	22.5	24.1	25.6	27.2	28.8	30.3	31.9	33.4	35	36.6	38.1	39.7	41.3	42.8	44.4	45.9	47.5	49.1	50.6	52.2	53.8	55.3	56.9
365	16.6	18.1	19.7	21.3	22.8	24.4	25.9	27.5	29.1	30.6	32.2	33.8	35.3	36.9	38.4	40	41.6	43.1	44.7	46.3	47.8	49.4	50.9	52.5	54.1	55.6	57.2
368	16.8	18.3	19.9	21.4	23	24.6	26.2	27.7	29.3	30.8	32.4	33.9	35.5	37.1	38.6	40.2	41.8	43.3	44.9	46.4	48	49.6	51.1	52.7	54.3	55.8	57.4

Better ear

235	240	245	250	255	260	265	270	275	280	285	290	295	300	305	310	315	320	325	330	335	340	345	350	355	360	365	368
50.6																											
50.9	52.5																										
51.3	52.8	54.4																									
51.6	53.1	54.7	56.3																								
51.9	53.4	55	56.6	58.1																							
52.2	53.8	55.3	56.9	58.4	60																						
52.5	54.1	55.6	57.2	58.8	60.3	61.9																					
52.8	54.4	55.9	57.5	59.1	60.6	62.2	63.8																				
53.1	54.7	56.3	57.8	59.4	60.9	62.5	64.1	65.6																			
53.4	55	56.6	58.1	59.7	61.3	62.8	64.4	65.9	67.5																		
53.8	55.3	56.9	58.4	60	61.6	63.1	64.7	66.3	67.8	69.4																	
54.1	55.6	57.2	58.8	60.3	61.9	63.4	65	66.6	68.1	69.7	71.3																
54.4	55.9	57.5	59.1	60.6	62.2	63.8	65.3	66.9	68.4	70	71.6	73.1															
54.7	56.3	57.8	59.4	60.9	62.5	64.1	65.6	67.2	68.8	70.3	71.9	73.4	75														
55	56.6	58.1	59.7	61.3	62.8	64.4	65.9	67.5	69.1	70.6	72.2	73.8	75.3	76.9													
55.3	56.9	58.4	60	61.6	63.1	64.7	66.3	67.8	69.4	70.9	72.5	74.1	75.6	77.2	78.8												
55.6	57.2	58.8	60.3	61.9	63.4	65	66.6	68.1	69.7	71.3	72.8	74.4	75.9	77.5	79.1	80.6											
55.9	57.5	59.1	60.6	62.2	63.8	65.3	66.9	68.4	70	71.6	73.1	74.7	76.3	77.8	79.4	80.9	82.5										
56.3	57.8	59.4	60.9	62.5	64.1	65.6	67.2	68.8	70.3	71.9	73.4	75	76.6	78.1	79.7	81.3	82.8	84.4									
56.6	58.1	59.7	61.3	62.8	64.4	65.9	67.5	69.1	70.6	72.2	73.8	75.3	76.9	78.4	80	81.6	83.1	84.7	86.3								
56.9	58.4	60	61.6	63.1	64.7	66.3	67.8	69.4	70.9	72.5	74.1	75.6	77.2	78.8	80.3	81.9	83.4	85	86.6	88.1							
57.2	58.8	60.3	61.9	63.4	65	66.6	68.1	69.7	71.3	72.8	74.4	75.9	77.5	79.1	80.6	82.2	83.8	85.3	86.9	88.4	90						
57.5	59.1	60.6	62.2	63.8	65.3	66.9	68.4	70	71.6	73.1	74.7	76.3	77.8	79.4	80.9	82.5	84.1	85.6	87.2	88.8	90.3	91.9					
57.8	59.4	60.9	62.5	64.1	65.6	67.2	68.8	70.3	71.9	73.4	75	76.6	78.1	79.7	81.3	82.8	84.4	85.9	87.5	89.1	90.6	92.2	93.8				
58.1	59.7	61.3	62.8	64.4	65.9	67.5	69.1	70.6	72.2	73.8	75.3	76.9	78.4	80	81.6	83.1	84.7	86.3	87.8	89.4	90.9	92.5	94.1	95.6			
58.4	60	61.6	63.1	64.7	66.3	67.8	69.4	70.9	72.5	74.1	75.6	77.2	78.8	80.3	81.9	83.4	85	86.6	88.1	89.7	91.3	92.8	94.4	95.9	97.5		
58.8	60.3	61.9	63.4	65	66.6	68.1	69.7	71.3	72.8	74.4	75.9	77.5	79.1	80.6	82.2	83.8	85.3	86.9	88.4	90	91.6	93.1	94.7	96.3	97.6	99.4	
58.9	60.5	62.1	63.6	65.2	66.8	68.3	69.9	71.4	73	74.6	76.1	77.7	79.3	80.8	82.4	83.9	85.5	87.1	88.6	90.2	91.8	93.3	94.9	96.4	98	99.6	100

*The axes are the sum of hearing levels at 500, 1000, 2000, and 3000 Hz. The sum for the worse ear is read at the side; the sum for the better ear is read at the bottom. At the intersection of the row for the worse ear and the column for the better ear is the hearing impairment (%).

Table 3. Relationship of Binaural Hearing Impairment to Impairment of the Whole Person.

% Binaural hearing impairment	% Impairment of the whole person	% Binaural hearing impairment	% Impairment of the whole person
0 - 1.7	0	50.0 - 53.1	18
1.8 - 4.2	1	54.2 - 55.7	19
4.3 - 7.4	2	55.8 - 58.8	20
7.5 - 9.9	3	58.9 - 61.4	21
10.0 - 13.1	4	61.5 - 64.5	22
13.2 - 15.9	5	64.6 - 67.1	23
16.0 - 18.8	6	67.2 - 70.0	24
18.9 - 21.4	7	70.1 - 72.8	25
21.5 - 24.5	8	72.9 - 75.9	26
24.6 - 27.1	9	76.0 - 78.5	27
27.2 - 30.0	10	78.6 - 81.7	28
30.1 - 32.8	11	81.8 - 84.2	29
32.9 - 35.9	12	84.3 - 87.4	30
36.0 - 38.5	13	87.5 - 89.9	31
38.6 - 41.7	14	90.0 - 93.1	32
41.8 - 44.2	15	93.2 - 95.7	33
44.3 - 47.4	16	95.8 - 98.8	34
47.5 - 49.9	17	98.9 -100.0	35

9.1c Equilibrium

Equilibrium, or orientation in space, is maintained by the visual, kinesthetic, and vestibular mechanisms.

Vertigo, or vestibular dysequilibrium, is a sense of movement that is perceived by the patient as "subjective," in the case of movement of self, or as "objective," in the case of movement of the environment. The movements may be described as a sense of spinning, pushing or pulling, or tilting of the visual environment with a change of head position.

Disturbances of equilibrium may be classified as follows: (1) abnormalities of gait not associated with vertigo; (2) giddiness or "lightheadedness" that is distinguished from vertigo by the absence of feelings of movement; and (3) vertigo that is produced by disorders of the vestibular mechanism and its central nervous system components, including the cerebral cortex, cerebellum, and brain stem, and by eye movements.

Permanent impairment may result from any disorder causing vertigo or disorientation in space. Three regulatory systems, ocular (visual), kinesthetic (proprioceptive), and vestibular are related to the vestibulo-ocular reflex. The evaluation of impairments of equilibrium may include consideration of one or more of these mechanisms.

Vestibular System

Permanent impairment can result from defects of the vestibular (labyrinthine) mechanism and its central connections. The defects are evidenced by loss of equilibrium produced by (1) loss of vestibular function or (2) disturbances of vestibular function.

Complete loss of vestibular function may be unilateral or bilateral. When the loss is unilateral, adequate central nervous system compensation may or may not occur. With total bilateral loss of vestibular function, equilibrium is totally dependent on the kinesthetic and visual systems, which usually are unable to compensate fully for movement or ambulation. Depending on the extent of adjustment, the percentage of permanent impairment of the whole person may range from 0% to 95%.

Disturbances of vestibular function are evidenced by vertigo (vestibular dysequilibrium) as defined above. Lightheadedness and abnormalities of gait *not* associated with vertigo are *not* defined here as being disturbances of vestibular function.

Vertigo may be accompanied by varying degrees of nausea, vomiting, headache, immobility, ataxia, and nystagmus. Movement may increase the vertigo and the accompanying signs and symptoms. Peripheral vestibular (labyrinthine) disorders are often associated with hearing loss and tinnitus. Vestibular disorders may result in temporary or permanent impairments. Evaluation of vestibular impairment should be performed when the condition is stable and maximum adjustment has been achieved, which generally is considered to occur months after resolution of the disease or injury.

For evaluation of those patients with permanent disturbances of the vestibular mechanism, the following classification has been developed. The various classes provide a means by which a physician can correlate the patient's residual capacity for the usual activities of daily living and the extent of the patient's permanent impairment. Use of this classification presupposes that the physician has established a firm diagnosis based on a carefully obtained history, thorough examination, and the use of appropriate objective tests, supplemented by sound clinical judgment. Vestibular disorders cause a dynamic set of signs and symptoms subject to peripheral nervous system and central nervous system compensatory mechanisms; therefore, final conclusions as to permanent impairment should be based on determination of the patient's condition after it is stable.

Criteria of Vestibular Impairment

Class 1: Impairment of the Whole Person, 0%.
A patient belongs in class 1 when (a) signs of vestibular dysequilibrium are present without supporting objective findings *and* (b) the usual activities of daily living can be performed without assistance.

Class 2: Impairment of the Whole Person, 1% to 10%. A patient belongs in class 2 when (a) signs of dysequilibrium are present with supporting objective findings *and* (b) the usual activities of daily living are performed without assistance, except for complex activities such as bicycle riding or certain types of demanding activities related to the patient's work, such as walking on girders or scaffolds.

Class 3: Impairment of the Whole Person, 10% to 30%. A patient belongs in class 3 when (a) signs of vestibular dysequilibrium are present with supporting objective findings *and* (b) the patient's usual activities of daily living cannot be performed without assistance, except for such simple activities as self-care, some household duties, walking, and riding in a motor vehicle operated by another person.

Class 4: Impairment of the Whole Person, 30% to 60%. A patient belongs in class 4 when (a) signs of vestibular dysequilibrium are present with supporting objective findings *and* (b) the activities of daily living cannot be performed without assistance, except for self-care.

Class 5: Impairment of the Whole Person, 60% to 95%. A patient belongs in class 5 when (a) signs of vestibular dysequilibrium are present with supporting objective findings *and* (b) the usual activities of daily living cannot be performed without assistance, except for self-care not requiring ambulation, *and* (c) confinement to the home or premises is necessary.

9.2 The Face

The face and its parts and structural components serve multiple functions. The portal for deglutition is the mouth and lips. Disturbances in function can result in drooling or inability to contain food or liquid while eating. The lips and mouth also serve in vocal articulation, adding intelligibility to speech. The nose and mouth are the portals of entry for respiration. Impairment may be a result of neurologic disorders, such as partial or complete paralysis of the lips; scar formation and contracture of the lips; or loss of tissue.

The skin of the face has varied functions, such as covering the body and acting as a physical barrier, resisting trauma, providing sensory perception, and regulating temperature and body fluids. More specific protective functions include covering the eye and its contents with the eyelid.

The face has a unique role in communication. No other part of the body serves as specific a function for personal identity and for the expression of thought and emotion. Facial expressions are an integral part of normal living postures. A degree of normalcy is needed for effective verbal and nonverbal communication. Facial anatomy contributes to identity, expression, and normal functioning and to the appearance of the forehead and cheeks; eyes, eyelids, and brows; lips and mouth; nose; and chin and neck.

In evaluation of permanent impairment from a disorder of the face, functional capacity as well as structural integrity should be considered. This section deals with permanent impairment as it relates only to the face's structural integrity. For loss of function involving other aspects of the functioning of the face, the reader should refer to the specific organ system involved. Loss of structural integrity can result from cutaneous disfigurement, such as that due to abnormal pigmentation or scars, or from loss of supporting structures, such as soft tissue, bone, or cartilage of the facial skeleton. Other information on cutaneous disfigurement appears in the chapter on the skin.

Criteria for Facial Impairment

Class 1: Impairment of the Whole Person, 0% to 5%. A patient belongs in class 1 when the facial abnormality is limited to a disorder of the cutaneous structures, such as visible scars or abnormal pigmentation. For other criteria, the reader may refer to Chapter 13 on the skin.

Class 2: Impairment of the Whole Person, 5% to 10%. A patient belongs in class 2 when there is loss of supporting structure of part of the face, with or without a cutaneous disorder. Depressed cheek, nasal, or frontal bones constitute class 2 impairments.

Class 3: Impairment of the Whole Person, 10% to 15%. A patient belongs in class 3 when there is absence of a normal anatomic part or area of the face. Loss of an eye, which should be evaluated as indicated in Chapter 8, or loss of part of the nose with the resulting cosmetic deformity, constitutes a class 3 impairment. Such impairments may be associated with impairments of other organ systems, for instance the visual system (Chapter 8) or the respiratory system (Chapter 5).

Class 4: Impairment of the Whole Person, 15% to 35%. A patient belongs in class 4 when facial disfigurement is so severe that it precludes social acceptance. Massive distortion of normal facial anatomy constitutes a class 4 impairment. The reader may refer to the chapter on skin impairments (p. 277) and to the chapter on mental and behavioral disorders (p. 291).

Facial Disfigurement

The face is such a prominent feature that it plays a critical role in the individual's physical, psychological, and emotional makeup. Facial disfigurement can affect all of these components and can result in social and vocational handicaps and even psychiatric impairment.

Disfigurement of the face can result from many causes, particularly burns, traumatic injury, surgery, infections, or dysplasia. Effects on individuals can vary tremendously. We recommend that "total disfigurement of the face" after treatment be deemed a 15% to 35% impairment of the whole person. For the assessment of impairment related to mental and behavioral aspects of disfigurement, the reader may refer to the chapter on mental and behavioral disorders (p. 291).

Facial disfigurement may be considered total if it is severe and grossly deforming of the face and features. Such disfigurement must involve at least the entire area between the brow line and the upper lip on both sides. Severe disfigurement above the brow line should be deemed to be, at a maximum, 1% impairment of the whole person. If disfigurement is severe below the upper lip, it may be deemed to be an 8% whole-person impairment. Specific, prominent facial disfigurements are estimated as shown in Table 4 (below).

Table 4. Facial Disfigurement and Impairments.*

Disfigurement	% Impairment of the whole person
Unilateral total facial paralysis	
Mild	1 - 4
Severe	5 - 19
Bilateral total facial paralysis	
Mild	5 - 19
Severe	20 - 45
Loss or deformity of outer ear	0 - 5
Loss of entire nose	25 - 50
Nasal distortion in physical appearance	0 - 5

*With these guidelines, reasonable impairment values can be placed on other facial disfigurements.

9.3 The Nose, Throat, and Related Structures

The nose, throat, and related structures include the following:

1. **The nasal region:** This consists of the external part of the nose, the nasal cavity, and the nasopharynx.

2. **The oral region:** This consists of the mouth and lips, teeth, temporomandibular joint, tongue, hard and soft palate, region of the palatine tonsil, and oropharynx.

3. **The neck and chest region:** This consists of the hypopharynx, larynx, trachea, esophagus, and bronchi.

The functions of these structures, and the order in which they will be discussed, are as follows: (1) respiration; (2) mastication and deglutition; (3) olfaction and taste; and (4) speech. Permanent impairment may result from a deviation from normal in any of the above functions, and, because of their close relationship, more than one structure may be involved.

9.3a Respiration

Respiration may be defined as the act or function of breathing, that is, the act by which air is inspired and expired from the lungs. The respiratory mechanism includes the lungs and the air passages; the latter includes the nares, nasal cavities, mouth, pharynx, larynx, trachea, and bronchi.

In this chapter, discussion of permanent impairments related to respiration is limited to defects of the air passages. The reader is referred to the chapter on the respiratory system (p. 153) for a discussion of impairments of the lower airways and lung parenchyma.

The most commonly encountered defect of the air passages is obstruction, which may be partial, as with stenosis, or complete, as with occlusion. Obstructions and other air passage defects are evidenced primarily by dyspnea or so-called unusual breathlessness. The "sleep apnea syndrome," which is considered in the chapter on respiratory impairments (p. 153), may be related to functional upper-airway obstruction.

Dyspnea is a cardinal factor that contributes to a patient's diminished capacity to carry out activities of daily living and to permanent impairment. This subjective complaint or symptom, which indicates an awareness of respiratory distress, usually is noted first and is most severe during exercise. When dyspnea occurs at rest, respiratory dysfunction probably is severe. Dyspnea may or may not be accompanied by related signs or symptoms.

Patients with air passage defects may be evaluated in accordance with the classification in Table 5 (p. 231). Permanent impairments involving obstructive sleep apnea should be evaluated with the criteria described in the chapter on the respiratory system (p. 153).

Table 5. Classes of Air Passage Defects.

Class 1: **0%-10% impairment of the whole person**	**Class 2:** **11%-29% impairment of the whole person***	**Class 3:** **30%-49% impairment of the whole person**	**Class 4:** **50%-89% impairment of the whole person**	**Class 5:** **90%+ impairment of the whole person**
A recognized air passage defect exists.	A recognized air passage defect exists.	A recognized air passage defect exists.	A recognized air passage defect exists.	A recognized air passage defect exists.
Dyspnea does *not* occur at rest.	Dyspnea does *not* occur at rest.	Dyspnea does *not* occur at rest.	Dyspnea occurs at rest, although patient is not necessarily bedridden.	Severe dyspnea occurs at rest; spontaneous respiration is inadequate. Respiratory ventilation is required.
Dyspnea *is not* produced by walking or climbing stairs freely, performance of other usual activities of daily living, stress, prolonged exertion, hurrying, hill climbing, recreation† requiring intensive effort, or similar activity.	Dyspnea *is not* produced by walking freely on the level, climbing at least one flight of ordinary stairs, or the performance of other usual activities of daily living. Dyspnea *is* produced by stress, prolonged exertion, hurrying, hill climbing, recreation except sedentary forms, or similar activity.	Dyspnea *is* produced by walking more than one or two blocks on the level or climbing one flight of ordinary stairs even with periods of rest; performance of other usual activities of daily living, stress, hurrying, hill climbing, recreation, or similar activity.	Dyspnea is aggravated by the performance of any of the usual activities of daily living beyond personal cleansing, dressing, grooming, or its equivalent.	
Examination reveals one or more of the following: partial obstruction of oropharynx, laryngopharynx, larynx, upper trachea (to fourth ring), lower trachea, bronchi, or complete obstruction of the nose (bilateral) or nasopharynx.	Examination reveals one or more of the following: partial obstruction of oropharynx, laryngopharynx, larynx, upper trachea (to fourth ring), lower trachea, bronchi, or complete obstruction of the nose (bilateral) or nasopharynx.	Examination reveals one or more of the following: partial obstruction of oropharynx, laryngopharynx, larynx, upper trachea (to fourth ring), lower trachea, or bronchi.	Examination reveals one or more of the following: partial obstruction of oropharynx, laryngopharynx, larynx, upper trachea (to fourth ring), lower trachea, or bronchi.	Examination shows partial obstruction of the oropharynx, laryngopharynx, larynx, upper trachea (to fourth ring), lower trachea, or bronchi.

*Patients with successful permanent tracheostomy or stoma should be rated at 25% impairment of the whole person.
†Prophylactic restriction of activity, such as strenuous competitive sport, does not exclude patient from class 1.

9.3b Mastication and Deglutition

The act of eating includes mastication and deglutition. Numerous conditions of nongastrointestinal origin, singly or in combination, may interfere with these functions.

Dysfunction of the temporomandibular joint may impede mastication, affect speech, cause lower facial deformity, and produce pain.[4-6] In this section, the effect of temporomandibular joint dysfunction on eating is considered; other effects may be considered in conjunction with parts of the *Guides* that deal with the nervous system or pain.

In accordance with the philosophy of the *Guides*, when mastication and deglutition are evaluated, the ability to eat should be stable and maximal rehabilitation should have been achieved. When mastication or deglutition is impaired, the imposition of dietary restrictions usually results. Such restrictions are the most objective criteria by which to evaluate permanent impairment of these functions. The relationship of the restrictions to impairments of mastication and deglutition are shown in Table 6 (at right).

Table 6. Relationship of Dietary Restrictions to Permanent Impairment.

Type of restriction	**% Impairment of the whole person**
Diet is limited to semisolid or soft foods	5 - 19
Diet is limited to liquid foods	20 - 39
Ingestion of food requires tube feeding or gastrostomy	40 - 60

9.3c Olfaction and Taste

Only rarely does complete loss of the closely related senses of olfaction and taste seriously affect an individual's performance of the usual activities of daily living. The rare case almost invariably involves occupational considerations and disabilities that are outside the scope of a physician's responsibility in the evaluation of permanent impairment.

For this reason, a single value of 3% impairment of the whole person is suggested for use in cases involving complete bilateral loss of either sense due to peripheral lesions. This value is to be *combined* with any other impairment of the patient by means of the Combined Values Chart (p. 322).

Detection by the patient of any odor or taste, even though he or she cannot name it, precludes a finding of permanent impairment.

9.3d Speech

In this chapter, speech is defined as the capacity to produce vocal signals that can be heard, understood, and sustained over a useful period of time. Speech ought to allow effective communication in the activities of daily living.

This chapter does not consider the causes and characteristics of abnormal speech. Rather, it considers how an impairment relates to the individual's ability or efficiency in using speech to make himself or herself understood in daily living activities. It is assumed that speech evaluation pertains to the production of voice and articulate speech and not to the language content or structure of the patient's communication. On the basis of these assumptions, the primary problem is estimating proficiency in the use of oral language or measuring the utility of speech as defined above. This section also considers esophageal speech.

At this time there is no single, acceptable, proven test that will measure objectively the degrees of impairment from the many varieties of speech disorders. Therefore, it is recommended that speech impairment be evaluated by examining the audibility, intelligibility, and functional efficiency of speech.

Audibility is based on the patient's ability to speak at a level sufficient to be heard. Intelligibility is based on the ability to articulate and to link phonetic units of speech with sufficient accuracy to be understood. Functional efficiency is based on the ability to produce a satisfactorily rapid rate of speaking and to sustain this rate over a useful period of time.

Other definable attributes of speech, such as voice quality, pitch, and melodic variation, are not evaluated except as they affect one of the three primary characteristics noted above.

A classification chart, oral reading paragraph, and examining procedures for use in estimating speech impairment are described below.

Classification Chart

Judgments as to the amount of impairment should be made with reference to the classes, percentages, and examples provided in the classification chart (Table 7, p. 233). The 15 categories in the chart suggest activities or situations with different levels of impairment. Data gathered from direct observation of the patient or from interviews should be compared with these categories, and values should be assigned on the basis of the specific impairments that are present.

Oral Reading Paragraph

The paragraph of 100 words entitled "The Smith House," which is composed of 10 sentences, provides a uniform means of comparing a speech sample of the patient with the performance of normal speakers (Table 8, p. 233). The phonetic elements of the paragraph are selected particularly for their relevance to the intelligibility of the patient's speech.

Examining Procedure

1. General Orientation

The examining physician should have normal hearing as defined in the earlier section in this chapter on hearing.

The setting of the examination should be a reasonably quiet room that approximates the noise level conditions of everyday living.

The examiner should base judgments of impairment on two kinds of evidence: (a) attention to and observation of the patient's speech in the office, for example, during conversation, during the interview, and while reading and counting aloud; and (b) reports pertaining to the patient's performance in everyday living situations. The reports or the evidence should be supplied by reliable observers who know the patient well. The standard of evaluation is the normal speaker's performance in average situations of everyday living. It is assumed in this context that an average speaker can usually perform according to the following criteria:

(a) Patient can talk in a loud voice when the occasion demands it.

(b) Patient can sustain phonation for at least 10 seconds after one breath.

(c) Patient can complete at least a 10-word sentence in one breath.

(d) Patient can form all of the phonetic units of American speech and join them together intelligibly.

(e) Patient can maintain a speech rate of at least 75 to 100 words per minute and sustain a flow of speech for a reasonable length of time. A speech rate of 125 words per minute enables a speaker to read about one 8½ x 11-inch page of double-spaced text in 2 minutes.

Table 7. Speech Impairment Criteria.

Classification	Audibility	Intelligibility	Functional efficiency
Class 1 0%-14% speech impairment	Can produce speech of intensity sufficient for *most* of the needs of everyday speech communication, although this sometimes may require effort and occasionally may be beyond patient's capacity.	Can perform *most* of the articulatory acts necessary for everyday speech communication, although listeners occasionally ask the patient to repeat, and the patient may find it difficult or impossible to produce a few phonetic units.	Can meet *most* of the demands of articulation and phonation for everyday speech communication with adequate speed and ease, although occasionally the patient may hesitate or speak slowly.
Class 2 15%-34% speech impairment	Can produce speech of intensity sufficient for *many* of the needs of everyday speech communication; is usually heard under average conditions; however, may have difficulty in automobiles, buses, trains, stations, restaurants, etc.	Can perform *many* of the necessary articulatory acts for everyday speech communication. Can speak name, address, etc. and be understood by a stranger, but may have numerous inaccuracies; sometimes appears to have difficulty articulating.	Can meet *many* of the demands of articulation and phonation for everyday speech communication with adequate speed and ease, but sometimes gives impression of difficulty, and speech may sometimes be discontinuous, interrupted, hesitant, or slow.
Class 3 35%-59% speech impairment	Can produce speech of intensity sufficient for *some* of the needs of everyday speech communication, such as close conversation; however, has considerable difficulty in such noisy places as listed above; the voice tires rapidly and tends to become inaudible after a few seconds.	Can perform *some* of the necessary articulatory acts for everyday speech communication; can usually converse with family and friends; however, strangers may find it difficult to understand the patient, who often may be asked to repeat.	Can meet *some* of the demands of articulation and phonation for everyday speech communication with adequate speed and ease, but often can sustain consecutive speech only for brief periods; may give the impression of being rapidly fatigued.
Class 4 60%-84% speech impairment	Can produce speech of intensity sufficient for *a few* of the needs of everyday speech communication; can barely be heard by a close listener or over the telephone, perhaps may be able to whisper audibly but has no louder voice.	Can perform a *few* of the necessary articulatory acts for everyday speech communication; can produce some phonetic units; may have approximations for a few words such as names of own family members; however, unintelligible out of context.	Can meet a *few* of the demands of articulation and phonation for everyday speech communication with adequate speed and ease, such as single words or short phrases, but cannot maintain uninterrupted speech flow; speech is labored, rate is impractically slow.
Class 5 85%-100% speech impairment	Can produce speech of intensity sufficient for *none* of the needs of everyday speech communication.	Can perform *none* of the articulatory acts necessary for everyday speech communication.	Can meet *none* of the demands of articulation and phonation for everyday speech communication with adequate speed and ease.

Table 8. Test Oral Reading Paragraph: The Smith House.

Larry and Ruth Smith have been married nearly 14 years. They have a small place near Long Lake. Both of them think there's nothing like the country for health. Their two boys would rather live here than any other place. Larry likes to keep some saddle horses close to the house. These make it easy to keep his sons amused. If they wish, the boys can go fishing along the shore. When it rains, they usually want to watch television. Ruth has a cherry tree on each side of the kitchen door. In June they enjoy the juice and jelly.

2. Specific Instructions

(a) Place the patient approximately 8 ft from the examiner.

(b) Interview the patient. This will permit observation of the patient's speech in ordinary conversation while pertinent historical information is obtained.

(c) Listen to the patient's speech as the patient reads aloud the short paragraph, "The Smith House" (Table 8, at left). For this exercise, have the patient's back toward the examiner, maintaining a separation of 8 ft.

Instruct the patient as follows: "You are to read this passage so I can hear you plainly. Be sure to speak so I can understand you."

(d) If additional reading procedures are required, simple prose paragraphs from a magazine may be used. A person who cannot read may be requested to give his or her name and address and name all the days of the week and months of the year. Additional evidence regarding the patient's rate of speech and ability to sustain it may be obtained by noting the time required to count to 100 by ones. Completion of this task in 60 to 75 seconds is accepted as normal.

(e) Record judgment of the patient's speech capacity with regard to each of the three columns of the classification chart (Table 7, above).

(f) The degree of impairment of speech is equivalent to the greatest percentage of impairment recorded in any one of the three columns of the classification chart.

For example, a patient's speech capacity is judged to be the following: audibility, 10% (class 1); intelligibility, 50% (class 3); and functional efficiency, 30% (class 2). The patient's speech impairment is judged to be equivalent to the greatest impairment, 50%.

According to Table 9 (below), an impairment of speech of 50% is judged to be an 18% impairment of the whole person.

Table 9. Speech Impairment Related to Impairment of the Whole Person.

% Speech impairment	% Impairment of the whole person	% Speech impairment	% Impairment of the whole person
0	0	50	18
5	2	55	19
10	4	60	21
15	5	65	23
20	7	70	24
25	9	75	26
30	10	80	28
35	12	85	30
40	14	90	32
45	16	95	33
		100	35

References

1. Noble WG. *Assessment of Hearing Loss and Handicap in Adults.* New York, NY: Academic Press; 1978.

2. American Academy of Otolaryngology Committee on Hearing and Equilibrium, and American Council of Otolaryngology Committee on the Medical Aspects of Noise. Guide for the evaluation of hearing handicap. *JAMA*. 1979;241:2055-2059.

3. American National Standards Institute. Specifications for Audiometers: *ANSI Standards* S3.6-1989. New York, NY: American National Standards Institute; 1989.

4. Kaplan AS, Assael LA, eds. *Temporomandibular Disorders: Diagnosis and Treatment.* Philadelphia, Pa: WB Saunders Co; 1991.

5. McNeil C, Rugh JD. Temporomandibular disorders: diagnosis, management, education, and reasearch. *J Am Dent Assoc.*1990;120:253-263.

6. Wilkes CH. Internal derangements of the temporomandibular joint: pathological variations. *Arch Otolaryngol Head Neck Surg.* 1989;115:469-477.

Chapter 10

The Digestive System

The purpose of this chapter is to provide criteria for evaluating permanent impairments of the digestive system. The digestive system includes the alimentary canal, liver, biliary tract, and pancreas. The oral cavity and pharynx are considered in the *Guides* chapter on the ear, nose, throat, and related structures. The impairments are expressed as estimates of the extent to which they hamper an individual's activities of daily living. The permanent impairments are evidenced by clinically established or objectively determined deviations from normal in the transport and assimilation of ingested food, the metabolism of nutrition, or the excretion of waste products.

Before using the information in this chapter, the reader is urged to review Chapters 1 and 2, which discuss the purposes of the *Guides* and the situations in which they are useful. Chapters 1 and 2 also discuss methods for examining patients and preparing reports. A medical evaluation report should include information such as that outlined below.

A. Medical Evaluation
- History of medical condition(s)
- Results of most recent clinical evaluation
- Assessment of current clinical status and statement of further medical plans
- Diagnosis

B. Analysis of Findings
- Impact of medical condition on life activities
- Explanation for concluding that the condition is stable, unlikely to change, and not amenable to further medical therapy
- Explanation for concluding that the individual is or is not likely to suffer further impairment by engaging in usual activities
- Explanation for concluding that accommodations or restrictions are or are not warranted

C. Comparison of Analysis with Impairment Criteria
- Description of clinical findings and how these findings relate to specific criteria
- Explanation of each impairment estimate
- Summary of impairment estimates
- Overall estimate of whole-person impairment

10.1 Desirable Weight

For the purpose of determining impairment resulting from digestive disorders, "desirable" weight may be defined as follows.

1. If the examiner is able to determine by history or from previous medical records a weight before onset of the patient's digestive disorder that the patient considers "usual and customary," the examiner should use that weight as the "desirable" weight from which any deviation is measured.

2. If the examiner is not able to determine by history or previous medical records a "usual and customary" weight that predated impairment, then the examiner should refer to a table of "desirable" weights and calculate deviations from the lower end of the table's range of desirable weights corresponding to the patient's sex, height, and body build.

Table 1 (p. 237) is recommended as a guide. Recently Willett et al[1] described a table of suggested weights for adults published by the US Department of Agriculture and the US Department of Health and Human Services. They criticized the table as being liberal in weight allowances.

For an obese person, the usual preimpairment weight may not be as physiologically desirable as the current weight. Thus, the examiner should use judgment in assessing the relative importance of weight loss.

10.2 Esophagus

Symptoms and signs of impairment include dysphagia, pyrosis or "heartburn," retrosternal pain, regurgitation, bleeding, and weight loss. One should be mindful that occasional, minor dyspepsia, "gas," and belching are within the experience of all normal persons.

Objective procedures useful in establishing esophageal impairment include, but are not limited to (1) imaging procedures, such as fluoroscopy and radiography employing contrast media, and computed tomography; (2) peroral endoscopy including cytologic study or biopsy; and (3) functional tests, such as manometry or measurement of intraesophageal pH.

The criteria for evaluating permanent impairment of esophageal function are those listed in Table 2 (p. 239).

Class 1: Impairment of the Whole Person, 0% to 10%

Example: A 44-year-old machinist complained of transient difficulty in swallowing, which had first occurred 9 months earlier while he was eating broiled lobster. Currently, symptoms referable to esophageal disease could not be elicited. His weight of 68.1 kg (150 lb) was within desirable limits for the man's height of 1.78 m (5 ft 10 in).

The man appeared healthy. His vital signs and results of physical examination were normal. A chest roentgenogram and electrocardiogram were normal. Barium swallow revealed a small, sliding hiatal hernia. Endoscopy disclosed no mucosal defect.

Diagnosis: Hiatal hernia, uncomplicated.

Impairment: 0% impairment of the whole person.

Comment: The symptoms are indicative of esophageal motor disorder, and a hiatal hernia is present, but these have not interfered with normal nutrition, nor have they impaired the man's ability to perform usual daily activities.

Class 2: Impairment of the Whole Person, 10% to 25%

Example: A 59-year-old woman, formerly employed as a nurse's aide, complained of having had almost daily retrosternal pain associated with difficult swallowing for 5 years. Her symptoms were less severe when she limited her diet to soft foods and were aggravated when she became upset, particularly at items of worry over the status of her husband, who was an invalid.

Physical examination showed a woman 1.7 m (5 ft 7 in) tall, of medium frame, who appeared older than her stated age. She weighed 53.6 kg (118 lb), which was within 10% of her usual weight of 58 kg (128 lb). Her blood pressure was 145/90 mm Hg. A chest roentgenogram and electrocardiogram were normal. Roentgenographic studies of the upper gastrointestinal tract showed a "corkscrew" configuration or "curling" of the esophagus, indicative of diffuse spasm. This diagnosis was confirmed by esophageal manometry. No mucosal defect was evident by endoscopy.

Diagnosis: Diffuse spasm of the esophagus.

Impairment: 15% impairment of the whole person.

Comment: The patient's symptoms were persistent, and she was obliged to restrict her diet. Her weight loss did not exceed 10% of the desirable level, and she was restrained only slightly in her daily activities.

Table 1. Desirable Weights by Sex, Height, and Body Build
(Indoor clothing weighing 2.3 kg [5 lb] for men and 1.4 kg [3 lb] for women; and shoes with 2.5-cm [1-in] heels).*

Men

Height in (cm)	Weight, lb (kg)		
	Small frame	Medium frame	Large frame
62(157)	128-134(58.0-60.7)	131-141(59.2-63.9)	138-150(62.5-67.8)
63(160)	130-136(59.0-61.7)	133-143(60.3-64.9)	140-153(63.5-69.4)
64(163)	132-138(60.0-62.7)	135-145(61.3-66.0)	142-156(64.5-71.1)
65(165)	134-140(60.8-63.5)	137-148(62.1-67.0)	144-160(65.3-72.5)
66(168)	136-142(61.8-64.6)	139-151(63.2-68.7)	146-164(66.4-74.7)
67(170)	138-145(62.5-65.7)	142-154(64.3-69.8)	149-168(67.5-76.1)
68(173)	140-148(63.6-67.3)	145-157(65.9-71.4)	152-172(69.1-78.2)
69(175)	142-151(64.3-68.3)	148-160(66.9-72.4)	155-176(70.1-79.6)
70(178)	144-154(65.4-70.0)	151-163(68.6-74.0)	158-180(71.8-81.8)
71(180)	146-157(66.1-71.0)	154-166(69.7-75.1)	161-184(72.8-83.3)
72(183)	149-160(67.7-72.7)	157-170(71.3-77.2)	164-188(74.5-85.4)
73(185)	152-164(68.7-74.1)	160-174(72.4-78.6)	168-192(75.9-86.8)
74(188)	155-168(70.3-76.2)	164-178(74.4-80.7)	172-197(78.0-89.4)
75(190)	158-172(71.4-77.6)	167-182(75.4-82.2)	176-202(79.4-91.2)
76(193)	162-176(73.5-79.8)	171-187(77.6-84.8)	181-207(82.1-93.9)

Women

Height in (cm)	Weight, lb (kg)		
	Small frame	Medium frame	Large frame
58(147)	102-111(46.2-50.2)	109-121(49.3-54.7)	118-131(53.3-59.3)
59(150)	103-113(46.7-51.3)	111-123(50.3-55.9)	120-134(54.4-60.9)
60(152)	104-115(47.1-52.1)	113-126(51.1-57.0)	122-137(55.2-61.9)
61(155)	106-118(48.1-53.6)	115-129(52.2-58.6)	125-140(56.8-63.6)
62(157)	108-121(48.8-54.6)	118-132(53.2-59.6)	128-143(57.8-64.6)
63(160)	111-124(50.3-56.2)	121-135(54.9-61.2)	131-147(59.4-66.7)
64(163)	114-127(51.9-57.8)	124-138(56.4-62.8)	134-151(61.0-68.8)
65(165)	117-130(53.0-58.9)	127-141(57.5-63.9)	137-155(62.0-70.2)
66(168)	120-133(54.6-60.5)	130-144(59.2-65.5)	140-159(63.7-72.4)
67(170)	123-136(55.7-61.6)	133-147(60.2-66.6)	143-163(64.8-73.8)
68(173)	126-139(57.3-63.2)	136-150(61.8-68.2)	146-167(66.4-75.9)
69(175)	129-142(58.3-64.2)	139-153(62.8-69.2)	149-170(67.4-76.9)
70(178)	132-145(60.0-65.9)	142-156(64.5-70.9)	152-173(69.0-78.6)
71(180)	135-148(61.0-66.9)	145-159(65.6-71.9)	155-176(70.1-79.6)
72(183)	138-151(62.6-68.4)	148-162(67.0-73.4)	158-179(71.6-81.2)

*Source: 1979 Body Build Study, Society of Actuaries and Association of Life Insurance Medical Directors of America, 1980.
Copyright © 1983, The Metropolitan Life Insurance Company. Courtesy *Statistical Bulletin*, Metropolitan Life Insurance Company.

Class 3: Impairment of the Whole Person, 25% to 50%

Example: A 49-year-old automobile mechanic complained of intermittent retrosternal pain, dysphagia, and nocturnal regurgitation with an occasional and partial remission during the past 5 years. Pain had become a less prominent feature, but dysphagia had become more troublesome. The man could swallow solid foods only if he also drank large volumes of liquids. Before the onset of his illness, he had weighed 81.7 kg (180 lb); now he weighed 70.4 kg (155 lb).

A physical examination indicated evidence of weight loss. With his height of 1.88 m (6 ft 2 in), the man appeared lanky and gaunt. The vital signs were normal. A chest roentgenogram showed widening of the mediastinum but no densities in the lung fields that might indicate aspiration. A barium swallow demonstrated a markedly dilated and tortuous esophagus that terminated in a filiform constriction. Endoscopy showed no mucosal defect. Dilation of the lower esophageal sphincter by bougie or balloon provided partial, temporary relief of dysphagia and was required about twice a year.

Diagnosis: Achalasia of the esophagus.

Impairment: 30% impairment of the whole person.

Comment: The patient's symptoms were persistent and progressive despite dietary limitation and esophageal dilatation; weight loss exceeded 10% of the desirable level. The impairment might be lessened if the patient could be persuaded to undergo surgical esophagomyotomy.

Class 4: Impairment of the Whole Person, 50% to 75%

Example: A 58-year-old former accountant, 1.78 m (5 ft 10 in) in height, had almost complete esophageal obstruction. Five years earlier he had required extensive resection of the lower esophagus and proximal stomach because of cancer. Although there was no evidence of tumor recurrence, the man's ability to eat was severely restricted by early satiety, and his swallowing was impaired by stenosing esophagitis. Surgical correction was unsuccessful. Currently, a gastrostomy tube was used for feeding. While the patient previously maintained a weight of 68.1 kg (150 lb), he now weighed only 49.9 kg (110 lb). Dilation of the strictured esophagus was required about once a month to accommodate saliva secretions.

Diagnosis: Stenosing esophagitis.

Impairment: 65% impairment due to stenosing esophagitis and 15% impairment due to gastrostomy, which *combine* to give a 70% impairment of the whole person (Combined Values Chart, p. 322).

Comment: Symptoms and signs of disease have progressed despite exhaustive treatment, and further therapy can only be palliative. The man's weight loss has exceeded 20% of the desirable level. His prognosis is poor.

10.3 Stomach and Duodenum

Symptoms and signs of impairment include nausea, vomiting, pain, bleeding, obstruction, diarrhea, weight loss, certain types of malassimilation, such as defective digestion or absorption, and nutritional deficiencies that may include hematologic and neurologic manifestations.

Objective procedures useful in establishing impairment of the stomach and duodenum include, but are not limited to (1) imaging techniques, such as fluoroscopy and roentgenography with contrast media, scintigraphy, and computed tomography; (2) peroral endoscopy, with biopsy and cytologic study; (3) gastric secretory tests; (4) tests of assimilation; and (5) stool examination.

Criteria for evaluating permanent impairment consequent to disease or injury of the stomach or duodenum are those listed in Table 2 (p. 239).

Class 1: Impairment of the Whole Person, 0% to 10%

Example: A 28-year-old schoolteacher complained of having episodic epigastric pain and burning during a 5-year period. He denied nausea, vomiting, hematemesis, or melena. His height was 1.8 m (5 ft 11 in), and his weight was 72.6 kg (160 lb). Barium meal examination showed a deformed duodenal bulb; there was no evidence of gastric retention or pyloric stenosis. Peroral endoscopy revealed the scar of a healed ulcer on the posterior wall of the first portion of the duodenum.

Diagnosis: Duodenal ulcer in remission.

Impairment: 5% impairment of the whole person.

Comment: Symptoms have been remittent, and the disease has been uncomplicated. Dietary restriction has not usually been necessary. Desirable weight and normal activities have been maintained.

Class 2: Impairment of the Whole Person, 10% to 25%

Example: A slight, 40-year-old male clerk had had intermittent ulcer symptoms during a period of 10 years. Bleeding had occurred on three occasions; blood replacement was required twice. He had had one episode of transient pyloric obstruction. The man repeatedly refused to consider a surgical remedy. To maintain any degree of symptomatic remission, he required continuing medical therapy. His height was 1.78 m (5 ft 8 in), and his weight was 59 kg (130 lb), which was 7% below desirable his weight. Upper gastrointestinal tract roentgenograms showed a marked clover-leaf deformity of the duodenal bulb with a 3-mm ulcer fleck.

Diagnosis: Active duodenal ulcer with a history of recurring complications.

Impairment: 15% impairment of the whole person.

Comment: The disease has been complicated, and symptoms have recurred despite medical therapy. The patient's performance of daily activities has been interrupted repeatedly. The patient has adamantly declined surgery, which might lessen the impairing condition.

Class 3: Impairment of the Whole Person, 25% to 50%

Example: A 50-year-old woman, who was a librarian, had undergone resection of the stomach distally 2 years earlier to remove the focus of multiple, dysplastic, adenomatous polyps. She now complained of episodes of lightheadedness, sweating, and palpitation that occurred 15 minutes after meals. The symptoms could be avoided partially by dietary restriction and by lying down. Since the operation, the woman's weight had dropped to approximately 15% below her desirable weight.

Physical examination showed the patient's weight to be 45.4 kg (100 lb) and her height, 1.6 m (5 ft 3 in). She had a well-healed scar on the upper abdomen; otherwise, the results of physical examination were unremarkable. Upper gastrointestinal tract roentgenograms showed evidence of 70% gastric resection and a patent, undistorted gastrojejunostomy.

Diagnosis: Postgastrectomy dumping syndrome.

Impairment: 30% impairment of the whole person.

Comment: The patient had symptoms that interfered with performance of her normal activities, despite dietary restriction. She was unable to maintain her weight within 10% of the desirable level.

Class 4: Impairment of the Whole Person, 50% to 75%

Example: A 62-year-old journalist had required a total gastrectomy 3 years earlier for removal of stomach cancer. An esophagoenterostomy (Hunt-Lawrence pouch) was constructed. After the operation he complained of anorexia and early satiety, and he sustained unrelenting weight loss and developed signs of nutritional deficiency. He was unable to work except for brief periods.

A physical examination showed a malnourished man who appeared older than his stated age. He was 1.75 m (5 ft 9 in) tall and weighed 52.7 kg (116 lb).

Table 2. Classes of Impairment of the Upper Digestive Tract (Esophagus, Stomach and Duodenum, Small Intestine, and Pancreas).

Class 1: **0%-9% impairment of the whole person**	**Class 2:** **10%-24% impairment of the whole person**	**Class 3:** **25%-49% impairment of the whole person**	**Class 4:** **50%-75% impairment of the whole person**
Symptoms or signs of upper digestive tract disease are present, or there is anatomic loss or alteration;	Symptoms and signs of organic upper digestive tract disease are present, or there is anatomic loss or alteration;	Symptoms and signs of organic upper digestive tract disease are present, or there is anatomic loss or alteration;	Symptoms and signs of organic upper digestive tract disease are present, or there is anatomic loss or alteration;
and	**and**	**and**	**and**
Continuous treatment is not required;	Appropriate dietary restrictions and drugs are required for control of symptoms, signs, or nutritional deficiency;	Appropriate dietary restrictions and drugs do not completely control symptoms, signs, or nutritional state;	Symptoms are not controlled by treatment;
and	**and**	**or**	**or**
Weight can be maintained at desirable level*;	Loss of weight below "desirable weight"* does not exceed 10%.	There is 10%-20% loss of weight below "desirable weight"* that is ascribable to a disorder of upper digestive tract.	There is greater than 20% loss of weight below the "desirable weight"* that is ascribable to disorder of upper digestive tract.
or			
There are no sequelae after surgical procedures.			

*Refer to Table 1.

His tongue was smooth and glistening. No masses were palpated in the vicinity of a healed, upper abdominal scar. There was slight pedal edema. Laboratory tests showed anemia and hypoproteinemia. An intact esophagojejunostomy with no mucosal defect was evident by roentgenography.

Diagnosis: Postoperative absence of the stomach with esophagojejunal anastomosis; secondary nutritional deficiency.

Impairment: 60% impairment due to total gastrectomy, which should be *combined* with an appropriate estimate for anemia impairment (see *Guides* chapter on the hematopoietic system) to determine the impairment of the whole person.

Comment: The patient's weight loss exceeded 20% of the desirable level, and there was evidence of marked nutritional deficiency. The patient was unable to perform normal living activities, and there was little prospect that his impairment could be lessened.

10.4 Small Intestine

Symptoms and signs of impairment include abdominal pain, diarrhea, steatorrhea, bleeding, obstruction, and weight loss, which often are associated with general debility and other extraintestinal manifestations.

Objective procedures useful in establishing impairment of the small intestine include, but are not limited to (1) fluoroscopy and roentgenography employing contrast media; (2) peroral endoscopy and mucosal biopsy; and (3) measures of intestinal assimilation, for example, tests for fecal fat content and urinary d-xylose excretion, carbon 14 breath test, and Schilling test.

Criteria for evaluating permanent impairment of small-intestine function are those listed in Table 2 (above).

Class 1: Impairment of the Whole Person, 0% to 10%

Example: Ten years earlier, a 35-year-old attorney, whose usual weight before illness had been 72.6 kg (160 lb), had required an abdominal operation because of recurrent and protracted fever, abdominal pain, and distention. Approximately 30 cm of the terminal ileum had been resected and an ileoascending colostomy constructed. The histologic findings in the resected specimen had been consistent with regional enteritis (Crohn's disease).

There was no recurrence of symptoms. The patient maintained a weight of 70.3 kg (155 lb) on an unrestricted diet. He had two or three soft stools daily. Laboratory findings included a normal hemogram and blood chemistry panel. Roentgenograms of the remaining small intestine and the ileocolic anastomosis were unremarkable.

Diagnosis: Partial, distal ileal resection (Crohn's disease).

Diagnosis: Partial, distal ileal resection (Crohn's disease).

Impairment: 0% impairment.

Comment: There have been no symptoms suggesting recurrence of intestinal disease, and during the 10 years after his operation the patient required no therapy. He maintained a nearly desirable weight and easily performed his usual activities.

Class 2: Impairment of the Whole Person, 10% to 25%

Example: A 64-year-old commercial artist had noted the onset of diarrhea, weight loss, and vague abdominal distress 5 years earlier. A macrocytic anemia was found, and extensive diverticulosis of the small intestine was evident by barium meal examination. Before the onset of her illness, the patient had weighed 54.4 kg (120 lb); her height was 1.55 m (5 ft 1 in). All symptoms cleared when she was given oral tetracycline and parenteral cyanocobalamin (vitamin B_{12}).

Two years ago, the patient had experienced mild diarrhea during several weeks, which again subsided with a course of tetracycline. Roentgengraphic examination showed persistence of numerous diverticula in the small intestine, which were even more prominent in the jejunum.

At present, the patient's nutritional state was normal, and her weight was maintained at 49.9 kg (110 lb). She had no untoward symptoms, and she enjoyed a relatively unrestricted diet. She required periodic intramuscular injections of cyanocobalamin.

Diagnosis: Diverticulosis of the small intestine; overgrowth of enteric bacterial flora.

Impairment: 15% impairment due to diverticulosis of the small intestine, which should be combined with an appropriate impairment estimate for anemia (see *Guides* chapter on the hematopoietic system) to determine impairment of the whole person.

Comment: This patient could perform the activities of daily living and her weight was unimpaired, but she was dependent on continuing therapy.

Class 3: Impairment of the Whole Person, 25% to 50%

Example: A 38-year-old community college instructor, 1.6 m (5 ft 3 in) in height, suffered from recurring diarrhea and loss of stamina. His weight had dropped from 59 to 49.9 kg (130 to 110 lb) after partial resection, 3 years earlier, of the distal ileum, which showed evidence of regional enteritis. In ensuing years, the patient had several bouts of partial intestinal obstruction, each subsiding with supportive therapy. Surgical reintervention was not required. Dietary restriction, vitamin supplements, antidiarrheal agents, and occasional corticosteroid therapy were needed to help the patient sustain an adequate health state.

At present, roentgenograms of the small intestine showed segmental distortion consistent with recurrent inflammation and edema.

Diagnosis: Recurrent regional enteritis, with intestinal malabsorption and recurring obstruction after ileal resection.

Impairment: 40% impairment of the whole person.

Comment: This patient functioned only marginally; his nutritional state was impaired, and his weight deficit exceeded 10% of the desirable level despite dietary adjustment and medication.

Class 4: Impairment of the Whole Person, 50% to 75%

Example: A 35-year-old department store saleswoman had developed life-threatening volvulus 1 year earlier. A major portion of her small bowel had become entrapped in adhesions, the consequence of a previous operation. Extensive resection of incarcerated and strangulated intestine was required. She was dependent on continuous dietary control and nutritional supplements and was frequently obliged to take medication to alleviate abdominal pain and diarrhea. Dehydration and electrolyte depletion necessitated repeated hospitalization. Diminished stamina permitted her to perform only essential activities of daily living.

At present, the patient's weight was relatively stable at 39.5 kg (87 lb), whereas it should have been at least 57.6 kg (127 lb) for her height of 1.65 m (5 ft 5 in) and her medium body frame. Tests confirmed that her intestinal absorptive capacity was sharply reduced. Otherwise the results of examination and other studies were normal.

Diagnosis: Intestinal malabsorption due to extensive small-bowel resection.

Impairment: 75% impairment of the whole person.

Comment: The patient's nutritional status was severely impaired by an irreversible defect of the small intestine. Her weight loss exceeded 20% of the desirable level, and her performance of daily activities was markedly limited.

Table 3. Classes of Colonic and Rectal Impairment.

Class 1: **0%-9% impairment of the whole person**	**Class 2:** **10%-24% impairment of the whole person**	**Class 3:** **25%-39% impairment of the whole person**	**Class 4:** **40%-60% impairment of the whole person**
Signs and symptoms of colonic or rectal disease are infrequent and of brief duration;	There is objective evidence of colonic or rectal disease or anatomic loss or alteration;	There is objective evidence of colonic or rectal disease or anatomic loss or alteration;	There is objective evidence of colonic or rectal disease or anatomic loss or alteration;
	and	**and**	**and**
and	There are mild gastrointestinal symptoms with occasional disturbances of bowel function, accompanied by moderate pain;	There are moderate to severe exacerbations with disturbance of bowel habit, accompanied by periodic or continual pain;	There are persistent disturbances of bowel function present at rest with severe persistent pain;
	and	**and**	**and**
Limitation of activities, special diet, or medication is not required;	Minimal restriction of diet or mild symptomatic therapy may be necessary;	Restriction of activity, special diet, and drugs are required during attacks;	Complete limitation of activity, continued restriction of diet, and medication do not entirely control symptoms;
and	**and**	**and**	**and**
No systemic manifestations are present and weight and nutritional state can be maintained at desirable level;	No impairment of nutrition results.	There are constitutional manifestations (fever, anemia, or weight loss).	There are constitutional manifestations (fever, weight loss, or anemia) present;
or			**or**
There are no sequelae after surgical procedures.			There is no prolonged remission.

10.5 Colon, Rectum, and Anus

Symptoms and signs of impairment of the colon, rectum, and anus include abdominal, pelvic, or perineal pain, disordered bowel action, tenesmus, fecal incontinence, bleeding, suppuration, and the appearance of hemorrhoids, fissures, and fistulas; systemic manifestations may include fever, weight loss, debility, and anemia.

Objective procedures useful in establishing impairment of the colon, rectum, and anus include, but are not limited to, (1) digital and endoscopic examination, including anoscopy, proctoscopy, sigmoidoscopy, and colonoscopy; (2) biopsy; (3) fecal microscopy and culture; and (4) fluoroscopy and roentgenography employing contrast media.

Criteria for evaluating impairment in function of the colon and rectum are those listed in Table 3 (above).

Class 1: Impairment of the Whole Person, 0% to 10%

Example: A 50-year-old woman, a part-time social worker, enjoyed generally good health except for a tendency, of several years' duration, to have mildly erratic bowel action with alternating constipation and diarrhea. Stools, while varying in consistency, were never known to contain abnormal materials. Proctosigmoidoscopy showed clear mucosa; barium enema examination outlined a normal colon with several diverticula in the sigmoid segment and enteric muscle spasm.

Diagnosis: (1) Irritable bowel syndrome; (2) diverticulosis coli.

Impairment: 0% impairment.

Comment: The symptoms, while occasionally annoying, have not interfered with the patient's necessary activities. She needed to make only a minor dietary adjustment.

Class 2: Impairment of the Whole Person, 10% to 25%

Example: A 28-year-old graduate student and part-time teaching assistant had a 10-year history of recurring ulcerative colitis. During exacerbations, she was troubled by moderate abdominal distress, diarrhea, and passage of blood-tinged stools. Colonoscopy showed varying degrees of granularity and punctate friability in the rectosigmoid mucosa; the remainder of the colon appeared normal by endoscopy. The patient had no fever or anemia, nor did she ever require hospitalization. Her symptoms remitted in response to a moderately restricted diet, antidiarrheal medication, and avoidance of unduly strenuous activity.

Diagnosis: Idiopathic ulcerative colitis, mild, limited to the rectosigmoid segment.

Impairment: 15% impairment of the whole person.

Comment: The disease was remittent, and the symptoms only occasionally interfered with necessary activity; symptomatic and supportive therapy adequately controlled the disease.

Class 3: Impairment of the Whole Person, 25% to 40%

Example: A 35-year-old computer programmer had had Crohn's disease since age 19 years. He had been hospitalized on several occasions, requiring intensive therapy, including transfusion of packed red blood cells to correct anemia.

The man had recurring diarrhea associated with cramping abdominal pain and occasional perianal suppuration with draining fistulas. He declined elective proctocolectomy. He managed to continue in his sedentary occupation on a limited schedule, but his weight remained 20% or more below the desirable level.

An examination and other studies disclosed lesions of Crohn's disease affecting the perineum, rectum, several colon segments, and the terminal ileum.

Diagnosis: Chronic, recurrent enterocolitis (Crohn's disease).

Impairment: 35% impairment attributable to enterocolitis, which should be *combined* with an appropriate impairment estimate for anemia to determine impairment of the whole person (Combined Values Chart, p. 322).

Comment: The disease, while remitting occasionally, interfered with the patient's pursuit of usual activities, especially work activities. He will require continuing close observation and treatment. His nutritional status was impaired.

Class 4: Impairment of the Whole Person, 40% to 60%

Example: A 42-year-old woman, formerly a buyer for a large department store, had a 15-year history of chronic ulcerative colitis, which limited her activity and required intensive treatment including an occasional blood transfusion. The result was increasing debility and nutritional deficiency. As a further complication of her inflammatory bowel disease, the patient developed jaundice and hepatomegaly.

Extensive and severe involvement of the colon was evident by barium enema examination and by colonoscopy. Results of liver function tests were severely abnormal, and liver biopsy confirmed a nonsuppurative cholangitic cirrhosis. Fever, anemia, and jaundice persisted. The patient declined the option of liver transplantation. In the opinion of her physician, surgery could not be considered as a therapeutic option because of the patient's general debility and advanced, complicated disease.

Diagnosis: (1) Chronic ulcerative colitis, severe; (2) sclerosing cholangitis with cirrhosis.

Impairment: 60% impairment due to ulcerative colitis, which should be *combined* with appropriate impairment estimates for the liver disorder and anemia (Combined Values Chart, p. 322) to determine the total whole-person impairment.

Criteria for evaluating permanent impairment of the anus are listed in Table 4 (p. 243).

Class 1: Impairment of the Whole Person, 0% to 10%

Example: Five years earlier, a 45-year-old security guard had had an acute pararectal abscess drained surgically. An anal fistula resulted, with recurrent bouts of acute infection and intermittent drainage. One year later, a fistulectomy had been performed. Since then there had been no further infection or drainage, nor had regular bowel activity been disturbed.

A medical examination showed a well-healed anal scar with slight distortion of the anal orifice but no weakness of the anal sphincter.

Diagnosis: Healed anal fistula.

Impairment: 0% impairment.

Comment: This man had documented anal disease that was appropriately and successfully treated. His daily activities were not impaired.

Class 2: Impairment of the Whole Person, 10% to 20%

Example: A 32-year-old woman, employed from time to time in a florist's shop, had had Crohn's colitis for 14 years, which usually was well controlled by medical therapy. However, during one exacerbation, a pararectal abscess developed that ruptured spontaneously and led to development of a chronically draining anal fistula. Later the patient developed a small rectovaginal fistula. Symptoms related to anal dysfunction occasionally recurred, but usually they were tolerably controlled by treatment. An attempt at surgical remedy of the anal fistula was deemed inadvisable because of the extent of disease elsewhere in the rectum and colon.

Diagnosis: Chronic anal fistula with moderate impairment of anal function, associated with Crohn's disease of the colon.

Table 4. Classes of Anal Impairment.

Class 1: 0%-9% impairment of the whole person	Class 2: 10%-19% impairment of the whole person	Class 3: 20%-35% impairment of the whole person
Signs of organic anal disease are present, or there is anatomic loss or alteration;	Signs of organic anal disease are present, or there is anatomic loss or alteration;	Signs of organic anal disease are present, and there is anatomic loss or alteration;
or	**and**	**and**
There is mild incontinence involving gas or liquid stool;	Moderate but partial fecal incontinence is present requiring continual treatment;	Complete fecal incontinence is present;
or	**or**	**or**
Anal symptoms are mild, intermittent, and controlled by treatment.	Continual anal symptoms are present and incompletely controlled by treatment.	Signs of organic anal disease are present, and severe anal symptoms unresponsive or amenable to therapy are present.

Impairment: 10% impairment due to the anal disorder, which is to be *combined* (Combined Values Chart, p. 322) with an appropriate percent for the colonic disease to determine the whole-person impairment.

Gynecologic evaluation for impairment due to the rectovaginal fistula should also be performed, and an appropriate whole-person impairment should be determined by using the Combined Values Chart.

Comment: Anal function has been impaired, but symptoms have been responsive to treatment when required. The patient's ability to perform normal activity has been only slightly impaired.

Class 3: Impairment of the Whole Person, 20% to 35%

Example: Ten years earlier, a 56-year-old truck driver had developed a pararectal abscess that had drained spontaneously. During the ensuing 3 years, infection had recurred, with opening of fistulous tracts in four other areas surrounding the anus. Surgical repair was undertaken in two stages, but this necessitated incision and excision of substantial portions of the anal sphincter muscle. Recovery was delayed by wound infections. Eventually the perineum healed, but the patient had no fecal control. Despite daily rectal irrigation, he soiled himself occasionally.

An examination disclosed complete functional loss of the anal sphincter mechanism.

Diagnosis: Anal incontinence due to complete loss of sphincter function.

Impairment: 25% impairment of the whole person.

Comment: The patient had uncontrollable fecal incontinence that was not amenable to further therapy.

10.6 Enterocutaneous Fistulas

Permanent enterocutaneous fistulas of the gastrointestinal tract, biliary tract, or pancreas, associated with diseases of these structures or their treatment, are evaluated as part of the organ system primarily involved. Permanent, surgically created stomas usually are provided to compensate for anatomic losses and to allow either ingress to or egress from the alimentary tract.

If a patient has a permanent, surgically created stoma, a percentage based on Table 5 (below) should be *combined* (Combined Values Chart, p. 322) with an estimate based on criteria related to the involved organ.

Table 5. Impairments from Surgically Created Stomas.

Created stoma	% Impairment of the whole person
Esophagostomy	10 - 15
Gastrostomy	10 - 15
Jejunostomy	15 - 20
Ileostomy	15 - 20
Colostomy	5 - 10

10.7 Liver and Biliary Tract

Symptoms and signs of hepatobiliary impairment include pain, nausea, vomiting, anorexia, loss of strength and stamina, reduced resistance to infection, altered immune response, jaundice, and pruritus. Complications of advanced liver disease include ascites and generalized ascites, portal venous hypertension leading to esophageal varices and hemorrhage, and metabolic disturbances leading to hepatic encephalopathy and renal failure.

Objective procedures useful in establishing hepatobiliary impairment include, but are not limited to, (1) ultrasonography; (2) contrast radiography, such as percutaneous and endoscopic cholangiography; (3) computed tomography and magnetic resonance imaging; (4) nuclide scintigraphy; (5) angiography; (6) liver biopsy and fine-needle aspiration; and (7) laboratory tests to assess the bile ducts and various functions of the liver.

Criteria for evaluating permanent impairment of the liver and biliary tract are listed in Table 6 (p. 245).

Class 1: Impairment of the Whole Person, 0% to 15%

Example: A 30-year-old construction worker with a history of excessive alcohol consumption had been hospitalized 5 years earlier because of severe delirium tremens, fever, and jaundice. A liver biopsy specimen showed extensive fatty metamorphosis with steatonecrosis, scattered inflammatory cell infiltration, and minimal periportal fibrosis. Since being released from the hospital, the patient abstained from alcohol, felt well, and exhibited normal vigor and appetite.

Physical examination showed a well-developed, muscular man with no evidence of jaundice or ascites. The liver edge was palpated 2 cm below the right costal margin. Liver function tests yielded values within the normal ranges, except for a serum aspartate aminotransferase (AST; formerly serum glutamic oxaloacetic transaminase) level of 45 U/L.

Diagnosis: History of acute alcoholic hepatitis and steatonecrosis, with residual slight hepatomegaly, probably due to fatty metamorphosis and portal fibrosis.

Impairment: 0% impairment.

Comment: The preexisting disease is well documented. Recovery has been satisfactory, and there is only minimal evidence of residual hepatic impairment. The man requires no treatment other than continued abstinence from alcohol, and he is able to engage fully in normal daily activities.

Class 2: Impairment of the Whole Person, 15% to 30%

Example: A 35-year-old plumber had had acute viral hepatitis 10 years earlier, with a protracted convalescence. Recently the disease had been quiescent; the patient had no visible icterus, ascites, or evidence of gastrointestinal tract bleeding. The man's strength and nutritional state were satisfactory, although his stamina was limited.

A physical examination showed that the patient was well nourished and well muscled. Several small telangiectases were seen on the left shoulder. A nontender, firm, rounded liver edge was palpated 4 cm below the right costal margin; the inferior margin of the spleen was palpated 1 cm below the left costal margin. Liver function tests indicated the following: serum bilirubin, 36 μmol/L (2.1 mg/dL); serum albumin, 40 g/L; serum globulin, 40 g/L; and serum AST, 70 U/L. The serum hepatitis B surface antigen and core antibody were positive. A liver biopsy specimen showed chronic active hepatitis without scarring.

Diagnosis: Chronic active hepatitis B.

Impairment: 15% impairment of the whole person.

Comment: There is documented evidence of chronic active hepatitis, but the patient can perform normal activities, although his stamina was reduced. Liver function was impaired to a slight to moderate degree.

Class 3: Impairment of the Whole Person, 30% to 50%

Example: A 48-year-old publishing executive had had what was described as acute hepatitis at age 18 years, followed by recurrent icteric illness at the ages of 22 and 30 years. In the past year his appetite declined; he became more easily fatigued, although he was still capable of limited desk work. His family had remarked on his sallow complexion.

On physical examination, the patient appeared chronically ill and perceptibly jaundiced. Scattered telangiectases were noted on his neck and upper thorax. Both liver and spleen were enlarged. No ascites or edema was evident. Laboratory studies included a normal urinalysis, hemogram with macrocytic indices, serum bilirubin level of 48 μmol/L (2.8 mg/dL), serum albumin level of 30 g/L, and serum alanine aminotransferase (formerly serum glutamic pyruvic transaminase) level of 180 U/L. Markers of specific viral infection were absent from the serum. A liver biopsy specimen showed chronic active hepatitis with extensive microlobular and macrolobular distortion of hepatic architecture.

Diagnosis: Non-A, non-B, chronic active hepatitis complicated by cirrhosis.

Impairment: 40% impairment of the whole person.

Comment: There is evidence of chronic, active, probably progressive, liver disease that has impaired the patient's capacity to perform normal activities.

Table 6. Classes of Liver and Biliary Tract Impairment.

Class 1: 0%-14% impairment of the whole person	Class 2: 15%-29% impairment of the whole person	Class 3: 30%-49% impairment of the whole person	Class 4: 50%-95% impairment of the whole person
Liver impairment			
There is objective evidence of persistent liver disease, even though no symptoms of liver disease are present and no history of ascites, jaundice, or bleeding esophageal varices within 3 years; **and** Nutrition and strength are good; **and** Biochemical studies indicate minimal disturbance in function; **or** Primary disorders of bilirubin metabolism are present.	There is objective evidence of chronic liver disease, even though no symptoms of liver disease are present and no history of ascites, jaundice, or bleeding esophageal varices within 3 years; **and** Nutrition and strength are good; **and** Biochemical studies indicate more severe liver damage than class 1.	There is objective evidence of progressive chronic liver disease, or history of jaundice, ascites, or bleeding esophageal or gastric varices within past year; **and** Nutrition and strength may be affected; **or** There is intermittent hepatic encephalopathy.	There is objective evidence of progressive chronic liver disease, or persistent jaundice or bleeding esophageal or gastric varices, with central nervous system manifestations of hepatic insufficiency; **and** Nutritional state is poor.
Biliary tract impairment			
There is occasional episode of biliary tract dysfunction.	There is recurrent biliary tract impairment irrespective of treatment.	There is irreparable obstruction of the bile tract with recurrent cholangitis.	There is persistent jaundice and progressive liver disease due to obstruction of the common bile duct.

Class 4: Impairment of the Whole Person, 50% to 95%

Example: A 55-year-old woman, formerly employed as a photographer's assistant, during a 5-year period had had repeated attacks of acute cholecystitis. Because of her religious beliefs, she refused to seek medical care. She had experienced increasingly frequent and severe bouts of right upper quadrant pain, nausea, vomiting, fever, jaundice, dark urine, and pruritus. She had been unable to work for more than a year. Laboratory tests yielded results consistent with biliary obstruction and advanced liver damage. A liver biopsy specimen showed advanced biliary cirrhosis. The woman declined any consideration of an invasive procedure that might alleviate her disease.

Diagnosis: Biliary cirrhosis, secondary to recurrent and progressive obstruction of bile ducts.

Impairment: 85% impairment of the whole person.

Comment: The patient sustained severe and irreparable impairment of liver and biliary tract function. Her capacity to perform normal activities has been gravely impaired.

10.8 Pancreas

Symptoms and signs of impairment of pancreatic function include, but are not limited to, pain, anorexia, nausea, vomiting, diarrhea, steatorrhea, weight loss, muscle wasting, jaundice, diabetes mellitus, and debility. Impairment due to *endocrine* disturbance related to the pancreas is considered in the *Guides* chapter on the endocrine system.

Objective procedures useful in establishing impairment of pancreatic function include, but are not limited to, (1) ultrasonography; (2) radiography, including plain or scout films of the abdomen, computed tomography, and endoscopic pancreatography; (3) guided fine-needle aspiration; (4) determination of plasma glucose level and glucose tolerance; (5) assay of pancreatic enzyme activity in blood, urine, and feces; (6) sweat electrolyte test; and (7) procedures such as the secretin test.

Criteria for evaluating impairment of pancreatic function are those listed in Table 2 (p. 239).

Class 1: Impairment of the Whole Person, 0% to 10%

Example: A 40-year-old bartender had had episodic epigastric pain associated with elevated serum amylase activity once or twice annually for the past

3 years. Despite a cholecystectomy for removal of gallstones 2 years ago, she was still subject to attacks of pain, often provoked by a large meal or by immoderately imbibing alcoholic beverages. A reduced-calorie diet corrected the patient's exogenous obesity but did not reduce her weight below a desirable level. No clinical or laboratory evidence of pancreatic insufficiency was present.

Diagnosis: Recurrent acute pancreatitis.

Impairment: 5% impairment of the whole person.

Comment: A preexisting disease was documented and treated appropriately. There was no current evidence of residual pancreatic impairment, and, despite occasional interruption by recurring symptoms, the patient was able to perform normal daily activities.

Class 2: Impairment of the Whole Person, 10% to 25%

Example: A 35-year-old farm worker was thrown against the steering wheel of his truck when it slid off a road. A few weeks later, while seeming to recover from his injuries, he noted increasing abdominal pain and distention. An expanding cyst of the pancreas was demonstrated by serial ultrasonography. Subtotal pancreatectomy was required to remove the cyst and allay the associated inflammatory reaction.

Fifteen months later, despite treatment with pancreatic enzyme supplements, the man had intermittent diarrhea with steatorrhea, and his stamina was notably diminished. He was 1.9 m (6 ft 3 in) tall and weighed 74.5 kg (164 lb), whereas his previous weight had been 81.7 kg (180 lb). He still experienced occasional epigastric and back pain. Tests showed no evidence of impaired glucose tolerance or diabetes.

Diagnosis: Status post subtotal pancreatectomy consequent to trauma, residual chronic pancreatitis, exocrine pancreatic insufficiency.

Impairment: 20% impairment of the whole person.

Comment: Pancreatic exocrine function was impaired, but the patient was able to maintain a weight within 10% of the desirable level. However, his capacity to perform normal activities was reduced.

Class 3: Impairment of the Whole Person, 25% to 50%

Example: A 45-year-old former salesperson had had unrelenting abdominal pain requiring medication for relief, after cholecystectomy and subtotal pancreatectomy to allay chronic pancreatitis. Dietary restriction and abstinence from alcohol did not lessen her symptoms. Insulin was needed daily for control of diabetes consequent to her operation. She was 1.73 m (5 ft 8 in) tall. She was unable to regain lost weight, even with the aid of pancreatic enzyme supplements. Her current weight was 15% below her desirable level of 61.3 kg (135 lb).

Diagnosis: Chronic, persistent pancreatitis.

Impairment: 40% impairment due to chronic pancreatitis, which should be *combined* (Combined Values Chart, p. 322) with an appropriate impairment estimate for diabetes to determine impairment of the whole person. Impairment related to diabetes mellitus is considered in the *Guides* chapter on the endocrine system.

Comment: Both exocrine and endocrine functions of the pancreas were impaired, and continuing treatment was necessary. The patient, despite treatment, was unable to bring her weight to within 10% of the desirable level.

Class 4: Impairment of the Whole Person, 50% to 76%

Example: A 47-year-old manufacturer's representative had noted, 13 months earlier, the onset of vague abdominal pain, weight loss, and uncharacteristic depression, which were followed by gradually deepening jaundice. Investigation had disclosed a cystic adenocarcinoma occupying most of the pancreas. Surgical eradication of the lesion had required total pancreatectomy and duodenectomy (Whipple operation). The patient now exhibited a malabsorption syndrome with steatorrhea, which was only partially relieved by pancreatic enzyme supplements. Diabetes mellitus that developed after the operation was "brittle" and controlled only with difficulty by repeated daily injections of insulin. The patient's weight declined since operation and was 25% below the desirable level. The man was barely able to perform essential daily activities.

Diagnosis: Pancreatic insufficiency consequent to total pancreatectomy.

Impairment: 70% impairment due to total pancreatic insufficiency, which is to be *combined* (Combined Values Chart, p. 322) with an appropriate impairment estimate for diabetes mellitus to determine impairment of the whole person (refer to *Guides* chapter on endocrine system).

Comment: This patient's capacity to perform normal activities was seriously impaired by total loss of the pancreas, and his debility was only partially alleviated by intensive treatment.

Table 7. Classes of Hernia-related Impairment.

Class 1: 0%-9% impairment of the whole person	Class 2: 10%-19% impairment of the whole person	Class 3: 20%-30% impairment of the whole person
Palpable defect in supporting structures of abdominal wall;	Palpable defect in supporting structures of abdominal wall;	Palpable defect in supporting structures of abdominal wall;
and	**and**	**and**
Slight protrusion at site of defect with increased abdominal pressure; readily reducible;	Frequent or persistent protrusion at site of defect with increased abdominal pressure; manually reducible;	Persistent, irreducible, or irreparable protrusion at site of defect;
or	**or**	**and**
Occasional mild discomfort at site of defect, but not precluding normal activity.	Frequent discomfort, precluding heavy lifting, but not hampering normal activity.	Limitation in normal activity.

10.9 Hernias of the Abdominal Wall

Symptoms and signs of abdominal wall impairment include discomfort or pain at or near the site of herniation, typically intermittent and often associated with postural changes or increased abdominal pressure; visible or palpable protrusion or swelling at the site of herniation, often appearing and disappearing depending on abdominal pressure; and more acute and intense pain due to complications, especially incarceration and strangulation of contained bowel or omentum.

Incisional hernias can be unsightly and annoying; other symptoms, if any, tend to be related to the size of the incisional hernia. Inguinal and femoral hernias typically are painful and entail a greater risk of grave complication. Most hernias of the abdominal wall are amenable to surgical correction.

Objective procedures useful in establishing impairment by hernias include, but are not limited to, (1) physical examination of abdominal wall; and (2) imaging by roentgenography or computed tomographic scan with or without the use of contrast media.

Criteria for evaluating permanent impairment due to herniation of the abdominal wall are listed in Table 7 (above).

Class 1: Impairment of the Whole Person, 0% to 10%

Example: A 60-year-old had woman required cholecystectomy 3 years earlier for relief of calculous biliary tract disease. Her postoperative course had been uneventful.

The oblique, right upper quadrant incision healed but left a palpable defect in the middle part. There remained a slight and visible protrusion at this site when the patient rose from a supine position. She had no pain or discomfort in the region of the scar, which she perceived as unsightly.

Diagnosis: Uncomplicated incisional hernia.

Impairment: 0% impairment.

Comment: The incisional hernia was asymptomatic and only mildly annoying to the patient. She is at no significant risk of a complication.

Class 2: Impairment of the Whole Person, 10% to 20%

Example: For several years a 50-year-old manager of an appliance store had been aware of a recurring protrusion in the right inguinal area when he strained or exerted increased intra-abdominal pressure. The protrusion had enlarged and entered the base of the scrotum but could be easily and painlessly reduced. The patient declined a recommended surgical repair and was willing to accept the preclusion of heavy lifting and the risk of a possible complication.

Diagnosis: Reducible right indirect inguinal hernia.

Impairment: 10% impairment of the whole person.

Comment: The patient was restricted in exertion but chose to live with his limitation. He was made aware of the possible consequences of an unrepaired inguinal hernia but declined operation. His normally sedentary activities were not impaired.

Class 3: Impairment of the Whole Person, 20% to 30%

Example: A 64-year-old man, nearing retirement from his job for 5 years as a branch bank manager, had recurrent, bilateral, inguinal hernias despite three previous attempts at repair, two on the right side and one on the left. The protrusions were only partially reducible and often caused discomfort. No complication had supervened. The patient was reluctant to submit to further attempts at repair.

Diagnosis: Recurrent bilateral inguinal hernias, after unsuccessful herniorrhaphy.

Impairment: 30% impairment of the whole person.

Comment: Despite repeated surgical repair, the inguinal hernias recurred and were only partially reducible. The patient felt obliged to wear a supporting device. He often experienced inguinal discomfort, and he was restricted in his normal activities.

References

1. Willett WC, Stampfer M, Manson JA, Van Itallie T. New weight guidelines for Americans: justified or injudicious. *Am J Clin Nutr.* 1991;53:1102-1103.

2. Berk JE, Haubrich WS, Kalser MH, Roth JLA, Schaffner F, eds. *Bockus' Gastroenterology.* 4th ed. Philadelphia, Pa: WB Saunders Co; 1985.

3. Miura S, Shikata J, Hasebe M, Kobayashi K. Long-term outcome of massive small bowel resection. *Am J Gastroenterol.* 1991;86:454-459.

4. Sherlock S, ed. *Diseases of the Liver and Biliary System.* 8th ed. Oxford, England: Blackwell Scientific Publications; 1988.

5. Sleisenger MH, Fordtran JS, eds. *Gastrointestinal Disease.* 4th ed. Philadelphia, Pa: WB Saunders Co; 1989.

6. Wyngaarden JB, Smith LH Jr, eds. *Cecil's Textbook of Medicine.* 18th ed. Philadelphia, Pa: WB Saunders Co; 1988.

Chapter 11

The Urinary and Reproductive Systems

This chapter provides criteria for evaluating the effects that permanent impairments of the urinary and reproductive systems have on the ability of individuals to perform their activities of daily living. The chapter discusses, in turn, (1) the upper urinary tract and urinary diversion; (2) the bladder; (3) the urethra; (4) the male reproductive organs; and (5) the female reproductive organs.

Before using the information in this chapter, the reader should peruse Chapters 1 and 2, which discuss the purpose of the *Guides* and the situations in which it is useful. Chapters 1 and 2 also discuss methods for examining patients and preparing reports. A medical evaluation report should include information such as that outlined below.

A. Medical Evaluation
- History of medical condition(s)
- Results of most recent evaluation
- Assessment of current clinical status and statement of further medical plans
- Diagnoses

B. Analysis of Findings
- Impact of medical condition(s) on life activities
- Explanation for concluding that the condition is stable and is unlikely to change
- Explanation for concluding that the individual is or is not likely to suffer further impairment by engaging in usual activities
- Explanation for concluding that accommodations or restrictions are or are not warranted

C. Comparison of Analysis with Impairment Criteria
- Description of clinical findings and how these findings relate to *Guides* criteria
- Explanation of each impairment rating or estimate
- Summary of impairment ratings
- Overall whole-person impairment rating or estimate

11.1 Upper Urinary Tract

The parenchyma of the kidneys produces urine, which is conducted by the renal calyces, pelves, and ureters to the urinary bladder. The kidney is an important homeostatic regulatory organ. The degree to which renal and conduit abnormalities may affect the whole person ranges from a clinically undetectable change to marked specific and generalized manifestations of deterioration of nephron reserves and urine transport.

Symptoms and signs of impairment of function of the upper urinary tract may include changes in micturition; edema; impairment of physical stamina; loss of weight and appetite; anemia; uremia; loin, abdominal, or costovertebral angle pain; hematuria; chills and fever; hypertension and its complications; abnormalities in the appearance of the urine or its sediment; and biochemical changes in the blood. Renal disease may be evidenced only by laboratory findings.

Objective Techniques Useful in Evaluation of the Upper Urinary Tract

Two clinically useful determinations of renal function, serum creatinine and the renal clearance of endogenous creatinine, can serve as guidelines for evaluating function of the upper urinary tract. The serum creatinine level is a good reflection of overall renal function. Under conditions of normal hydration, the serum creatinine level should be 133 μmol/L (1.5 mg/dL) or less.

The glomerular filtration rate, which measures renal clearance of endogenous creatinine, gives a quantitative estimate of the total functioning nephron population. The reliability of clearance tests of renal function is improved by longer periods of urine collection; therefore, measurement of the 24-hour endogenous creatinine clearance should be used. The normal ranges of creatinine clearance are 130 to 200 L/24 h (90 to 139 mL/min) in men and 115 to 180 L/24 h (80 to 125 mL/min) in women.

If there are discrepancies in these two tests, it may be desirable to perform additional investigations, such as metabolic studies, tests of concentrations of electrolytes and other chemicals in serum and urine, urine osmolalities, urinalyses, urine cultures, radiologic investigations, isotope renograms, and renal computed tomographic scans. Assessment of parenchymal disfiguration and conduit abnormality may require diagnostic procedures, such as endoscopy with study of one or both kidneys, biopsy, arteriography, uroradiography, computed tomography, or magnetic resonance imaging.

Criteria for Evaluating Impairment of the Upper Urinary Tract

The creatinine clearance is the most accurate reflection of renal function and will quantitate the degree of functional impairment of the upper urinary tract (Table 1, p. 251).

From a physiologic point of view, an individual with one kidney may have no actual impairment of renal function; nevertheless, with that condition there exists an absence or loss of the normal safety factor that may be of potential significance in evaluating impairment. The individual with one kidney, regardless of cause, should be considered to have a *10% whole-person impairment* because of the loss of an essential organ. This percentage would be *combined* with the estimate for any other permanent impairment; the Combined Values Chart (p. 322) would be used.

Deterioration of renal function requiring either peritoneal dialysis or hemodialysis indicates severe impairment in the range of a class 4 impairment, or 65% to 90% (Table 1, p. 251). Successful renal transplantation may result in marked improvement of renal function to the level of a class 2 impairment, or 15% to 30% of function. However, transplant recipients require continuous observation and medication, which may add to their impairment. For this reason, and at the discretion of the evaluating physician, 0% to 5% may be added to the final estimate of renal function impairment.

Furthermore, impairment related to complications of the disease or therapy, such as cushingoid changes and osteoporosis, should be evaluated as they arise, and appropriate percentages should be *combined* with the final renal impairment estimate by means of the Combined Values Chart (p. 322).

Class 1: Impairment of the Whole Person, 0% to 15%
A patient belongs in class 1 when (1) diminution of upper urinary tract function is present, as evidenced by creatinine clearance of 75 to 90 L/24 h (52 to 62.5 mL/min); *or* (2) intermittent symptoms and signs of upper urinary tract dysfunction are present that do not require continuous treatment or surveillance (Table 1, p. 251).

Example 1: When a 22-year-old man was 12 years of age, he had developed backache, fever, hematuria, headache, and hypertension during an epidemic of hemolytic streptococcal tonsillitis. At that time he was edematous and oliguric, and renal functions were depressed. The urine contained numerous red blood cells and red blood cell casts, and he passed 2.4 g of protein per 24 hours in the urine. Creatinine clearance was 72 L/24 h (50 mL/min). After a severe illness, the patient improved and was well except for microscopic hematuria that finally cleared. Six months after the illness, the creatinine clearance had been 130 L/24 h (90 mL/min).

Current studies revealed a healthy man with no evidence of renal disease by biopsy and urinalysis and a creatinine clearance of 158 L/24 h (110 mL/min).

Diagnosis: A healthy man with kidneys that are completely recovered from poststreptococcal acute glomerulonephritis.

Impairment: 0% impairment of the whole person.

Example 2: A 40-year-old man had an acute episode of renal colic and later passed a small urinary calculus. He had had two previous episodes of renal colic with spontaneous passage of urinary calculi. Excretory urograms were normal, and no evidence of metabolic disease was present. Results of urine, creatinine clearance, and phenolsulfonphthalein studies were within normal limits.

Diagnosis: Recurrent renal calculi.

Impairment: 5% impairment of the whole person.

Table 1. Upper Urinary Tract Impairments.

Class 1: **0%-14% impairment of the whole person**	**Class 2:** **15%-34% impairment of the whole person**	**Class 3:** **35%-59% impairment of the whole person**	**Class 4:** **60%-95% impairment of the whole person**
Diminution of upper urinary tract function is present as evidenced by creatinine clearance of 75-90 L/24 h (52-62.5 mL/min);	Diminution of upper urinary tract function is present as evidenced by creatinine clearance of 60-75 L/24 h (42-52 mL/min);	Diminution of upper urinary tract function is present as evidenced by creatinine clearance of 40-60 L/24 h (28-42 mL/min);	Diminution of upper urinary tract function is present as evidenced by creatinine clearance below 40 L/24 h (28 mL/min);
or	**or**	**or**	**or**
Intermittent symptoms and signs of upper urinary tract dysfunction are present that do not require continuous treatment or surveillance.	Although creatinine clearance is greater than 75 L/24 h (52 mL/min), symptoms and signs of upper urinary tract disease or dysfunction necessitate continuous surveillance and frequent treatment.	Although creatinine clearance is 60-75 L/24 h (42 to 52 mL/min), symptoms and signs of upper urinary tract disease or dysfunction are incompletely controlled by surgical or continuous medical treatment.	Although creatinine clearance is 40-60 L/24 h (28-42 mL/min), symptoms and signs of upper urinary tract disease or dysfunction persist despite surgical or continuous medical treatment.

Class 2: Impairment of the Whole Person, 15% to 35%

A patient belongs in class 2 when (1) diminution of upper urinary tract function is present as evidenced by creatinine clearance of 60 to 75 L/24 h (42 to 52 mL/min); *or* (2) symptoms and signs of upper urinary tract disease or dysfunction require continuous surveillance and frequent treatment, although creatinine clearance is greater than 75 L/24 h (52 mL/min).

Example 1: A 45-year-old man with a history of nephritis as a child underwent an emergency appendectomy and drainage of an appendiceal abscess. Despite an adequate urine output during the postoperative period, the serum creatinine level rose to 248 μmol/L (2.8 mg/dL). The man's convalescence was prolonged, but the anemia subsided and his stamina returned to normal.

Twelve months after the appendectomy, the patient felt well and was able to engage in most of his usual daily activities. The urine showed a trace of protein (0.75 g/24 h). Excretory urograms showed no architectural abnormality; creatinine clearances ranged from 60 to 70 L/24 h (42 to 49 mL/min).

Diagnosis: Asymptomatic but persistent proteinuria after childhood nephritis aggravated by surgery years later.

Impairment: 15% impairment of the whole person.

Example 2: A 50-year-old woman had had a successful operation for a parathyroid adenoma. She continued to have periodic attacks of pyelonephritis occasioned by residual calculi in both kidneys, and she passed stones sporadically. The infrequent clinical attacks of pyelonephritis responded to antibiotics. The symptoms of urinary tract infection were controlled by continuous medication. The creatinine clearance was stable at approximately 65 L/24 h (45 mL/min). The bilateral pyelocaliceal deformities and the size of the kidneys as delineated by excretory urography had not changed appreciably in a 3-year period.

Diagnosis: Renal calculi and bilateral chronic pyelonephritis.

Impairment: 30% impairment due to upper urinary tract impairment, which is *combined* by means of the Combined Values Chart (p. 322) with an appropriate value for parathyroid impairment to estimate whole-person impairment.

Example 3: A 52-year-old man had had surgical reconstruction of his left lower ureter because of severe damage to its function from retroperitoneal fibrosis. Despite apparently normal architecture and function of the left kidney, vesicoureteral reflux could be demonstrated, and repeated attacks of pyelonephritis occurred when antibacterial medication was discontinued. The creatinine clearance was 100 L/24 h (69 mL/min). Since the left kidney was normal in appearance and showed no deterioration of function, no surgical intervention was contemplated.

Diagnosis: Active unilateral chronic pyelonephritis secondary to vesicoureteral reflux.

Impairment: 15% impairment of the whole person.

Example 4: A 28-year-old man with progressive chronic glomerulonephritis developed marked azotemia and oliguria requiring hemodialysis. Successful renal transplantation with a kidney from his mother resulted in good renal function with a creatinine clearance of 108 L/24 h. The patient received maintenance treatment with azathioprine and prednisone and required close observation for development of osteoporosis.

Diagnosis: Functioning renal transplant.

Impairment: 25% impairment of the whole person due to renal disease and the need for continuous medication.

Comment: If secondary infection or other complication develops because of the immunosuppressive therapy, the patient should be reevaluated; any permanent impairment percent related to a complication would be *combined* with the estimate for renal impairment by means of the Combined Values Chart (p. 322).

Class 3: Impairment of the Whole Person, 35% to 60%

A patient belongs in class 3 when (1) diminution of upper urinary tract function is present, as evidenced by creatinine clearance of 40 to 60 L/24 h (28 to 42 mL/min); *or* (2) symptoms and signs of upper urinary tract disease or dysfunction are incompletely controlled by surgical or continuous medical treatment, although creatinine clearance is 60 to 75 L/24 h (42 to 52 mL/min).

Example 1: A 52-year-old woman complained of chronic fatigue. On examination, she was found to have elevation of the serum creatinine level and moderate anemia. There was no clear-cut history of nephritis. A renal biopsy specimen showed diffuse glomerulonephritis. A high-dose excretory urogram delineated contracted kidneys with normal pyelocaliceal architecture. Results of urine culture were negative; creatinine clearance was 50 L/24 h (35 mL/min).

Diagnosis: Chronic glomerulonephritis with renal atrophy.

Impairment: 60% impairment due to upper urinary tract impairment, which is to be *combined* by means of the Combined Values Chart (p. 322) with an appropriate percent value for the anemia to determine the total impairment.

Example 2: A 48-year-old man had calculi in the minor calices of both kidneys. He had a history of multiple endoscopic and open surgical procedures for stone removal. He had marked diminution in the size of one kidney and bilateral pyelographic architectural changes as a result of previous surgical procedures and recurrent pyelonephritis. Despite continuous antibacterial medication, the urine remained infected, and periodic episodes of chills, fever, and back pain occurred. Creatinine clearance was 65 L/24 h (45 mL/min).

Diagnosis: Renal calculi with bilateral recurrent pyelonephritis.

Impairment: 50% impairment of the whole person.

Example 3: A 48-year-old man was injured in an automobile crash and developed hematuria. A physical examination showed his blood pressure to be 150/90 mm Hg, and radiologic studies showed that his left kidney was damaged. All other findings were normal. The man was kept at bed rest in a hospital for a week and then discharged.

About 16 months later the man began to complain of severe headaches. The blood pressure was found to be 240/160 mm Hg, and malignant hypertensive retinopathy was noted. Investigation revealed a creatinine clearance of 40 L/24 h (28 mL/min) and definite evidence of left renovascular hypertension. The left kidney was removed. Biopsy specimens from the right kidney showed malignant hypertensive changes. The histologic examination of the left kidney showed ischemia and juxtaglomerular hypertrophy.

After surgery the patient's blood pressure fell to 170/110 mm Hg, and during the next 6 months it leveled off at 155/95 mm Hg. The eyegrounds showed grade II changes (Keith-Wagner classification), and creatinine clearance rose slowly to level off at 58 L/24 h (40 mL/min).

Diagnosis: Left nephrectomy for malignant hypertensive vascular disease.

Impairment: 55% impairment due to arteriolar nephrosclerosis and 10% impairment due to nephrectomy, which *combine* (Combined Values Chart, p. 322) to give an estimate of 60% impairment of the urinary system; the 60% impairment should be combined with an appropriate value for the cardiovascular impairment to determine whole-person impairment.

Class 4: Impairment of the Whole Person, 60% to 95%

A patient belongs in class 4 when (1) diminution of upper urinary tract function is present, as evidenced by creatinine clearance below 40 L/24 h (28 mL/min); *or* (2) symptoms and signs of upper urinary tract disease or dysfunction persist despite surgical or continuous medical treatment, although creatinine clearance is 40 to 60 L/24 h (28 to 42 mL/min).

Example 1: A 44-year-old man with a family history of polycystic renal disease experienced sudden flank pain and noted gross hematuria. During the 2 years preceding the acute episode, the man's serum creatinine level had increased from 707 to 884 μmol/L (8 to 10 mg/dL), and he was maintained on a protein-restricted diet. Until the current episode, he was working regularly and was relatively asymptomatic.

Results of a physical examination were normal. Renal evaluation disclosed that the creatinine clearance was 35 L/24 h (24 mL/min). Endoscopy and retrograde urograms showed bilateral deformities characteristic of polycystic renal disease.

Diagnosis: Bilateral polycystic renal disease; advanced renal insufficiency.

Impairment: 70% impairment of the whole person.

Example 2: A young woman became anuric after severe abruptio placentae. A percutaneous renal biopsy was performed. The histologic diagnosis was renal cortical necrosis, and periodic courses of peritoneal dialysis were instituted. After 49 days of anuria and then oliguria, the urine output increased; on the 60th day the serum creatinine level, which at the start of the illness had been 1945 μmol/L (22 mg/dL), began to fall without peritoneal dialysis. Twelve months after the anuria episode, the patient performed most activities of daily living despite severely compromised renal function. The creatinine clearance leveled off at 11.5 L/24 h (8 mL/min).

Diagnosis: Renal cortical necrosis; severe chronic renal failure.

Impairment: 75% impairment of the whole person.

Example 3: A 56-year-old woman with chronic progressive glomerulonephritis was severely anemic, azotemic, and oliguric and required hemodialysis twice weekly. For 1 or 2 days after treatment she felt well and was able to perform her duties in the workplace and care for her home. On the days just before dialysis she was nauseated, lethargic, and edematous.

Diagnosis: Severe chronic renal failure.

Impairment: 80% to 90% impairment of the whole person.

Comment: The woman's renal failure and the refractory anemia justify the high impairment percent estimate.

11.2 Urinary Diversion

Permanent, surgically created forms of urinary diversion are usually provided to compensate for anatomic losses and to allow for egress of urine. They are evaluated as a part of, and in conjunction with, the assessment of the involved portion of the urinary tract.

Irrespective of how well these diversions function in the preservation of renal integrity and the disposition of urine, the following values for the diversions (Table 2) should be combined with those determined under the criteria previously given for the urinary tract.

Table 2. Impairment from Urinary Diversion.

Type of diversion	% Impairment of the whole person
Ureterointestinal	10
Cutaneous ureterostomy	10
Nephrostomy	15

Example 1: A 56-year-old man with bilateral nephrostomies because of obliterative, fibrotic, ureteral disease, a condition of at least 5 years' duration, had renal calculi removed. An attempt to reconstitute normal conduit function through surgery was unsuccessful. Urinary infection could not be eradicated, and the patient complained of hematuria when the nephrostomy tubes were changed and of occasional episodes of fever and flank pain. He continued to engage in most activities of daily living. The creatinine clearance was 50 L/24 h (35 mL/min).

Diagnosis: Pyeloureteral disease requiring bilateral nephrostomy diversion.

Impairment: 65% impairment due to pyeloureteral disease and 15% impairment due to bilateral nephrostomies, which *combine* to give 70% impairment of the whole person (Combined Values Chart, p. 322).

Example 2: A 52-year-old woman had no evidence of recurrent cancer 7 years after anterior pelvic exenteration and ureteroileostomy for carcinoma of the cervix. She had calculi removed from both kidneys, and she experienced periodic episodes of pyelonephritis, even while taking continual medication. Radiologic changes suggesting pyelonephritis were present. The creatinine clearance was 60 L/24 h (24 mL/min).

Diagnosis: Ureteroileostomy, urinary diversion, and chronic bilateral pyelonephritis.

Impairment: 65% impairment due to bilateral pyelonephritis, 10% impairment due to ureteroileostomy, and 55% impairment due to pelvic exenteration; that is, excision of bladder, lower ureters, uterus, cervix, vagina, fallopian tubes, and ovaries, which *combine* to an estimated 85% whole-person impairment (Combined Values Chart, p. 322).

11.3 Bladder

The bladder is a voluntarily controllable reservoir for urine that normally permits the patient to retain urine for several hours. Symptoms and signs of impairment of function of the bladder may include urinary frequency, pain with voiding (dysuria), incontinence, retention of urine, hematuria, pyuria, passage of urinary calculi, and a suprapubic mass. Objective techniques useful in evaluating function of the bladder include but are not limited to cystoscopy, cystography, voiding cystourethrography, cystometry, uroflowmetry, urinalysis, and urine cultures.

Criteria for Evaluating Permanent Impairment of the Bladder

When evaluating permanent impairment of the bladder, the status of the upper urinary tract must also be considered. The appropriate impairment values for both should be *combined* by means of the Combined Values Chart (p. 322) to determine renal system impairment.

Class 1: Impairment of the Whole Person, 0% to 15%

A patient belongs in class 1 when the patient has symptoms and signs of bladder disorder requiring intermittent treatment and normal functioning between the episodes of malfunctioning.

Example: A 41-year-old woman had been treated with radium for uterine fibroids 20 years earlier. Recent episodes of urinary tract bleeding caused by post-irradiation telangiectasia of the bladder required emergency hospitalization and blood vessel fulguration with the patient under anesthesia. The episodes occurred at intervals ranging from 1 to 2 weeks to 6 months. Between attacks, the findings from blood and urine studies were normal. After each episode, the patient was able to resume usual activities within 7 days.

Diagnosis: Post-irradiation telangiectasia of the bladder.

Impairment: 10% impairment of the whole person.

Class 2: Impairment of the Whole Person, 15% to 25%

A patient belongs in class 2 when (1) there are symptoms or signs of a bladder disorder requiring continuous treatment; *or* (2) there is good bladder reflex activity, that is, storage of urine, but no voluntary control.

Example 1: A 35-year-old woman developed such progressive and painful urinary frequency that she was voiding at intervals of 10 to 15 minutes day and night. A diagnosis of interstitial cystitis was established, and the usual treatment of bladder dilation with various agents was ineffective. The upper urinary tract was normal and was uninfected. After a cystectomy and ureteroileostomy, the woman was able to resume her normal activities.

Diagnosis: Contracted, fixed bladder requiring urinary diversion.

Impairment: 20% impairment due to urinary diversion procedure after removal of the bladder.

Example 2: A 42-year-old man with chronic renal infection resistant to antibiotic therapy developed severe cystitis requiring him to empty his bladder at intervals of less than 30 minutes and the use of a urine collecting device. The man's general physical condition was good, but his urine contained numerous white blood cells and a few red blood cells. He refused urinary diversion through a surgical procedure. He could not retain his urine long enough to permit him to perform the usual activities of daily living.

Diagnosis: Chronic cystitis.

Impairment: 20% impairment due to cystitis, which should be *combined* (Combined Values Chart, p. 322) with an appropriate percent for the upper urinary tract disorder to determine the whole-person impairment.

Class 3: Impairment of the Whole Person, 25% to 40%

A patient belongs in class 3 when the bladder has poor reflex activity, that is, there is intermittent dribbling and no voluntary control.

Example: A 52-year-old man had a radical retropubic prostatectomy for localized carcinoma of the prostate. His postoperative course was uneventful; he was sent home on the 6th postoperative day, and his catheter was removed on the 14th postoperative day. His further convalescence was uneventful. He continued to have intermittent loss of urine when he coughed, sneezed, or lifted a heavy object. He had no incontinence during normal sedentary activities. Repeat evaluation, including urodynamics, showed no neurologic abnormality.

Diagnosis: Stress urinary incontinence after radical retropubic prostatectomy.

Impairment: 25% due to stress urinary incontinence, which required the patient to wear protective padding during normal work activities.

Class 4: Impairment of the Whole Person, 40% to 60%
A patient belongs in class 4 when there is no reflex or voluntary control of the bladder, that is, there is continuous dribbling of urine.

Example: A 35-year-old workman fell from the roof of a building, suffering a compression fracture of the lumbar spine and contusion of the lower lumbar spinal cord. He was initially paraplegic, but with surgical debridement and rehabilitation he recovered the use of his lower extremities. He was, however, left with a cauda equina neurologic deficit, that is, anesthesia of the perineum and perirectal area and total urinary incontinence. The man elected not to undergo implantation of an artificial urinary sphincter and instead elected to wear an external condom catheter.

Diagnosis: Neurogenic bladder impairment.

Impairment: 50% impairment due to total loss of urinary control.

11.4 Urethra

In the female, the urethra is a urinary conduit containing a voluntary sphincter. In the male, the urethra possesses a voluntary sphincter and propulsive muscles and is a conduit for urine and seminal ejaculations.

Symptoms and signs of impairment of function of the urethra include dysuria, diminished urinary stream, urinary retention, incontinence, extraneous or ectopic openings, periurethral mass or masses, and diminished urethral caliber.

Objective techniques useful in evaluating function of the urethra include, but are not limited to, urethroscopy, urethrography, cystourethrography, endoscopy, and cystometrography.

Criteria for Evaluating Permanent Impairment of the Urethra

When evaluating permanent impairment of the urethra, one must also consider the status of the upper urinary tract and bladder. Impairments for the parts of the urinary system should be *combined* by means of the Combined Values Chart (p. 322) to estimate whole-person impairment.

Class 1: Impairment of the Whole Person, 0% to 10%
A person belongs in class 1 when symptoms and signs of a urethral disorder are present that require intermittent therapy for control.

Example: As a result of an injury 2 years earlier, a 27-year-old man had a urethral stricture that required dilation every few weeks. Between dilations he was free of symptoms, and he had symptoms only as the urethra gradually constricted. There was no upper urinary tract infection.

Diagnosis: Traumatic urethral stricture.

Impairment: 5% impairment of the whole person.

Class 2: Impairment of the Whole Person, 10% to 20%
A patient belongs in class 2 when there are symptoms and signs of a urethral disorder that cannot be effectively controlled by treatment.

Example 1: A 23-year-old man experienced considerable laceration of the ventral surface of the penis that created a surgically uncorrectable fistula. He was able to perform most activities of daily living, but he could not void normally. He could ejaculate during sexual intercourse, but he was unable to make his wife pregnant.

Diagnosis: Urethral fistula.

Impairment: 15% impairment due to the urethral fistula and 10% impairment due to impaired sexual function, which *combine* to a 24% whole-person impairment (Combined Values Chart, p. 322).

Example 2: A 31-year-old man was struck by a motor vehicle and had a pelvic fracture, fracture dislocation of the symphysis, laceration of the prostatomembranous urethra, and laceration of the bulbomembranous urethra. The pelvic fracture was stabilized, and it healed. The urethral lacerations were repaired, but postoperative fibrosis resulted in extensive urethral strictures that could not be corrected with further procedures. Two years later the patient required frequent urethral dilations to void, and he had chronic urinary tract infection with ascending pyelonephritis secondary to the urethral obstruction and frequent urethral instrumentation. The man's creatinine clearance declined to 65 L/24 h (45 mL/min).

Diagnosis: Traumatic urethral stricture with chronic pyelonephritis.

Impairment: 20% impairment due to urethral stricture and 25% impairment due to upper urinary tract damage, which *combine* to a 40% impairment of the whole person (Combined Values Chart, p. 322).

Example 3: A 21-year-old factory worker was crushed between a forklift and a wall. His bony pelvis was fractured, his urethra was totally severed at the apex of the prostate, and his perineum was severely lacerated. Immediate reconstructive urethral surgery was unsuccessful, and 1 year after the injury a ureterosigmoidostomy was necessary, which resulted in hydronephrosis of the right kidney and repeated urinary tract infections. The diversion was converted to an ileal conduit, and renal infections occurred only sporadically thereafter.

At examination, the worker was found to be impotent. The pelvic fracture was healed, and there was no musculoskeletal impairment. Because of occasional urinary tract infections, the man periodically was unable to attend meetings and conferences and pursue some recreational activities. Creatinine clearance was 70 L/24 h (49 mL/min).

Diagnosis: Severed urethra, hydronephrosis with recurrent urinary tract infections, impotence.

Impairment: 20% impairment due to the severed urethra, 30% impairment due to upper urinary tract impairment, 10% impairment due to ureteroileostomy, 30% impairment due to upper urinary tract impairment, and 30% impairment due to loss of sexual function, which *combine* to give a 65% impairment of the whole person (Combined Values Chart, p. 322).

11.5 Male Reproductive Organs

The male reproductive organs include the penis, scrotum, testes, epididymides, spermatic cords, prostate, and seminal vesicles. The impairment percentages of the male reproductive organs are given in the following sections for men 40 to 65 years old. The percentages may be increased by 50% for men below the age of 40 years and decreased by 50% for those over the age of 65 years. For instance, a 50% increase of a 20% impairment equals a 30% impairment.

11.5a Penis

The penis has sexual functions of erection and ejaculation and urinary functions. The latter are discussed in the section on the urethra (p. 255).

The symptoms and signs of impairment of function of the penis include abnormalities of erection and sensation and partial or complete loss of the penis.

Criteria for Evaluating Permanent Impairment of the Penis

When evaluating impairment of the penis, it is necessary to consider impairment of both the sexual and the urinary functions. The degree of impairment of sexual function should be determined in accordance with the criteria that follow, and this estimate should be *combined* by means of the Combined Values Chart (p. 322) with the appropriate percentage for estimated impairment of urinary function to determine the whole-person impairment. The criteria in this part may be used to estimate impairment related to the use of a penile implant.

Objective techniques useful in evaluating function of the penis include, but are not limited to, penile tumescence studies, Doppler ultrasound evaluations of penile blood flow, dynamic cavernosometry and cavernosography, and angiography.

Class 1: Impairment of the Whole Person, 0% to 10%
A patient belongs in class 1 when sexual function is possible, but there are varying degrees of difficulty of erection, ejaculation, or sensation.

Example: A 32-year-old man suffered a compressive injury to the penile shaft. Healing occurred with partial cicatrization of the left mid-corpus cavernosum. A bow-string curvature to the left occurred during erections. Sensation and ejaculation were normal, but pain resulted if intercourse were not undertaken carefully.

Diagnosis: Posttraumatic fibrosis of left mid-corpus cavernosum.

Impairment: 9% impairment of the whole person, which takes into consideration the patient's age.

Class 2: Impairment of the Whole Person, 10% to 19%
A patient belongs in class 2 when sexual function is possible and there is sufficient erection, *but* ejaculation and sensation are impaired.

Example: A 28-year-old man suffered a fractured pelvis with wide separation of the symphysis pubis, perivesical and periprostatic hematomas, and a tear of the prostatomembranous urethra. The injuries were corrected with reconstructive surgery, and there was no subsequent urinary difficulty. Erection and intercourse were possible, but penile sensation and ejaculation were absent.

Diagnosis: Posttraumatic ejaculatory dysfunction and penile anesthesia.

Impairment: 15% impairment of the whole person, which includes consideration for the patient's age.

Class 3: Impairment of the Whole Person, 20%
A patient belongs in class 3 when no sexual function is possible.

Example: An 18-year-old man suffered traumatic dislocation of the penis. Corporeal repair and urethoplasty preserved genital appearance and urethral function, but erection was not possible. Doppler flow studies showed markedly diminished penile arterial blood flow.

Diagnosis: Posttraumatic vascular and neurologic penile insufficiency.

Impairment: 30% of the whole person, which considers the patient's age by addition of 50% of the 20% whole-person impairment.

11.5b Scrotum

The scrotum covers, protects, and provides a suitable environment for the testes.

Symptoms and signs of impairment of function of the scrotum include pain, enlargement, lack of testicular mobility, inappropriate location of the testes, and masses.

Objective techniques useful in evaluating function of the scrotum include, but are not limited to, observation, palpation, testicular examination, and scrotal ultrasound.

Criteria for Evaluating Permanent Impairment of the Scrotum

Class 1: Impairment of the Whole Person, 0% to 10%
A patient belongs in class 1 when there are symptoms and signs of scrotal loss or disease and there is no evidence of testicular malfunction, although there may be testicular malposition.

Example: A 38-year-old man had an injury resulting in loss of all scrotal skin. Split-thickness skin graft reconstruction gave a good cosmetic result. At examination there was no evidence of testicular malfunction, but testicular mobility was affected, and the patient experienced discomfort during exercise and in certain positions.

Diagnosis: Ablation of scrotal skin; split-thickness skin graft reconstruction of the scrotum.

Impairment: 5% impairment of the whole person, which considers the patient's age.

Class 2: Impairment of the Whole Person, 10% to 20%
A patient belongs in class 2 when (1) there are symptoms and signs of architectural alteration or disease such that the testes must be implanted in other than a scrotal position to preserve testicular function, and pain or discomfort is present with activity; *or* (2) there is total loss of the scrotum.

Example: A 50-year-old man suffered extensive burns of the lower extremities, genitals, and abdomen. Skin grafting to the abdomen and lower extremities was satisfactory; however, it was necessary to transplant the testicles to subcutaneous pouches in the thighs to permit adequate skin coverage of the scrotal area.

Diagnosis: Burn ablation of the scrotum.

Impairment: 15% impairment of the whole person.

Class 3: Impairment of the Whole Person, 20% to 35%
A patient belongs in class 3 when there are signs and symptoms of scrotal disease that are uncontrolled by treatment and limit the patient's physical activities.

Example: A 55-year-old man underwent high-dose external beam radiation therapy to his pelvis for carcinoma of the prostate. Five years later he was apparently cured of the cancer, but he had marked lymphedema of the penis and scrotum for which there was no effective treatment. The large size of his genitals and the weeping skin severely limited physical activities.

Diagnosis: Postirradiation lymphedema of penile and scrotal skin.

Impairment: 30% impairment of the whole person due to persisting symptoms, lack of effective therapy, and limitation of physical activity.

11.5c Testes, Epididymides, and Spermatic Cords

The testes produce spermatozoa, synthesize male steroid hormones, and provide the appearance and "psychological badge" of maleness. The epididymides and spermatic cords transport the spermatozoa.

Signs and symptoms of impairment of function of the testes, epididymides, and spermatic cords include local or referred pain; tenderness and change in size, contour, position, and texture; and abnormalities of testicular hormones and seminal fluid.

Objective techniques useful in evaluating function of the testes, epididymides, and spermatic cords include, but are not limited to, vasography, ultrasound, lymphangiography, spermatic arteriography and venography, biopsy, semen analysis, and studies of follicle-stimulating, ketosteroid, and hydroxysteroid hormones.

Criteria for Evaluating Permanent Impairment of the Testes, Epididymides, and Spermatic Cords

Class 1: Impairment of the Whole Person, 0% to 10%
A patient belongs in class 1 when (1) symptoms and signs of testicular, epididymal, or spermatic cord disease are present and there is anatomic alteration; *and* (2) continuous treatment is not required; *and* (3) there are no abnormalities of seminal or hormonal function; *or* (4) a solitary testis is present.

Example: A 36-year-old man had repeated episodes of epididymal orchitis as a result of recurrent prostatitis. He had symptoms of discomfort between attacks and clinical evidence of chronic epididymitis. He did not want vas deferens ligations, because he had normal seminal fluid and might want to beget children.

Diagnosis: Chronic epididymitis secondary to chronic prostatitis.

Impairment: 5% impairment due to epididymitis and 5% impairment due to prostatitis, which take into consideration the patient's age and *combine* to a 10% whole-person impairment (Combined Values Chart, p. 322).

Class 2: Impairment of the Whole Person, 10% to 15%
A patient belongs in class 2 when (1) symptoms and signs of testicular, epididymal, or spermatic cord disease are present and there is anatomic alteration; *and* (2) frequent or continuous treatment is required, or treatment is not possible; *and* (3) there are detectable seminal or hormonal abnormalities.

Example: A 30-year-old man had had bilateral mumps orchitis 2 years before the current examination and, subsequently, bilateral testicular atrophy. Earlier he had fathered two children, but he currently was unable to make his wife pregnant. A basic examination showed no abnormality; semen analysis revealed marked oligospermia.

Diagnosis: Oligospermia.

Impairment: 14% impairment of the whole person.

Class 3: Impairment of the Whole Person, 15% to 20%
A patient belongs in class 3 when trauma or disease produces bilateral anatomic loss of the primary sex organs, or there is no detectable seminal or hormonal function of these organs.

Example: A 17-year-old boy was injured by a farm machine, sustaining amputation of the scrotum and its contents. He was examined 2 years later when his condition was stable.

Diagnosis: Traumatic orchiectomy.

Impairment: Estimates are 20% impairment due to gonadal loss and 15% impairment due to scrotal loss, which consider the patient's young age, and 5% impairment due to lack of an endocrine gland; these values *combine* to give an estimated 35% impairment of the whole person (Combined Values Chart, p. 322).

11.5d Prostate and Seminal Vesicles

The prostate and seminal vesicles are involved with transport and nutritional modification of, and maintaining an adequate environment for, spermatozoa and semen. Impairments associated with urinary functions of the parts of the urethra involved with these organs are discussed in the part of this chapter on the urethra (p. 255).

Symptoms and signs of impairment of function of the prostate and seminal vesicles include local or referred pain; tenderness; changes in size and texture; disturbances in function of spermatic cords, epididymides, and testes; oligospermia; hemospermia; and urinary tract abnormalities.

Objective techniques useful in evaluating function of the prostate and seminal vesicles include but are not limited to urography, endoscopy, prostatic ultrasonography, vasography, biopsy, examination of prostatic secretions, and analysis of hormone excretion patterns.

Criteria for Evaluating Permanent Impairment of the Prostate and Seminal Vesicles

Class 1: Impairment of the Whole Person, 0% to 10%
A patient belongs in class 1 when (1) symptoms and signs of prostatic or seminal vesicular dysfunction or disease are present; *and* (2) anatomic alteration is present; *and* (3) continuous treatment is not required.

Example: A 42-year-old man had had many episodes of acute prostatitis in the past 10 years and some episodes of mild perineal discomfort that required pain medication.

Diagnosis: Chronic prostatitis with acute febrile episodes.

Impairment: 5% impairment of the whole person.

Class 2: Impairment of the Whole Person, 10% to 15%
A patient belongs in class 2 when (1) frequent severe symptoms and signs of prostatic or seminal vesicular dysfunction or disease are present; *and* (2) anatomic alteration is present; *and* (3) continuous treatment is required.

Example: After drainage of a prostatic abscess 15 months earlier, a 34-year-old man had continuous symptoms and signs of prostatitis, which he could tolerate only with the constant use of antibacterial medications. At examination he had perineal pain, a low-grade fever, and hemospermia.

Diagnosis: Recurrent acute and chronic prostatitis.

Impairment: 14% impairment of the whole person, which includes allowance for the patient's age.

Class 3: Impairment of the Whole Person, 15% to 20%
A patient belongs in class 3 when there has been ablation of the prostate seminal vesicles. This occurs almost exclusively with extirpative surgery for prostatic carcinoma. The impairments estimated for loss of the prostate and seminal vesicles should be *combined* with those for sexual dysfunction or urinary incontinence if those conditions are present. The Combined Values Chart (p. 322) is used.

11.6 Female Reproductive Organs

The female reproductive organs include the vulva, clitoris, vagina, cervix, uterus, fallopian tubes, and ovaries. The degree of impairment of the female reproductive system is influenced by age, and especially by whether the woman is in the childbearing age group. The physiologic differences of premenopausal and postmenopausal women are considered in establishing the criteria in this chapter for evaluating and estimating impairments of the female's reproductive organs.

11.6a Vulva and Vagina

The vulva has cutaneous, sexual, and urinary functions. The urinary function has been discussed in the part of this chapter on the urethra. The vagina has a sexual function and serves as a birth passageway. The clitoris is an erectile organ that has an important role in sexual functioning.

Symptoms and signs of impairment of function of the vulva and vagina include loss or altered sensation; loss of lubrication; complete or partial absence; presence of vulvovaginitis; vulvitis; vaginitis; cicatrization; ulceration; stenosis; atrophy or hypertrophy; neoplasia or dysplasia; difficulty with sexual intercourse, urination, or vaginal delivery; and secondary effects on underlying perineal structures.

Criteria for Evaluating Permanent Impairment of the Vulva and Vagina

Class 1: Impairment of the Whole Person, 0% to 15%
A patient belongs in class 1 when (1) symptoms and signs of disease or deformity of the vulva or vagina are present that do not require continuous treatment; *and* (2) sexual intercourse is possible; *and* (3) the vagina is adequate for childbirth if the patient is premenopausal.

Example: An obese 38-year-old married woman, who had given vaginal birth to three living children, experienced recurrent chronic dermatitis of the genitocrural area. At intervals, she required treatment for intense pruritus and active dermatitis. Her discomfort was more marked during warm and humid weather. Laboratory cultures for fungal infection were negative. The patient did not have diabetes mellitus. There was remission of symptoms when her weight was controlled, when she avoided tight clothing, and when she observed careful hygienic measures. Satisfying sexual intercourse was possible if precautions were observed to avoid excessive vulval irritation.

Diagnosis: Dermatitis of the vulva, intertrigo.

Impairment: 0% impairment of whole person.

Class 2: Impairment of the Whole Person, 15% to 25%
A patient belongs in class 2 when (1) symptoms and signs of disease or deformity of the vulva or vagina are present that require continuous treatment; *and* (2) sexual intercourse is possible only with some degree of difficulty; *and* (3) the premenopausal patient has limited potential for vaginal delivery.

Example: A 34-year-old married woman developed a rectovaginal fistula after vaginal delivery of her second child. This was corrected surgically, but the woman developed severe vaginal stenosis. She required intermittent dilatation of the vagina under anesthesia and the continuous use of vaginal creams. These measures made sexual intercourse possible, but it was painful and the patient lacked sexual sensation and enjoyment. A third pregnancy ended with a cesarean section because vaginal delivery was deemed hazardous.

Diagnosis: Severe postoperative vaginal stenosis.

Impairment: 20% impairment of the whole person, which includes consideration for the patient's age.

Class 3: Impairment of the Whole Person, 25% to 35%
A patient belongs in class 3 when (1) symptoms and signs of disease or deformity of the vulva or vagina are present that are not controlled by treatment; *and* (2) sexual intercourse is not possible; *and* (3) vaginal delivery is not possible for the premenopausal patient.

Example: A 30-year-old woman with two children had invasive squamous cell carcinoma of the cervix treated with radiation therapy. She subsequently developed a vesicovaginal fistula, rectovaginal fistula, and severe vaginal stenosis. The vaginal depth was 2 cm, and a sinus tract 5 mm in diameter led to the cervix; mucus, feces, and urine were discharged through the sinus. Sexual intercourse was impossible, and pregnancy seemed impossible.

Diagnosis: Vesicovaginal fistula, rectovaginal fistula, and severe vaginal stenosis.

Impairment: Vaginal impairment was estimated to be 35%, which includes consideration for the patient's age; this was *combined* by means of the Combined Values Chart (p. 322) with appropriate estimates for the bladder and rectal impairments to determine the whole-person impairment.

11.6b Cervix and Uterus

The cervix serves as a passageway for spermatozoa and menstrual blood, maintains closure of the uterus during pregnancy, and serves as a portion of the birth canal during vaginal delivery. The uterus is influenced by hormones that are elaborated by the ovaries or administered exogenously. It serves as the organ of menstruation, a means of transportation of spermatozoa, and the container of the products of fertilization. The uterus supplies the power for the first and third stages of labor and, in part, for the second stage.

Symptoms and signs of impairment of function of the cervix and uterus include abnormalities of menstruation, fertility, pregnancy, or labor; excessive size, stenosis, or atresia of the cervical canal; cervical incompetence during pregnancy; noncyclic hemorrhage; uterine displacement; dysplasia; and neoplasia.

Objective techniques useful in evaluating function of the cervix and uterus include, but are not limited to, cervical mucous studies; vaginal, cervical, and intrauterine cytologic smears; biopsy; probing and measuring with calibrated sounds; radiologic studies using radiopaque contrast media; blood and urine hormone studies; basal body temperature recordings; studies of sperm concentration, mobility, and viability; dilation and curettage of the uterus; microscopic study of the endometrium; gynecography; laparoscopy; computed tomography; magnetic resonance imaging; hysteroscopy; ultrasound placental localization techniques; and intra-amniotic pressure studies.

Criteria for Evaluating Permanent Impairment of the Cervix and Uterus

Class 1: Impairment of the Whole Person, 0% to 15%
A patient belongs in class 1 when (1) symptoms and signs of disease or deformity of the cervix or uterus are present that do not require continuous treatment; *or* (2) cervical stenosis, if present, requires no treatment; *or* (3) the postmenopausal patient has anatomic loss of the cervix or uterus.

Example 1: A 22-year-old married woman had experienced menarche at age 14 years. Her menstrual periods lasted 3 days and were of normal volume, and no noncyclic bleeding occurred. Pelvic examination revealed slight asymmetry of the uterus, and an interior smooth, nontender mass 4 cm in diameter projected from the uterus. Ultrasound confirmed the presence of a leiomyoma.

After 1½ years of marriage, during which no contraceptives were used, the woman became pregnant. There was no growth of the leiomyoma during pregnancy and no pain associated with the tumor. The patient was delivered of a healthy infant weighing 12.6 kg (5 lb 12 oz) at 38 weeks. Menstrual periods after delivery averaged 32 days between cycles and were normal in volume and duration.

Diagnosis: Asymptomatic subserosal uterine leiomyoma.

Impairment: 0% impairment of the whole person.

Example 2: A 60-year-old married woman who had had a vaginal hysterectomy 20 years previously for adenomyosis developed vaginal vault prolapse. She noted pelvic pressure and a large bulge protruding from the vulva. Clinical examination disclosed vaginal vault prolapse without significant rectocele, cystocele, or descent of the uterine-vaginal angle. The patient preferred a nonoperative approach to remedying the bulge, and a doughnut pessary was placed. This reduced the vaginal prolapse, and the patient's symptoms resolved. She changed the pessary twice weekly and used a povidone-iodine douche to diminish vaginal discharge.

Diagnosis: Posthysterectomy vaginal vault prolapse.

Impairment: 10% impairment of the whole person.

Class 2: Impairment of the Whole Person, 15% to 25%

A patient belongs in class 2 when (1) symptoms and signs of disease or deformity of the cervix or uterus are present that require continuous treatment; *or* (2) cervical stenosis, if present, requires periodic treatment.

Example: As the result of conization of the cervix, a para-2, 30-year-old woman developed partial stenosis of the cervix and incomplete retention of menstrual blood. Because of prolongation of menstruation and dysmenorrhea, cervical dilation was necessary at 2- to 4-month intervals.

After 2 years the woman became pregnant. Her infant was delivered by cesarean section at 38 weeks, before the onset of labor, because of abruptio placentae. After the delivery she continued to require cervical dilation at 2-month intervals.

Diagnosis: Incomplete cervical stenosis.

Impairment: 15% impairment of the whole person.

Class 3: Impairment of the Whole Person, 25% to 35%

A patient belongs in class 3 when (1) symptoms and signs of disease or deformity of the cervix or uterus are present that are not controlled by treatment; *or* (2) cervical stenosis is complete; *or* (3) the premenopausal woman has anatomic or complete functional loss of the cervix or uterus.

Example 1: As a result of the vaginal delivery of a large infant after a long, difficult labor, a 34-year-old woman suffered severe prolapse of the uterus, which required surgical repair of the anterior and posterior vaginal walls, extensive amputation of the cervix, and posterior fixation of the uterus by plication of the broad ligaments. With careful management, three subsequent pregnancies were achieved, each of which ended in spontaneous abortion between 12 and 16 weeks' gestation, the result of premature dilation of the cervix. Objective evidence that there was almost no cervix indicated that a repair of the incompetent cervix was impossible.

Diagnosis: Partial absence of cervix and cervical incompetence.

Impairment: 30% impairment of the whole person.

Example 2: A 28-year-old gravida-0 woman had stage IB invasive squamous cell carcinoma of the cervix. She underwent radical hysterectomy with pelvic lymphadenectomy. The ovaries were conserved, and no lymph nodes were positive for metastatic disease.

Diagnosis: Absence of the uterus in a reproductive-age patient secondary to treatment of invasive squamous cell carcinoma of the cervix.

Impairment: 30% impairment of the whole person.

11.6c Fallopian Tubes and Ovaries

The fallopian tubes transport ova and spermatozoa. The ovaries develop and release ova and elaborate sex and reproductive hormones.

Symptoms and signs of impairment of function of the fallopian tubes and ovaries include vaginal bleeding or discharge; stenosis or obstruction of the fallopian tubes; abnormal morphologic characteristics; a pelvic mass; neoplasm; absent, infrequent, or abnormal ovulation; abnormal elaboration of hormones; and menstrual dysfunction.

Objective techniques useful in evaluating the function of the fallopian tubes and ovaries include, but are not limited to, cervical and vaginal cytologic smears, pelvic roentgenography, hysterosalpingography, gynecography, ovarian biopsy, blood and urine hormonal assays, ultrasound, computed tomography, magnetic resonance imaging, laparoscopy, and basal body temperature studies.

Criteria for Evaluating Permanent Impairment of the Fallopian Tubes and Ovaries

Any associated endocrine impairment should be evaluated in accordance with the criteria set forth in the *Guides* chapter on the endocrine system (p. 263).

Class 1: Impairment of the Whole Person, 0% to 15%
A patient belongs in class 1 when (1) symptoms and signs of disease or deformities of the fallopian tubes or ovaries are present that do not require continuous treatment; *or* (2) only one fallopian tube or ovary is functioning in a premenopausal patient; *or* (3) there is bilateral loss of function of the fallopian tubes or ovaries in a postmenopausal patient.

Example: A 28-year-old married woman failed to become pregnant after 6 years of marriage, even though contraceptives were not used and sexual intercourse was of average frequency. The woman had experienced menses every 40 to 60 days since menarche at age 12 years. After a hysterosalpingogram revealed bilateral tubal patency and the husband's semen analysis indicated a normal sperm count, clomiphene citrate was administered to induce ovulation. The woman conceived in her second cycle and was delivered of a healthy infant at term.

Diagnosis: Irregular ovulation secondary to hypothalamic-pituitary dysfunction.

Impairment: 5% impairment of the whole person.

Class 2: Impairment of the Whole Person, 15% to 25%
A patient belongs in class 2 when symptoms and signs of disease or deformity of the fallopian tubes or ovaries are present that require continuous treatment, but tubal patency persists and ovulation is possible.

Example: A 27-year-old woman who had borne two children developed increasing pain secondary to severe pelvic endometriosis. She had a laparotomy for resection of bilateral ovarian endometriomas, resection and fulguration of peritoneal implants, and presacral neurectomy. A normal pregnancy ensued that resulted in the birth of a healthy infant. After breast-feeding for 14 months, the patient developed pelvic pain secondary to recurrent endometriosis. This required intermittent medical therapy for suppression of the chronic, recurring pain.

Diagnosis: Recurrent pelvic endometriosis requiring intermittent medical therapy to control pain.

Impairment: 20% impairment of the whole person.

Class 3: Impairment of the Whole Person, 25% to 35%
A patient belongs in class 3 when (1) symptoms and signs of disease or deformity of the fallopian tubes or ovaries are present, and there is a total loss of tubal patency or total failure to produce ova in the premenopausal years; *or* (2) bilateral loss of the fallopian tubes or ovaries occurs in a premenopausal patient.

Example: A 32-year-old mother of two children had severe pelvic infection. Diagnostic studies indicated total proximal and distal occlusion of the fallopian tubes and the presence of bilateral 6-cm hydrosalpinx. A bilateral salpingectomy was performed.

Diagnosis: Bilateral salpingectomy.

Impairment: 30% impairment of the whole person.

References

1. Cassidy MJD, Beck RM. Renal functional reserve in live related kidney donors. *Am J Kidney Dis.* 1988;11:468-472.

2. Danforth DN ed. *Textbook of Obstetrics and Gynecology.* 5th ed. Philadelphia, Pa: JB Lippincott Co; 1986.

3. Schena FP, Cameron JS. Treatment of proteinuric idiopathic glomerulo-nephritides in adults: a retrospective survey. *Am J Med.* 1988;85:315-326.

4. Shabsigh R, Fishman IJ, Quesada ET, Seale-Hawkins CK, Dunn JK. Evaluation of vasculogenic erectile impotence using duplex ultrasonography. *J Urol.* 1989;142:1469-1474.

5. Walsh PC, ed. *Campbell's Urology.* 5th ed. Philadelphia, Pa: WB Saunders Co; 1986.

Chapter 12

The Endocrine System

The purpose of this chapter is to provide physicians with criteria they can use to evaluate permanent impairment of the endocrine system. The endocrine system is composed of the hypothalmic-pituitary complex, thyroid, parathyroids, adrenals, islet tissue of the pancreas, and gonads. These ductless glands secrete hormones that regulate the activity of organs or tissues of the body. Examples of such regulation include control of growth, bone structure, sexual development and function, metabolism, and electrolyte balance. The various endocrine glands are usually interdependent, and a disorder of one gland may be reflected by dysfunction in one or more of the other endocrine glands, which, in turn, may affect other body systems. This possibility should be considered when the individual's permanent impairment is evaluated.

Impairments involving the endocrine system usually result from altered hormone secretion by one or more endocrine glands or the elaboration of hormonal substances by nonendocrine tissue. Dysfunction may be associated with morphologic changes in the endocrine gland(s) involved, such as atrophy, hypertrophy, hyperplasia, or neoplasia; or there may be no demonstrable morphologic changes. Injuries of the glands also can cause impairment.

The specific causes of abnormal secretion are not considered in this chapter. Rather, the chapter focuses on the limitations that continued endocrine dysfunction engenders, considering these especially in terms of the patient's performance of daily activities.

When an endocrine disorder results in *decreased* secretion of a hormone, it is generally possible to replace the hormone with either oral or parenteral medication. In many instances, this results in virtual normalization of body physiology, except, of course, for the inability to secrete the hormone. Apart from the need to take the medication on an ongoing basis, decreased secretion does not result in any impairment. In other cases, replacement hormone cannot be given in a way that completely mimics physiologic hormone secretion, and therefore the patient may be impaired permanently, in terms of either normal activity or ability to respond to stress.

Endocrine deficiencies may be associated with impairments of other organ systems. Such deficiencies should be evaluated in accordance with the criteria in the appropriate *Guides* chapters; the impairment rating of any other body system would be *combined* with that based on this chapter, with the Combined Values Chart (p. 322) used to determine the estimated whole-person impairment.

Disorders resulting in *increased* secretion of a hormone often can be effectively treated, and the patient therefore would not have a permanent impairment. In some cases, treatment may leave the patient with a reduced ability to secrete the hormone, and impairment would be evaluated accordingly. When hypersecretion cannot be effectively treated, the guidelines in this chapter can be used to evaluate impairment.

Neoplasms of the endocrine glands may produce nonhormonal permanent impairments manifested by pain or by effects involving other body systems. Such impairments should be evaluated with the criteria set forth in the *Guides* chapters concerning the respective body systems. It is recognized that, in addition to the abnormalities discussed in this chapter, others may occur that involve the endocrine system. If such abnormalities produce permanent impairment and guidance from this book is lacking, the physician should attempt to assign an impairment percentage reflecting the degree of the impairment.

The focus of this chapter is evaluation of physical impairment that may result from endocrine dysfunction. Since many endocrine abnormalities produce cosmetic or psychiatric abnormalities, the evaluator may wish to consider the criteria for psychiatric impairments discussed in Chapter 14.

Before using the information in this chapter, the reader is urged to read Chapters 1 and 2 and the Glossary, which provide a general discussion of the purpose of the *Guides* and the situations in which they are useful. Chapters 1 and 2 also discuss methods of evaluating patients and preparing reports. A medical evaluation report should include information such as that shown below.

A. Medical Evaluation
- History of medical condition(s)
- Results of most recent clinical evaluation
- Assessment of current clinical status and statement of further medical plans
- Diagnoses

B. Analysis of Findings
- Impact of medical condition(s) on life activities
- Explanation for concluding that the condition is stable and unlikely to change
- Explanation for concluding that the individual is or is not likely to suffer further impairment by engaging in usual activities
- Explanation for concluding that accommodations or restrictions are or are not warranted

C. Comparison of Analysis with Impairment Criteria
- Description of clinical findings and how these findings relate to specific criteria
- Explanation of each impairment estimate
- Summary of all impairment estimates
- Overall whole-person impairment estimate

12.1 Hypothalamic-Pituitary Axis

The intimate relationship between the hypothalamus and the pituitary requires that they be regarded as a unit. The hypothalamus produces chemical factors, such as releasing and inhibitory hormomes, that influence anterior pituitary function and factors that serve as hormones in their own right, such as antidiuretic hormone (ADH) and oxytocin.

The anterior lobe of the pituitary gland produces trophic hormones that control the activity of the thyroid gland (thyrotropin), the adrenal gland (corticotropin), and the gonads (luteinizing hormone [LH] and follicle-stimulating hormone [FSH]). Growth hormone (GH) is responsible for growth before epiphyseal closure and soft-tissue growth after closure and contributes to glucose homeostasis. Prolactin is necessary for lactation.

The posterior lobe of the pituitary is an extension of hypothalamic neurons. Antidiuretic hormone regulates the fluid balance of the body through its ability to influence the excretion of water. The actions of oxytocin, especially in the male, are not well understood.

Permanent impairments due to altered function of the thyroid gland, adrenal glands, and gonads are discussed in subsequent sections of this chapter.

Symptoms and Signs of Impairment of the Hypothalamic-Pituitary Axis

Hypothalamic and pituitary diseases can cause impairments through structural abnormalities or through alterations in hormone production. Structural changes resulting in visual field abnormalities, temporal lobe seizures, frontal lobe abnormalities, headaches, obstructive hydrocephalus, or nonendocrine hypothalamic dysfunction are considered in the chapter on the nervous system (p. 139).

Hypersecretion by the anterior lobe may be manifested by (1) prolactin hypersecretion resulting from a microadenoma or macroadenoma (prolactinoma), the most common cause; (2) GH hypersecretion caused by a pituitary adenoma; or (3) corticotropin hypersecretion leading to adrenocortical hyperfunction.

Prolactin excess results in hypogonadism, which in women may lead to amenorrhea or oligomenorrhea, infertility, varying degrees of estrogen deficiency, decreased libido, and galactorrhea, and in men, to decreased libido, impotence, or infertility. Impairment from prolactin excess is equivalent to gonadotropic deficiency of the appropriate end organ, that is, secondary ovarian failure in women and testicular failure in men. Gonadal failure is discussed further in the reproductive section of this chapter.

Growth hormone hypersecretion results in gigantism before epiphyseal closure and in acromegaly in the adult. The manifestations of acromegaly include enlargment of the hands and feet, coarseness of facial features, and prognathism. Fatigue and increased perspiration are common symptoms. Acromegaly of long duration leads to morbidity from degenerative arthritis and to shortened life expectancy resulting from increased mortality from cardiovascular disease. Growth hormone excess may lead to glucose intolerance or may precipitate or exacerbate diabetes mellitus.

Hyposecretion of anterior lobe hormones may cause isolated or multiple hormone deficiences known as hypopituitarism. The deficiencies may be partial or complete. In childhood, hypopituitarism may be genetic, congenital due to infiltrative disease, related to a craniopharyngioma or adenoma, or of unknown cause. In the adult years, pituitary tumors, infarction (especially postpartum infarction), and surgical or radiotherapeutic interventions are the most common causes.

Hypopituitarism that begins in childhood leads to short stature, failure to enter puberty, and symptoms of thyroid and cortisol deficiency. In adults, hypopituitarism results in hypogonadism, manifested by impotence, and thyroid hormone and cortisol deficiency; women may have amenorrhea. Postpartum pituitary infarction results in an inability to lactate. Hypopituitarism in a person with diabetes results in decreasing insulin requirements. Pallor, fatigue, lethargy, weight loss, and weakness also are common.

Hyperfunction of the posterior lobe, which causes the syndrome of inappropriate antidiuretic hormone secretion (SIADH), may result from a variety of central nervous system disorders. However, SIADH is rarely permanent. Inability of the kidneys to secrete a water load leads to hyponatremia if water intake is not restricted. Fatigue and lethargy progressing to confusion, coma, and seizures may result, depending on the degree of hyponatremia.

Hypofunction of the posterior lobe results in ADH deficiency and diabetes insipidus. Hypofunction usually stems from diseases involving the hypothalamus or pituitary stalk, and less commonly from diseases of the pituitary gland itself. The hypofunction may be hereditary, or it may be related to trauma, surgery, metastatic tumors, craniopharyngioma, histiocytosis X, or other conditions. If thirst is normal, diabetes insipidus is mostly an inconvenience because of polyuria, polydipsia, and nocturia. If thirst is impaired because of concomitant hypothalamic disease, then severe hypernatremia may result, leading to mental depression or coma.

Objective Techniques in Evaluating Function of the Hypothalamic-Pituitary Axis

Structural abnormalities are evaluated by computed tomography (CT), roentgenograms of the sella turcica, and magnetic resonance (MR) imaging. Angiography occasionally is required. Evaluation of visual fields may be needed; this is considered in the *Guides* chapter on the visual system.

Hormonal function must be assessed, and this is often done by stimulation or suppression testing. In children, roentgenography to determine bone age is useful; the age according to roentgenography may be compared with that according to physical examination, including height.

Growth hormone deficiency is assessed by measuring GH in the blood after stimulation testing with exercise, insulin, levodopa, arginine, or other agents. Corticotropin deficiency is assessed by measuring serum corticotropin and cortisol levels and by stimulation testing with insulin or metyrapone.

The diagnosis of secondary hypothyroidism (pituitary and hypothalamic hypothyroidism) is made by demonstrating low concentrations of thyroid hormones without elevation of the thyrotropin level. In this circumstance, CT scanning or MR imaging and tests of pituitary function, including measurement of thyrotropin secretion after injection of protirelin, are needed to determine whether the hypothalamus or the pituitary is responsible. Secondary gonadal insufficiency, that is, hypogonadotropic hypogonadism, requires the demonstration of end organ failure, with low testosterone level in men and low estrogen levels in women, and low or normal levels of the gonadotropins, LH and FSH.

Insufficiency of ADH requires the documentation of urine hyposmolality in the face of a stimulus to urine concentration, usually water restriction. Subsequently, an increase in urine osmolality in response to ADH administration must be demonstrated. Prolactin deficiency is documented by low basal levels of the hormone and its failure to increase after injection of protorelin, chlorpromazine, or other stimulating agent.

Growth hormone excess is documented by failure to suppress GH concentration after a glucose load. Prolactin excess is documented by measurement of elevated basal levels. Inappropriate secretion of ADH is documented by hyponatremia with inappropriately elevated urine osmolality, in the presence of normal cardiac, renal, adrenal, and thyroid function.

Criteria for Evaluating Permanent Impairment of the Hypothalamic-Pituitary Axis

The assessment of permanent impairment of the whole person from disorders of the hypothalamic-pituitary axis requires evaluation of (1) primary abnormalities related to GH, prolactin, or ADH; (2) secondary abnormalities in other endocrine glands, such as thyroid, adrenal, and gonads; and (3) structural and functional disorders of the central nervous system caused by anatomic abnormalities of the pituitary.

The physician must evaluate each disorder separately, using the guidelines in this or other chapters, such as those on the nervous system, visual system, or mental and behavioral disorders. The estimated impairments of the various organ systems then should be *combined* by means of the Combined Values Chart (p. 322).

Class 1: Impairment of the Whole Person, 0% to 15%

A patient with hypothalamic-pituitary disease belongs in class 1 when the disease can be controlled effectively with continuous treatment. As discussed in the introduction to this chapter, many patients who are well controlled with medication may be considered to have no impairments. But if a patient does not take the medication, any degree of impairment may result.

Example: A 19-year-old man developed severe thirst and increased frequency of urination after head trauma occurred in a motor vehicle crash 15 months earlier. His fluid intake and output ranged from 4 to 7 L/d. Nocturia occurred three to six times, and thirst during the night was marked. His general health was excellent, except for fatigue related to interrupted sleep.

On initial assessment, serum osmolality was 292 mOsm/kg and serum sodium concentration was 142 mEq/L; urine osmolality was 120 mOsm/kg, and specific gravity was 1.003. There was no glycosuria. An attempt at water deprivation led to severe thirst with a serum osmolality of 302 mOsm/kg and urine osmolality of 150 mOsm/kg. After an initial ADH injection, urine osmolality rose to 450 mOsm/kg and urine volume diminished.

The patient was placed on a regimen of desmopressin acetate (DDAVP), 0.1 mL twice daily by nasal spray. On this regimen he felt well, and his urine output was well controlled. Symptoms recurred if a dose of DDAVP was missed. No other endocrine disease was found, and he was able to carry out ordinary daily activities.

Diagnosis: Traumatic diabetes insipidus controlled by treatment.

Impairment: 5% impairment of the whole person.

Class 2: Impairment of the Whole Person, 15% to 25%

A patient with hypothalamic-pituitary disease belongs in class 2, when the related symptoms and signs are inadequately controlled by treatment.

Example: A 57-year-old man developed fatigue, hyperhidrosis, headaches, carpal tunnel syndrome, and enlargement of his hands, feet, and nose. He also complained of pain in his knees and back and decreased libido. He was found to have an enlarged sella turcica with suprasellar extension of a pituitary tumor; there were no visual field abnormalities. His GH level of 575 ng/mL was markedly elevated.

Despite an attempt at surgical excision and ionizing radiation therapy, the patient's GH level remained elevated at 100 ng/mL. He was unable to tolerate bromocriptine therapy. His testosterone level was low, but thyroid and adrenal function remained normal. His headaches were relieved, but symptoms of fatigue, excess perspiration, and joint discomfort continued. Libido improved with bimonthly injections of testosterone. The carpal tunnel syndrome required surgical therapy.

Diagnosis: Acromegaly, moderately severe, inadequately controlled by therapy.

Impairment: 15% impairment resulting from acromegaly and 5% impairment from testosterone deficiency, which *combine* to 19% impairment of the whole person (Combined Values Chart, p. 322).

Class 3: Impairment of the Whole Person, 25% to 50%

A patient with hypothalamic-pituitary disease belongs in class 3 when severe symptoms and signs persist despite treatment.

Example: A 55-year-old man had been seen initially at age 45 years because of an enlarged sella turcica. Evaluation revealed a testosterone deficiency and no suprasellar extension of the tumor. The patient was not treated and was lost to follow-up. Several years later he was hospitalized with complaints of excruciating headache, visual loss, and impotence.

Physical examination showed that his beard was markedly diminished and he had a female escutcheon. Testing of visual fields showed nearly complete loss of vision in the left eye and a temporal field defect in the right eye with macular involvement. A skull roentgenogram revealed a massively enlarged sella turcica. A CT scan showed extensive suprasellar growth of the tumor with a suggestion of hemorrhage into the tumor.

The patient underwent emergency transsphenoidal pituitary decompression under coverage with glucocorticoids. After the decompression, visual acuity in the left eye was limited to finger counting, and the temporal field loss in the right eye remained. The preoperative prolactin concentration was 1000 ng/mL, and postoperatively the prolactin level remained elevated at 660 ng/mL.

In the postoperative period, the patient received a course of ionizing radiation to the sella turcica. Subsequent evaluation revealed an elevated prolactin concentration of 280 ng/mL, low testosterone concentration, deficient cortisol response to hypoglycemia, and decreased thyroid function. Vision was unchanged, and mild headaches persisted. The patient was unable to tolerate bromocriptine. Despite testosterone administration, the patient remained impotent.

Diagnosis: Prolactin-secreting pituitary adenoma with pituitary apoplexy, secondary panhypopituitarism, and partial blindness.

Impairment: 10% impairment resulting from pituitary dysfunction, 10% impairment from secondary adrenal dysfunction, and 5% impairment from secondary testosterone deficiency, which *combine* to 23% impairment from endocrine dysfunction; 33% impairment from loss of visual acuity; and 10% impairment from persistent headache. These impairments *combine* to give 53% impairment of the whole person (Combined Values Chart, p. 322).

12.2 Thyroid

The thyroid gland, through its secretion of hormones, influences the metabolic rate of many organ systems. Hypersecretion and hyposecretion of thyroid hormones cause impairments.

Hypersecretion by the thyroid gland results in hyperthyroidism and may be manifested by nervousness, weight loss, heat intolerance, goiter, tachycardia, palpitation, diarrhea, tremor, and muscle weakness. Eye changes, such as exophthalmos, may be present.

Hyposecretion by the thyroid gland results in hypothyroidism and may be manifested by lethargy, slowing of mental processes, weakness, cold intolerance, dry skin, constipation, and myxedema. Late complications include myocardial insufficiency, effusions into body cavities, and coma. Hypothyroidism in infancy may be associated with failure of physical and mental development.

Objective Techniques in Evaluating Function of the Thyroid

These include, but are not limited to, determination of (1) circulating thyroid hormone levels, including total thyroxine, free thyroxine, triiodothyronine, and free triiodothyronine; (2) circulating pituitary thyrotropin level measured by a sensitive assay; (3) radioiodine uptake of the thyroid gland; and (4) radiotriiodothyronine resin or red blood cell uptake. The nature of thyroid nodules is often best evaluated by needle aspiration or biopsy.

Criteria for Evaluating Permanent Impairment of the Thyroid

Hyperthyroidism is not considered to be a cause of permanent impairment, because the hypermetabolic state in practically all patients can be corrected by treatment. However, the ophthalmopathy seen in some cases of hyperthyroidism may persist after treatment of the thyrotoxic state and result in permanent cosmetic disfigurement or visual impairment. These conditions should be evaluated as described in the chapters on the ear, nose, throat, and related structures and the visual system.

Hypothyroidism, in most instances, can be controlled satisfactorily by the administration of thyroid medication. Occasionally, because of associated disease in other organ systems, full hormone replacement may not be possible.

Class 1: Impairment of the Whole Person, 0% to 15%

A patient belongs in class 1 when (1) continuous thyroid therapy is required for correction of the thyroid insufficiency or for maintenance of normal thyroid anatomy *and* (2) there is no objective physical or laboratory evidence of inadequate replacement therapy.

Example: In a 45-year-old woman with symptoms of mild hypothyroidism of 2 years' duration, the diagnosis of lymphoepithelial goiter (Hashimoto's thyroiditis) was made after needle biopsy. She required daily therapy with 0.20 mg of levothyroxine to maintain a normal-sized thyroid, although the symptoms of hormone deficiency were relieved by a lower dose.

Diagnosis: Hashimoto's thyroiditis controlled by treatment.

Impairment: 5% impairment of the whole person.

Class 2: Impairment of the Whole Person, 15% to 25%

A patient belongs in class 2 when (1) symptoms and signs of thyroid disease are present, or there is anatomic loss or alteration, *and* (2) continuous thyroid hormone replacement therapy is required for correction of the confirmed thyroid insufficiency, *and* (3) the presence of a disease process in another body system permits only partial replacement of the thyroid hormone.

Example: A 65-year-old man had severe hypothyroidism of 16 months' duration, with pronounced mental slowing, loss of memory, and apathy. He also had severe coronary artery disease with angina pectoris that could be precipitated by walking only 50 ft. The total thyroxine level was 0.5 mg/dL, and that of thyrotropin was 100 mU/mL. Repeated trials and careful adjustment of doses of levothyroxine indicated that a dose larger than 0.05 mg/d caused aggravation of the angina. Significant debility due to hypothyroidism persisted.

Diagnosis: Partially treated hypothyroidism.

Impairment: 20% impairment resulting from hypothyroidism, which is to be *combined* with an appropriate value for the cardiovascular impairment to determine impairment of the whole person. However, if the cardiovascular disease were treated, for instance, by angioplasty or bypass surgery, it might be possible to replace the thyroid hormone level fully, in which case the degree of impairment would need to be reevaluated.

12.3 Parathyroids

The secretion of parathyroid hormone from the four parathyroid glands regulates the levels of serum calcium and phosphorus, which are essential to the proper functioning of the skeletal, digestive, renal, and nervous systems. The major abnormalities of the glands include hyperfunction, hypofunction, and carcinoma.

Symptoms and Signs of Impairment of Function of the Parathyroids

Hypersecretion of parathyroid hormone, or hyperparathyroidism, may be due to the hyperfunctioning of one gland, as with an adenoma, or that of all four glands, as with hyperplasia, or may result from a parathyroid carcinoma. Manifestations of this condition include lethargy, constipation, nausea, vomiting, and polyuria, and, in extreme cases, bone pain, renal calculi, renal failure, and coma.

Hyposecretion of parathyroid hormone, or hypoparathyroidism, may be due to inadvertent removal of the parathyroid glands during thyroidectomy, surgical excision for the treatment of hyperparathyroidism, or unknown causes. Manifestations include chronic tetany, paresthesias, and seizures, and especially in idiopathic cases, cataracts, chronic moniliasis of the skin, alopecia, and hypofunction of other endocrine organs. Idiopathic hypoparathyroidism may be associated with hypothyroidism, diabetes mellitus, adrenal insufficiency, hypogonadism, or pernicious anemia.

Objective Techniques in Evaluating Parathyroid Function

Techniques of evaluating parathyroid gland function include determinations of serum calcium, phosphorus, albumin, creatinine, and parathyroid hormone levels, calcium concentration in urine, and urinary cyclic adenosine monophosphate response to intravenously administered parathyroid hormone. Intravenous pyelography, skeletal roentgenography, and bone density studies may be useful.

Criteria for Evaluating Permanent Impairment of the Parathyroids

In most cases of hyperparathyroidism, surgical treatment results in correction of the primary abnormality, although secondary symptoms and signs may persist, such as renal calculi or renal failure. The latter signs should be evaluated according to criteria in the chapter on the urinary and reproductive systems. If surgery fails, or if the patient cannot undergo surgery, long-term therapy may be necessary, in which case the permanent impairment may be classified according to the criteria in Table 1 (below).

Table 1. Impairments Related to Hyperparathyroidism.

Severity	% Impairment of the whole person
Symptoms and signs easily controlled with medical therapy	0 - 14
Persistent mild hypercalcemia with mild nausea and polyuria	15 - 29
Severe hypercalcemia with nausea and lethargy	30 - 90

Hypoparathyroidism is a chronic condition of variable severity that requires long-term medical therapy in most cases. The degree of severity determines the estimated degree of permanent impairment, as Table 2 (p. 269) indicates.

Table 2. Impairments Related to Hypoparathyroidism.

Severity	% Impairment of the whole person
Symptoms and signs easily controlled by medical therapy	0 - 9
Intermittent hypercalcemia or hypocalcemia; symptoms more frequent than with above category, despite careful medical attention	10 - 20

12.4 Adrenal Cortex

The adrenal cortex synthesizes and secretes adrenocortical hormones. These hormones participate in the regulation of electrolyte and water metabolism and in the intermediate metabolism of carbohydrate, fat, and protein. They also affect inflammatory response, cell membrane permeability, and antigen-antibody reactions, and they play a role in the development and maintenance of secondary sexual characteristics.

Impairment may result from either hypersecretion or hyposecretion of the cortical hormones. Such abnormalities may be associated with dysfunction of another endocrine gland, for instance, the pituitary. If this occurs, the adrenal impairment and the impairment related to the other gland are both evaluated, and the two whole-person impairments are *combined* by means of the Combined Values Chart (p. 322).

Symptoms and Signs of Impairment of Function of the Adrenal Cortex

Hypersecretion of adrenocortical hormones results from hyperplasia or from benign or malignant tumors of the adrenal cortex. The symptoms and signs of adrenocortical disease may arise from hypersecretion of one or more of the following hormones: (1) glucocorticoids, (2) mineralocorticoids, (3) androgens, and (4) estrogens. In some instances, there may be hypersecretion of hormones in one category and hyposecretion of those in another.

Iatrogenic Cushing's syndrome secondary to nonphysiologic doses of glucocorticoids administered for systemic diseases such as bronchial asthma, systemic lupus erythematosus, or rheumatoid arthritis is the most common condition related to adrenal hormonal excess.

Among the diseases caused by hypersecretion of the adrenocortical hormones are Cushing's syndrome, the adrenogenital syndrome, and primary aldosteronism. Hypersecretion of the adrenal cortex caused by hyperplasia may be associated either with a tumor of the anterior pituitary gland or with a malignant tumor that arises outside the endocrine system and causes ectopic corticotropin secretion.

Hyposecretion of adrenocortical hormones may be primary, resulting from surgical removal or destruction of the adrenals, as with Addison's disease, or secondary, resulting from decreased production of corticotropin. Therapy is guided by the number of hormonal deficiencies, which may be single, as in hypoaldosteronism, or multiple, as in adrenocortical destruction. One normal adrenal gland can compensate for the loss of the other.

Objective Techniques in Evaluating Function of the Adrenal Cortex

These techniques include (1) measurement of adrenocortical hormones in the urine, such as free cortisol and aldosterone, and of hormones in the plasma, such as cortisol and aldosterone; (2) measurement of corticotropin, serum electrolytes, plasma glucose, and creatinine; (3) measurement of the effects of suppression and stimulation of adrenocortical function; and (4) roentgenography of the adrenal glands, CT scanning, MR imaging, arteriography, and venography of the skull.

Criteria for Evaluating Permanent Impairment of the Adrenal Cortex

Hypoadrenalism is a lifelong condition that requires long-term replacement therapy with glucocorticoids and/or mineralocorticoids for proven hormonal deficiencies. Evaluation of improvement may be difficult, because a person may be fully functional on an everyday basis while taking replacement medication but not be able to respond properly to the stress of fever, trauma, infection, or very warm weather. This impaired ability to respond to stress needs careful consideration. Impairments should be classified according to Table 3 (below).

Table 3. Impairments Related to Hypoadrenalism.

Severity	% Impairment of the whole person
Symptoms and signs controlled with medical therapy	0 - 14
Symptoms and signs controlled inadequately, especially during acute illnesses	15 - 29
Severe symptoms of adrenal crisis during major illnesses*	30 - 90

*This would be considered a permanent impairment only if the episodes recurred and could not be controlled with therapy.

Hyperadrenocorticism caused by the chronic side effects of nonphysiologic doses of glucocorticoids, that is, iatrogenic Cushing's syndrome, is related to dosage and duration of treatment and may cause osteoporosis, hypertension, diabetes mellitus, and the catabolic effects that result in protein myopathy, striae, and easy bruising. Permanent impairments may range from 0% to 100%, depending on the severity and chronicity of the disease process for which the steroids are given. Impairments from diseases of the pituitary-adrenal axis should be estimated according to Table 4 (below).

Table 4. Impairments Related to Hyperadrenocorticism.*

Severity	% Impairment of the whole person
Minimal, as with hyperadrenocorticism that is surgically corrected by removal of a pituitary or adrenal adenoma or due to moderate pharmacologic doses of glucocorticoids	0 - 14
Moderate, as with bilateral hyperplasia that is treated with medical therapy or adrenalectomy or due to large pharmacologic doses of glucocorticoids	15 - 39
Severe, as with aggressively metastasizing adrenal carcinoma	Variable†

*This table should be used to evaluate impairments resulting from general effects of adrenal steroids, such as myopathy, easy bruising, and obesity. The estimated percentages should be *combined* with those related to specific impairments, such as diabetes or fractures due to osteoporosis, by means of the Combined Values Chart (p. 322).

†The degree of estimated impairment will depend on the effects of the tumor on other organ systems; appropriate *Guides* chapters should be consulted.

12.5 Adrenal Medulla

The adrenal medulla synthesizes and secretes primarily epinephrine, which functions in the regulation of blood pressure and cardiac output and, to some extent, affects the intermediate metabolism of the body. The adrenal medulla is usually not essential to the maintenance of life or well-being. Hence, its absence does not constitute a permanent impairment.

Hyperfunction of the adrenal medulla may be caused by pheochromocytomas or, rarely, by hyperplasia of the chromaffin cells. Pheochromocytomas may arise at any site in the body that has sympathetic nervous tissue. The presence of a pheochromocytoma is usually associated with paroxysmal or sustained hypertension. Approximately 10% of pheochromocytomas are malignant. Pheochromocytomas may be multiple in an individual and may occur in families in association with medullary carcinoma of the thyroid and hyperplasia of the parathyroid; this constitutes the syndrome of multiple endocrine neoplasms.

Objective Techniques in Evaluating the Function of the Adrenal Medulla

These techniques include (1) measurement of unmetabolized urinary catecholamines, including total catecholamines, epinephrine, and norepinephrine, and of their degradation products in urine, vanillylmandelic acid and metanephrines; (2) measurement of the plasma catecholamines, epinephrine, norepinephrine, and dopamine; and (3) radiography of the adrenals, including arteriography, venography, CT scanning, and MR imaging.

Criteria for Evaluating Permanent Impairment of the Adrenal Medulla

Permanent impairment related to a pheochromocytoma may be classified by means of Table 5 (below).

Table 5. Permanent Impairment Related to Pheochromocytomas.

Severity	% Impairment of the whole person
Minimal, as when the duration of hypertension has not led to cardiovascular disease and a benign tumor can be removed surgically	0 - 14
Moderate, as with an inoperable malignant pheochromocytoma; the signs and symptoms of catecholamine excess can be controlled with blocking agents	15 - 29
Severe, as with a widely metastatic malignant pheochromocytoma, in which symptoms of catecholamine excess cannot be controlled	30 - 90

12.6 Pancreas (Islets of Langerhans)

Insulin and glucagon are among the hormones secreted by the islets of Langerhans. Both hormones are required for the maintenance of normal metabolism of carbohydrates, lipids, and proteins. Permanent impairment may result from a deficiency or an excess of either hormone. Removal of normal pancreatic tissue during the resection of an islet cell neoplasm does not constitute an endocrine impairment if, after the operation, the patient's carbohydrate tolerance is normal.

Symptoms and Signs of Impairment of Function of the Pancreatic Islets

Abnormalities of islet cell function may be manifested by high plasma glucose levels, as in diabetes mellitus, or by low plasma glucose levels, as in hypoglycemia. Diabetes mellitus is classified into two main groups: insulin-dependent (type I) diabetes and non-insulin-dependent (type II) diabetes. People with insulin-dependent diabetes mellitus, if untreated, will worsen to have stupor, coma, and then death. This type of diabetes mellitus usually begins in young persons, but it may occur at any age. People with non-insulin-dependent diabetes generally are more than 40 years old and are overweight.

The main complications of diabetes mellitus and their associated impairments are (1) retinopathy, causing visual impairment; (2) nephropathy, causing renal impairment; (3) arteriosclerosis, causing arteriosclerotic heart disease and cerebrovascular and peripheral vascular disease; and (4) neuropathy.

Hypogycemia occasionally causes impairment. Hypoglycemia may result from excessive insulin that either is produced endogenously or administered by injection. Hypoglycemia may be manifested by weakness, sweating, tachycardia, headache, muscular incoordination, blurred vision, loss of consciousness, and convulsions. Prolonged hypoglycemia or repeated severe attacks of hypoglycemia may lead to mental deterioration.

Objective Techniques in Evaluating Impairments Related to Diabetes Mellitus

These techniques include, but are not limited to, (1) determination of fasting and postprandial plasma glucose levels; (2) determination of hemoglobin A_{1c} level; (3) measurements of levels of cholesterol and other lipids; (4) electrocardiogram or cardiac stress testing; (5) ophthalmologic examination; (6) tests of renal and bladder function, including measurement of urine protein; tests of urinary "microalbumin" may detect diabetic nephropathy at an early stage and predict future impairment, but they do not give additional information about the patient's current status; (7) Doppler testing of the peripheral circulation; (8) roentgenograms of the chest, gastrointestinal tract, pelvis, or extremities, including arteriograms; and (9) neurologic testing.

It is useful to examine the results from blood glucose testing done by the patient at home, because this gives an additional measure of the degree of glucose control. However, these measurements may be manipulated by the patient, and therefore they are less objective than laboratory methods.

Much of the impairment that results from diabetes is related to the complications of diabetes. Therefore, the examiner must always not only determine the presence or absence of retinopathy, neuropathy, and other signs, but also evaluate the other systems that may be involved. Impairments of other systems would be expressed as whole-person impairments and then *combined* with an impairment percent resulting from instability of glucose control by means of the Combined Values Chart (p. 322).

Criteria for Evaluating Permanent Impairment Related to Diabetes Mellitus

Permanent impairment from diabetes mellitus can be evaluated by the following criteria.

Class 1: Impairment of the Whole Person, 0% to 5%

A patient with diabetes mellitus belongs in class 1 if he or she has non-insulin-dependent (type II) diabetes mellitus that can be controlled by diet. The person may or may not have evidence of diabetic microangiopathy, as indicated by the presence of retinopathy or albuminuria greater than 30 mg/dL.

Example 1: Medical examinations during a 2-year period disclosed 1+ glucosuria in a moderately obese 40-year-old man. Fasting plasma glucose level was 160 mg/dL on two occasions. Retina examination showed no diabetic retinopathy, and there was no albumin in the urine. After 3 months on a special diet, the man's weight was normal, and his fasting plasma glucose level was 110 mg/dL.

Diagnosis: Non-insulin-dependent (type II) diabetes mellitus controlled by diet, without evidence of diabetic microangiopathy.

Impairment: 0% impairment of the whole person.

Example 2: An obese 45-year-old woman had an elevated fasting plasma glucose level on an initial evaluation, and a physical examination 14 months later disclosed retinal microaneurysms and "dot and blot" hemorrhages. There was no impairment of vision.

Diagnosis: Non-insulin-dependent (type II) diabetes mellitus with early diabetic retinopathy.

Impairment: 5% impairment of the whole person.

Class 2: Impairment of the Whole Person, 5% to 10%

A patient belongs in this classification when there is a diagnosis of non-insulin-dependent (type II) diabetes mellitus; *and* when satisfactory control of the plasma glucose level requires both a restricted diet and hypoglycemic medication, either an oral agent or insulin. Evidence of microangiopathy, as indicated by retinopathy or by albuminuria of greater than

30 mg/dL, may or may not be present. If retinopathy has led to visual impairment, this must be evaluated as described in the chapter on the visual system.

Example 1: Several years ago, a 55-year-old man had developed the signs and symptoms of non-insulin-dependent (type II) diabetes mellitus. Examination at that time disclosed no retinopathy or proteinuria. Although he lost weight on a prescribed diet, the plasma glucose level could not be maintained within normal limits on that diet. When the patient was on a restricted diet and was taking an oral agent, his fasting serum glucose level was 120 mg/dL, and his glycohemoglobin level was 9.5% (normal, 6.0% to 8.5%).

Diagnosis: Non-insulin-dependent (type II) diabetes mellitus reasonably well controlled by diet and oral agent.

Impairment: 5% impairment of the whole person.

Example 2: A 50-year-old man had had non-insulin-dependent (type II) diabetes mellitus for 5 years. At the onset of the disease, he had a fasting plasma glucose level of 190 mg/dL when on a restricted diet and taking an oral hypoglycemic agent. Four years ago, his right leg was amputated above the knee because of severe peripheral vascular disease leading to gangrene of the foot.

At present, the man adheres to a prescribed diet and takes 16 U of isophane insulin daily. On this regimen, the fasting plasma glucose level is 125 to 140 mg/dL. The patient has no symptoms, nor does he have glucosuria or acetonuria. The glycohemoglobin concentration is 10.8%.

Diagnosis: Non-insulin-dependent (type II) diabetes mellitus with complications, requiring insulin to control hyperglycemia. Plasma glucose level is fairly well controlled by diet and one daily injection of insulin.

Impairment: 10% impairment resulting from non-insulin-dependent (type II) diabetes mellitus and 36% impairment from a midthigh amputation above the knee joint, which *combine* to give 42% impairment of the whole person (Combined Values Chart, p. 322).

Class 3: Impairment of the Whole Person, 10% to 20%
A patient belongs in this class when insulin-dependent (type I) diabetes mellitus is present with or without evidence of microangiopathy.

Example 1: A 33-year-old woman had had insulin-dependent (type I) diabetes mellitus for 5 years. She originally presented with polyuria, polydipsia, and weight loss, and with a plasma glucose level of 400 mg/dL and marked ketonuria. The condition was satisfactorily controlled with a prescribed diet and an injection of insulin before both breakfast and dinner. Meals and insulin had to be taken at prescribed times to maintain adequate glycemic control. There was no evidence of microangiopathy.

Diagnosis: Insulin-dependent (type I) diabetes mellitus satisfactorily controlled by insulin and diet.

Impairment: 15% impairment of the whole person.

Example 2: A 40-year-old woman had onset of insulin-dependent (type I) diabetes mellitus 20 years earlier, when she had experienced polydipsia, polyuria, weight loss, and plasma glucose level of 350 mg/dL. At present, the condition is satisfactorily controlled with diet and a daily injection of insulin. Ophthalmologic examination discloses that background retinopathy is present.

Diagnosis: Insulin-dependent (type I) diabetes mellitus with diabetic microangiopathy and no visual impairment.

Impairment: 20% impairment of the whole person.

Example 3: A 45-year-old man had had insulin-dependent (type I) diabetes mellitus for 25 years. He had proliferative retinopathy, an elevated creatinine level, and a diminished creatinine clearance. The plasma glucose level was controlled by a mixture of isophane and regular insulin given twice daily, 12 U before breakfast and 6 U before dinner. Ophthalmologic examination showed 70% impairment of vision of the right eye and 63% impairment in the left, which *combine* to give 55% impairment of the visual system (Chapter 8, Table 6, p. 218).

Diagnosis: Insulin-dependent (type I) diabetes mellitus with complications; plasma glucose level is satisfactorily controlled by diet and insulin.

Impairment: 20% impairment from diabetes mellitus, and 55% impairment of the visual system, which should be *combined* by means of the Combined Values Chart (p. 322) and then *combined* with a whole-person impairment estimate for the urinary system to determine total permanent impairment.

Class 4: Impairment of the Whole Person, 20% to 40%
A patient belongs in class 4 when the patient has the diagnosis of insulin-dependent (type I) diabetes mellitus, and when hyperglycemia or hypoglycemia occurs frequently despite the conscientious efforts of both the patient and the physician.

Example 1: A 24-year-old man had had labile insulin-dependent (type I) diabetes mellitus for 10 years. His physical activities varied greatly from day to day. Despite adherence to a prescribed diet that included between-meal and bedtime snacks, and despite a carefully planned insulin program with both morning and evening injections, results of home plasma glucose tests varied greatly, and at times severe insulin reactions occurred without warning. The man was 10% underweight but showed no clinical or laboratory evidence of complications.

Diagnosis: Insulin-dependent (type I) diabetes mellitus, not adequately controlled by diet and insulin.

Impairment: 35% impairment of the whole person.

Example 2: A 35-year-old woman had had poorly controlled insulin-dependent (type I) diabetes mellitus for 15 years. Although fasting plasma glucose level was often greater than 200 mg/dL, and the urine usually contained glucose, severe hypoglycemic reactions occurred unpredictably several times a week. The patient was malnourished on a 3000-kcal diet, and she took injections of 30 U of insulin zinc suspension before breakfast and 10 U of insulin zinc suspension before supper. She became fatigued easily and complained of burning foot pain and of difficulty in walking. Vibratory sensation and deep tendon reflexes were absent below the knees. Examination of the fundi disclosed numerous microaneurysms, but there was no visual impairment.

Diagnosis: Insulin-dependent (type I) diabetes mellitus with complications, not adequately controlled by diet and insulin.

Impairment: 40% impairment resulting from diabetes mellitus and 15% impairment from peripheral neuropathy, which *combine* to 49% impairment of the whole person (Combined Values Chart, p. 322).

Objective Techniques in Evaluating Impairments Related to Hypoglycemia

These techniques include, but are not limited to, (1) measurement of plasma glucose after overnight or longer periods of fasting on several occasions; (2) roentgenograms of the skull, chest, and abdomen; (3) tests of liver function; and (4) tests of adrenocortical and pituitary gland function. Documented hypoglycemia requires a detailed medical evaluation to determine the specific cause.

Criteria for Evaluating Permanent Impairments Related to Hypoglycemia

These criteria are as follows.

Class 1: Impairment of the Whole Person, 0% to 5%

A patient has class 1 impairment when surgical removal of an islet cell adenoma results in complete remission of the symptoms and signs of hypoglycemia, and there are no postoperative sequelae.

Example: The wife of a 45-year-old man noted that increasingly often her husband had a bad temper on arising, but that his outlook improved after breakfast. The man did not use alcohol or tobacco. Late one morning while at work, the man suddenly became agitated and lost consciousness. On emergency admission to a hospital, his plasma glucose level was 20 mg/dL. The man remained weak and irritable before breakfast, despite a high carbohydrate intake that included a large feeding at bedtime. His fasting plasma glucose level never exceeded 35 mg/dL. Plasma insulin, C-peptide, and proinsulin levels were elevated during the hypoglycemic episodes.

An abdominal examination and a chest roentgenogram disclosed no abnormalities, and pituitary, adrenal, and liver functions were normal. During an operation, a small insulinoma, later found to be benign, was excised from the head of the pancreas. After a 3-month recovery period, the patient remained without symptoms.

Diagnosis: Benign functioning islet cell adenoma (insulinoma), with remission after excision.

Impairment: 0% impairment of the whole person.

Class 2: Impairment of the Whole Person, 5% to 50%

A patient with symptoms and signs of hypoglycemia has class 2 impairment, which ranges from 5% to 50%, depending on the degree of control obtained with diet and medications, other coexisting conditions, and on how the condition affects daily activities.

Example: A 55-year-old man developed alarming personality changes during a period of a few weeks and had a seizure. A diagnosis of insulinoma was made. Laparotomy revealed a large islet cell adenocarcinoma in the tail of the pancreas with metastases in the liver. The spleen and the main tumor mass were resected. The man experienced no impairment of hepatic function, and recovery from surgery was uneventful except for persistence of mild fasting hypoglycemia.

The hypoglycemia responded well to frequent feedings of a high-protein, high-carbohydrate diet and 40 mg of prednisone taken daily. Ten months after returning to work, the patient still had occasional transient mental lapses, during one of which the plasma glucose level was 28 mg/dL. When the daily dosage of prednisone was increased to 60 mg, the symptomatic hypoglycemia improved, but the manifestations of Cushing's syndrome became more prominent.

Diagnosis: Metastatic islet cell adenocarcinoma with incomplete control of symptoms.

Impairment: 50% impairment resulting from the pancreatic malignant neoplasm and hypoglycemia and 10% impairment from steroid-induced Cushing's syndrome; because they involve different parts of the endocrine system, these impairment values are *combined*, giving 55% impairment of the whole person (Combined Values Chart, p. 322).

12.7 The Gonads

The gonads produce spermatozoa or ova and also produce sex hormones that affect physical and sexual development and behavior. The interstitial cells of the testes produce male hormones. The most significant hormones of the ovaries are estrogen from the follicles and progesterone from the corpora lutea. Changes in function of the gonads can be produced by tumors, trauma, infection, scarring, and surgical removal. Gonadal function may vary with changes in the pituitary-hypothalamic axis.

Symptoms and Signs of Impairment of Function of the Gonads

Precocious puberty in boys results in early, rapid growth and accelerated skeletal maturation. Occasionally a tendency toward this condition is familial. Precocious puberty in girls may be caused by an ovarian tumor, but usually a cause is not found; the condition can result in accelerated skeletal maturation. Some ovarian tumors may cause masculinization. Certain ovarian conditions produce heavy and irregular menstrual periods.

Testicular hypofunction results in eunuchism or a eunuchlike condition. Symptoms are diminished sexual function, failure to develop or maintain secondary sexual characteristics, and, if there is onset before adolescence, growth of the body beyond the usual age because of delayed epiphyseal closure. Patients with this condition usually lack endurance and strength.

Ovarian hypofunction, with onset before adolescence, may be characterized by primary amenorrhea, poor development of secondary sexual characteristics, and growth beyond the usual age because of delayed maturation of the skeleton. Menopause is a natural occurrence in older women, but it also may follow surgical removal of the ovaries. It may be accompanied by such symptoms as hot flashes, irritability, fatigue, and headaches. Osteoporosis and other changes may occur during later years.

Objective Techniques in Evaluating Function of the Gonads

These techniques include, but are not limited to, (1) measurements of plasma gonadotropins, testosterone, estrogen, and progesterone, and occasionally 17-ketosteroids in the urine; (2) radiographic determinations of bone age in children and adolescents; (3) evaluation of sella turcica size by CT scan or MR imaging; (4) sex chromatin and chromosome studies; (5) testicular biopsy; (6) semen examination; (7) vaginal cytologic examination; (8) culdoscopy or laparoscopy; (9) endometrial biopsy; (10) ovarian biopsy; and (11) pelvic ultrasound in women.

Criteria for Evaluating Permanent Impairment of the Gonads

A patient with anatomic loss or alteration of the gonads that results in an absence, or an abnormally high level, of gonadal hormones would have 0% to 5% impairment of the whole person. Impairment resulting from inability to reproduce, and other impairments associated with gonadal dysfunction, should be evaluated in accordance with the criteria set forth in the chapter on the urinary and reproductive systems (p. 249).

Example 1: A 13-year-old girl complained of severe menorrhagia during the preceding 18 months. She had experienced vaginal bleeding since the age of 9 years, at which time breast development began and pubic hair appeared. Also at that time, there was a growth spurt that slowed and stopped during her 13th year. On physical examination her height was 4 ft 11 in (150 cm).

The girl's bone age was 17 years, and it seemed unlikely that she would grow taller. Urinary gonadotropin values were in the low-normal range, while levels of urinary estrogens were elevated. The right ovary was enlarged to about five times its normal size. The ovary was removed surgically and was found to contain a benign granulosa cell tumor. The left ovary was the size of an infant's and without visible follicles. A year after the operation, the patient had regular, normal menses.

Diagnosis: Precocious puberty caused by granulosa cell tumor of the ovary.

Impairment: 0% impairment resulting from precocious puberty. The impairment of the whole person would be determined by the loss of one ovary. Short stature is not considered an impairment.

Example 2: A 31-year-old man complained of lack of sexual development and function, a high-pitched voice, and having no beard. He was tall and had relatively long arms and legs. The penis was tiny, and the scrotum and testes were small. The bone age was 18 years, the plasma testosterone level was 70 ng/mL, and the plasma gonadotropin level was low.

The man responded well to continuous treatment with testosterone. The penis became larger, and there was adequate sexual functioning. He had an increase in body and facial hair, and his voice became deeper.

Diagnosis: Hypogonadotropic hypogonadism.

Impairment: 5% impairment of the whole person.

12.8 Mammary Glands

The mammary glands make, store, and secrete milk. Absence of the mammary glands does not cause impairment of the whole person in males, but in females it will prevent nursing. In some endocrine disorders, there may be galactorrhea in females and gynecomastia in males. Gynecomastia in males may be accompanied by galactorrhea.

A female patient of childbearing age with absence of the breasts, a patient with galactorrhea sufficient to require the use of absorbent pads, and a male patient with painful gynecomastia that interferes with the performance of daily activities would each have 0% to 5% impairment of the whole person. If there were a coexisting psychiatric impairment, the whole-person impairment would be greater.

12.9 Metabolic Bone Disease

Metabolic bone disease, such as osteoporosis, vitamin D-resistant osteomalacia, and Paget's disease, may require continuous therapy. These conditions, unless accompanied by pain, skeletal deformity, or peripheral nerve involvement, are estimated to be 0% impairments. When continuous hormone and mineral therapy gives complete relief of symptoms, impairment of the whole person may be considered to be 0% to 3%. When continuous therapy is required to relieve pain, and the activities of daily living are restricted because of pain, the estimate should be 5% to 15% impairment of the whole person.

Impairment from pain, which may result from spinal collapse or other complications of metabolic bone disease, is discussed in the chapters on the musculoskeletal system and pain. In general, the impairment percents shown in the *Guides* chapters make allowance for the pain that may accompany the impairing conditions. Any associated loss of motion should be evaluated in accordance with the criteria set forth in the chapter on the musculoskeletal system.

Example: A 68-year-old woman had severe osteoporosis of the axial skeleton and, to a lesser extent, of the extremities. She had considerable local pain with motion of the back and spine, along with some generalized backache and spasm related to partial collapse of T4 and T12. Pain persisted despite prolonged therapy with anabolic agents, estrogens, vitamin D, and calcium.

Diagnosis: Postmenopausal osteoporosis with incomplete symptomatic control and collapse of thoracic vertebrae.

Impairment: 15% impairment of the whole person, which should be *combined* by means of the Combined Values Chart (p. 322) with the estimated impairment percentage related to any musculoskeletal system impairment.

References

1. Wilson JD, Foster DW, eds. *Williams Textbook of Endocrinology.* 7th ed. Philadelphia, Pa: WB Saunders Co; 1985.

2. Felig P, Baxter J, Broadus A, Frohman L. *Endocrinology and Metabolism.* 2nd ed. New York, NY: McGraw-Hill Book Co; 1987.

3. Marble A, Krall LP, Bradley RF, Christlieb AR, Soeldner JS, eds. *Joslin's Diabetes Mellitus.* 12th ed. Philadelphia, Pa: Lea & Febiger; 1985.

4. Levin ME, O'Neal LW, eds. *The Diabetic Foot.* 3rd ed. St Louis, Mo: CV Mosby Co; 1983.

5. Davidson JK, ed. *Clinical Diabetes Mellitus: A Problem-Oriented Approach.* 2nd ed. New York, NY: Thieme Medical Publishers; 1991.

Chapter 13

The Skin

This chapter provides criteria for evaluating the effects of permanent impairments of the skin and its appendages. These are considered especially in terms of the effects they may have on an individual's ability to carry out daily activities, including those related to employment.

Before using the information in this chapter, the reader should study Chapters 1 and 2 and the Glossary (p. 315), which discuss the general purpose of the *Guides*, the situations in which they are useful, basic definitions, and recommended methods for evaluating impairments. An impairment evaluation report, as explained in Chapter 2, should include information such as that shown below.

A. Medical Evaluation
- History of medical condition
- Results of most recent medical evaluation
- Assessment of current medical status and statement of further medical plans
- Diagnosis

B. Analysis of Findings
- Impact of medical condition on life activities
- Explanation for concluding that the condition is stable and unlikely to change
- Explanation for concluding that the individual is or is not likely to suffer further impairment by engaging in usual activities
- Explanation for concluding that accommodations or restrictions related to the impairment are or are not warranted

C. Comparison of Analysis with Impairment Criteria
- Description of clinical findings and how these findings relate to *Guides* criteria
- Explanation of each estimated impairment
- List of all impairment percentages
- Estimated whole-person impairment percentage

13.1 Structure and Functions

The components of the skin and its functions are shown in Table 1 (p. 278). The functions of the skin include (1) providing a protective covering; (2) participating in sensory perception, temperature regulation, fluid regulation, electrolyte balance, immunobiologic defenses, and resistance to trauma; and (3) regenerating the epidermis and its appendages.

Protective skin functions include, for example, barrier defenses against damage by chemical irritants and allergic sensitizers, invasion by microorganisms, and injuries by ultraviolet light. Temperature regulation involves the proper function of the sweat glands and the small blood vessels. The barrier defense against fluid loss is related to the intactness of the stratum corneum.

Permanent impairment of the skin is defined as any anatomic or functional abnormality or loss that persists after medical treatment and rehabilitation and

Table 1. Structure and Functions of the Skin.*

Structure or component	Function	Perturbations
Epidermis		
Stratum corneum	Barrier against microorganisms, chemicals, water loss	Infection, contact dermatitis, xerosis
Squamous and basal cells	Stratum corneum regeneration, wound repair	Squamous or basal cell carcinoma, ulceration
Melanocytes	Protection from ultraviolet radiation	Vitiligo, sunburn, hyperpigmentation, melanoma
Langerhans cells	Immune surveillance	Allergic contact dermatitis
Dermis		
Blood vessels and mast cells	Nutrition, thermoregulation, vasodilation	Ulceration, heat stroke, urticaria (contact, systemic), hand-arm vibration syndrome
Lymphatics	Immune surveillance, lymphatic circulation	Lymphedema
Nerve tissue	Sensory perception	Neuropathies, pain, itching, sensory changes
Connective tissue	Protection from trauma; wound repair	Hypertrophic and atrophic scars, scleroderma
Eccrine (sweat) glands	Thermoregulation	Heat intolerance
Sebaceous glands	Synthesis of skin surface lipids	Acne, chloracne, xerosis
Hair	Insulation, outward appearance	Folliculitis, alopecia
Nails	Manipulation of small objects	Paronychia, dystrophy, onycholysis, difficulty with grasping

*Modified from Mathias,[5] Table 10-7, p. 138.

after a length of time sufficient to permit regeneration and other physiologic adjustments. A permanent impairment is unlikely to change in the near future. Impairments may relate, for instance, to immunobiologic defenses against microorganisms or to alterations of sensory perception because of a systemic disorder. Because the degree of a permanent impairment may change, the patient's impairment should be reevaluated at appropriate intervals.

Evaluations of cutaneous impairment must consider abnormalities of function of the skin's components as well as losses of function. Evaluation is usually possible through the exercise of sound clinical judgment based on a detailed medical history, a thorough physical examination, and the judicious use of diagnostic procedures. Laboratory aids include such procedures as patch, open, scratch, intracutaneous, and serologic tests for allergy; Wood's light examinations and cultures and scrapings for bacteria, fungi, and viruses; and biopsies.

13.2 Methods of Evaluating Impairment

In evaluation of a permanent impairment related to a skin disorder, the actual functional loss should be the prime consideration, although the extent of the cosmetic involvement also may be important. Impairments of other body systems, for instance, behavioral problems, restriction of motion or ankylosis of joints, and respiratory, cardiovascular, endocrine, or gastrointestinal tract disorders, may be associated with skin impairments. When there is a permanent impairment of more than one body system, the extent of whole-person impairment related to each system should be evaluated, and the estimated impairment percentages should be *combined* using the Combined Values Chart (p. 322) to determine the person's total impairment.

Manifestations of skin disorders may be influenced by physical and chemical agents that a patient may encounter. Avoidance of these agents, perhaps by changing occupation, might alleviate the skin disorder. Nonetheless, the presence of the disorder should be recognized, and it should be evaluated in accordance with the criteria below.

In determining the appropriate impairment class (Table 2, p. 280) for an affected individual, the physician should primarily consider the impact of the skin condition on the individual's daily activities. Likewise, the frequency and complexity of needed medical treatment may vary considerably. Both the frequency and the intensity of signs or symptoms, as well as the frequency and complexity of the needed medical treatment, may be used to determine the appropriate percentage and estimate within any impairment class. In general, the more frequent and intense the symptoms and the more frequent and complex the medical treatment, the higher the estimated impairment percentage should be.

Impairment estimates or ratings for the skin generally should be expressed in whole numbers ending in 0 or 5, except for class 1 estimates, for which smaller increments may occasionally be justified.

This chapter includes several examples of impairment in each class to assist the physician in arriving at appropriate estimates of impairment percentages.

13.3 Pruritus

Pruritus is a subjective, unpleasant sensation and symptom that provokes the desire to scratch or rub and is frequently associated with cutaneous disorders. Pruritus is closely related to pain and is mediated by pain receptors and pain fibers when they are weakly stimulated. The itching sensation may be intolerable. Like pain, pruritus may be defined as a unique complex made up of afferent stimuli interacting with the emotional or affective state of the individual and modified by the individual's past experience and present state of mind.

The sensation of pruritus has two elements, peripheral neural stimulation and central nervous system reaction, that are extremely variable in makeup and time. The first element may vary from the absence of sensation to an awareness that stimuli are producing either a usual or an unusual sensation. The second element is modified by the person's state of attentiveness, past experience, motivation at the moment, and stimuli such as exercise, sweating, and changes in temperature.

In evaluating pruritus associated with skin disorders, the physician should consider (1) how the pruritus interferes with the individual's performance of the activities of daily living, including occupation; and (2) to what extent the description of the pruritus is supported by objective skin findings, such as lichenification, excoriation, or hyperpigmentation. Subjective complaints of itching that cannot be substantiated objectively may require referral or consultation.

13.4 Disfigurement

Disfigurement is an altered or abnormal appearance. This may be an alteration of color, shape, or structure, or a combination of these. Disfigurement may be a residual of injury or disease, or it may accompany a recurrent or ongoing disorder. Examples of disfigurement include giant pigmented nevi, nevus flammeus, cavernous hemangioma, and alterations in pigmentation.

With disfigurement there is usually no loss of body function and little or no effect on the activities of daily living. Nevertheless, disfigurement may impair by causing social rejection or an unfavorable self-image with self-imposed isolation, life-style alteration, or other behavioral changes. If impairment due to disfigurement does exist, it is usually manifested by a change in behavior, such as withdrawal from social contacts, in which case it would be evaluated in accordance with the criteria in the *Guides* chapter on mental and behavioral conditions.

Impairments related to disfigurement or altered pigmentation should be evaluated in accordance with the criteria given in Table 2 (p. 280) and described later in this chapter. Descriptions of disfigurement are enhanced by good color photographs showing multiple views of the defects. The probable duration and the permanency of the disfigurement should be estimated.

The possibility of improving the condition through medical or surgical therapy, and the extent to which it can be concealed cosmetically, as with hairpieces, wigs, or cosmetics, should be described in writing and depicted with photographs if possible.

13.5 Scars and Skin Grafts

Scars are cutaneous abnormalities that result from the healing of burned, traumatized, or diseased tissue, and they represent a special type of disfigurement. Scars should be described by giving their dimensions in centimeters and by describing their shape, color, anatomic location, and any evidence of ulceration; depression or elevation, which relates to whether they are "atrophic" or "hypertrophic"; texture, which relates to whether they are soft and pliable or hard and indurated, thin or thick, and smooth or rough; and attachment, if any, to underlying bone, joints, muscles, or other tissue. Good color photographs with multiple views of the defect enhance the description of scars.

The tendency of a scar to disfigure should be considered in evaluating whether an impairment due to the scar is permanent. Another consideration is whether the scar can be changed, made less visible, or concealed. Function may be restored without improving appearance, and appearance may be improved without altering function.

Table 2. Impairment Classes and Percents for Skin Disorders*

Class 1: **0%-9% impairment**	**Class 2:** **10%-24% impairment**	**Class 3:** **25%-54% impairment**	**Class 4:** **55%-84% impairment**	**Class 5:** **85%-95% impairment**
Signs and symptoms of skin disorder are present or only intermittently present;	Signs and symptoms of skin disorder are present or intermittently present;	Signs and symptoms of skin disorder are present or intermittently present;	Signs and symptoms of skin disorder are *constantly* present;	Signs and symptoms of skin disorder are *constantly* present;
and	**and**	**and**	**and**	**and**
There is no limitation or limitation in the performance of *few* activities of daily living, although exposure to certain chemical or physical agents might increase limitation temporarily;	There is limitation in the performance of *some* of the activities of daily living;	There is limitation in the performance of *many* of the activities of daily living;	There is limitation in the performance of *many* of the activities of daily living that may include intermittent confinement at home or other domicile;	There is limitation in the performance of *most* of the activities of daily living, including occasional to constant confinement at home or other domicile;
and	**and**	**and**	**and**	**and**
No treatment or intermittent treatment is required.	Intermittent to constant treatment may be required.	Intermittent to constant treatment may be required.	Intermittent to constant treatment may be required.	Intermittent to constant treatment may be required.

*The signs and symptoms of disorders in classes 1 and 2 may be intermittent and not present at the time of examination. The impact of the skin disorder on daily activities should be the primary consideration in determining the class of impairment. The frequency and intensity of signs and symptoms and the frequency and complexity of medical treatment should guide the selection of an appropriate impairment percentage and estimate within any class (see chapter introduction).

Skin grafts may be used to replace skin losses resulting from trauma or disease. Grafts commonly lack hair, lubrication, pliability, and sensation and demonstrate altered pigmentation. These changes affect the function and appearance of the site where the graft is placed. The altered lubrication, pliability, and sensation may result in diminished protection against microorganisms and diminished resistance to mechanical, chemical, and thermal trauma. The altered appearance may be significant, if the area involves exposed parts such as the dorsum of the hand, the face, or the neck.

If a scar involves the loss of sweat gland function, hair growth, nail growth, or pigment formation, the effect of such a loss on the performance of daily living activities should be evaluated.

Burns and scars may be evaluated according to the criteria in this chapter, with special consideration of the impact of the injury on the patient's daily activities. When the impairment resulting from a burn or scar is based on peripheral nerve dysfunction or loss of range of motion, it may be evaluated according to the criteria in *Guides* Chapters 3 and 4, provided appropriate guidelines exist in those chapters. If chest-wall excursion were limited, or if there were behavioral changes secondary to disfigurement, the chapters on the respiratory system or mental and behavioral conditions would be consulted.

If other chapters also were used to estimate the impairment from a patient's skin disorder, the skin disorder evaluation would *exclude* consideration of the components evaluated with those chapters. If impairment from a skin disorder is to be considered along with a component based on any other organ system, both components first must be expressed as whole-person impairment percents and then *combined* using the Combined Values Chart (p. 322).

13.6 Patch Testing—Performance, Interpretation, and Relevance

Patch testing is not a substitute for an adequately detailed history. Nevertheless, when properly performed and interpreted, patch testing can make a significant contribution to the diagnosis and management of contact dermatoses.

The physician must be aware that patch testing can yield false-positive and false-negative results. Selecting the proper concentration of the suspected chemical, vehicle, site of application, and type of patch is critical in assuring the validity of the procedure. Making such selections and determining the relevance of the test results require considerable skill and experience.

A positive or negative patch test result should not be accepted at face value until the details of the testing procedures have been evaluated. Although appropriate test concentrations and vehicles have been established for many common sensitizers, for most chemicals in existence there are no established vehicle and concentration standards. Further details about patch testing and its pitfalls are discussed in standard texts, some of which are listed at the end of this chapter.

13.7 Criteria for Evaluating Permanent Impairment of the Skin

Class 1: Impairment of the Whole Person, 0% to 10%
A patient belongs in class 1 when (1) signs or symptoms of a skin disorder are present or only intermittently present; *and* (2) there is no limitation, or limitation in the performance of *few* activities of daily living, although exposure to certain chemical or physical agents might increase limitation temporarily; *and* (3) no treatment or intermittent treatment is required.

Example 1: A 48-year-old white man had been involved with the manufacturing of silver nitrate for 20 years. Five years ago he noted bluish discoloration of the inner canthi of his eyes, which progressed so that presently his sclerae, face, and arms were decidedly bluish and the unexposed skin showed a slightly bluish tint. Although the man was aware of these changes, they did not bother him. There was no loss of function or impairment in the performance of daily activities, and otherwise his health was good.

Physical examination disclosed the changes of the eyes described above and bluish pigmentation in the posterior nasal passages and around the turbinates and the fauces. The remainder of the physical examination was normal. Results of laboratory studies were normal, except that biopsy of the skin of the arm confirmed the diagnosis of argyria.

Diagnosis: Argyria.

Impairment: 0% impairment of the whole person.

Comment: If impairment from cosmetic disfigurement existed, it would be manifested by behavioral changes, which would be evaluated in accordance with the criteria set forth in the *Guides* chapter on mental and behavioral conditions.

Example 2: A 62-year-old man developed a lichenoid, purpuric dermatosis of the legs 3 years ago, and a biopsy was performed. He experienced no pruritus, and he received specific medication. Six months later an incomplete, annular, infiltrative lesion causing no symptoms developed in the right antecubital fossa. A biopsy established the diagnosis of mycosis fungoides. Results of thorough blood studies and bone marrow and liver biopsies were normal. The lesion responded completely to 300 rad (3 Gy) of x-ray therapy.

Diagnosis: Mycosis fungoides.

Impairment: 0% impairment of the whole person.

Comment: Mycosis fungoides (cutaneous T-cell lymphoma) is a slowly progressive malignant neoplasm that may recur, which may lead to increasing impairment.

Example 3: A 27-year-old man who worked for a small paint manufacturing company developed acute contact dermatitis of the hands and arms. He related the onset of the illness and exacerbations to the preparation of batches of latex paint. Patch testing revealed a strong allergic reaction to 0.1% petrolatum mixture of a nonmercurial preservative, 2-n-4-isothiazolin-3-1, which was used by the company in its latex paints. The patient was unable to avoid latex paint completely, and his dermatitis continued. When he left the company to seek other employment, the dermatitis resolved.

Diagnosis: Allergic contact dermatitis caused by a preservative.

Impairment: 0% impairment of the whole person.

Comment: The preservative to which the worker was allergic was manufactured for use in latex paints. While it was used widely in the paint manufacturing industry, it was not used in other industries where the worker might come into contact with it. He had no limitation in the performance of daily activities, and therefore his impairment was estimated at 0%. However, he might have been considered disabled under some state workers' compensation statutes.

Example 4: A 38-year-old woman sustained a 7 x 12-cm second-degree flame burn to her forearm, which healed spontaneously. She had no complaints, and there was no interference with daily living activities. Physical examination disclosed a 7 x 12-cm depigmented area of the arm, but the healed skin demonstrated normal pliability, lubrication, and sensation.

Diagnosis: Scarring caused by thermal burn.

Impairment: 0% impairment of the whole person.

Example 5: A 52-year-old janitor had episodes of transient dermatitis of the hand from the detergents he used in wet-work duties during a 13-year period. About 10 years ago, depigmentation developed on the sides of most of his fingers and over the dorsums of the hands and distal forearms. Recently, other areas of depigmentation became apparent on the upper torso and thighs. A physical examination confirmed these changes.

The janitor used a germicidal disinfectant that contained para-tertiary butyl phenol (TBP). Patch tests revealed a 2+ reaction to TBP 1% in petrolatum but not to other common industrial allergens. A month after the tests were performed, the site of the positive patch test became depigmented. Ultraviolet light therapy in combination with oral methoxsalen (PUVA therapy) failed to stimulate repigmentation during a 1-year period. Covering with cosmetics was unsatisfactory.

The janitor also was required to perform outdoor maintenance work. Sunburn frequently occurred in the areas of his skin that lacked pigmentation. Early actinic changes with wrinkling, bruising, and scaling of the skin were present. His increased susceptibility to sunburning required the regular use of protective suncreens for outdoor work and other activities. Otherwise he had no impairment in performing activities of daily living.

Diagnosis: Allergic contact dermatitis and occupational leukoderma caused by a phenolic chemical, TBP.

Impairment: 5% impairment of the whole person.

Comment: This impairment estimate does not consider any impairment of the man's self-image or of social relationships, nor the effects these impairments might have on his future life—including his employment. Any behavioral changes, if present, would be evaluated in accordance with the criteria in the *Guides* chapter on mental and behavioral disorders (p. 291).

Example 6: A 25-year-old woman, who performed outdoor utility repairs, sustained a thermal burn on the left side of the face and arm. She required a 6 x 10-cm skin graft to the left forearm. She complained that numbness in the graft interfered with certain nonspecialized hand activities. She experienced intermittent pain of the left ear when she was outdoors in cold weather, especially when temperatures were below 20°F.

The pain constituted an annoyance that required warming of the ear with a cap or the placement of something warm over the area. Because of the hypopigmentation at the burn sites, she was required to wear sunscreen with a high sun protection factor. The atrophy and scaling of the left forearm required the regular use of a moisturizer.

Physical examination disclosed that the forearm graft was completely healed, showed only a protective reaction, and was atrophic and scaly. There was normal range of motion. The remainder of the skin on the left forearm and that of the left side of the face, including the ear, was hypopigmented, and its sensation was normal.

Diagnosis: Skin graft and hypopigmentation secondary to thermal burn.

Impairment: 5% impairment of the whole person.

Comment: The patient's numbness was related to the residual effects of the burn and graft and was not related to a peripheral nerve injury. Accordingly, neurologic assessment of the peripheral nerves was not necessary.

Example 7: A 35-year-old woman had a 10-year history of chronic urticaria (hives). She had never had life-threatening angioedema, nor had she needed to go to an emergency room because of related symptoms. Without treatment, the woman had urticarial lesions on the hands, face, or trunk daily, involving 10% to 20% of the body surface. When the lesions were on the hands, the swelling interfered with driving or with grasping objects. When the lesions were present, she had severe itching that interfered with sleep, sexual relations, and ability to concentrate on her work and housekeeping activities.

Physical examination, performed when the patient was taking a nonsedating oral antihistamine, indicated that the patient was free of urticarial lesions. Laboratory testing indicated 12% eosinophils in the blood smear (200 white blood cells counted).

Diagnosis: Chronic urticaria.

Impairment: 5% impairment due to urticaria.

Comment: With present treatment, the patient had no limitation in her daily activities. However, if the patient were treated with a sedating antihistamine, there might be limitation of her ability to perform certain activities, such as driving or participation in group activities, and the estimated impairment might need to be increased. Further, such treatment might have an impact on the patient's employability for certain jobs, a factor in disability. These considerations are discussed in Chapter 2 and the Glossary.

If a change in therapy became necessary, or if therapy at some future time no longer controlled the urticaria, a reevaluation would be indicated. For example, on the basis of the information given above, if the patient's urticaria could not be controlled, the estimated impairment due to her skin disease would be 20%.

Class 2: Impairment of the Whole Person, 10% to 25%

A person belongs in class 2 when (1) signs and symptoms of a skin disorder are present or intermittently present; *and* (2) there is limitation in the performance of *some* of the activities of daily living; *and* (3) intermittent to constant treatment may be required.

Example 1: A 28-year-old woman developed an eczematous eruption beneath the wedding ring on the fourth finger of her left hand shortly after the birth of her first child 6 years earlier. The eruption gradually spread to involve areas on several fingers of both hands, despite treatment and avoidance of the use of jewelry. The eruption persisted for several months, then subsided slowly. A severe flare-up of hand dermatitis occurred after the birth of a second child 2 years later.

At present, a chronic, low-grade dermatitis persisted despite special precautions. Intermittent treatment was required to control the dermatitis. The patient had no history of eczema, hay fever, or asthma, and no family history of atopy. Her general health was good, but the chronic hand dermatitis caused intermittent discomfort and limitation in the performance of some activities of daily living, such as dishwashing, childcare, and grasping.

Results of a physical examination and basic laboratory studies were normal except for scarring and lichenification. Patch tests performed with various food, household, cosmetic, and diagnostic and therapeutic materials were nonreactive.

Diagnosis: Chronic dermatitis of the hands, due to undetermined factors.

Impairment: 10% impairment of the whole person.

Comment: Although the patient's chronic dermatitis caused impairment of some daily activities and merited placement in functional class 2, the intermittent nature of the symptoms and the need for treatment warranted an impairment estimate of only 10%, at the lower end of the class 2 impairment range.

Example 2: A 43-year-old construction worker suffered a second-degree burn of the anterior part of the neck, which healed with hypertrophic scar formation involving an estimated 1% of the skin surface. The scar was quite susceptible to ultraviolet light, so the man had to wear sun blockers when he was outdoors. In addition, the scar was easily irritated and lacked durability, so he was unable to wear clothes that rubbed on his neck. He had intermittent episodes of itching and burning confined to the scarred areas, which temporarily caused him to stop all activities for periods of 5 to 10 minutes.

A physical examination indicated that the scar was raised, red, and hard and contrasted markedly with the adjacent normal skin. There was limitation of flexion and extension of the neck.

Diagnosis: Hypertrophic scar secondary to thermal burn; limitation of neck motion.

Impairment: 10% impairment of the whole person.

Comment: The skin impairment should be *combined* using the Combined Values Chart (p. 322) with the estimated impairment due to loss of motion of the neck (refer to *Guides* chapter on musculoskeletal system).

Example 3: A 25-year-old man who had a family history of "eczema" and "hay fever" had had a recurrent pruritic eruption since the age of 1 month, when it was characterized by oozing lesions of the face, scalp, neck, and upper extremities. A diagnosis of infantile eczema was made shortly after onset. As a boy he had had periods of relatively complete remission, but even during these periods, lichenified patches in his antecubital, popliteal, and neck areas persisted. Exacerbations were severe during high school years and increased in frequency during college.

For the past several years, the man had suffered exacerbations approximately once per month, lasting 7 to 10 days and involving the shoulders, arms, hands, legs, and trunk. The exacerbations could be brought on by cold weather, sudden changes in environmental temperature, or stressful situations at home. During the exacerbations, the eczema limited some activities of daily living, and he had difficulty sleeping, washing dishes, and concentrating on his work as an accountant. During remissions, the lichenified dermatitis persisted in the antecubital and popliteal fossae and at the sides of the neck, but this was a minimal annoyance and did not significantly limit daily activities.

The eczema required intermittent application of topical steroid creams during relative remissions. When it flared up, constant application of topical steroids was required, as were antihistamines and oatmeal starch baths. Systemic steroids were required once per year to induce remissions.

Results of a physical examination with basic laboratory studies were normal, except that lichenified areas appeared at the lateral aspects of the neck and in the creases of the arms and legs.

Diagnosis: Atopic dermatitis.

Impairment: 15% impairment of the whole person.

Comment: Excerbations of atopic dermatitis may be precipitated by a variety of excitants. The estimated impairment, 15%, is based on occasional interference with some activities of daily living. The frequency and severity of the signs and symptoms and the need for, and complexity of, medical treatment merit an estimate near the middle of class 2.

Example 4: A 30-year-old white man was employed in a rare-metals refining plant. He was inadvertently splashed with concentrated liquid zirconium chloride over the face, scalp, and neck. He was immediately washed and then taken to the hospital, where he remained for 2 days. Healing and epithelialization occurred without complications. He returned to work 22 days after the episode.

Months after the incident, the man noted that depigmentation of the splashed areas had begun to occur. He noted that the depigmented areas sunburned easily, causing considerable discomfort and restricting his ability to work outdoors or pursue other outdoor activities. Regular application of a sunscreen was necessary. Whenever the patient operated a hot kiln or approached a furnace, the heat caused a marked stinging sensation within the affected skin areas, which was so intense that he had to stop all activities for 10 to 15 minutes until the pain subsided. Also, muscle twitching occurred within affected areas. Similar episodes might be provoked by hot showers or extremely warm days. Occasional muscle twitching and severe discomfort might occur within the affected areas and wake the patient from sleep once or twice a week. The patient experienced considerable embarrassment when attempting to explain his disfigurement, and he avoided many kinds of social activities in which he previously had participated.

A physical examination 1 year later showed that there had been no change in the patient's pigment loss, hyperesthesia, and intolerance to sunlight and warmth. There were well-demarcated areas of depigmentation on the right side of the face, extending from behind the right ear to the center of the face, and from the midtemple area of the scalp to the chin. There were smaller areas of depigmentation on the left side of the neck and behind the right ear. The maximum dimensions of the depigmented areas on the right side of the face were 16 x 11 cm. There were narrow collars of hyperpigmentation around the depigmented areas. Neurologic examination indicated that all of the depigmented areas were hypersensitive to cold, heat, pinprick, and touch, and for some of these areas, low-temperature stimuli were mistakenly identified as "hot" and "burning."

Diagnosis: Zirconium chloride burn and leukoderma with residual skin dysfunction.

Impairment: 20% impairment of the whole person.

Comment: The percentage of cutaneous impairment is based on the limitation of some activities of daily living. The frequent occurrence of intense signs and symptoms, which precludes the performance of various activities, merits a rating at the upper end of class 2 impairment. If effective medical treatment were available that could reduce the frequency and intensity of the signs and symptoms, then the estimated impairment percentage could be reduced. The behavioral changes exhibited by this patient should be evaluated according to the criteria described in the *Guides* chapter on mental and behavioral disorders (p. 291); any psychiatric impairment would increase the skin-related impairment.

Example 5: A 40-year-old woman purchased a sculptured-nail kit consisting of liquid methylmethacrylate monomer and powdered methylmethacrylate polymer. When mixed and applied to the fingernails according to directions, the chemicals formed a paste, which hardened to clear plastic resembling artificial nails. The woman's nails initially were normal, but she eventually developed swelling and redness of the eponychial and paronychial areas with severe pain and paresthesia of all fingers. She lost the nails on all 10 fingers. When the acute inflammatory process subsided, the woman underwent patch testing and a positive result was found to 5% methylmethacrylate monomer in olive oil.

The patient was observed for several years, during which time none of her fingernails regrew. The nail beds were exposed and keratinized, and the paronychial areas continued to be swollen and tender. The paresthesia persisted, although the woman long before had stopped using the sculptured nail kit. She complained of difficulty grasping, cold sensitivity, burning, tingling, and a "pins and needles" sensation, especially when picking up small objects such as coins.

The woman also had difficulty with other nonspecialized hand activities, which aggravated the symptoms and increased the paresthesia of the fingers. She typically applied adhesive bandages over petroleum jelly to her nail beds and wore gloves most of her waking hours. She was anxious and depressed and required an occasional psychiatric consultation.

Diagnosis: Chemically induced nail dystrophy and anonychia.

Impairment: 20% impairment due to chemically induced nail dystrophy, which is to be *combined* using the Combined Values Chart (p. 322) with an appropriate value for the paresthesia (see the part on the hand in the *Guides* chapter on the musculoskeletal system) to estimate the whole-person impairment. A mental and behavioral impairment (Chapter 14, p. 291) might further increase the estimate.

Class 3: Impairment of the Whole Person, 25% to 55%
A patient belongs in class 3 when (1) signs and symptoms of the skin disorder are present or intermittently present; *and* (2) there is limitation in the performance of *many* of the activities of daily living; *and* (3) intermittent to constant treatment may be required.

Example 1: A 45-year-old man had had a persistent pruritic dermatitis involving the ankles, forearms, and hands, and occasionally the face and neck, for 6 years. The skin over these parts was excoriated and lichenified. He had had recurrent bouts of pyogenic infection, and on occasion regional lymph nodes had become swollen and tender.

At the time of onset, the man's work as a nurseryman included general greenhouse activity, such as planting, weeding, watering, fertilizing, and spraying with numerous pesticides and antifungal agents. Some of the chemicals were found to be primary irritants. The man's dermatitis initially responded to topical therapy and the avoidance of irritants, but the condition would flare up after reexposure. Eventually, the symptoms did not subside with avoidance of incriminated agents and changing jobs, and neurodermatitis or the "itch-scratch syndrome" ensued. Warm environments, sweating, and stress provoked episodes of severe itching. The man had no history of a previous dermatologic problem.

Three years before examination, the patient began to have episodes of headache and memory loss and to note periods of tenseness and apprehension accompanied by nausea and vomiting. He was treated intermittently for the mental disturbances, and there was little improvement of the neurodermatitis.

The patient had not engaged in nursery work for the past 3 years. He found it difficult to tolerate other kinds of work, claiming that they made his dermatitis worse. He was gainfully employed no more than 6 months during the year. At home he was unable to perform household maintenance chores and to participate in social and recreational activities, and he experienced difficulty sleeping.

A physical examination disclosed the signs described above.

Diagnosis: Persistent neurodermatitis secondary to occupational contact dermatitis.

Impairment: 30% impairment due to the skin disorder, which is to be increased by an amount that is proportional to the estimated mental and behavioral impairment (see Chapter 14).

Example 2: A 28-year-old man had had acne vulgaris, hydradenitis suppurativa, and dissecting cellulitis of the scalp for the past 12 years. The condition only temporarily improved with conventional methods of treatment, which included topical and systemic antibiotics, intralesional corticosteroids, aspiration, marsupialization, using zinc sulfate, and two courses of isotretinoin. During the past 5 years he developed large cystic lesions, mainly involving the posterior scalp, face, neck, upper trunk, axilla, and inguinal area. The lesions were accompanied by fever and aching joints.

The man's skin was severly scarred. The large lesions on his back, chest, and scalp and in the inguinal area made it difficult for him to rest comfortably in warm weather. In the warm environment of the workplace and especially in the summer, clothing irritated his skin, causing a flaring of the cysts and sinuses. Sweating also aggravated the disorder. He had difficulty sleeping, participating in social and recreational activities, and maintaining regular employment.

Physical examination demonstrated the presence of inflamed cystic lesions located as described above. The white blood cell count was 22,000/mm^3.

Diagnosis: Acne conglobata; hydradenitis suppurativa; dissecting cellulitis of the scalp; severe scar formation.

Impairment: 30% impairment of the whole person.

Example 3: A 44-year-old man sustained burns to the dorsum of both hands and both feet, which required grafting. The grafts healed well, but the man was bothered by dryness and cracking, and the grafts were easily injured by minor trauma and noxious chemicals. He bathed and shampood with gloves on, because water and soap irritated his hands. He also had trouble grasping his toothbrush, comb, or writing instrument because of the cracking, decreased sensation, and stiffness of the skin. His feet were uncomfortable in leather shoes, and he wore cloth shoes. He had to use moisturizers constantly.

A physical examination disclosed that the grafts on the patient's hands and feet were dry, somewhat atrophic, and stiff.

Diagnosis: Scarring due to thermal burns.

Impairment: 30% impairment of the whole person.

Example 4: A 45-year-old white man developed an eczematous eruption on his left hand and arm during the spring 4 years ago. The eruption was treated effectively by admitting him to the hospital and giving topical medications. After he was discharged, the condition flared up, involving the right side of his face and neck and the left forearm to the bottom of his workshirt sleeve. The eruption responded incompletely to treatment but subsided in the fall. It returned the next spring but subsided during the winter.

During the next 2 years, up until the time of his impairment assessment, the eruption persisted perennially and was characterized as being erythematous and slightly scaling, with distinct borders and confluent patches involving the face, neck, and arms. It was learned that the eruption on the exposed area subsided to some degree when the man was away from work, but it flared up within a day after his return, even on the night shift. He worked in the warehouse of a paper box factory and handled only printed paper cartons. The work areas were illuminated exclusively by banks of fluorescent tubes contained in low-hanging fixtures.

A medical examination disclosed evidence of chronic dermatitis. There were no positive reactions from extensive patch tests with materials from the patient's work, home, or personal activities, or from those on the standard screening tray. The minimal erythema dose was significantly decreased. Photopatch tests with halogenated salicylanilides and fragrances were negative. However, within 6 hours after he was exposed to 5 minutes of light from an 8-W fluorescent bulb, severe erythema and edema developed in the exposed area. Five days later, this area was eczematous. Results of tests for urinary porphyrins were within normal limits.

It was determined that the patient experienced severe photosensitivity. He had marked exacerbations of the persistent eruption when exposed to sunlight, even through window glass, and he could not go out during daylight hours or remain in rooms with natural light coming through the windows. He noted that the skin eruption was aggravated by exposure to light from fluorescent light sources. Thus, he was precluded from entering into many normal employment and social activities. He used topical corticosteroid medications on a continuing basis to maintain control, but even with the physician's care he could not eradicate the skin eruption, which remained itchy and unsightly.

Diagnosis: Persistent light reactor, with reactions elicited and aggravated by ultraviolet light and fluorescent light.

Impairment: 40% impairment of the whole person.

Example 5: About 22 months earlier, a 35-year-old man had developed a persistently sore mouth. An examination revealed many eroded lesions of the tongue and oral mucous membranes. The patient subsequently noted the appearance of vesicles and bullae over the face, trunk, and extremities. A diagnosis of pemphigus vulgaris was confirmed by laboratory studies. Oral corticosteroids were administered in high doses to control the disease.

The patient continued to have persistent blisters and erosions that resulted in chronic, unremitting pain on swallowing or attempting to speak. He was unable to eat solid foods, brush his teeth, speak above a whisper, or sleep at night. Because of the severity of the erosions and the skin fragility involving his mouth, trunk, and genital area, he was unable to have sexual intercourse. Azathioprine therapy was added to the high-dose corticosteroid regimen, but control of the disease was limited. The complex therapy for his illness required frequent visits to the physician for checkups and laboratory monitoring.

A physical examination disclosed infected bullae of the mouth and trunk and increased systolic blood pressure. Laboratory studies indicated leukopenia, believed to be the result of the therapy.

Diagnosis: Pemphigus vulgaris.

Impairment: 45% impairment.

Comment: The patient had interference with many activities of daily living because of the lesions and pain of pemphigus. Therapy led to leukopenia, which also should be evaluated in terms of impairment (see *Guides* chapter on hematopoietic system). The whole-person impairments of several organ systems would be *combined* using the Combined Values Chart (p. 322).

Example 6: A 22-year-old woman entered the hospital with fever, malaise, arthralgia, painful hands and feet, and marked erythema, bullae, and edema of the face and the back areas not covered by her bathing suit. She also had tender, red legs with several small ulcers, and she complained of abdominal pain and nausea. The acute episode had been precipitated by a trip to the seashore, where she had sunbathed for several hours.

A physical examination disclosed that the patient had erythema, edema, and scaling of exposed body areas; generalized annular, atrophic plaques involving the trunk; and atrophic plaques and bullae on her palms and soles. The liver was tender to palpation, and there was an apical systolic murmur. Funduscopic examination showed perivascular hemorrhages and fluffy exudates. Laboratory tests indicated hemolysis, leukopenia, hypocomplementemia, hyperglobulinemia, albuminuria, hematuria, a positive result of a lupus erythematosus cell test, and high antinuclear antibody titer.

Steroid therapy was begun, and the patient's condition responded well. However, the hematuria and albuminuria persisted, and maintenance steroid therapy was necessary. She remained tired most of the time, especially after slight exertion. Hydroxychloroquine and, later, dapsone therapy was begun for the severe cutaneous involvement with only partial improvement of lesions on the palms and soles. She continued to have considerable difficulty with grasping, standing, and walking.

Diagnosis: Systemic lupus erythematosus.

Impairment: 50% impairment due to lupus erythematosus, which is to be *combined* using the Combined Values Chart (p. 322) with appropriate impairment estimates related to the other involved systems, the hematopoietic, urinary, and visual systems.

Class 4: Impairment of the Whole Person, 55% to 85%
A patient belongs in class 4 when (1) signs and symptoms of a skin disorder are *constantly* present; *and* (2) there is limitation in the performance of *many* of the activities of daily living, which may include intermittent confinement at home or other domicile; *and* (3) intermittent to constant treatment may be required.

Example 1: A 55-year-old man, who had been employed for 30 years as a parts clerk at a construction company warehouse, severely injured his right leg in a crash that occurred during working hours. The injury was followed by a deep-vein thrombophlebitis of the right leg that required 6 months of total or partial bed rest in a hospital and at home.

After recovery the man began to work for a chemical company. He wore an elastic stocking, but his right leg began to swell more and more each day. Four days after starting work, he spilled a can of caustic drain cleaner, causing second- and third-degree burns over 20% of the right lower leg. He was hospitalized for 12 weeks until the burn healed, leaving a scar but no thickening or contracture.

After 4 months, the man returned to work at the chemical company, but in spite of using elastic support stockings and diuretics, the leg edema became intolerable. He was unable to stay on his feet for more than 4 hours at a time without significant swelling and discomfort. He began to develop stasis dermatitis with ulceration. Periodic treatment with Unna paste boots and occasional admissions to the hospital healed the ulcers only temporarily. He began to experience sleeplessness, and he could tolerate clothing over the leg only for 1 or 2 hours. After 5 years at the chemical company, he quit work and applied for workers' compensation benefits, alleging total disability. Thereafter he had to be hospitalized because of sepsis and persisting cellulitis.

At the time of evaluation, the patient had pitting edema of the right leg below the knee. A hypopigmented, atrophic, hyperesthetic scar extended from the midthigh to the ankle and from the anterior midline around the thigh to the posterior midline. There was altered perception of pain and touch such that the slightest stimulation of the skin in the area of the scar was associated with marked discomfort. The dysesthesia was so severe that the patient could not tolerate clothing rubbing the scar. He had a 4 x 5-cm ulcer with a granulating base over the right medial malleolus. The surrounding skin was erythematous, and the patient had difficulty with weight-bearing because of pain from the ulcer.

Diagnosis: Postthrombophlebitis syndrome with stasis dermatitis and ulceration; scar formation secondary to chemical burn.

Impairment: 55% impairment of the whole person.

Comment: Future episodes of phlebitis, cellulitis, and ulceration are to be expected. Diligent medical care will be required indefinitely. In similar cases, a physician might be asked to apportion a percentage of the whole-person impairment to the crash injury and to the burn. Apportionment is discussed in Chapters 1 and 2 and the Glossary (p. 315).

Example 2: Raynaud's phenomenon had first been observed in a 38-year-old construction worker about 5 years previously. Four years ago, the worker had noted difficulty in swallowing, and then he had developed swelling and tightening of the skin of the fingers, with gradually worsening ulcerations on several digits of both hands. Dressing and feeding became progressively more difficult.

The patient had impairment of a number of the activities of daily living. He had to chop up his food to swallow it. He had difficulty with self-care and personal hygiene, including brushing his teeth, combing his hair, and dressing himself. He was unable to grasp hammers and screwdrivers at work because of the pain associated with finger ulcerations. On outdoor jobs in the winter, he had to carry a hand warmer and stop work frequently because of severe Raynaud's phenomenon. He had difficulty climbing a ladder and grasping the rungs.

A physical examination showed that the patient had increased pigmentation with telangiectasia, primarily on the face, forearms, and dorsal surface of his hands. He had a pinched facial appearance, and the skin over most of the body was hidebound and not easily movable. The chest excursion was limited. The fingers were held in flexion, and the patient had ulcerations on the distal phalanges of both index fingers. He was unable to extend his fingers because of stiffness, tightness, and pain.

The patient's weight was 20% below his desirable weight. A complete blood cell count was within normal limits, except for an erythrocyte sedimentation rate of 40 mm/h. Other findings were normal, except that roentgenographic examinations showed mild esophageal stenosis and disturbed peristaltic activity.

Diagnosis: Acrosclerotic scleroderma, mild stenosis of the esophagus, and flexion deformities of fingers with chronic ulcerations.

Impairment: 55% impairment due to scleroderma, which should be *combined* using the Combined Values Chart (p. 322) with appropriate impairment estimates for stenosis of the esophagus and flexion deformities.

Example 3: A 32-year-old white man was first admitted to the hospital because of a widespread pustular eruption associated with an acute conjunctivitis and severe arthritis of all joints of the hands, wrists, knees, ankles, and toes. The man stated that he had been in good health until 2 months before admission, when he had developed an erythematous, scaly eruption of the pretibial areas, which spread to involve the upper extremities and hand. He then developed pain, swelling, and erythema of the knees and a sterile urethral discharge. The joints of the hands and feet were warm, red, and tender, with minimal swelling. Findings from a skin biopsy specimen were compatible with exudative psoriasis. He was treated with topical therapy, with no response, but his condition improved with systemic steroids and cytotoxic agents. At the time of discharge, the diagnosis was thought to be Reiter's syndrome, keratoderma blennorrhagica, or pustular psoriasis with psoriatic arthritis.

The man was rehospitalized 3 months later with an acute and severe exacerbation of his skin eruption, with severe pain, swelling, and deformity of all joints of his extremities. A skin biopsy specimen again was diagnostic of exudative psoriasis. Radiographic examination of the hands and wrists demonstrated marked demineralization of the carpal bones, the proximal and distal heads of the metacarpals, and the phalanges. Joint space narrowing and periosteal reactions were present in the metacarpal bones of both hands. Flexion deformities were present in both hands.

Oral doses of methotrexate only partially controlled the disease. The patient continued to have periodic flareups of arthritis and psoriasis that required hospitalization. Exacerbations of the disease with generalized pustulation involving the trunk, palms, and soles made it difficult for him to care for himself, stand, sit, walk, and drive. He had difficulty with grasping and tactile discrimination at work, and he was unable to have sexual intercourse.

Diagnosis: Pustular psoriasis with psoriatic arthritis.

Impairment: 60% impairment due to psoriasis, which should be *combined* using the Combined Values Chart (p. 322) with appropriate impairment estimates for limitations of joint motion and for any other involved organ system.

Comment: The clinical features of Reiter's syndrome and pustular psoriasis may overlap. Both may relapse and adversely affect the activities of daily living.

Example 4: A 25-year-old man had suffered burns over 85% of the total body surface area and smoke inhalation 3 years previously. Some areas healed spontaneously, and some required skin grafting. The man developed respiratory distress during the acute phase, which responded to pulmonary treatment. However, he could not work with heavy equipment, because his skin was fragile, dried, and cracked. When exposed to warm environments, the man became hot and dizzy because he was unable to perspire. He had marked difficulty with writing, walking, and nonspecialized hand activities, because of scar formation that caused pain and decreased ranges of motion. His ability to participate in group activities was greatly limited. He had no sexual relations after the injury and became short of breath with physical activity.

A physical examination disclosed that 85% of his body had healed atrophic scars, healed hypertrophic scars, and minimally atrophic skin grafts and donor sites. Several of the healed atrophic areas were depigmented, including some on the cheeks and the backs of the hands. There was partial destruction of the left ear, and the fingernails were distorted. He had a diminished range of motion of both hands.

Diagnosis: Extensive scarring due to thermal burns.

Impairment: 60% impairment of the whole person.

Comment: The skin (burn) impairment should be *combined* (Combined Values Chart, p. 322) with whole-person impairments due to loss of motion (Chapter 3) and pulmonary dysfunction (Chapter 5) and adjusted to consider any mental and behavorial impairment present (Chapter 14).

Example 5: A 56-year-old man was admitted to the hospital because of a generalized pruritic eruption. His condition had begun 20 years earlier with pruritic patches on the back and extremities. Despite topical therapy, the eruption gradually became generalized, and many patches became infiltrated plaques. Recently, nodular lesions and tumors developed. Past treatment included topical nitrogen mustard, PUVA, photophoresis, and electron beam therapy.

A physical examination showed a generalized eruption consisting of erythematous, scaly plaques, some of which were quite firm. There were many excoriations on the trunk and extremities and foul-smelling and draining nodular tumors on the face, palms, and soles. Palpable axillary and inguinal lymph nodes were present.

Laboratory tests were normal, except that examination of a skin biopsy specimen and an axillary lymph node confirmed the diagnosis of mycosis fungoides.

The patient was given a cytotoxic agent intravenously daily for 5 days, followed by oral doses of the same cytotoxic agent. The eruption was not controlled with the cytotoxic agent and radiation therapy. He was confined to his home and was unable to care for himself, walk, travel, grasp, or participate in sexual activity.

Diagnosis: Mycosis fungoides.

Impairment: 75% impairment of the whole person.

Comment: Tumor-stage, widespread mycosis fungoides requires close medical surveillance. Morbidity is considerable, and the prognosis is poor. There is interference with some activities of daily living, and most patients die within 2 to 5 years.

Class 5: Impairment of the Whole Person, 85% through 95%

A patient belongs in Class 5 when (1) signs and symptoms of skin disorder are *constantly* present; *and* (2) there is limitation in the performance of *most* of the activities of daily living, including occasional to constant confinement at home or other domicile; *and* (3) intermittent to constant treatment may be required.

Example 1: A 12-year-old girl had had photophobia for 8 years. At the age of 5 years, she had developed marked pigmentation of the sun-exposed areas of the face, chest, arms, and legs. Since then, she developed generalized freckling of the skin, several areas of telangiectasia, and multiple basal and squamous cell epitheliomas. The condition was progressing in severity, and the patient required continuous observation and treatment. She had been confined to the home for the past year.

A physical examination showed all of the signs described above. Basic laboratory findings were normal, and results of fecal and urinary porphyrin studies were negative.

Diagnosis: Xeroderma pigmentosum.

Impairment: 85% impairment of the whole person.

Comment: Xeroderma pigmentosum is a progressive disease, and the ultimate impairment approaches 100%, a fatal devolution. Metastatic carcinoma from squamous cell carcinomas or malignant melanoma may develop.

Example 2: A 19-year-old man had bullous lesions that had developed shortly after birth and had been present continuously since then, except for very minor and short remissions. Bullae appeared after the slightest trauma and, at times, without apparent trauma, and healed with severe scarring. The man requires continuous hospitalization.

Examination showed that the man's fingers were tapered stumps. Bullae were present constantly in the mouth and pharnyx and probably extended to the epiglottis. His weight was 40% below the desirable weight for his height. Roentgenography showed a stricture of the esophagus.

Diagnosis: Epidermolysis bullosa dystrophica.

Impairment: 95% impairment due to epidermolysis bullosa dystrophica, which is to be *combined* (Combined Values Chart, p. 322) with impairment estimates for the stricture of the esophagus and the fingers to determine the impairment of the whole person.

Comment: This autosomal recessive disorder is one of the most impairing of all hereditary diseases, and impairment approaches 100% and death. An impairment related to mental and behavioral factors may be present.

References

1. Adams RM. *Occupational Skin Disease.* 2nd ed. Philadelphia, Pa: WB Saunders Co; 1990.

2. *The Cosmetic Benefit Study.* Washington, DC: The Cosmetic, Toiletry and Fragrance Association; 1978.

3. Key MM. Confusing compensation cases. *Cutis.* 1967;3:965-969.

4. Maibach HI, ed. *Occupational and Industrial Dermatology.* 2nd ed. Chicago, Ill: Year Book Medical Publishers; 1987.

5. Fisher AA. Permanent loss of fingernails from sensitization and reaction to acrylics in a preparation designed to make artificial nails. *J Dermatol Surg Oncol.* 1980;6:70-71.

6. Mathias CGT. The skin. In: Zenz C, ed. *Occupational Medicine.* 2nd ed. Chicago, Ill: Year Book Medical Publishers; 1988.

7. Taylor JS, ed. Occupational dermatoses. *Dermatol Clin North Am.* 1988;6:1-129.

8. Engrav LH, Covey MH, Dutcher KD, et al. Impairment, time out of school, and time off from work after burns. *Plast Reconstr Surg.* 1987;79:927-934.

9. Finlay AY, Khru GK, Luscombe DK, Salek MS. Validation of sickness impact profile and psoriasis disability index in psoriasis. *Br J Dermatol.* 1990;123:751-756.

10. Sheretz EF, Storrs FJ. Occupational contact dermatitis. In: Rosenstock L, Cullen M, eds. *Textbook of Clinical Occupational and Environmental Medicine.* Philadelphia, Pa: WB Saunders Co; in press.

11. Nethercott JR, Gallant C. Disability due to occupational contact dermatitis. *Occup. Med.* 1986; 1:199-204.

Chapter 14

Mental and Behavioral Disorders

This chapter discusses impairments due to mental disorders and considers behavioral impairments that may complicate any condition. Fundamental principles relating to impairments, their assessment, and the methods underlying the *Guides* are discussed in Chapters 1 and 2 and the Glossary (p. 315). The reader should peruse these parts before undertaking an impairment evaluation.

A medical impairment evaluation report performed according to the *Guides* should include information such as that shown below.

A. Medical Evaluation
- History of mental and behavioral disorder(s)
- Results of most recent clinical evaluation
- Assessment of current clinical status and statement of further medical plans
- Diagnosis

B. Analysis of Findings
- Impact of mental condition on normal life activities
- Explanation for concluding that the condition has been present for several months, is stable, and is unlikely to change
- Explanation for concluding that the individual is or is not likely to suffer impairment by engaging in usual activities
- Explanation for concluding that accommodations or restrictions related to the impairment are or are not warranted

C. Comparison of Analysis with Impairment Criteria
- Description of clinical findings and how these findings relate to the impairment and *Guides* criteria
- Description of the effect of impairment on the individual's ability to function
- Estimate of the severity of the impairment

Basic Principles

Three principles, described below, are central to assessing mental impairment.

1. The diagnosis is among the factors to be considered in assessing the severity and possible duration of the impairment, but it is not the sole criterion.

2. Motivation for improvement may be a key factor in the outcome of an individual's impairment.

3. Assessing impairment requires a thorough review of the history of the impairment, its treatment, and attempts at rehabilitation.

Some of the material in this chapter is taken from Social Security Administration (SSA) regulations that were developed with the advice of a knowledgeable working group.[1] In the SSA regulations there are three underlying concepts: (1) a medically determinable impairment must exist; (2) the impairment must result in an inability to work; and (3) the impairment must be expected to last for at least 12 months.

The SSA's "Listing"[1] for mental disorders conforms to the terminology of *Diagnostic and Statistical Manual of Mental Disorders, Revised Third Edition* (*DSM-III-R*)[2] terminology and is divided into eight broad categories. The Listing describes the criteria that must be met if the person may be said to "meet the Listing" and thus be unable to engage in work. For example, the first of the eight categories deals with schizophrenic, paranoid, and other psychotic disorders. To meet the Listing, the claimant must satisfy criteria that are arranged in a menu format somewhat like that of *DSM-III-R*.[2]

The group A criteria are symptoms, and in addition to satisfying them, the claimant must satisfy group B criteria, which are expressed in terms of ability to function in various settings (see Section 14.3, p. 293). Alternatively, the claimant may meet group C criteria by exhibiting a specified duration of the disorder with frequent deterioration or inability to function outside of highly supportive living situations. For detailed information, the reader should consult the SSA Listing,[1] which is available through state agencies responsible for disability determinations or the SSA.

The *Guides* is also useful in conjunction with other approaches. These may be different from the *Guides*' approach and definitions. The *Guides* user should become familiar with the guidelines and approaches of the system within which the evaluation is being performed. Meyerson and Fine[3] reviewed and discussed aspects of disability evaluation systems. The Glossary (p. 315) considers programs, regulations, and procedures of the SSA.

14.1 Diagnosis of Impairment

Diagnostic Systems

The *Diagnostic and Statistical Manual of Mental Disorders, Revised Third Edition*,[2] commonly known as *DSM-III-R*, is a widely accepted classification system for mental disorders. It is similar to another system, the International Classification of Diseases (ICD), which also is in widespread use.[4] The criteria for mental disorders include a wide range of signs, symptoms, and impairments. Most mental disorders are characterized by one or more impairments. However, an individual may have a mental or behavioral impairment without meeting the criteria specified in *DSM-III-R* or the ICD.

The *DSM-III-R* calls for a multiaxial evaluation. Each of five axes refers to a different class of information. The first three axes constitute the official diagnostic evaluation. These include the clinical syndromes and the conditions that are the focus of treatment (axis I); the personality and developmental disorders (axis II); and the physical disorders and conditions that may be relevant to understanding and managing the care of the individual (axis III). Axis IV, referring to psychosocial stressors, and axis V, referring to adaptive functioning, may be particularly important for assessing impairment severity.

In some individuals it is not possible to make a determination on the basis of the available information. Under these circumstances the examiner should not feel obligated to provide an opinion about which he or she is uncertain but should seek and review relevant information from additional sources, such as medical and employment records, before rendering an opinion.

Specific Impairments

In judging the degree of mental impairment it is important to recognize that there are various types of mental disorders, each of which, like a physical disorder, has its own natural course and unique characteristics. It is apparent that some serious mental disorders are chronic. The term "remission," rather than "cure," is used to indicate an individual's improvement. The remission may be intermittent, long-term, or short-term, and it may occur in stages rather than all at once. Degrees of impairment may vary considerably among patients, and the severity of an impairment is not necessarily related to the diagnosis. Indeed, the diagnosis per se is of limited relevance to an objective assessment of a psychiatric impairment, because the words do not provide sufficient insight into the nature of the impairment.

An episode of depression that follows a stressful life event, for instance, often is a short-term, self-limiting illness that clears up when the stressful situation is relieved. Other affective disorders have their own patterns of recurrence and chronicity and often respond well to therapeutic interventions. Somatic and psychological treatment and adequate supervision are important in all affective disorders, because of the risk of suicide.

The schizophrenias are usually chronic disorders; the onset may be insidious and recognized only in retrospect. Certain organic disorders such as traumatic brain injury and life-long mental retardation are persistent and chronic, and treatment consists of minimizing the response to the pathophysiologic changes. For some patients, achieving a degree of capability and habilitation may be the goal.

The types of mental dysfunction in the various psychiatric disorders are curiously similar regardless of the specific diagnosis. Just as "fever" and "pain" are seen in different kinds of somatic illnesses, so "anxiety" and "hostility" may be observed in different kinds of mental disorders.

14.2 Evidence of Mental Impairment

The following recommendations for documentation draw heavily on the "Listing of Mental Impairments" in regulations from the SSA.[1] The SSA's evaluation system and most other systems require the existence of an impairment that is established and documented by medical evidence relating to signs, symptoms, and results of laboratory tests, including psychological tests. In general, the diagnosis of a mental disorder should be justified by the history, signs, and symptoms, and a diagnosis according to *DSM-III-R* should be given. If there is uncertainty about the exact diagnosis, the differential diagnosis should be discussed.

The methodology of the *Guides* requires that the presence of a mental disorder be documented primarily on the basis of reports from accepted professional sources, such as psychiatrists, psychologists, psychiatric nurses, psychiatric social workers, and health professionals in hospitals and clinics. Adequate descriptions of functional limitations should be obtained from these sources and, if possible, from programs in which the individual has been observed over a period of time. Data gathered during a period of years are particularly useful.

The individual's own description of his or her functioning and limitations is an important source of information. The presence of a mental disorder does not automatically rule out the individual as a reliable source of information. Information from nonmedical sources, such as family members and others who have knowledge of the patient, may be useful in indicating the level of functioning and the severity of the impairment.

Information from medical and nonmedical sources may be used to obtain detailed descriptions of the individual's activities of daily living, social functioning, concentration, persistence, pace, and ability to tolerate increased mental demands (stress). This information may be available from professionals in community mental health centers, day-care centers, and sheltered workshops, and it also can be provided by family members. If the descriptions from these sources are insufficiently detailed or in conflict with the observed clinical picture or the reports of others, it is necessary to resolve the inconsistencies. Also, any gaps in the history should be explained.

An individual's level of functioning may vary considerably over time. The level of functioning at a specific time may seem relatively adequate or, conversely, rather poor. Proper evaluation of an impairment must take into account variations in the level of functioning with time in arriving at a determination of severity. Thus, it is important to obtain evidence over a sufficiently long period before the date of examination. This evidence should include treatment notes, hospital discharge summaries, work evaluations, and rehabilitation progress notes if they are available.

An individual may have worked or have attempted to work when there was a question about impairment. The individual's efforts may have been independent, or the work may have been in conjunction with a community mental health or other sheltered program and of short or long duration. Information concerning the individual's behavior during the attempt, and the circumstances surrounding termination of the work effort, are particularly useful in determining the individual's ability to function in a work setting and with others. Results of work evaluations and rehabilitation programs can be significant sources of data concerning impairments affecting work capabilities.

The results of well-standardized psychological tests, such as the Wechsler Adult Intelligence Scale, the Minnesota Multiphasic Personality Inventory-2, the Rorschach Psychodiagnostic Inkblot Test, and the Thematic Apperception Test, may be useful in establishing the existence of a mental disorder. For example, the Wechsler Adult Intelligence Scale is useful in establishing mental retardation. Broad-based neuropsychological assessments using, for example, the Halstead-Reitan or the Luria-Nebraska batteries may be useful in determining deficiencies in brain functioning, particularly in individuals with subtle signs such as those that may be seen in traumatic brain injuries.

Taking a standardized test requires concentration, persistence, and pacing; thus, observing individuals during the testing process may provide useful information. The description of test results should include the objective findings, a description of what occurred during the testing, and the test results. A report of intellectual assessment should include a discussion of whether the obtained intelligence quotient (IQ) score is considered to be valid and consistent with the individual's impairment and degree of functional limitation.

14.3 Assessing Impairment Severity

The system of the SSA is recommended for assessing the severity of mental impairments. Although by definition under that system an impairment arising from a mental disorder must be severe enough to cause inability to work, it should be understood that the severity of a mental disorder does not necessarily equate with the inability to work. For instance, an individual with a serious illness, such as a delusional disorder, may be able to work in certain settings.

The SSA suggests four aspects or areas for assessing the severity of mental impairments[1]: (1) limitations in activities of daily living; (2) social functioning; (3) concentration, persistence, and pace; and (4) deterioration or decompensation in work or worklike settings. Also, independence, appropriateness, and effectiveness of activities should be considered. The four aspects of functional limitation are discussed below.

1. Activities of daily living include such activities as self-care, personal hygiene, communication, ambulation, travel, sexual function, sleep, and social and recreational activities. Any limitations in these activities should be related to the mental disorder rather than to such factors as lack of money or lack of transportation. In the context of the individual's overall situation, the quality of these activities is judged by their independence, appropriateness, effectiveness, and sustainability. It is necessary to define the extent to which the individual is capable of initiating and participating in these activities independent of supervision or direction.

What is assessed is not simply the number of activities that are restricted, but the overall degree of restriction or combination of restrictions. For example, a person who can cook and clean might be considered to have marked restriction of daily activities, if he or she were too fearful to leave the home to shop or go to the physician's office.

2. Social functioning refers to an individual's capacity to interact appropriately and communicate effectively with other individuals. Social functioning includes the ability to get along with others, such as family members, friends, neighbors, grocery clerks, landlords, or bus drivers. Impaired social functioning may be demonstrated by a history of altercations, evictions, firings, fear of strangers, avoidance of interpersonal relationships, social isolation, or similar events or characteristics. It is helpful to give specific examples illustrating the impaired functioning.

Strength in social functioning may be documented by an individual's ability to initiate social contact with others, communicate clearly with others, and interact and actively participate in group activities. Cooperative behavior, consideration for others, awareness of others' sensitivities, and social maturity also need to be considered. Social functioning in work situations may involve interactions with the public, responding to persons in authority such as supervisors, or being part of a team.

It is not only the number of aspects in which social functioning is impaired that is significant, but also the overall degree of interference with a particular aspect or combination of aspects. For example, a hostile, uncooperative person who is tolerated by local storekeepers and neighbors may have marked restriction in overall functioning, because antagonism and hostility are not acceptable in the workplace or in social contexts.

3. Concentration, persistence, and pace are called "task completion" in proposed SSA Rules.[5] These refer to the ability to sustain focused attention long enough to permit the timely completion of tasks commonly found in work settings. In activities of daily living, concentration may be reflected in terms of ability to complete everyday household tasks. Deficiencies in concentration, persistence, and pace are best noted from previous work attempts or from observations in worklike settings, such as day-treatment centers and incentive work programs. Describing specific examples of the patient's capabilities is useful. Major impairments of these abilities can often be assessed through direct psychiatric examinations or psychological testing. However, mental status examinations or psychological test data alone should not be considered adequate to describe fully the patient's concentration and sustained ability to perform work tasks.

Concentration and mental status may be assessed by such tasks as subtracting 7s serially from 100. In psychological tests of intelligence or memory, concentration is assessed through tasks requiring short-term memory or tasks that must be completed within established time limits.

In evaluating fitness for work, capability may be assessed by the completion of such tasks as filing index cards, locating telephone numbers, and disassembling and reassembling objects. Strengths and weaknesses in mental concentration may be described in terms of frequency of errors, the time it takes to complete the task, and the extent to which assistance is required to complete the task. A person who appears to concentrate adequately during a mental status examination or a psychological test might not do so in a setting more like that of the working world.

4. Deterioration or decompensation in work or worklike settings refers to repeated failure to adapt to stressful circumstances. In the face of such circumstances the individual may withdraw from the situation or experience exacerbation of signs and symptoms of a mental disorder; that is, decompensate and have difficulty maintaining activities of daily living, continuing social relationships, and completing tasks. Stresses common to the work environment include attendance, making decisions, scheduling, completing tasks, and interacting with supervisors and peers. It is useful to give examples of decompensation and the stresses that might have brought it about.

In assessing the *stress* tolerance of the individual, the examiner should be mindful of the following issues. First, "stress" may be defined with reference to an objective ("reasonable man") standard in some systems and a more subjective standard in others. Second, the circumstances of a given case might suggest a prophylactic preclusion from certain types of tasks or work settings; for example, a patient with symptoms of posttraumatic stress disorder dating from a robbery and assault might require a prophylactic preclusion from jobs involving contact with the general public or handling large sums of money. In another case, a "personality clash" between the individual and his or her supervisor might require only that the individual be precluded from working with the particular supervisor.

Under the SSA system, the medical reviewer may need to determine the residual functional capacity, a multidimensional description of work-related abilities retained by the individual in spite of medical impairment. The residual functional capacity involves four capacities related to the main aspects or areas described previously. The four capacities are indicated below.

1. *Understanding and memory* relate to the ability to remember procedures related to work; to understand and remember short and simple instructions; and to understand and remember detailed instructions.

2. *Sustained concentration and persistence* relate to the ability to carry out short, simple instructions; carry out detailed instructions; maintain attention and concentration for extended periods; perform activities within a schedule; maintain regular attendance and be punctual within customary tolerances; sustain an ordinary routine without special supervision; work with or near others without being distracted; make simple work-related decisions; complete a normal workday and workweek without interruptions from psychologically based symptoms; and perform at a consistent pace without an unreasonable number of and unreasonably long rest periods.

3. *Social interaction* involves the ability to interact appropriately with the general public; ask simple questions or request assistance; accept instructions and respond appropriately to criticism from supervisors; get along with coworkers and peers without distracting them or exhibiting behavioral extremes; maintain socially appropriate behavior; and adhere to basic standards of neatness and cleanliness.

4. *Adaptation* is the ability to respond appropriately to changes in the work setting; to be aware of normal hazards and take appropriate precautions; to use public transportation and travel to and within unfamiliar places; to set realistic goals; and to make plans independently of others.

14.4 Additional Considerations

Particular problems often arise in evaluating mental impairments of individuals who have long histories of repeated hospitalizations or prolonged outpatient care with supportive therapy and medication. Individuals with chronic psychotic disorders commonly have their lives structured in such a way as to minimize stress and reduce their signs and symptoms. Such individuals may be more impaired in terms of work capability than their signs and symptoms indicate. The results of a single examination may not adequately describe the ability of a such person to function in a sustained way. Thus, it is necessary to review information pertaining to the individual's functioning at times of increased stress.

Effects of Structured Settings

Particularly in cases involving long-standing mental disorders, overt symptoms may be controlled or attenuated by psychosocial factors, such as placement in a hospital, halfway house, board and care facility, or similar environment. These highly structured and supportive settings may greatly reduce the mental demands placed on an individual. With lowered mental demands, overt signs and symptoms of the underlying mental disorder may be minimized; however, the individual's ability to function outside of the structured setting may not have changed. The evaluator of an individual whose symptoms are controlled in the structured setting must consider the individual's ability to function independently of that setting.

Effects of Medication

Attention must be given to the effects of medication on the individual's signs, symptoms, and ability to function. Although psychoactive medications may control certain signs or symptoms, such as hallucinations, impaired attention span, restlessness, or hyperactivity, the treatment may not affect all limitations imposed by the mental disorder. If an individual's symptoms are attenuated by psychoactive medications, the evaluator should focus particular attention on limitations that may persist. Those limitations should be used as measures of the impairment's severity.

Psychoactive medications used to treat some mental illnesses may cause drowsiness, blunted affect, or unwanted effects involving various body systems. Medications that are necessary to control such symptoms as hallucinations may cause a decrease in motivation and level of activity. These side effects should be considered in evaluating the overall severity of the individual's impairment and ability to function. As explained in Chapter 2, the evaluator may need to provide an impairment estimate for the drug's side effect.

Effects of Rehabilitation

Of paramount importance to the evaluator is the degree of vocational limitation of the impaired individual, which may range from minimal to total. The severity of an impairment may change with the course of the illness, and when the individual needs less medical care, vocational skills may be intact, or the individual may have limitations that may or may not be reversible. The evaluator should judge the possible duration of the impairment that remains, whether remission is likely to be fast or slow, whether it will be partial or total, and whether the impairment is likely to remain stable or to change. These considerations should contribute to the examiner's judgment about the degree of impairment.

Rehabilitation is a sine qua non in the treatment of most patients who have recovered or are recovering from the acute phase of a mental disorder, especially a major mental disorder. Even if it is not possible to effect total remission, an outcome may be considered worthwhile if the individual has been able to move from one degree of impairment to a lesser degree.

For some persons, lack of motivation seems to be a major feature of a continuing impairment. However, many patients who undergo proper rehabilitative measures, including some who have organic illnesses, achieve improvements in functioning. But determining permanent impairment is often imprecise, and rarely is there certainty that it exists. The use of the "impairment" label tends to be pessimistic, providing an adverse prediction that may be self-fulfilling. However, the tendency for physicians and others to minimize psychiatric impairments must also be considered; this may lead to failure to refer patients for potentially helpful rehabilitative measures.

An important aspect of rehabilitation is the recognition that an individual who is taking certain types of medication may be able to sustain a satisfactory degree of functioning, whereas without medication he or she might fail to do so. For instance, there may be only a slight problem in the thinking process while the patient is taking a suitable medication, but a severe one if the patient is not taking medication.

Another consideration is that an employer needs the assurance that a worker who is taking the proper medication and is in an appropriate job can avoid injury to himself or herself and to coworkers. An analogy is seen in the care and treatment of a worker who has seizures: in such an instance, informing and educating the patient, family, employer, and coworkers are vital and should be a part of the rehabilitation process.

Just as there are degrees of impairment, total rehabilitation may not be possible. To use an example from physical medicine, it is essentially impossible for an amputated leg to be replaced, and the affected individual cannot hope to regain perfect, preinjury ambulation. However, a well-fitted prosthesis, accompanied by practice and training, can greatly improve the individual's ability to walk. If, in addition, the individual obtains suitable transportation, he or she may be restored to full gainful employment. If normal ambulation is a job requirement, an employer might be able to provide an alternative position or modify existing tasks so that they can be performed by an amputee making skillful use of a prosthesis.

Although the analogy between the loss of a limb and the loss of capability resulting from a mental disorder has limitations, it is important to recognize that impairment from a mental disorder may be just as real and severe as the impairment resulting from an injury or other illness. The link between motivation and recovery may need strengthening in individuals who are impaired by either physical or mental illnesses. This task falls especially on rehabilitationists and psychiatrists. But others can assist: an employer's providing alternative tasks or modifying existing work conditions may be an important part of restoring vocational ability to a patient with mental illness, to one recovering from an injury, or to a patient who has elements of both mental and physical illness.

14.5 Special Impairment Categories

Each of the systems of assessing impairments and disabilities recognizes some types of mental disorders and rejects others as causes of mental impairment. There is controversy about substance dependence disorders and personality disorders and especially about antisocial personality disorders. Adjustment disorders also present a dilemma to the evaluator. These are characterized by abnormal emotional responses to stressful life events, which resolve in a short time when the stressor is removed. Some authorities do not consider these responses to be medical impairments.

Substance Abuse

Controversy has been associated with the various systems for determining impairments and disabilities associated with substance abuse. Under past SSA regulations, documenting a disability required that certain complications or conditions known to be associated with substance abuse be present, and that their levels of severity match those for organic mental disorders, peripheral neuropathies, liver damage, gastritis, pancreatitis, or seizures.

Current SSA policy for determining disability related to substance addiction disorders is a modification of the Listing[1] and permits a substance addiction disorder in and of itself to be a disabling "impairment." Once a substance addiction impairment is established, a finding of disability will depend on the severity and duration of the impairment and the individual's remaining functional capacity. An impaired or lost ability to control the use of addictive substances does not in and of itself establish disability, and, as with any impairment, a diagnosis alone cannot be the basis for determining the presence of a disability. Rather, the basis is the severity of the individual's functional limitations.

Proposed SSA rules would evaluate substance abuse disorders in the same way as with other mental disorders.[4] The disorders would meet the listings if they result in at least *two* of the following: (1) marked restrictions in activities of daily living; (2) marked difficulties in maintaining social functioning; (3) marked difficulties in completing tasks in a timely manner because of deficiencies in concentration, persistence, and pace; and (4) repeated episodes of decompensation and loss of adaptive functioning, averaging three times per year, with each episode lasting 2 or more weeks.

Personality Disorders

Proposed SSA rules would handle personality disorders in much the same way as was described above for psychoactive substance dependence disorders. The disorder would meet the Listing[1] if a pathologic behavior pattern of severity prescribed in the rules resulted in marked difficulties in at least two of the four aspects described above, that is, activities of daily living, social functioning, task completion, and episodes of decompensation.

Mental Retardation

Under Social Security Disability Insurance, childhood benefits apply to dependent, disabled, adult children of an insured parent who dies, retires, or is disabled. Disability benefits are not payable to the children until age 18 years, and to qualify, the children's disabilities must begin before age 22 years. Under the Supplemental Security Income Program, disabled children under 18 years old are eligible, and there is no minimum age. The definition of disability for children is that there must be "an impairment or impairments of comparable severity to that which is considered disabling for an adult." Since a child is not expected to work, vocational factors are not considered.

The child's impairment must meet the criteria specified in the Listing,[1] with normal growth and development being a prime consideration. Under the Listing, mental retardation and autism require the presence of mental incapacity evidenced by dependence on others for personal needs, such as toileting, eating, dressing, or bathing, and an inability to follow directions, which precludes tests of intellectual functioning, or a valid verbal performance or full-scale IQ of 59 or less, or a score of 60 through 69 along with physical or mental impairment affecting daily activities, social functioning, or concentration, persistence, and pace.

Pain

The assessment of impairment due to pain, especially in circumstances in which the complaint exceeds what is expected on the basis of medical findings, is complex and controversial. While pain is discussed in the chapter on pain (p. 303) and elsewhere in this book, it is germane also to the consideration of mental and behavioral disorders. Mental illness may distort the perception of pain. Pain may be part of a somatic delusion in a patient with a major depression or a psychotic disorder. Pain may become the object of an obsessive preoccupation, or it may be the chief complaint in a conversion disorder.

The essential feature of somatoform pain disorder in *DSM-III-R* is preoccupation with pain in the absence of physical findings that adequately account for the pain and its intensity. In the past, this syndrome has been called "psychogenic pain disorder" or "idiopathic pain disorder," but these terms are often used more loosely to describe any complaint of pain that is greater than the physician expects for the average patient who has the same physical findings. The physician should recognize that anxiety and depression almost always magnify pain, and vice versa. The disorders with *impaired pain perception* are easier to evaluate than cases in which the pain is said to have a psychogenic component.

Establishing that pain is or is not a symptom of a mental impairment may be a difficult and complex task. Pain that presents only as a symptom of a mental disorder is rare. The following guidelines may be useful in determining whether pain is a symptom of a mental impairment. (1) All possible somatic causes of the pain have been eliminated by careful, comprehensive medical examinations. (2) Some significant emotional stressor has occurred in the patient's life that may have acted as a triggering agent, and the stressor and the pain have occurred in a reasonable sequence. (3) Evidence exists of a mental disorder other than a conversion-related one, and the pain may be a symptom of the former; for example, delusional pain may occur in a patient who has a subtle paranoid disorder.

Assessing impairment related to pain is difficult, and the process is not as clearly and precisely defined as with some kinds of impairments. Therefore, determinations about difficult and borderline cases in this category should be made through a multidisciplinary, multispecialty approach, in which physicians who are knowledgeable about the different body systems are involved as needed.

Malingering

Although malingering is thought to be rare, the physician should be aware of this possibility when evaluating impairments. The possibility of obtaining monetary awards and still avoiding work increases the likelihood of malingering. Malingering may arise with mental disorders or with nonpsychiatric conditions.

Certain symptoms, such as headache, low-back pain, peripheral neuralgia, and vertigo, are notoriously difficult to assess. Conditions that have more of an organic basis, such as appendicitis, a fracture, or pregnancy, tend to be more amenable to objective diagnostic studies than are psychiatric and neurologic complaints. Psychiatric disorders have not been rewarded financially as well as other conditions. Malingerers with supposed psychiatric conditions may be seen in circumstances involving the avoidance of an unpleasant duty or requirement, such as going to jail or entering military service.

Rather than giving outright fabrications, individuals may consciously or unconsciously exaggerate the symptoms of a disorder in the clinical or the impairment evaluation setting. Malingering or exaggeration of symptoms may be suspected when the individual's symptoms are vague, ill-defined, overdramatized, inconsistent, or not in conformity with signs and symptoms known to occur. In this situation, results of the physical and mental status examinations and other data and information of the evaluation may be inconsistent with the nature and intensity of the patient's complaints.

Circumstances in which an unusual number of ill-defined complaints occur in a circumscribed group, perhaps in a setting of poor morale or conflict, also may be viewed with suspicion. But the most appropriate approach for the examining physician is one of clinical neutrality, the application of standard interview and diagnostic procedures, and, if warning signs appear, a careful investigation that includes multidisciplinary evaluation and psychological testing as appropriate. A recent text considered malingering more fully.[6]

Motivation

Assessing motivation is difficult, because lack of motivation may be difficult to distinguish from mental impairment. When is an individual lacking energy, concentration, and initiative "depressed," and when is the individual "unmotivated?" Ultimately, making this distinction requires a clinical judgment, which should be aided by a careful investigation of the individual's efforts and accomplishments before the onset of the alleged impairment and a search for associated signs and symptoms of common mental disorders.

Motivation is a link between impairment and disability. For some people, poor motivation is a major cause of poor functioning. An individual's underlying character may be important in determining whether he or she is motivated to benefit from rehabilitation. Personality characteristics usually remain unchanged throughout life. However, internal events and psychological reactions can influence the course of illness. An individual who tends to be dependent may become more dependent as the illness proceeds, and one who is inclined to act impulsively may develop a pattern of antisocial behavior. Indeed, the development of a pathologic character trait may become more pronounced and significant than the illness in negating motivation for improved functioning.

Thus, as explained in Chapter 1 and the Glossary, the degree of disability in the social and vocational contexts is not necessarily the same as the degree of impairment. The loss of function may be greater or less than the impairment might imply, and the individual's performance may fall short of, or exceed, that usually associated with the impairment. Here the complex issue of "secondary gain" arises, which involves not only the amount of a financial award, but also the individual's life-style. The individual's motivation to recover and be self-sufficient will either diminish or enhance the quality of life in terms of social, vocational, and other activities. Impairment may lead to an almost total or to a minimal disability, depending on motivational factors. Although some clues may appear in the individual's clinical or family history, these are likely to be only suggestive.

When considering the total background and underlying character and value system of the individual, the evaluator must not ignore the educational levels and financial resources of family members. The evaluator should assess the usefulness of family influences, and if rehabilitation efforts are to be made, the evaluator and the patient may find benefit in the participation of one or more family members.

14.6 Format of the Report

The following general format for impairment reports has been adapted from that recommended by the SSA.[7] The content of the report may vary, depending on the system for which the report is being prepared. An impairment report based on the *Guides* also should include the main features of the Report of Medical Evaluation form shown in Chapter 2 (p. 11).

General Observations

1. How did the patient come to the examination, alone or accompanied? From what distance and by what transportation mode? If the patient came by automobile, who drove?

2. Note the patient's appearance: dress, grooming, appearance of invalidism.

3. Describe the patient's attitude and degree of cooperation.

4. Identify the informant and estimate his or her reliability. Ask if the patient has taken drugs or psychoactive substances within the past 24 to 48 hours, which might affect examination results.

Medical History

Describe the patient's general physical health. Describe significant past illnesses and injuries; ask about head injuries and residua. Describe hospitalizations for nonpsychiatric causes, diagnoses, durations, operations. Obtain information on human immunodeficiency virus (HIV) and sexually transmitted disease (STD) risk factors and exposures.

Describe current use of medication for nonpsychiatric causes and regimens; describe use of tobacco, alcohol, caffeine, and other drugs. Inquire about allergies.

Present Illness

Provide a detailed description of the pertinent history of the mental disorder and a detailed description of the individual's statement of the current complaint. Include (1) the date of onset, date when the patient became unable to work, description of how the disorder interferes with work, and information about outcome of attempts to resume work; (2) a description of the patient's daily activities, interests, and habits.

Hospitalization for Mental Illness

Obtain information on location, inclusive dates, duration, and status on admission. Describe therapy given and condition on discharge. Describe the results of psychological tests and other studies, such as electroencephalogram and radiographic studies.

Outpatient or Other Treatment

If treatment was given for a mental disorder, state the source of treatment, date, duration, and condition of the patient when first seen. Describe the type of therapy and response; if medications were used, list the drugs, dosages, and results. Describe the patient's condition when last seen.

Personal and Family History

Include a biographic description of the patient's relevant educational, social, military, marital, and occupational adjustment in terms of ability to conform to social standards, hold employment, advance in career, and adjust to supervisors and coworkers. Ask about mental illness in the family and conditions that may have familial or hereditary basis.

Assessment of Severity

Describe in detail the severity of limitations imposed by the disorder in the following four respects, giving examples.

1. Activities of daily living, including adaptive activities, such as cleaning, shopping, cooking, taking public transportation, paying bills, maintaining a residence, caring for self, grooming, using the telephone and directory, using the post office, and working.

2. Social functioning and ability to get along with others, including family members, friends, neighbors, grocery clerks, landlords, and others of the public. Social functioning in work situations may involve responding appropriately to persons in authority and cooperative behavior toward coworkers.

3. Concentration, persistence, and pace (task completion); this refers to the patient's ability to sustain focused attention long enough to permit the completion of everyday tasks in the workplace or home. Describe deficiencies in concentration, persistence, and pace that have been observed at work or in worklike settings. Include relevant information from the mental status examination and from psychological testing.

4. Deterioration or decompensation in worklike settings; describe failures to adapt to stressful circumstances that cause the individual either to withdraw from the situation or to experience signs and

symptoms and difficulties with activities of daily living, social relationships, and concentration, persistence, and pace. Describe any decompensation at work, which might involve decisions, attendance, schedules, completing tasks, interactions with supervisors, and interactions with peers.

Mental Status
Provide a description of the following: (1) patient's attitude and behavior; (2) stream of conversation and psychomotor activity (provide examples); (3) mood, affect, and emotional reactions; (4) content of special preoccupations (give verbatim examples); (5) sensorium, orientation, memory, and intellectual resources (provide examples); and (6) psychological testing (summarize tests used and results).

Diagnosis
Use current American Psychiatric Association nomenclature and the five axes of the multiaxial evaluation.[2]

14.7 A Method of Evaluating Psychiatric Impairment

There is no available empiric evidence to support any method for assigning a percentage of impairment of the whole person, but the following approach to estimating the extent of mental impairments is offered as a guide. Not everyone who has a mental or behavioral disorder is totally limited or totally impaired. Many individuals have specific limitations that do not preclude all of life's activities; on the other hand, there are individuals with less than chronic, but still unremitting, impairments who are severely limited in some areas of function. These impairments, too, are of concern.

Medically determinable impairments in thinking, affect, intelligence, perception, judgment, and behavior are assessed by direct observation, formal mental status examination, and neuropsychological testing. Translating specific impairments directly and precisely into functional limitations, however, is complex and poorly understood; for example, current research finds little relationship between psychiatric signs and symptoms such as those identified during a mental status examination, and the ability to perform competitive work.

To bridge the gap between impairment and disability, the group that advised the SSA on disability due to mental impairment identified the four categories of functional limitations discussed earlier (Section 14.3, p. 293). These categories tend to be complex social impairments that may be directly related to work or to other pursuits, such as recreation or caring for a family. Yet there is no specific medical test for any one of the categories. The physician's observations made during the medical examination should be incorporated into the evaluation together with other relevant observations, including those pertaining to carrying out activities of daily living, social functioning, concentration, persistence and pace, and adaptation.

The Table (p. 301) provides a guide for rating mental impairment in each of the four areas of functional limitation on a five-category scale that ranges from no impairment to extreme impairment. The following are recommended as anchors for the categories of the scale. "None" means no impairment is noted in the function; "mild" implies that any discerned impairment is compatible with most useful functioning; "moderate" means that the identified impairments are compatible with some but not all useful functioning; "marked" is a level of impairment that significantly impedes useful functioning. Taken alone, a "marked" impairment would not completely preclude functioning, but together with marked limitation in another class, it might limit useful functioning. "Extreme" means that the impairment or limitation is not compatible with useful function.

Extreme impairment in carrying out activities of daily living implies complete dependency on another person for care. In the sphere of social functioning, extreme impairment implies that the individual engages in no meaningful social contact, as with a patient in a withdrawn, catatonic state. An extreme limitation in concentration, persistence, and pace means that the individual cannot attend to conversation or any productive task at all; this might be seen in a person in an acute confusional state or in a person with a complete loss of short-term memory.

A person who cannot tolerate any change at all in routines or in the environment, or one who cannot function and who decompensates when schedules change in an otherwise structured environment, has an extreme limitation of adaptive functioning and an extreme psychiatric impairment. Such an individual might have a psychotic episode if a meal is not served on time or might have a panic attack when left without a companion in any situation.

In the ordinary individual, extreme impairment in only one class would be likely to preclude the performance of any complex task, such as one involving recreation or work. Marked limitation in two or more spheres would be likely to preclude

Table. Classification of Impairments Due to Mental and Behavioral Disorders.

Area or aspect of functioning	Class 1: No impairment	Class 2: Mild impairment	Class 3: Moderate impairment	Class 4: Marked impairment	Class 5: Extreme impairment
Activities of daily living Social functioning Concentration Adaptation	*No* impairment is noted	Impairment levels are compatible with *most* useful functioning	Impairment levels are compatible with *some,* but not all, useful functioning	Impairment levels *significantly impede* useful functioning	*Impairment levels preclude* useful functioning

performing complex tasks without special support or assistance, such as that provided in a sheltered environment. An individual who was impaired to a moderate degree in all four categories of functioning would be limited in ability to carry out many, but not all, complex tasks. Mild and moderate limitations reduce overall performance but do not preclude performance.

Translating these guidelines for rating individual impairment on ordinal scales into a method for assigning percentage of impairments, as if valid estimates could be made on precisely measured interval scales, cannot be done reliably. One cannot be certain that the difference in impairment between a rating of mild and moderate is of the same magnitude as the difference between moderate and marked. Furthermore, a moderate impairment does not imply a 50% limitation in useful functioning, and an estimate of moderate impairment in all four categories does not imply a 50% impairment of the whole person.

Physicians, of course, must often make judgments based more on clinical impressions than on accurate, objective, analytic empiric evidence. In those circumstances in which it is essential to make an estimate, the ordinal or numeric scale might be of some general use. For instance, one might assume that the extreme estimate of 95% to 100% mental impairment implies a state like that of coma, which is the most extreme impairment of central nervous system functioning and consciousness. Approaching 100% impairment of the whole person, according to the *Guides,* is considered to be approaching death.

Eventually, research may disclose direct relationships between medical findings and percentages of mental impairment. Until that time, the medical profession must refine its concepts of mental impairment, improve its ability to measure limitations, and continue to make clinical judgments.

Comment on Lack of Percents in This Edition

The decision not to use percentages for estimates of mental impairment in this fourth edition of the *Guides* was made only after considerable thought and discussion. The second edition (1984) provided ranges of percentages for estimating such impairment. Mental functions, such as intelligence, thinking, perception, judgment, affect, and behavior, were considered to fall into five classes, and the ranges were given as follows: normal, 0% to 5%; mild impairment, 10% to 20%; moderate impairment, 25% to 50%; moderately severe impairment, 55% to 75%; and severe impairment, more than 75%. Ability to carry out daily activities was estimated as follows: class 1, self-sufficient; class 2, needs minor help; class 3, needs regular help; class 4, needs major help; and class 5, quite helpless. From estimates of the individual's functioning, a whole-person impairment estimate could be made.

The procedure for the second edition was highly subjective. The third edition (1988) did not list percentages but instead provided the same classes of impairment as the fourth edition. There are some valid reasons to use ranges of percents for mental impairments. If this were done, the chapter on mental disorders would be consistent with *Guides* chapters for the other organ systems. Another point is that various systems for estimating disability have developed ranges of percentages; if such estimates were not provided in the *Guides,* the material in the *Guides* on mental disorders might be ignored. This would increase the likelihood that estimates would be made inconsistently in the various jurisdictions.

A more persuasive argument is that, unlike the situations with some organ systems, there are no precise measures of impairment in mental disorders. The use of precentages implies a certainty that does not exist, and the percentages are likely to be used inflexibly by adjudicators, who then are less likely to take into account the many factors that influence mental and behavioral impairment. Also, because no data exist that show the reliability of the impairment percentages, it would be difficult for *Guides* users to defend their use in administrative hearings. After considering this difficult matter, the Committee on Disability and Rehabilitation of the American Psychiatric Association advised *Guides'* contributors against the use of percentages in the chapter on mental and behavioral disorders of the fourth edition.

Example: A 27-year-old single woman was referred for evaluation of mental impairment. She had a 9-year history of chronic paranoid schizophrenia. She had not worked for longer than 2 months at a time since dropping out of business college at the age of 19 years. The young woman had lived at home and had been cared for and supported financially by her aging parents, who recently moved to a retirement community. For the past 3 months she had been living in a cooperative apartment and she had shown some ability to care for herself. However, she constantly needed to be reminded to bathe, take her medications, and complete the household chores.

The young woman had little self-confidence and did not engage independently in any activities, including cooking; however, when someone insisted that she cook, she was able to do so. Once she initiated a task, she was able to complete it in a timely manner. She had no friends and never initiated a conversation, and when she was approached or prodded she became terrified and occasionally abusive. The woman remained paranoid and said that "everyone is in my mind." Her attention span was limited to 25 to 30 minutes, and she frequently "blocked" in her speech and was unable to complete a thought.

Although the woman had been in a hospital only twice, she frequently stopped taking her neuroleptic medications, which were generally effective in controlling her delusions and hallucinations. During two periods when she was employed, she became overwhelmed by the pressures of work deadlines, blamed coworkers for slowing her down, stopped taking her medications, and needed intensive treatment. She handled some changes in her environment well but had considerable difficulty with deadlines and time constraints and with separation from her family.

A complete medical evaluation was performed, and there were no positive physical or laboratory findings. A mental status examination confirmed the history and findings described above.

Impairment: The evaluator believed the young woman's activities of daily living and social functioning were markedly impaired, and her ability to concentrate, maintain a reasonable pace, and adapt to change were moderately impaired. The evaluator believed that in more demanding social or vocational situations the woman would be markedly impaired in concentration and adaptation.

The evaluator concluded that, overall, the young woman had marked mental or psychiatric impairment (class 4).

References

1. Social Security Administration. Federal Old-Age, Survivors and Disability Insurance. *Listing of Impairments, Mental Disorders: Final Rule (Listing).* 20 CFR Part 404 (Reg No. 4) 50(167), *Federal Register* 1985:35038-35070. The Listing and other guidance appear also in: *Disability Evaluation Under Social Security.* Baltimore, Md: Social Security Administration; February 1986. Publication No. 64-039.

2. American Psychiatric Association, Committee on Nomenclature and Statistics. *Diagnostic and Statistical Manual of Mental Disorders, Revised Third Edition.* Washington, DC: American Psychiatric Association; 1987.

3. Meyerson A, Fine T. *Psychiatric Disability: Clinical, Legal, and Administrative Dimensions.* Washington, DC: American Psychiatric Press; 1987.

4. World Health Organization. *Manual of the International Statistical Classification of Diseases, Injuries, and Causes of Death: International Classification of Diseases (ICD).* Geneva, Switzerland: World Health Organization; 1978.

5. Social Security Administration. Federal Old-Age, Survivors and Disability Insurance. *Listing of Impairments, Mental Disorders in Adults: Proposed Rules. Federal Register,* July 18, 1991, vol 56, No. 138.

6. Meyerson A. Malingering. In: Kaplan H, Sadock B, eds. *Textbook of Psychiatry.* 5th ed. New York, NY: Williams & Wilkins; 1989.

7. Social Security Administration. *Consultative Examinations—Guide for Physicians.* Baltimore, Md: Social Security Administration; 1985. SSA publication 64-025.

Chapter 15

Pain

Pain is endemic in the United States population, yet knowledge and understanding about this complex entity and its determinants, diagnosis, and treatment are only rudimentary. This is especially true of chronic pain. Thus, any discussion of permanent impairment because of pain will be problematic as well as controversial. The difficulties that physicians experience in dealing with pain are based, in part, on the following characteristics and perceptions.

1. Pain encompasses a multifaceted concept that transcends the traditional medical model of disease based on pathogenesis at the tissue or organ level. A perceptive concept of pain includes consideration of cognitive, behavioral, environmental, and ethnocultural variables as well as pathophysiologic factors.

2. Pain is subjective, and its presence cannot be validated or measured objectively. People tend to view pain complaints with suspicion and disbelief, as with complaints of fatigue. A report of the Social Security Administration in 1987 averred that it is impossible to understand the pain that another person is suffering.[14]

3. Impairment due to pain has not been well defined. No consensus exists about the occurrence of pain in healthy people, nor is there information about its occurrence by age group.

The medical, social, and economic consequences of pain are enormous. A national survey reported in a 1987 Institute of Medicine monograph indicated that about 6% of visits to physicians are for new pain, and a telephone survey disclosed that about 14% of persons 18 to 65 years old have pain for more than 1 month per year.[12] Data from the United States and other nations indicate that at least half of all persons experience moderate pain during their lives.

The federal government has recognized the impact of pain. The Secretary of the US Department of Health and Human Services in 1985 formed a commission on the evaluation of pain, which concluded that chronic pain is not a psychiatric disorder. The commission recommended further study of the subject by the Institute of Medicine.[12] Currently, the Social Security Administration is supporting an investigation to assess the validity of criteria for identifying individuals with chronic pain.

15.1 Basic Assumptions

The *Guides* is intended to provide a standard method of analysis for evaluation of impairing conditions. Fundamental to the *Guides* is that it applies only to *permanent* impairments, which are defined as those that are stable and unlikely to change in future months because of medical or surgical therapy. Permanent impairments are considered further in Chapter 1 and the Glossary (p. 315).

In general, the impairment percents given in the tables and figures applicable to permanent impairments of the various organ systems include allowances for the pain that may occur with those impairments.

In considering pain, it is prudent to list the following assumptions.

1. Pain evaluation does not lend itself to strict laboratory standards of sensitivity, specificity, and other scientific criteria.

2. Chronic pain is not measurable or detectable on the basis of the classic, tissue-oriented disease model.

3. Pain evaluation requires acknowledging and understanding a multifaceted, biopsychosocial model that transcends the usual, more limited disease model.

4. Pain impairment estimates are based on the physician's training, experience, skill, and thoroughness. As with most medical care, the physician's judgment about pain represents a blend of the art and science of medicine, and the judgment must be characterized not so much by scientific accuracy as by procedural regularity.

The important task of evaluating impairment due to pain is difficult but not impossible. Physicians initially may feel uncomfortable evaluating pain, but they regularly employ similar methods and approaches in arriving at diagnostic and therapeutic judgments. Physicians generally are comfortable making decisions on the basis of probabilities backed up by experience and stated in terms of reasonable medical certainty. Pain should be evaluated by physicians who are conversant with the disorder.

15.2 Definitions

Pain is ubiquitous. Pain is usually regarded as a warning signal that alerts the organism to potential tissue damage. Indeed, life without pain is hardly conceivable and would result in irrevocable harm. Yet, strangely, there is no consensus as to a meaningful definition of pain.

The International Association for the Study of Pain defines pain as "an unpleasant sensory and emotional experience with actual or potential tissue damage [that is] described in terms of such damage." The Commission on the Evaluation of Pain defines pain as a "complex experience, embracing physical, mental, social and behavioral processes, which comprises the quality of life of many individuals." Another definition views pain as an unpleasant subjective perception in the context of tissue damage.

Embodied in the definitions above are the following concepts. Pain is subjective and cannot be measured objectively. Pain evokes negative psychologic reactions, such as fear, anxiety, and depression. Pain is perceived consciously and is evaluated in the light of past experiences. People usually regard pain as an indicator of physical harm, despite the fact that pain can exist without tissue damage, and tissue damage can exist without pain.

15.3 Pain, Impairment, and Disability

The *Guides* defines impairment as the loss, loss of use, or derangement of any body part, system, or function. Thus, impairment is defined on an anatomic, physiologic, or psychological basis. This definition operates at the organ level and presumes a disease model that involves endogenous systems and generally is independent of the external milieu. In this narrow context, it would be difficult to consider pain an impairment.

But the *Guides* interprets the definition of impairment to involve also interfering with the individual's performance of daily activities (see Glossary). In this broader context, impairment is at the level of the individual, is based on an illness model, and is viewed as being dependent on personal needs and the demands of the external milieu. In this context, pain may be viewed as an impairment that should be assessed according to the individual's residual functional capacity. Chronic pain and pain-related behavior are not, per se, impairments, but they should trigger assessments with regard to ability to function and carry out daily activities.

These concepts and definitions are blurred by the operational definitions and demands in different venues dealing with pain, impairment, and disability. The Social Security Administration, for instance, gives credence to pain only insofar as it relates to an underlying physical or mental impairment (see Glossary). Workers' compensation programs vary from state to state in their constraints and procedures. The US Department of Veterans Affairs generally does not consider pain, except as a manifestation of a physical or mental impairment. Private disability insurance programs tend to recognize pain as an exacerbating factor, if there is an underlying physical or mental impairment.

Related Concepts

Disease: This is a pathologic process or disorder at the tissue or organ system level.

Illness: This is an adverse, unhealthy process or disorder that affects the individual. An illness must be viewed in the context of both the external and internal milieu and transcends pathogenicity at the tissue level.

Nociception: This is the perception of pain resulting from a noxious stimulus to a nociceptor. Complex neurochemical and neuroelectrical processes transmit pain impulses from the site of injury along the peripheral, autonomic, and central nervous systems.

Modulation: Transmission of pain impulses along multisynaptic pathways can result in significant alteration of the quality and intensity of the stimulus. Modulation occurs in the central nervous system.

Perception: Conscious awareness or recognition of pain is governed by the cerebral cortex. The pain impulse is evaluated through association pathways, and it may be identified as "suffering." The emotional content of the evaluation depends on such factors as the individual's personality characteristics and value system, cognitive awareness, experiences, education, and ethnocultural background. Pain is viewed as an unpleasant experience, and the emotional content frequently consists of feelings of fear, anxiety, frustration, and depression. The fear of pain may be more devastating than the pain itself.

Response: The individual's response to perceived pain depends on multiple factors in the internal and external milieu. The response involves the central nervous system and the autonomic nervous system, is involuntary as well as voluntary, and may be appropriate or inappropriate. Before the pain response, the pain experience of the individual is unknown to others. The pain response provides a "window" through which others can discern and evaluate the individual's pain experience.

Suffering: This is a state of severe distress associated with events that threaten the individual's intactness. Suffering may or may not be associated with pain. Suffering and pain are distinct entities.

Malingering: This is the conscious and deliberate feigning of an illness or disability. Malingering is discussed in the *Guides* chapter on mental and behavioral disorders (p. 291).

Functional capacity evaluation: This involves examining an individual as the individual performs activities in a structured setting. It does not necessarily reflect what the individual *should be able* to do, but rather what the individual *can* do or *is willing* to do at a given time. Functional capacity depends especially on motivation, cognitive awareness, behavioral factors, and sincerity of effort, and these characteristics have a major impact on the functional capacity assessment (FCA).

The functional capacity assessment, which is performed by or under the supervision of the physician, varies according to the physician's training, experience, skill, competence, and understanding of the assessment processes. A great need exists for a valid, accurate, reliable, and relevant instrument for performing the FCA, one that is based on the full range of abilities and activities of normal persons.

15.4 Classification and Models

Classifying pain in a multiaxial context is important from both a conceptual and an operational perspective. Several models are proposed: a functional classification depending on neuropsychiatric considerations; a clinical classification depending on pathogenesis; and an operational or interactive classification depending upon a biopsychosocial concept. The models are not necessarily mutually exclusive: a patient seen in the office or clinic might have pain encompassing aspects of several of the models.

Neuropsychiatric Model

Nociceptive or somatic pain results from actual or impending tissue damage. This pain represents the usual and most frequent acute pain experience. Pain arising from peripheral or visceral tissues is defined within established neuroanatomic and neurophysiologic processes. Usually the pain is limited, easily diagnosed, short-lived, and readily treated. This type of pain occurs with a fractured bone, skin laceration or angina pectoris.

Neurogenic or central pain encompasses neuropathic and deafferentation pain. This pain results from spontaneous excitation within the central, peripheral, or autonomic nervous system and in the absence of any specific noxious painful stimuli. Making the diagnosis and evaluating this type of pain may be difficult, and the pain may be persistent and refractory to effective treatment. Examples include peripheral neuropathy, trigeminal neuralgia, and phantom limb pain.

Psychogenic pain is a psychiatric disorder that is part of such conditions as somatization disorder, thought disorder, mood disorder, and hypochondriasis.[1] Psychogenic pain should not be confused with chronic pain syndrome, which is *not* considered to be a mental disorder. Confusion arises because the chronic pain syndrome often is associated with emotional problems, such as depression and anxiety, which occur frequently in mental disorders.

Significant mind-body interrelationships exist with both the chronic pain syndrome and psychogenic pain. A useful diagnostic test is to ask the question, "Would the individual have pain if the mental disorder were absent?"

Pathogenesis Model

Primary pain is related to tissue trauma or physiologic disruption, either nociceptive or neurogenic. The link between the stimulus generating the pain and the resulting perception of pain is direct. The pain usually is acute and self-limiting. Examples include pain resulting from an acute sprain or renal lithiasis.

Secondary pain usually is the result of adverse pain behavior or ineffective medical treatment (iatrogenesis). Secondary pain arises not from the primary pain stimulus, but as the patient's reaction to the result of the primary pain problem. Secondary pain is likely to be persistent and difficult to manage. Examples of secondary pain include pain resulting from the treatment of a malignant neoplasm with surgery, radiation, or chemotherapy; pain resulting from substance abuse and dependency; and pain resulting from prolonged inactivity and deconditioning.

Biopsychosocial Model

Acute pain serves as an alerting mechanism that protects the individual. Acute pain usually is nociceptive, primary, and short-lived, and its psychosocial consequences are minimal. The perception of the pain and the individual's behavior and capability after the episode generally are commensurate with the noxious stimulus. The pain abates as healing occurs. Usually, acute pain is associated with conditions that are short-lived and self-limiting; thus, estimates of permanent impairment according to *Guides* criteria are not indicated.

Recurrent acute pain is a more complex subject than acute pain. This category involves the episodic painful sensations that occur in chronic disorders, such as the arthritides, trigeminal neuralgia, and some types of headache. Recurrent acute pain may be nociceptive or neurogenic, primary or secondary. Recurrent acute pain should not be confused with chronic pain, because the determinants are greatly different, especially the pathophysiologic ones.

The significance, evaluation, and medical management of recurrent acute pain are basically the same as for acute pain. However, the emphasis is on palliation and management and not on cure. Prognosis depends on the availability of effective treatment for the underlying pathologic process. Impairment is a function of the underlying disease process as modified by the superimposed pain and the patient's makeup.

Cancer-related pain, which frequently is referred to as chronic, intractable pain, represents one of the broadest syntheses of pain models because of the nature of the causative process. The pain may be nociceptive or neurogenic; primary or secondary; acute, recurrent, or chronic. Combinations of these varieties may occur. Understandably, significant psychological states often are at play in individuals with cancer. Fear, anxiety, depression, anger, denial, and other manifestations add dramatically to the patient's perception and interpretation of the pain experience.

In patients with cancer who have pain, the diagnosis and treatment usually have been accomplished as well as is possible. The goal of pain management is to provide a comfortable and dignified life. The basis of treatment includes the use of opioid and nonopioid analgesics, other pharmaceuticals, surgical intervention, and behavior modification techniques, including biofeedback, hypnosis, and relaxation therapy.

Chronic pain represents the nidus of the chronic pain syndrome. Chronic pain may be referred to as "chronic benign pain" to differentiate it from the pain related to a malignant neoplasm. Pain of long duration is properly referred to as "persistent pain," with the term "chronic pain" being reserved for the devastating and recalcitrant type with major psychosocial consequences. In this chapter, the term "chronic pain" is synonymous with "chronic pain syndrome." Under the *Guides* definitions, persistent pain may exist in the absence of chronic pain, but chronic pain always presumes the presence of persistent pain.

Chronic pain represents a malevolent and destructive force and generally is considered to be useless. Chronic pain is a self-sustaining, self-reinforcing, and self-regenerating process. It is not a symptom of an underlying acute somatic injury, but rather a destructive illness in its own right. It is an illness of the whole person and not a disease caused by the pathologic state of an organ system. Chronic pain is persistent, long-lived, and progressive. Pain perception is markedly enhanced. Pain-related behavior becomes maladaptive and grossly disproportional to any underlying noxious stimulus, which usually has healed and no longer serves as an underlying pain generator.

Chronic pain that is not recognized and properly treated results in a deterioration of coping mechanisms. Under such circumstances, limitations of functional capacity are apt to occur. The patient's maladaptive behavior may have medical, social, and economic consequences that greatly outweigh any somatic components of the illness. These consequences may include despair, alienation from family and society, loss of job, isolation, invalidism, and suicidal thoughts. Yet, chronic pain is not a psychiatric disorder.

Chronic pain may result from inappropriate management of acute pain. It is not possible to predict the course of a patient's condition from inception of the noxious stimulus to the development of the complete chronic pain syndrome. However, there is some evidence relating the development of chronic pain to emotional abuse, sexual abuse, physical abuse, substance abuse, or abandonment by the primary caregiver. A history of childhood sexual or physical abuse is a common theme among female patients with chronic pain. Early detection and prompt, effective intervention require a high index of suspicion and are essential to effective management.

15.5 Dynamic Interrelationships of Models

It is important to recognize that changing interrelationships exist among the biologic, psychological, and socioeconomic components and modifiers of pain (Fig. 1, at right). The devastating, stultifying economic and social impacts of chronic pain are well known. The psychological impact is manifested by depression, withdrawal, anxiety, and other mood disorders, and the biologic consequences are beginning to be explored. Animal studies demonstrate that neuroendocrine changes related to pain, which involve the thalamic-pituitary axis and the limbic system, can alter behavior. Other experimental studies indicate that persistent pain may result in increased morbidity and mortality.

In considering the various pain classifications and models, it is important to recognize the ascending order: tissue, organ, and organism. Disorders affecting tissues and organ systems result in symptoms and disease, and acute and recurrent pain can be viewed in this context. Disorders affecting the individual as a whole result in illnesses, such as those that characterize chronic pain. Regarding pain and its interrelated determinants, it is wise to consider Dr. William Osler's maxim, "It is not nearly as important what illness a patient has, as what patient has the illness."

Figure 1. Biopsychosocial Modifiers of Pain.

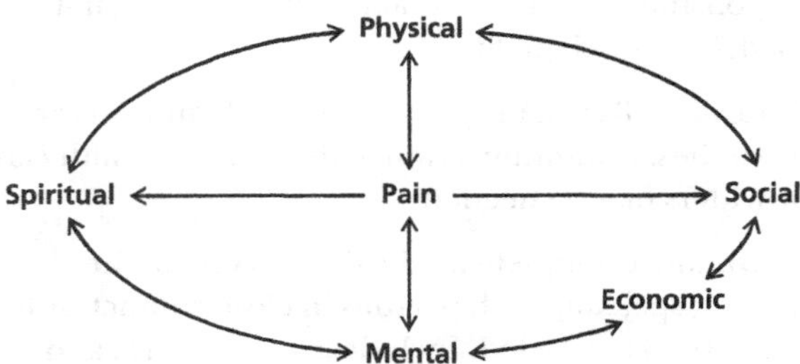

15.6 Clinical Assessment

Assessing the magnitude of the patient's pain and pain-related impairment requires a multidisciplinary approach based on the biopsychosocial model. In general, the assessment calls for the traditional approach of the physician. However, assessing chronic pain is a complex and lengthy process that usually requires hours if not days to complete. In difficult cases, it may be appropriate to enlist the aid of physicians specializing in pain medicine.

The *Guides* Chapter 2 describes in general terms the methods that should be used to evaluate and estimate the extent of impairments. The following steps should guide the examination of a patient with a complex pain problem. Some important information, for instance, that is described in steps 4, 5, and 6 below ideally will be available to the evaluator because of others' examinations and studies. It is the physician's responsibility to ensure that the information, if it is used, is of good quality.

1. Review all available medical records and diagnostic studies. Communication with previous health care providers may be needed.

2. Obtain a complete medical history from the patient, speaking with persons in close contact with the patient as needed. Include a family, work, and social activities history. List affected daily activities (See p. 313).

3. Document all current complaints and the pain history. The pain history should include a description of onset, location, quality, progression, character, intensity, variability, frequency, duration, migration pattern, precipitating and aggravating factors, epiphenomena, treatment, medications, and other interventions used and results.

4. Perform a complete physical and neurologic examination.

5. Arrange appropriate ancillary studies, for instance, roentgenographic, magnetic resonance imaging, and electromyographic studies.

6. Psychological testing is an integral part of evaluating pain. Using the Minnesota Multiphasic Personality Inventory has become standard. Other instruments include the Cornell Medical Index Health Questionnaire, McGill Pain Questionnaire, Beck and Zung Depression Indices, and Westhaven-Yale Multidimensional Pain Inventory.

7. Formulate a diagnostic impression based on the accumulated information. This assessment should refer to the cause and classification of the pain, description of the biopsychosocial impact, and prognosis.

8. Estimate the extent of the pain and impairment using the procedures described in Section 15.9 (p. 311) and other parts of the *Guides* as appropriate.

Diagnostic Characteristics (the Eight *Ds*) of Chronic Pain

The presence of two or more of the following characteristics should be considered to establish a presumptive diagnosis of chronic pain syndrome.

1. *Duration*: In the past, the term "chronic pain" has been applied to pain of greater than 6 months' duration; however, current opinion is that the chronic pain syndrome can be diagnosed as early as 2 to 4 weeks after its onset. Prompt evaluation and treatment are essential.

2. *Dramatization*: Patients with chronic pain display unusual verbal and nonverbal pain behavior. Words used to describe the pain are emotionally charged, affective, and exaggerated. Patients may exhibit maladaptive, theatrical behavior, such as moaning, groaning, gasping, grimacing, posturing, or pantomiming.

3. *Diagnostic Dilemma*: Patients tend to have extensive histories of evaluations by multiple physicians. The patient has undergone repeated diagnostic studies, despite which the clinical impressions tend to be vague, inconsistent, and inaccurate.

4. *Drugs:* Substance dependence and abuse involving drugs and alcohol is a frequent concomitant. Patients are willing recipients of multiple drugs, which may interact adversely. Often they consume excessive amounts of prescribed drugs.

5. *Dependence:* These patients become dependent on their physicians and demand excessive medical care. They expect passive types of physical therapy over long time periods, but these provide no lasting benefit. They become dependent on their spouses and families and relinquish all domestic and social responsibilities.

6. *Depression:* The condition is characterized by emotional upheaval. Patients tend to have psychological test results that suggest depression, hypochondriasis, and hysteria. Cognitive aberrations give way to unhappiness, depression, despair, apprehension, irritability, and hostility. Coping mechanisms are severely impaired. Low self-esteem results in impaired self-reliance and increased dependence on others.

7. *Disuse:* Prolonged, excessive immobilization results in secondary pain of musculoskeletal origin. Self-imposed splinting may be validated by misguided medical directives to be "cautious," and this can result in progressive muscular dysfunction and generalized deconditioning. The secondary pain further aggravates and perpetuates the reverberating pain cycle.

8. *Dysfunction:* Having lost adequate coping skills, patients with chronic pain begin to withdraw from the social milieu. They disengage from work, drop recreational endeavors, tend to alienate friends and family, and become increasingly isolated, eventually restricting their activities to the bare essentials of life. Bereft of social contacts, rebuffed by the medical system, and deprived of adequate financial means, the patient becomes an invalid in the broadest sense: physical, emotional, social, and economic.

The physician should suspect the presence of the chronic pain syndrome if a patient does not respond to appropriate medical care within a reasonable period of time, or if the patient's verbal or nonverbal pain behavior greatly surpasses the usual response to a given noxious stimulus.

15.7 Treatment

Pain, including persistent and chronic pain, need not be a progressive, destructive force. But physicians who specialize in pain medicine consider chronic pain to represent a failure of traditional medical approaches that is characterized by repeated diagnostic studies, excessive use of medicines, prolonged use of passive physical therapy modalities, prolonged immobilization, and unwise surgical intervention. All of these approaches only perpetuate and augment the syndrome.

Nonmedical factors also may have substantial roles in chronic pain conditions. The authoritative commission on pain in 1987 noted that there are many ways to reward illness behavior and provide disincentives for recovery. From the patient's standpoint, pain can provide the rationalization for quitting an unpleasant job or provide a useful attention-getting device. Pain also may lead to expectation of financial gain through an illness-compensation system.

Chronic Pain

Effective treatment of persistent and chronic pain recognizes it as a multifaceted illness, rather than as a localized disease process. The focus of treatment is on management rather than cure. Management requires a multidisciplinary effort that is carried out at a comprehensive pain center on an inpatient or outpatient basis. The goals should be clearly defined and articulated. These include an increase in functional capacity and a decrease in dependencies on medication and medical care providers.

Pain-oriented behavior usually can be decreased. Although pain perception often is not diminished, the significance of pain to the patient can be reduced. Return to the work force is highly desirable, and this can be achieved in about one half of treated patients. A return of the work ethic in the patient with chronic pain depends on many variables, including character traits, personality, ethnic and cultural background, the presence of support systems, motivation, and satisfaction with the position held before the event that gave rise to the condition.

Effective management incorporates the three major pathways indicated below.

Rehabilitation: This includes physical rehabilitation, with mobilization, stretching, and strengthening exercises; and rehabilitation in terms of medical and psychological factors, including those that involve vocation, social relationships, and use of medications.

Behavior modification: This may include operant conditioning and relaxation therapy.

Cognitive therapy: This includes helping the patient understand and revamp thought processes aided by knowledgeable persons in medicine, psychiatry, and psychology. Patients with chronic pain must "take control" again and become responsible for their lives.

15.8 Estimating Impairment

If the patient's pain or pain-related condition is to be evaluated under the criteria of the *Guides*, by definition it must be one that is stable and unlikely to change in the future despite therapy (see Glossary, p. 315). Pain is a subjective perception. Usually no exact relationships exist among the degree of pain, extent of pathologic change, and extent of impairment.

Decreased ability to carry out daily activities may be one result of pain-related impairment. This decreased ability is *not* merely a function of verbal behavior. An individual who complains of constant pain but who has no objectively validated limitations in daily activities has *no* impairment. The proper test is not "Does this daily activity cause pain?" but rather "Can the patient perform this daily activity?"

Evaluating functional capacity (p. 305) is the process of assessing the patient's ability to carry out the activities necessary for daily living. There is no universally accepted standard, method, or instrument for evaluating functional capacity. Rather, functional capacity evaluation depends on medical experience and judgment. The process is a comprehensive, multidimensional assessment of the individual's capabilities, considering biologic, psychological, and social aspects of the individual's condition. This type of evaluation is more complex and difficult than estimating an impairment using anatomic or physiologic measures.

The validity of a functional capacity evaluation depends on the capability of the physician or the trained examiner acting under the physician's purview. The Visual Analogue Scale, a linear scale used to grade pain from 1 to 10 depending on severity, may be useful in determining pain intensity, but it must not be the primary criterion. The physician's judgment must be based on reasonable certainty. The goal should be to achieve precision, replicability, and interobserver agreement, not necessarily absolute accuracy.

Assessment Content

A comprehensive pain assessment includes clinical assessment (Section 15.7, p. 310); classification (Section 15.4, p. 305); and description of the effects of the pain on performing daily activities (functional capacity evaluation). In estimating the extent of pain-related impairment, the following criteria should be observed.

1. Acute pain is not a "permanent impairment."

2. Psychogenic pain is a mental disorder that should be evaluated according to the chapter on mental and behavioral disorders (p. 291).

3. Recurrent acute pain is likely to be classified as primary and nociceptive or neurogenic. Such pain relates clearly to well-defined diseases or pathologic entities.

4. Chronic pain (chronic pain syndrome) is likely to be classified as secondary pain. Chronic pain in the absence of objectively validated diseases or impairments, such as those that are described in the *Guides*, should be evaluated on a multidisciplinary basis by physicians with a special interest and background in pain medicine and considering the effects of the pain on the patient's ability to carry out daily activities. The Pain Intensity-Frequency Grid (Fig. 2, at right) should be used to describe the degree of impairment resulting from this disorder.

Figure 2. Pain Intensity-frequency Grid.

		Frequency			
		Intermittent	Occasional	Frequent	Constant
Intensity	Minimal				
	Slight				
	Moderate				
	Marked				

The Pain Intensity-frequency Grid (Fig. 2, above) should be interpreted according to the guidelines below. The physician should indicate in the impairment report in which category of the grid the pain impairment lies. In some instances, an impairment percent applicable to the patient's pain may be determined, if the condition causing the pain can itself be evaluated according to the criteria applicable to a particular organ system as with example 3 (p. 313).

Intensity

Minimal: The pain is annoying, but it has not been documented medically to have caused appreciable diminution in an individual's capacity to carry out daily activities. The pain does not interfere with sleep, and it requires only *occasional* use of nonnarcotic medication.

Slight: The pain is tolerated by the individual but has been documented medically to cause diminution in an individual's capacity to carry out *some* specified daily activities. The pain may interfere with sleep. Nonnarcotic medication may be consumed regularly, and occasional narcotic medication may be required.

Moderate: The pain has been documented medically to result in *extensive diminution* in an individual's capacity to carry out specific activities of daily living. The pain may be tolerable, but it interferes with sleep. It frequently requires use of narcotic medication, or it may require invasive procedures. Recreation and socialization are severely limited.

Marked: The pain precludes carrying out *most* activities of daily living. Sleep is disrupted. Recreation and socialization are impossible. Narcotic medication or invasive procedures are required and may not result in complete pain control.

Frequency

Intermittent: The pain has been documented medically to occur less than one fourth of the time when the individual is awake.

Occasional: The pain has been documented medically to occur between one fourth and one half of the time when the individual is awake.

Frequent: The pain has been documented medically to occur between one half and three fourths of the time when the individual is awake.

Constant: The pain has been documented medically to occur between three fourths and all of the time when the individual is awake.

15.9 Headache

Head, neck, and facial pain disorders, in this section referred to as headache disorders, possess some features that distinguish them from other painful disorders. Generally, however, these common disorders may be considered in terms of the same model.

The *primary headache disorders* include migraine, cluster headache, and tension-type headache. The *secondary headache disorders* are those that are associated with a variety of organic causes and with an identifiable, distinct pathologic process, of which head pain is a symptom. More than 300 organic disorders are capable of producing secondary headaches. However, more than 90% of headaches requiring medical attention are the result of one or more of the primary headache disorders.

Headache may present either in an intermittent, recurring fashion or in a persistent, constant form. Though headaches such as migraine are generally intermittent and periodic, they may evolve or transform to a state of constancy. Similarly, headaches secondary to organic processes may begin intermittently and then evolve to a more constant form.

Pathogenesis

Whereas muscular and vascular disturbance have been considered in the past to be the fundamental physiologic alterations causing primary headache disorders, current concepts of headache pathogenesis hold that these disorders arise from disturbances within the central nervous system. Supporting this neurogenic concept of migraine is the frequent presence of premonitory symptoms suggesting hypothalmic dysfunction; the presence of focal neurologic disturbances that cannot be explained solely by cerebral blood flow alterations; the accompanying features that include autonomic and systemic dysfunction; evidence concerning alteration of serotonin function; encephalographic alterations indicating neuronal disturbances during attacks; and the presence of inflammation within the trigeminal nerve vascular system that is induced by nervous system alterations.

Other evidence of this concept is that the primary headache disorders often improve with the use of pharmaceuticals and other therapeutic approaches that influence serotonin function independent of direct vascular or muscular effects.

Migraine

Migraine embodies an increasing variety of headache presentations, which range from typical, characteristic, periodic attacks to a daily persistent form. There is growing support for a concept suggesting that migraine represents a broad clinical spectrum. At one extreme are patients with an occasional intermittent migraine with aura, and at the other extreme are those with daily persistent pain similar to the traditional types of chronic tension-type headache.

Migraine may be defined as a complex neurophysiologic disorder characterized by episodic and progressive attacks of head pain with numerous neurologic, autonomic, systemic, and psychophysiologic disturbances. There is increasing recognition of migraine's capacity to transform or evolve from intermittent attacks to daily or almost daily head pain. This variant form most recently has been termed transformational migraine, progressive migraine, or pernicious migraine. Migraine is considered to be inherited as an autosomal dominant trait with incomplete penetrance.

Subclassifications of migraine reflect specific migraine syndromes and include ophthalmoplegic migraine, hemiplegic migraine, aphasic migraine, and retinal migraine. Major and sometimes prolonged disturbances of brain-stem function may occur with migraine, including dizziness with or without vertigo and disequilibrium; nausea, vomiting, diarrhea, and anorexia; loss of consciousness; sudden mood change; and dramatic disturbances, such as stupor, confusion, and ataxia.

Tension-type Headache

Many clinicians experienced with headache believe that tension-type headache represents a variant form of migraine. There is a significant overlap between the symptoms of tension-type headache and those of migraine, and a large number of patients with tension-type headache suffer superimposed periodic migraine.

Cluster Headache
Cluster headache is a devastating and painful affliction in which attacks of one-half hour to 1½ hours occur daily for weeks, months, or years at a time. Up to eight or more attacks may occur per day. The term "cluster headache" was originally used to describe the clustering or sequence of bouts of attacks in which the headache cycle occurred for a period of time, usually several months, and then remitted for a quiescent period referred to as the interim. A chronic form of cluster headache without an interim now is recognized.

Primary Headache Frequency Patterns
Three patterns of primary headache occur, as shown below, and these are independent of the specific diagnosis. Complex or mixed forms of headache may occur, in which varying intensities and frequencies of one form occur with superimposed features of another form.

1. Minimal, slight, moderate, and marked headache may occur in intermittent, occasional, frequent, or constant forms.

2. Cycles or episodes of the above may occur, lasting moments, hours, days, weeks, months, or years, which are followed by periods of complete or almost complete remission.

3. Constant and persistent pain of varying intensity may last years, decades, or a lifetime.

Chronic Pain
Chronic, intractable pain embodies a condition in which a malevolent and destructive influence occurs. Headache that evolves into chronic pain is a self-sustaining process and does not reflect an underlying acute somatic injury. Rather, the headache is a disorder in its own right and is chronic, long-lived, and progressive. The patient's pain perception is markedly enhanced, the pain behavior becomes maladaptive and counterproductive, and both behavior and perception are greatly disproportional to any identifiable underlying noxious stimulation.

Clinical Features Distinguishing Headache Illnesses from Other Painful Disorders
Many of the headache illnesses are accompanied by dramatic, often strokelike clinical phenomena that can be even more disruptive and disabling than the pain experience itself. Moreover, functioning in patients with headache syndromes often is compromised by the effects of excessively used sedative medications prescribed or taken to treat the headache.

Many headache symptoms persist beyond the period of pain itself or can occur hours or days in advance of an attack. After the acute episode, a period of mental dullness, fatigue, and somnolence occurs, which is similar to that seen in the postictal phase of an epileptic seizure.

Diagnostic and Therapeutic Considerations
Because the presence or suspected presence of a primary headache disorder does not exclude the presence of a separate, comorbid, distinct pathologic process that might be responsible for secondary headache, broad and careful diagnostic measures are required both initially and periodically. Moreover, in the presence of an intense pharmacotherapeutic program, the monitoring of blood levels of the pharmaceutical agent, organ responses, and cardiac status is required for safety. Screening studies are necessary to determine the safety of drug administration, and other measures may be required.

Determining Impairment
Impairment related to headache pain should be estimated according to the procedures described in Section 15.8 (p. 309) for evaluating other types of pain. It is important to remember that assessing *permanent* impairment refers to assessing a condition that is stable and unlikely to change in future months despite medical or surgical therapy. The vast majority of patients with headache will not have permanent impairments.

Examples of Evaluating Pain

Example 1: A 34-year-old man injured his back while lifting a heavy object; this injury was an L4 to L5 disk herniation causing radiculopathy. He had an operation for removal of the disk and had good pain relief for 3 weeks. He then developed constant low-back pain and burning pain radiating down the right leg to the toes. During the succeeding 2 years, he was under the care of a neurosurgeon, an orthopedic surgeon, and a neurologist, and the diagnoses of arachnoiditis and neuritis were made.

The man required the use of narcotics, anti-inflammatory drugs, and antidepressants, but these did not relieve his pain. He could not participate in recreational activities or sit long enough to drive, and he required assistance to put on his shoes and socks.

Diagnosis: Arachnoiditis; neuritis; disk herniation at L4 to L5.

Impairment: 10% whole-person impairment from a herniated disk, DRE lumbosacral category III (p. 110); pain impairment due to frequent pain of moderate intensity.

Comment: The man's pain, which followed the primary insult and a surgical procedure, and his inability to perform some daily living activities established the presence of chronic pain syndrome. Any peripheral nerve impairment other than that due to the L4 to L5 lesion should be determined by referring to criteria in Section 3.1 or 3.2 of Chapter 3 (pp. 15 and 75), and the whole-person impairment percent should be *combined* with the spine impairment percent (Combined Values Chart, p. 322).

Example 2: A 47-year-old woman bumped the dorsum of her right hand as she was stocking shelves at work. Within 24 hours, the hand became swollen and painful. Roentgenograms disclosed no fracture. Within a week of the injury, the hand had become red, swollen, and hot, and she was unable to tolerate stimulation of any kind of the affected part. A physician made the diagnosis of reflex sympathetic dystrophy. The patient underwent a series of stellate ganglion blocks, which did not provide lasting relief.

A year after the injury, the patient had a surgical sympathectomy, which did not relieve the pain. An examination showed that the woman held her right hand in a protected fashion guarded by the left hand. The history indicated that she could not perform domestic tasks and that she had to rely on family members to assist with dressing, hygiene, and most daily activities. She also no longer took part in social activities. She described her pain as being intense and constant and would not allow anyone to touch the affected limb.

Diagnosis: Reflex sympathetic dystrophy; impairment due to constant, marked pain.

Impairment: Impairment due to constant, marked pain.

Comment: The patient became totally focused on her pain, her life was consumed by the pain, and she was incapable of performing most daily activities.

An impairment percent related to the causalgia may be determined according to criteria in Chapter 3, Section 3.1 (p. 15) for impairment of hand and wrist motion and sensation.

Example 3: A 55-year-old executive developed trigeminal neuralgia affecting the maxillary and mandibular branches of the trigeminal nerve. The pain initially diminished with carbamazepine therapy, but after 2 years it recurred. It then became persistent, despite large doses of carbamazepine combined with baclofen and clonazepam and the adjunctive use of acupuncture. Chewing, swallowing, and toothbrushing initiated paroxysms of pain. If the man spoke cautiously, he could avoid pain most of the time. He could not go to work because of the attacks. He was unwilling to submit to surgical intervention.

Diagnosis: Trigeminal neuralgia.

Impairment: Impairment due to intermittent pain of marked severity.

Comment: The man's attacks were infrequent but severe, even though they lasted only a few minutes. The patient believed the attacks prevented his working, which required that he almost continuously converse in person or by telephone.

In this instance, a whole-person impairment percent may be derived by referring to the impairment criteria for cranial nerve V (Chapter 4, p. 139).

References

1. American Psychiatric Association, Committee on Nomenclature and Statistics. *Diagnostic and Statistical Manual of Mental Disorders, Revised Third Edition.* Washington, DC: American Psychiatric Association; 1987.

2. Aronoff GM, ed. *Evaluation and Treatment of Chronic Pain.* Baltimore, Md: Urban & Schwarzenberg; 1985.

3. Barber J, Adrian C, eds. *Psychological Approaches to the Management of Pain.* New York, NY: Brunner-Mazel Inc; 1982.

4. Berde CB. Psychosocial aspects of chronic pain and the elderly. *Int Assoc Stud Pain Newslett.* January-February 1992:2-4.

5. Cavalieri F, Salaffi F, Ferracioli GF. Relationship between physical impairment, psychological variables and pain in rheumatoid disability: an analysis of their relative impact. *J Clin Exp Rheumatol.* 1991;9:47-50.

6. Cousins MJ, Phillips GD, eds. *Acute Pain Management.* New York, NY: Churchill Livingstone; 1986.

7. Gildenberg PL, DeVaul RA, eds. *The Chronic Pain Patient: Evaluation and Management.* Basel, Switzerland: S Karger AG; 1985.

8. Guyer DW, Wiltse LL, Eskay ML, Guyer BH. The long range prognosis of arachnoiditis. *Spine.* 1989;14:1332-1341.

9. Helme RD, Katz B, Gibson S, Corvan T. Can psychometric tools be used to analyze pain in a geriatric population? *Clin Exp Neurol.* 1989;26:113-117.

10. Millard RW. The functional assessment screening questionnaire: application for evaluating pain-related disability. *Arch Phys Med Rehabil.* 1989;70:303-307.

11. Murdrick NR. Predictors of disability among mid-life men and women: difference by severity of impairment. *J Community Health.* 1988;13:70-84.

12. Osterweis M, Kleinman A, Mechanic D, eds. *Pain and Disability: Clinical Behavioral and Public Policy Perspectives. Report of the Institute of Medicine Committee on Pain, Disability and Chronic Illness Behavior.* Washington, DC: National Academy Press; 1987.

13. Reesor KA, Craig KD. Medically incongruent chronic back pain: physical limitations, suffering and ineffective coping. *Pain.* 1988;32:35-45.

14. *Report of the Commission on the Evaluation of Pain, US Department of Health and Human Services, Social Security Administration (SSA) Office of Disability.* Washington, DC: Social Security Administration; March 1987. Publication 64-031.

15. Rigby AS, Rudolfer SM, Badley EM, Brayshaw NC. The relationship between impairment and disability in arthritis: an application of the theory of generalized linear models. *Int Disabil Stud.* 1989;11:84-88.

16. Rosen JC, Grubman JA, Bevins T, Frymoyer JW. Musculoskeletal status and disability of MMPI profile sub-groups among patients with low back pain. *Health Psychol.* 1987;6:581-598.

17. Ryley JF, Ahern DK, Follick MJ. Chronic pain and functional impairment: assessing beliefs about their relationship. *Arch Phys Med Rehabil.* 1988;69:579-582.

18. Spektor S. Chronic pain and pain-related disabilities. *J Disabil.* 1990;1:98-102.

19. States JD, Viano DC. Injury impairment and disability scales to assess the permanent consequences of trauma. *Accident Anal Prev.* 1990;22:151-160.

20. Turk DC, Rudy TE, Stieg RL. The disability determination dilemma: toward a multi-axial solution. *Pain.* 1988;34:217-229.

21. Vasudevan SV. Impairment, disability and functional capacity assessment. In: Turk DC, Melzack R, eds. *Handbook of Pain Assessment.* New York, NY: Guilford Press; 1992.

22. Vasudevan SV. The relationship between pain and disability: an overview of the problem. *J Disabil.* 1991;2:44-53.

23. Vasudevan SV, Monsein M. Evaluation of function and disability in the patient with chronic pain. In: Raj PP, ed. *Practical Management of Pain.* 2nd ed. St Louis, Mo: Mosby-Year Book Inc; 1992.

24. Von Korff M, Dworkin SF, Le Resche I. Graded chronic pain status: an epidemiological evaluation. *Pain.* 1990;40:279-291.

25. Waddell G, Plowsky I, Bond MR. Clinical assessment and interpretation of abnormal illness behavior in low back pain. *Pain.* 1989;31:41-53.

Glossary

Definitions related to impairment assume importance, because terms associated with impairment evaluations may have special meanings in a legal context beyond their usual meanings in medical communications. This glossary provides a guide to the terms that should be used in reporting, analyzing, understanding, and discussing impairment evaluations and estimates carried out according to *Guides* criteria. It also defines important terms in the fields of disability, workers' compensation, and short- and long-term disability and considers Social Security System disability determinations and the Americans with Disabilities Act of 1992.

Terms Used in Assessments According to *Guides*

1. Impairment: Impairment is the loss, loss of use, or derangement of any body part, system, or function.

Permanent impairment is impairment that has become static or well stabilized with or without medical treatment and is not likely to remit despite medical treatment.

A permanent impairment is considered to be unlikely to change substantially and by more than 3% in the next year with or without medical treatment. If an impairment is not *permanent,* it is inappropriate to characterize it as such and evaluate it according to *Guides* criteria.

Evaluation of permanent impairment is acquisition and analysis of information, including clinical evaluation, that is carried out according to Chapters 1 and 2 and other applicable parts of the *Guides.*

Impairment rating consists of analyzing data accumulated in the course of an impairment evaluation and comparing those data with *Guides* criteria to estimate the extent of the impairment. Impairment ratings prepared according to *Guides* criteria are *estimates* of impairment.

Impairment reporting is explaining the information acquired in the course of evaluating, analyzing, and estimating the extent of an impairment. An impairment report should be prepared according to the procedures described in Chapter 2 and other applicable parts of the *Guides.*

2. Apportionment: This is an estimate of the degree to which each of various occupational or nonoccupational factors may have caused or contributed to a particular impairment. For each alleged factor, two criteria must be met:

a. The alleged factor *could have caused* or contributed to the impairment, which is a medical determination (see "causation," p. 316).

b. In the case in question, the factor *did cause* or contribute to the impairment, which usually is a nonmedical determination. The physician's analysis and explanation of causation is significant.

3. Clinical Evaluation: This is the collection of data by a physician or other health care professional for the purposes of assessing the health status of an individual, formulating a medical management plan, and implementing a course of treatment. The data include information obtained by history; findings obtained from a physical examination; and findings from laboratory and other types of tests and diagnostic procedures, including roentgenograms, electrocardiograms, blood tests and chemistry studies, and tests of excreta and body fluids.

4. Disfigurement: This is an altered or abnormal color, shape, or structure of a visible body part. Disfigurement may be the result of an injury or disease, or it may accompany a recurring or chronic disease or disorder of function. Disfigurement may produce social rejection, impairment of self-image with self-imposed isolation, alteration of life-style, or other adverse changes.

5. Intensity and Frequency: The intensity and frequency of an individual's symptoms or signs may be graded as shown below.

Intensity

a. *Minimal:* The symptoms or signs are annoying but have not been documented medically to cause appreciable diminution in an individual's capacity to carry out daily activities.

b. *Slight:* The symptoms or signs are tolerated by the individual and have been documented medically to cause *some* diminution in an individual's capacity to carry out activities of daily living.

c. *Moderate:* The symptoms or signs have been documented medically to cause *serious* diminution in an individual's capacity to carry out activities of daily living.

d. *Marked:* The symptoms or signs *preclude carrying out* activities of daily living.

Frequency

a. *Intermittent:* The symptoms or signs have been documented medically to occur less than one fourth of the time when the patient is awake.

b. *Occasional:* The symptoms or signs have been documented medically to occur between one fourth and one half of the time when the patient is awake.

c. *Frequent:* The symptoms and signs have been documented medically to occur between one half and three fourths of the time when the patient is awake.

d. *Constant:* The symptoms and signs occur between three fourths and all of the time when the patient is awake.

6. Medically Documented: This means that hospital and medical office records and ancillary records, such as those involving physiotherapy and occupational therapy, collected over a period of time, reflect a medical history and medical findings that support a diagnosis meeting established medical criteria and calling for medical management that is consistent with accepted principles and practice.

To meet the above criteria, the medical records must contain entries that show an appropriately complete initial evaluation; follow-up visits at appropriate intervals describing the interval history, current findings on examination, and the individual's response to treatment; vigorous use of medication and other treatment modalities if indicated; results of timely diagnostic tests and procedures; and appropriate referral for medical specialty evaluation. The records should document behavior of both the patient and the physician reflecting appropriate concern regarding the impact of the medical condition on the patient's daily activities.

7. Daily Living Activities: An impairment estimate based on *Guides* criteria is intended, among other purposes, to be an estimate of the degree to which an individual's capacity to carry out daily activities has been diminished.

The Table (p. 317) indicates some of the activities of daily living.

Aggravation, Recurrence, Causation, Disability, Workers' Compensation, and Employability

1. Aggravation: This means that a physical, chemical, or biologic factor, which may or may not be work related, contributed to the worsening of a preexisting medical condition or infirmity in such a way that the degree of permanent impairment increased by more than 3%.

Causation means that a physical, chemical, or biologic factor contributed to the occurrence of a medical condition. To decide that a factor alleged to have caused or contributed to the occurrence or worsening of a medical condition has, in fact, done so, it is necessary to verify both of the following.

a. The alleged factor *could have caused* or contributed to worsening of the impairment, which is a medical determination.

b. The alleged factor *did cause* or contribute to worsening of the impairment, which is a nonmedical determination.

In many benefit systems, causation and aggravation must be verified before awards are made. In contrast to traumatic injuries, which often can be

Table. Activities of Daily Living, with Examples.

Activity	Example
Self-care, personal hygiene	Bathing, grooming, dressing, eating, eliminating
Communication	Hearing, speaking, reading, writing, using keyboard
Physical activity	*Intrinsic:* Standing, sitting, reclining, walking, stooping, squatting, kneeling, reaching, bending, twisting, leaning
	Functional: Carrying, lifting, pushing, pulling, climbing, exercising
Sensory function	Hearing, seeing, tactile feeling, tasting, smelling
Hand functions	Grasping, holding, pinching, percussive movements, sensory discrimination
Travel	Riding, driving, traveling by airplane, train, or car
Sexual function	Participating in desired sexual activity
Sleep	Having a restful sleep pattern
Social and recreational activities	Participating in individual or group activities, sports, hobbies

related to an event that occurred at a particular time and place, the role of occupational or environmental factors in causing or aggravating disorders of the various body systems is difficult to document.

Documentation of "aggravation" or "causation" will depend in large measure on the acquisition, review, and analysis of existing office and hospital records dating from the onset of the condition and including the initial evaluation for the condition; the results of tests or diagnostic procedures showing when and how the individual's health was affected by an alleged physical, chemical, or biologic factor; and the results of occupational or environmental surveys, tests, or analyses. These include the following.

a. Records of medical office or hospital visits that were specifically attributable to the injury or disease caused by alleged exposure to one or more factors and for which the individual was treated.

b. Medical office or hospital records that show the individual suffered or is likely to suffer injury or harm as a result of the exposure.

c. Reports of results of tests or diagnostic procedures showing specific sensitivity to a factor to which the individual was exposed.

d. Reports of the results of an environmental survey or analysis showing the nature and intensity of factors to which the individual was exposed.

e. Reports of the results of an analysis defining the minimal levels of exposure to a factor likely to cause injury or harm to the individual and discussion of the medical basis for the conclusions.

f. Reports of the results of an analysis that indicates the individual was exposed in some place to factors to which he or she is sensitive, at intensities or durations equal to or greater than those to which the individual would have been exposed elsewhere, except that a physician or other responsible person restricted the exposure.

g. Records containing an explanation of the medical basis for any conclusion that the individual experienced, or is likely to experience, progression or worsening of the condition as a result of continued exposure to physical, chemical, or biologic factors.

Aggravation may involve both occupational and nonoccupational disorders in the following ways.

a. An occupational disorder may be aggravated by a supervening nonoccupational disorder.

b. An occupational disorder may be aggravated by a supervening occupational condition arising out of and in the course of employment by the same employer.

c. An occupational disorder may be aggravated by a supervening industrial condition arising out of and in the course of employment by a different employer.

d. An occupational disorder may be aggravated by a preexisting nonoccupational condition.

e. An occupational disorder may aggravate a preexisting nonoccupational condition.

2. Recurrence: A recurrence requires no identifiable incident as a trigger to the medical condition in question; rather, the patient has a resumption of symptoms or signs that can be related to the previously existing medical condition or injury.

3. New Injury: With a new injury, an identifiable new incident must be shown to have caused the injury. If it is thought that a preceding factor or situation, such as one related to an illness or occupation, might have had a role in the injury's development, then the causation must be established as described above.

4. Disability: Disability is a decrease in, or the loss or absence of, the capacity of an individual to meet personal, social, or occupational demands, or to meet statutory or regulatory requirements.

Permanent disability occurs when the degree of capacity becomes static or well stabilized and is not likely to increase despite continuing use of medical or rehabilitative measures. Disability may be caused by medical impairment or by nonmedical factors.

Evaluation or rating of disability is a nonmedical assessment of the degree to which an individual does or does not have the capacity to meet personal, social, occupational, or other demands, or to meet statutory or regulatory requirements.

5. Illness, Disease: An illness may be considered to be the summation of the physical, mental, and other kinds of factors that are involved in an individual's less than optimal health status. A disease may be considered to be the specific pathophysiologic processes involved, which give rise to the individual's signs and symptoms and their progression.[1]

6. Employability: This is the capacity of an individual to meet the demands of a job and the conditions of employment associated with that job as defined by an employer, with or without accommodation.

7. Employability Determination: This is an assessment by management of the individual's capacity, with or without accommodation, to meet the demands of a job and the conditions of employment. The management carries out an assessment of performance capability to estimate the likelihood of performance failure and the likelihood of incurring liability in case of human failure. If either likelihood is too great, then the employer may not consider the individual employable in the job.

8. Medical Determination Related to Employability: This is the process of evaluating the relationship of an individual's health to the demands of a specific job as described by the employer, such as demands for performance, reliability, integrity, endurance, or prolonged service. The physician must ensure that the medical evaluation is complete and detailed enough to draw valid conclusions with respect to the individual's capability of meeting the job's demands and carrying out essential job functions.

The physician's tasks are to (1) identify impairments that could affect performance and determine whether or not the impairments are permanent; and (2) identify impairments that could lead to sudden or gradual incapacitation, further impairment, injury, transmission of a communicable disease, or other adverse occurrence.

In estimating the risk factors, the physician should indicate whether or not the individual represents a greater risk to the employer than someone without the same medical condition and should indicate the limits of the physician's ability to predict the likelihood of an untoward occurrence.

9. Risk, Hazard: A *risk* represents the probability of an adverse event; a risk must be weighed together with the consequences of the adverse event. An individual's activities or characteristics, and biologic, physical, or chemical factors, may increase the risk of morbidity or mortality.

A *hazard* is a potential source of danger; to a woman contemplating crossing the Atlantic Ocean in a rowboat, the Atlantic presents a serious hazard. Excessive numbers of coliform bacteria or *Shigella dysenteriae* in the public water supply present a hazard to a city.

10. Possibility, Probability: These are terms that refer to the likelihood or chance that an injury or illness was caused or aggravated by a particular factor. "Possibility" sometimes is used to imply a likelihood of less than 50%; "probability" sometimes is used to imply a likelihood of greater than 50%.

Social Security Disability Determinations

Although the Social Security system predated the first *Guides* edition and is not based on the *Guides*, a description of the system is included here to compare and contrast the ways in which medical information is used under each approach. The Social Security Administration (SSA) has national responsibility under Public Law 74-271 for the administration of both the Social Security disability insurance program (title II) and the supplemental security income (SSI) program (title XVI). Every person who pays into Social Security contributes to the Social Security Disability Trust Fund.

The title II program provides cash benefits to disabled workers and their dependents who have contributed to the trust fund through the FICA tax on their earnings. A person qualifies under the title II program because of financial need. The title XVI program provides for a minimum income for the needy, aged, blind, and disabled. Under that program, financial need is indicated by limitation of income and resources to a level that is equal to or less than an amount specified in the law.

Definitions and Terms

Under the title II and title XVI programs, the definitions of disability are essentially the same. The law defines disability as "the inability to engage in any substantial gainful activity by reason of any medically determinable physical or mental impairment that can be expected to result in death or has lasted or can be expected to last for a continuous period of not less than 12 months (Section 223 [d] [1] [A]). The law may apply to infants and children as well as adults. In terms of the law, a person is either disabled or not disabled.

To meet the definition of disability, an individual's impairment or combination of impairments must be of such severity that he or she not only is unable to do the work previously done, but also cannot perform any other kind of substantial gainful work considering the individual's age, education, and work experience (Section 223 [d] [2] [A]). Substantial gainful work means any work that involves significant and productive physical or mental activities and is performed for pay or profit to a specified level, currently $500 for disabled persons and $850 for blind persons.

The term "medically determinable physical or mental impairment" means that the impairment may be either physical or mental but it must be an impairment that can be demonstrated by the symptoms, signs, and laboratory findings reported by acceptable medical sources, which include licensed physicians.

Medical Basis of Disability

To qualify for payments under either the title II or the title XVI program, an individual must have a "medically determinable" impairment. This is defined as an impairment that has demonstrable anatomic, physiologic, or psychological abnormalities. Abnormalities that manifest themselves only as symptoms do not qualify.

Signs are defined as anatomic, physiologic, or psychological abnormalities that can be observed by using medically acceptable techniques. Laboratory findings are manifestations of anatomic, physiologic, or psychological phenomena that are demonstrable by replacing or extending the perceptiveness of the observer's senses; they include chemical, electrophysiologic, roentgenographic, and psychological tests.

Listing of Impairments

Under the Social Security System, there is a sequence in evaluating disability claims that reflects the requirements of the law and regulations. This step-by-step procedure is known as the "sequential evaluation process." Initial steps in the process include a determination as to whether the claimant's impairments meet or equal any impairment in the Listing of Impairments.

The Listing of Impairments is organized by body system as a set of medical evaluation criteria. For each body system, the medical evaluation criteria include key concepts used in evaluating impairments and a description of the type of medical evidence needed. The Listing is divided into two parts. Part A contains medical criteria that apply to persons 18 years old and older. These criteria also may be applied to impairments of persons less than 18 years old, if the disease process has a similar effect on adults and younger persons. Part B contains medical criteria that apply only to evaluating the impairments of persons under age 18 years.

The medical evaluation criteria in the Listing describe impairments in terms of specific signs, symptoms, and laboratory findings that are presumed to be severe enough to keep an individual from working for a year or longer or, in the case of a child, performing age-appropriate activities. The Listing describes more than 100 common diseases and disorders, which are so serious or life-threatening that if the claimant meets one of them and is not engaging in substantial gainful activity, he or she is deemed to be disabled.

If an individual has an impairment that does not meet the specific criteria described in the Listing but has an impairment equal in severity to a listed impairment, and is not engaging in substantial gainful activity, he or she is presumed to meet the definition of disability. Under the SSA system, no claimant is denied a determination of disability solely on the basis of not meeting or equaling the criteria of the Listing.

Collection of Medical Evidence

For a medical report to furnish the SSA with sufficient medical evidence, it should include (1) medical history; (2) clinical findings, such as results of a physical or mental status examination; (3) laboratory findings; (4) diagnosis based on signs and symptoms; (5) the treatment prescribed, with response and prognosis; and (6) a medical source statement based on the source's own findings.

The medical evidence, including clinical and laboratory findings, should be complete and detailed enough to allow SSA personnel to make the disability determination. In addition, the report should enable them to determine the nature and limiting effects of the impairment(s), its probable duration, and the claimant's remaining capacity to engage in work-related physical or mental activities.

The medical source statement, noted above, details what the claimant can do despite his or her impairment(s). It should describe such work-related activities as sitting, walking, lifting, carrying, hearing, speaking, and traveling. In cases involving mental impairments, the SSA must have a statement about the claimant's capacity for understanding and memory; sustained concentration and persistence; social interaction; and adaptation.

Under the Social Security Act, disability is defined strictly in economic terms and ability to work, while in the *Guides*, disability is defined in terms of an individual's capacity to meet personal, social, recreational, occupational, and other demands.

The Americans with Disabilities Act

This section provides background on the Americans with Disabilities Act (ADA) and compares and contrasts the concepts of the *Guides* with those of the Act. The provisions of the ADA governing employment-related decisions (title I) became effective on July 26, 1992, for private-sector organizations that employ 25 or more employees. Because the intent of the ADA is to compel organizations to employ qualified individuals with "disabilities," it is likely that physicians will experience an increasing demand for giving guidance to employers with respect to an individual's "disability" status. In addition, there will be questions regarding performance capability, acceptability of risk to oneself or others, the need for accommodation, and the type of accommodation that may be warranted. It is important to recognize that *none* of these is a medical issue.

The following definitions are based on the concepts of *EEOC Title I Regulations and Interpretive Appendix* (29 CFR 1630).

1. Accommodation means modification of a job or workplace that enables a "disabled" employee to meet the same job demands and conditions of employment required of any other employee in the same, or a similar, job. Accommodation need be considered only with respect to the essential functions of a job. *Reasonable accommodation* means accommodation that does not result in undue cost or hardship to the employer.

2. Disability means a physical or mental impairment that substantially limits one or more of the major life activities of the individual; or a record of such an impairment; or being regarded as having such an impairment.

3. Essential functions of a job means the fundamental duties of the employment position that the disabled individual seeks or holds. Essential functions may be understood to be those elements of a job such that failure in one or more of the elements would be cause for removal from the job. "Essential functions" do not include marginal functions.

4. Major life activities means such functions as caring for oneself, performing manual tasks, walking, seeing, hearing, speaking, breathing, learning, and working. A list of daily activities appears earlier in the Glossary (Table, p. 317).

5. Physical or mental impairment means the following:

a. Any physiologic disorder or condition, cosmetic disfigurement, or anatomic loss affecting one or more of the following body systems: neurologic, musculoskeletal, special sense organs, respiratory (including speech organs), cardiovascular, reproductive, digestive, genitourinary, hemic and lymphatic, skin, and endocrine systems; or

b. Any mental or psychological disorder, such as mental retardation, organic brain syndrome, emotional or mental illness, and specific learning disabilities.

6. Substantially limits means the following:

a. The person is unable to perform a major life activity that the average person in the general population can perform; or

b. The person is significantly restricted as to the conditions, manner, or duration under which he or she can perform a particular major life activity, compared to the conditions, manner, or duration under which the average person can perform the same activity.

The ADA uses the term "disability," and its use of the concept is similar to the concept of "impairment" used in the *Guides*. It is important to note, however, that under the ADA, identification of an individual with a "disability" does not depend on the results of a *medical* evaluation. An individual may be identified as having a disability if there is a record of an impairment that has substantially limited one or more major life activities or, of greater concern, if the individual *is regarded as having* a disability.

In carrying out and reporting the results of an impairment evaluation, it is essential that the physician distinguish carefully between an impairment that is documented in accordance with *Guides* criteria and a presumed impairment that is based on nonmedical factors. Clearly, a question exists as to whether or not an impairment based on *Guides* criteria automatically will constitute a "record" of an ADA-covered disability or signify that the individual is "regarded" as having such a disability.

"Accommodation" is *not* a medical matter. Accommodation is the result of an employer's decision regarding modifications of a job or workplace that are "reasonable" with respect to the employer's cost and the degree of hardship imposed. The physician may be able to help an employer understand the relationships between a medical impairment, the demands made of an individual in the workplace, and the individual's capabilities. The physician also can help the employer explore the need for accommodation. But it is not appropriate for the physician to recommend a specific accommodation.

Once the employer determines it is appropriate to accommodate an individual's disability and redefines the job or workplace, the physician's role is to answer the following question: "Is there a medical reason to believe it is not feasible or appropriate to assign these [specified] tasks and duties to this person under these [specified] working conditions?"

Reference

1. Luck JV Jr, Florence DW. A brief history and comparative analysis of disability systems and impairment rating guides. *Orthoped Clin North Am.* 1988;19:839-844.

Combined Values Chart

The values are deriv.d from the formula A+B (1–A)=*combined* value of A and B, where A and B are the decimal equivalents of the impairment ratings. In the chart all values are expressed as percents. To *combine* any two impairment values, locate the larger of the values on the side of the chart and read along that row until you come to the column indicated by the smaller value at the bottom of the chart. At the intersection of the row and the column is the combined value.

For example, to combine 35% and 20% read down the side of the chart until you come to the larger value, 35%. Then read across the 35% row until you come to the column indicated by 20% at the bottom of the chart. At the intersection of the row and column is the number 48. Therefore, 35% *combined* with 20% is 48%. Due to the construction of this chart, the larger impairment value must be identified at the side of the chart.

If three or more impairment values are to be combined, select any two and find their combined value as above. Then use that value and the third value to locate the combined value of all. This process can be repeated indefinitely, the final value in each instance being the combination of all the previous values. In each step of this process the larger impairment value must be identified at the side of the chart.

Note: If impairments from two or more organ systems are to be *combined* to express a whole-person impairment, each must first be expressed as a whole-person impairment percent.

	1	**2**	**3**	**4**	**5**	**6**	**7**	**8**	**9**	**10**	**11**	**12**	**13**	**14**	**15**	**16**	**17**	**18**	**19**	**20**	**21**	**22**	**23**	**24**	**25**	**26**	**27**	**28**	**29**	**30**	**31**	**32**	**33**	**34**	**35**	**36**	**37**	**38**	**39**	**40**	**41**	**42**	**43**	**44**	**45**	**46**	**47**	**48**	**49**	**50**
1	2																																																	
2	3	4																																																
3	4	5	6																																															
4	5	6	7	8																																														
5	6	7	8	9	10																																													
6	7	8	9	10	11	12																																												
7	8	9	10	11	12	13	14																																											
8	9	10	11	12	13	14	14	15																																										
9	10	11	12	13	14	14	15	16	17																																									
10	11	12	13	14	15	15	16	17	18	19																																								
11	12	13	14	15	15	16	17	18	19	20	21																																							
12	13	14	15	16	16	17	18	19	20	21	22	23																																						
13	14	15	16	16	17	18	19	20	21	22	23	23	24																																					
14	15	16	17	17	18	19	20	21	22	23	23	24	25	26																																				
15	16	17	18	18	19	20	21	22	23	24	24	25	26	27	28																																			
16	17	18	19	19	20	21	22	23	24	24	25	26	27	28	29	29																																		
17	18	19	19	20	21	22	23	24	24	25	26	27	28	29	29	30	31																																	
18	19	20	20	21	22	23	24	25	25	26	27	28	29	29	30	31	32	33																																
19	20	21	21	22	23	24	25	25	26	27	28	29	30	30	31	32	33	34	34																															
20	21	22	22	23	24	25	26	26	27	28	29	30	30	31	32	33	34	34	35	36																														
21	22	23	23	24	25	26	27	27	28	29	30	30	31	32	33	34	34	35	36	37	38																													
22	23	24	24	25	26	27	27	28	29	30	31	31	32	33	34	34	35	36	37	38	38	39																												
23	24	25	25	26	27	28	28	29	30	31	31	32	33	34	35	35	36	37	38	38	39	40	41																											
24	25	26	26	27	28	29	29	30	31	32	32	33	34	35	35	36	37	38	38	39	40	41	41	42																										
25	26	27	27	28	29	30	30	31	32	33	33	34	35	36	36	37	38	39	39	40	41	42	42	43	44																									
26	27	27	28	29	30	30	31	32	33	33	34	35	36	36	37	38	39	39	40	41	42	42	43	44	45	45																								
27	28	28	29	30	31	31	32	33	34	34	35	36	36	37	38	39	39	40	41	42	42	43	44	45	45	46	47																							
28	29	29	30	31	32	32	33	34	34	35	36	37	37	38	39	40	40	41	42	42	43	44	45	45	46	47	47	48																						
29	30	30	31	32	33	33	34	35	35	36	37	38	38	39	40	40	41	42	42	43	44	45	45	46	47	47	48	49	50																					
30	31	31	32	33	34	34	35	36	36	37	38	38	39	40	41	41	42	43	43	44	45	45	46	47	48	48	49	50	50	51																				
31	32	32	33	34	34	35	36	37	37	38	39	39	40	41	41	42	43	43	44	45	45	46	47	48	48	49	50	50	51	52	52																			
32	33	33	34	35	35	36	37	37	38	39	39	40	41	42	42	43	44	44	45	46	46	47	48	48	49	50	50	51	52	52	53	54																		
33	34	34	35	36	36	37	38	38	39	40	40	41	42	42	43	44	44	45	46	46	47	48	48	49	50	50	51	52	52	53	54	54	55																	
34	35	35	36	37	37	38	39	39	40	41	41	42	43	43	44	45	45	46	47	47	48	49	49	50	51	51	52	52	53	54	54	55	56	56																
35	36	36	37	38	38	39	40	40	41	42	42	43	43	44	45	45	46	47	47	48	49	49	50	51	51	52	53	53	54	55	55	56	56	57	58															
36	37	37	38	39	39	40	40	41	42	42	43	44	44	45	46	46	47	48	48	49	49	50	51	51	52	53	53	54	55	55	56	56	57	58	58	59														
37	38	38	39	40	40	41	41	42	43	43	44	45	45	46	46	47	48	48	49	50	50	51	51	52	53	53	54	55	55	56	57	57	58	58	59	60	60													
38	39	39	40	40	41	42	42	43	44	44	45	45	46	47	47	48	49	49	50	50	51	52	52	53	54	54	55	55	56	57	57	58	58	59	60	60	61	62												
39	40	40	41	41	42	43	43	44	44	45	46	46	47	48	48	49	49	50	51	51	52	52	53	54	54	55	55	56	57	57	58	59	59	60	60	61	62	62	63											
40	41	41	42	42	43	44	44	45	45	46	47	47	48	48	49	50	50	51	51	52	53	53	54	54	55	56	56	57	57	58	59	59	60	60	61	62	62	63	63	64										
41	42	42	43	43	44	45	45	46	46	47	47	48	49	49	50	50	51	52	52	53	53	54	55	55	56	56	57	58	58	59	59	60	60	61	62	62	63	63	64	65	65									
42	43	43	44	44	45	45	46	47	47	48	48	49	50	50	51	51	52	52	53	54	54	55	55	56	57	57	58	58	59	59	60	61	61	62	62	63	63	64	65	65	66	66								
43	44	44	45	45	46	46	47	48	48	49	49	50	50	51	52	52	53	53	54	54	55	56	56	57	57	58	58	59	60	60	61	61	62	62	63	64	64	65	65	66	66	67	68							
44	45	45	46	46	47	47	48	48	49	50	50	51	51	52	52	53	54	54	55	55	56	56	57	57	58	59	59	60	60	61	61	62	62	63	64	64	65	65	66	66	67	68	68	69						
45	46	46	47	47	48	48	49	49	50	51	51	52	52	53	53	54	54	55	55	56	57	57	58	58	59	59	60	60	61	62	62	63	63	64	64	65	65	66	66	67	68	68	69	69	70					
46	47	47	48	48	49	49	50	50	51	51	52	52	53	54	54	55	55	56	56	57	57	58	58	59	60	60	61	61	62	62	63	63	64	64	65	65	66	67	67	68	68	69	69	70	70	71				
47	48	48	49	49	50	50	51	51	52	52	53	53	54	54	55	55	56	57	57	58	58	59	59	60	60	61	61	62	62	63	63	64	64	65	66	66	67	67	68	68	69	69	70	70	71	71	72			
48	49	49	50	50	51	51	52	52	53	53	54	54	55	55	56	56	57	57	58	58	59	59	60	60	61	62	62	63	63	64	64	65	65	66	66	67	67	68	68	69	69	70	70	71	71	72	72	73		
49	50	50	51	51	52	52	53	53	54	54	55	55	56	56	57	57	58	58	59	59	60	60	61	61	62	62	63	63	64	64	65	65	66	66	67	67	68	68	69	69	70	70	71	71	72	72	73	73	74	
50	51	51	52	52	53	53	54	54	55	55	56	56	57	57	58	58	59	59	60	60	61	61	62	62	63	63	64	64	65	65	66	66	67	67	68	68	69	69	70	70	71	71	72	72	73	73	74	74	75	75

Combined Values Chart (continued)

	1	2	3	4	5	6	7	8	9	10	11	12	13	14	15	16	17	18	19	20	21	22	23	24	25	26	27	28	29	30	31	32	33	34	35	36	37	38	39	40	41	42	43	44	45	46	47	48	49	50
51	51	52	52	53	53	54	54	55	55	56	56	57	57	58	58	59	59	60	60	61	61	62	62	63	63	64	64	65	65	66	66	67	67	68	68	69	69	70	70	71	71	72	72	73	73	74	74	75	75	76
52	52	53	53	54	54	55	55	56	56	57	57	58	58	59	59	60	60	61	61	62	62	63	63	64	64	64	65	65	66	66	67	67	68	68	69	69	70	70	71	71	72	72	73	73	74	74	75	75	76	76
53	53	54	54	55	55	56	56	57	57	58	58	59	59	60	60	61	61	61	62	62	63	63	64	64	65	65	66	66	67	67	68	68	69	69	69	70	70	71	71	72	72	73	73	74	74	75	75	76	76	77
54	54	55	55	56	56	57	57	58	58	59	59	60	60	60	61	61	62	62	63	63	64	64	65	65	66	66	66	67	67	68	68	69	69	70	70	71	71	71	72	72	73	73	74	74	75	75	76	76	77	77
55	55	56	56	57	57	58	58	59	59	60	60	60	61	61	62	62	63	63	64	64	64	65	65	66	66	67	67	68	68	69	69	69	70	70	71	71	72	72	73	73	73	74	74	75	75	76	76	77	77	78
56	56	57	57	58	58	59	59	60	60	60	61	61	62	62	63	63	63	64	64	65	65	66	66	67	67	67	68	68	69	69	70	70	71	71	71	72	72	73	73	74	74	74	75	75	76	76	77	77	78	78
57	57	58	58	59	59	60	60	60	61	61	62	62	63	63	63	64	64	65	65	66	66	66	67	67	68	68	69	69	69	70	70	71	71	72	72	72	73	73	74	74	75	75	75	76	76	77	77	78	78	79
58	58	59	59	60	60	61	61	61	62	62	63	63	63	64	64	65	65	66	66	66	67	67	68	68	68	69	69	70	70	71	71	71	72	72	73	73	74	74	74	75	75	76	76	76	77	77	78	78	79	79
59	59	60	60	61	61	61	62	62	63	63	64	64	64	65	65	66	66	66	67	67	68	68	68	69	69	70	70	70	71	71	72	72	73	73	73	74	74	75	75	75	76	76	77	77	77	78	78	79	79	80
60	60	61	61	62	62	62	63	63	64	64	64	65	65	66	66	66	67	67	68	68	68	69	69	70	70	70	71	71	72	72	72	73	73	74	74	74	75	75	76	76	76	77	77	78	78	78	79	79	80	80
61	61	62	62	63	63	63	64	64	65	65	65	66	66	66	67	67	68	68	68	69	69	70	70	70	71	71	72	72	72	73	73	73	74	74	75	75	75	76	76	77	77	77	78	78	79	79	79	80	80	81
62	62	63	63	64	64	64	65	65	65	66	66	67	67	67	68	68	68	69	69	70	70	70	71	71	72	72	72	73	73	73	74	74	75	75	75	76	76	76	77	77	78	78	78	79	79	79	80	80	81	81
63	63	64	64	64	65	65	66	66	66	67	67	67	68	68	69	69	69	70	70	70	71	71	72	72	72	73	73	73	74	74	74	75	75	76	76	76	77	77	77	78	78	79	79	79	80	80	80	81	81	82
64	64	65	65	65	66	66	67	67	67	68	68	68	69	69	69	70	70	70	71	71	72	72	72	73	73	73	74	74	74	75	75	76	76	76	77	77	77	78	78	78	79	79	79	80	80	81	81	81	82	82
65	65	66	66	66	67	67	67	68	68	69	69	69	70	70	70	71	71	71	72	72	72	73	73	73	74	74	74	75	75	76	76	76	77	77	77	78	78	78	79	79	79	80	80	80	81	81	81	82	82	83
66	66	67	67	67	68	68	68	69	69	69	70	70	70	71	71	71	72	72	72	73	73	73	74	74	75	75	75	76	76	76	77	77	77	78	78	78	79	79	79	80	80	80	81	81	81	82	82	82	83	83
67	67	68	68	68	69	69	69	70	70	70	71	71	71	72	72	72	73	73	73	74	74	74	75	75	75	76	76	76	77	77	77	78	78	78	79	79	79	80	80	80	81	81	81	82	82	82	83	83	83	84
68	68	69	69	69	70	70	70	71	71	71	72	72	72	72	73	73	73	74	74	74	75	75	75	76	76	76	77	77	77	78	78	78	79	79	79	80	80	80	80	81	81	81	82	82	82	83	83	83	84	84
69	69	70	70	70	71	71	71	71	72	72	72	73	73	73	74	74	74	75	75	75	76	76	76	76	77	77	77	78	78	78	79	79	79	80	80	80	80	81	81	81	82	82	82	83	83	83	84	84	84	85
70	70	71	71	71	72	72	72	72	73	73	73	74	74	74	75	75	75	75	76	76	76	77	77	77	78	78	78	78	79	79	79	80	80	80	81	81	81	81	82	82	82	83	83	83	84	84	84	84	85	85
71	71	72	72	72	72	73	73	73	74	74	74	74	75	75	75	76	76	76	77	77	77	77	78	78	78	79	79	79	79	80	80	80	81	81	81	81	82	82	82	83	83	83	83	84	84	84	85	85	85	86
72	72	73	73	73	73	74	74	74	75	75	75	75	76	76	76	76	77	77	77	78	78	78	78	79	79	79	80	80	80	80	81	81	81	82	82	82	82	83	83	83	83	84	84	84	85	85	85	85	86	86
73	73	74	74	74	74	75	75	75	75	76	76	76	77	77	77	77	78	78	78	78	79	79	79	79	80	80	80	81	81	81	81	82	82	82	82	83	83	83	84	84	84	84	85	85	85	85	86	86	86	87
74	74	75	75	75	75	76	76	76	76	77	77	77	77	78	78	78	78	79	79	79	79	80	80	80	81	81	81	81	82	82	82	82	83	83	83	83	84	84	84	84	85	85	85	85	86	86	86	86	87	87
75	75	76	76	76	76	77	77	77	77	78	78	78	78	79	79	79	79	80	80	80	80	81	81	81	81	82	82	82	82	83	83	83	83	84	84	84	84	85	85	85	85	86	86	86	86	87	87	87	87	88
76	76	76	77	77	77	77	78	78	78	78	79	79	79	79	80	80	80	80	81	81	81	81	82	82	82	82	82	83	83	83	83	84	84	84	84	85	85	85	85	86	86	86	86	87	87	87	87	88	88	88
77	77	77	78	78	78	78	79	79	79	79	80	80	80	80	80	81	81	81	81	82	82	82	82	83	83	83	83	83	84	84	84	84	85	85	85	85	86	86	86	86	86	87	87	87	87	88	88	88	88	89
78	78	78	79	79	79	79	80	80	80	80	80	81	81	81	81	82	82	82	82	82	83	83	83	83	84	84	84	84	84	85	85	85	85	85	86	86	86	86	87	87	87	87	87	88	88	88	88	89	89	89
79	79	79	80	80	80	80	80	81	81	81	81	82	82	82	82	82	83	83	83	83	83	84	84	84	84	84	85	85	85	85	86	86	86	86	86	87	87	87	87	87	88	88	88	88	88	89	89	89	89	90
80	80	80	81	81	81	81	81	82	82	82	82	82	83	83	83	83	83	84	84	84	84	84	85	85	85	85	85	86	86	86	86	86	87	87	87	87	87	88	88	88	88	88	89	89	89	89	89	90	90	90
81	81	81	82	82	82	82	82	83	83	83	83	83	83	84	84	84	84	84	85	85	85	85	85	86	86	86	86	86	87	87	87	87	87	87	88	88	88	88	88	89	89	89	89	89	90	90	90	90	90	91
82	82	82	83	83	83	83	83	83	84	84	84	84	84	85	85	85	85	85	85	86	86	86	86	86	87	87	87	87	87	87	88	88	88	88	88	88	89	89	89	89	89	90	90	90	90	90	90	91	91	91
83	83	83	84	84	84	84	84	84	85	85	85	85	85	85	86	86	86	86	86	86	87	87	87	87	87	87	88	88	88	88	88	88	89	89	89	89	89	89	90	90	90	90	90	90	91	91	91	91	91	92
84	84	84	84	85	85	85	85	85	85	86	86	86	86	86	86	87	87	87	87	87	87	88	88	88	88	88	88	88	89	89	89	89	89	89	90	90	90	90	90	90	91	91	91	91	91	91	92	92	92	92
85	85	85	85	86	86	86	86	86	86	87	87	87	87	87	87	87	88	88	88	88	88	88	88	89	89	89	89	89	89	90	90	90	90	90	90	90	91	91	91	91	91	91	91	92	92	92	92	92	92	93
86	86	86	86	87	87	87	87	87	87	87	88	88	88	88	88	88	88	89	89	89	89	89	89	89	90	90	90	90	90	90	90	90	91	91	91	91	91	91	91	92	92	92	92	92	92	92	93	93	93	93
87	87	87	87	88	88	88	88	88	88	88	88	89	89	89	89	89	89	89	89	90	90	90	90	90	90	90	91	91	91	91	91	91	91	91	92	92	92	92	92	92	92	92	93	93	93	93	93	93	93	94
88	88	88	88	88	89	89	89	89	89	89	89	89	90	90	90	90	90	90	90	90	91	91	91	91	91	91	91	91	91	92	92	92	92	92	92	92	92	93	93	93	93	93	93	93	93	94	94	94	94	94
89	89	89	89	89	90	90	90	90	90	90	90	90	90	91	91	91	91	91	91	91	91	91	92	92	92	92	92	92	92	92	92	93	93	93	93	93	93	93	93	93	94	94	94	94	94	94	94	94	94	95
90	90	90	90	90	91	91	91	91	91	91	91	91	91	91	92	92	92	92	92	92	92	92	92	92	93	93	93	93	93	93	93	93	93	93	94	94	94	94	94	94	94	94	94	94	95	95	95	95	95	95
91	91	91	91	91	91	92	92	92	92	92	92	92	92	92	92	92	93	93	93	93	93	93	93	93	93	93	93	94	94	94	94	94	94	94	94	94	94	94	95	95	95	95	95	95	95	95	95	95	95	96
92	92	92	92	92	92	92	93	93	93	93	93	93	93	93	93	93	93	93	94	94	94	94	94	94	94	94	94	94	94	94	94	95	95	95	95	95	95	95	95	95	95	95	95	96	96	96	96	96	96	96
93	93	93	93	93	93	93	93	94	94	94	94	94	94	94	94	94	94	94	94	94	94	95	95	95	95	95	95	95	95	95	95	95	95	95	95	96	96	96	96	96	96	96	96	96	96	96	96	96	96	97
94	94	94	94	94	94	94	94	94	95	95	95	95	95	95	95	95	95	95	95	95	95	95	95	95	96	96	96	96	96	96	96	96	96	96	96	96	96	96	96	96	96	97	97	97	97	97	97	97	97	97
95	95	95	95	95	95	95	95	95	95	96	96	96	96	96	96	96	96	96	96	96	96	96	96	96	96	96	96	96	96	97	97	97	97	97	97	97	97	97	97	97	97	97	97	97	97	97	97	97	97	98
96	96	96	96	96	96	96	96	96	96	96	96	96	97	97	97	97	97	97	97	97	97	97	97	97	97	97	97	97	97	97	97	97	97	97	97	97	97	98	98	98	98	98	98	98	98	98	98	98	98	98
97	97	97	97	97	97	97	97	97	97	97	97	97	97	97	97	97	98	98	98	98	98	98	98	98	98	98	98	98	98	98	98	98	98	98	98	98	98	98	98	98	98	98	98	98	98	98	98	98	98	99
98	98	98	98	98	98	98	98	98	98	98	98	98	98	98	98	98	98	98	98	98	98	98	98	98	99	99	99	99	99	99	99	99	99	99	99	99	99	99	99	99	99	99	99	99	99	99	99	99	99	99
99	99	99	99	99	99	99	99	99	99	99	99	99	99	99	99	99	99	99	99	99	99	99	99	99	99	99	99	99	99	99	99	99	99	99	99	99	99	99	99	99	99	99	99	99	99	99	99	99	99	100
	1	**2**	**3**	**4**	**5**	**6**	**7**	**8**	**9**	**10**	**11**	**12**	**13**	**14**	**15**	**16**	**17**	**18**	**19**	**20**	**21**	**22**	**23**	**24**	**25**	**26**	**27**	**28**	**29**	**30**	**31**	**32**	**33**	**34**	**35**	**36**	**37**	**38**	**39**	**40**	**41**	**42**	**43**	**44**	**45**	**46**	**47**	**48**	**49**	**50**

Combined Values Chart (continued)

	51	52	53	54	55	56	57	58	59	60
51	76									
52	76	77								
53	77	77	78							
54	77	78	78	79						
55	78	78	79	79	80					
56	78	79	79	80	80	81				
57	79	79	80	80	81	81	82			
58	79	80	80	81	81	82	82	82		
59	80	80	81	81	82	82	82	83	83	
60	80	81	81	82	82	82	83	83	84	84
61	81	81	82	82	82	83	83	84	84	84
62	81	82	82	83	83	83	84	84	84	85
63	82	82	83	83	83	84	84	84	85	85
64	82	83	83	83	84	84	85	85	85	86
65	83	83	84	84	84	85	85	85	86	86
66	83	84	84	84	85	85	85	86	86	86
67	84	84	84	85	85	85	86	86	86	87
68	84	85	85	85	86	86	86	87	87	87
69	85	85	85	86	86	86	87	87	87	88
70	85	86	86	86	87	87	87	87	88	88
71	86	86	86	87	87	87	88	88	88	88
72	86	87	87	87	87	88	88	88	89	89
73	87	87	87	88	88	88	88	89	89	89
74	87	88	88	88	88	89	89	89	89	90
75	88	88	88	89	89	89	89	90	90	90
76	88	88	89	89	89	89	90	90	90	90
77	89	89	89	89	90	90	90	90	91	91
78	89	89	90	90	90	90	91	91	91	91
79	90	90	90	90	91	91	91	91	91	92
80	90	90	91	91	91	91	91	92	92	92
81	91	91	91	91	91	92	92	92	92	92
82	91	91	92	92	92	92	92	92	93	93
83	92	92	92	92	92	93	93	93	93	93
84	92	92	92	93	93	93	93	93	93	94
85	93	93	93	93	93	93	94	94	94	94
86	93	93	93	94	94	94	94	94	94	94
87	94	94	94	94	94	94	94	95	95	95
88	94	94	94	94	95	95	95	95	95	95
89	95	95	95	95	95	95	95	95	95	96
90	95	95	95	95	96	96	96	96	96	96
91	96	96	96	96	96	96	96	96	96	96
92	96	96	96	96	96	96	97	97	97	97
93	97	97	97	97	97	97	97	97	97	97
94	97	97	97	97	97	97	97	97	98	98
95	98	98	98	98	98	98	98	98	98	98
96	98	98	98	98	98	98	98	98	98	98
97	99	99	99	99	99	99	99	99	99	99
98	99	99	99	99	99	99	99	99	99	99
99	100	100	100	100	100	100	100	100	100	100

	61	62	63	64	65	66	67	68	69	70
61	85									
62	85	86								
63	86	86	86							
64	86	86	87	87						
65	86	87	87	87	88					
66	87	87	87	88	88	88				
67	87	87	88	88	88	89	89			
68	88	88	88	88	89	89	89	90		
69	88	88	89	89	89	89	90	90	90	
70	88	89	89	89	90	90	90	90	91	91
71	89	89	89	90	90	90	90	91	91	91
72	89	89	90	90	90	90	91	91	91	92
73	89	90	90	90	91	91	91	91	92	92
74	90	90	90	91	91	91	91	92	92	92
75	90	91	91	91	91	92	92	92	92	93
76	91	91	91	91	92	92	92	92	93	93
77	91	91	91	92	92	92	92	93	93	93
78	91	92	92	92	92	93	93	93	93	93
79	92	92	92	92	93	93	93	93	93	94
80	92	92	93	93	93	93	93	94	94	94
81	93	93	93	93	93	94	94	94	94	94
82	93	93	93	94	94	94	94	94	94	95
83	93	94	94	94	94	94	94	95	95	95
84	94	94	94	94	94	95	95	95	95	95
85	94	94	94	95	95	95	95	95	95	96
86	95	95	95	95	95	95	95	96	96	96
87	95	95	95	95	95	96	96	96	96	96
88	95	95	96	96	96	96	96	96	96	96
89	96	96	96	96	96	96	96	96	97	97
90	96	96	96	96	97	97	97	97	97	97
91	96	97	97	97	97	97	97	97	97	97
92	97	97	97	97	97	97	97	97	98	98
93	97	97	97	97	98	98	98	98	98	98
94	98	98	98	98	98	98	98	98	98	98
95	98	98	98	98	98	98	98	98	98	99
96	98	98	99	99	99	99	99	99	99	99
97	99	99	99	99	99	99	99	99	99	99
98	99	99	99	99	99	99	99	99	99	99
99	100	100	100	100	100	100	100	100	100	100

	71	72	73	74	75	76	77	78	79	80
71	92									
72	92	92								
73	92	92	93							
74	92	93	93	93						
75	93	93	93	94	94					
76	93	93	94	94	94	94				
77	93	94	94	94	94	94	95			
78	94	94	94	94	95	95	95	95		
79	94	94	94	95	95	95	95	95	96	
80	94	94	95	95	95	95	95	96	96	96
81	94	95	95	95	95	95	96	96	96	96
82	95	95	95	95	96	96	96	96	96	96
83	95	95	95	96	96	96	96	96	96	97
84	95	96	96	96	96	96	96	96	97	97
85	96	96	96	96	96	96	97	97	97	97
86	96	96	96	96	97	97	97	97	97	97
87	96	96	96	97	97	97	97	97	97	97
88	97	97	97	97	97	97	97	97	97	98
89	97	97	97	97	97	97	97	98	98	98
90	97	97	97	97	98	98	98	98	98	98
91	97	97	98	98	98	98	98	98	98	98
92	98	98	98	98	98	98	98	98	98	98
93	98	98	98	98	98	98	98	98	99	99
94	98	98	98	98	99	99	99	99	99	99
95	99	99	99	99	99	99	99	99	99	99
96	99	99	99	99	99	99	99	99	99	99
97	99	99	99	99	99	99	99	99	99	99
98	99	99	99	99	100	100	100	100	100	100
99	100	100	100	100	100	100	100	100	100	100

	81	82	83	84	85	86	87	88	89	90
81	96									
82	97	97								
83	97	97	97							
84	97	97	97	97						
85	97	97	97	98	98					
86	97	97	98	98	98	98				
87	98	98	98	98	98	98	98			
88	98	98	98	98	98	98	98	99		
89	98	98	98	98	98	98	99	99	99	
90	98	98	98	98	99	99	99	99	99	99
91	98	98	98	99	99	99	99	99	99	99
92	98	99	99	99	99	99	99	99	99	99
93	99	99	99	99	99	99	99	99	99	99
94	99	99	99	99	99	99	99	99	99	99
95	99	99	99	99	99	99	99	99	99	100
96	99	99	99	99	99	99	99	100	100	100
97	99	99	99	100	100	100	100	100	100	100
98	100	100	100	100	100	100	100	100	100	100
99	100	100	100	100	100	100	100	100	100	100

	91	92	93	94	95	96	97	98	99
91	99								
92	99	99							
93	99	99	100						
94	99	100	100	100					
95	100	100	100	100	100				
96	100	100	100	100	100	100			
97	100	100	100	100	100	100	100		
98	100	100	100	100	100	100	100	100	
99	100	100	100	100	100	100	100	100	100

Index

In this index, specific disorders that are mentioned only to illustrate evaluation for a larger class of impairments or for an organ system are denoted by the phrase "case report/example."

A

D

E

F

G

H

I

O

P

T

W

X

Z